Mayo Clinic
Gastrointestinal Imaging Review

Mayo Clinic
Gastrointestinal Imaging Review

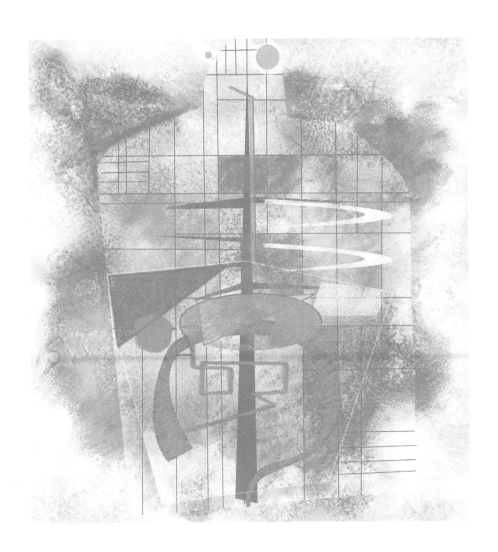

C. Daniel Johnson, M.D.
Grant D. Schmit, M.D.

MAYO CLINIC SCIENTIFIC PRESS
TAYLOR & FRANCIS GROUP

ISBN 0-8493-9795-2

For order inquiries, contact Taylor & Francis Group, 6000 Broken Sound Parkway NW, Suite #300, Boca Raton, FL 33487, www.taylorandfrancis.com.

Catalog record is available from the Library of Congress

Care has been taken to confirm the accuracy of the information presented and to describe generally accepted practices. However, the authors, editors, and publisher are not responsible for errors or omissions or for any consequences from application of the information in this book and make no warranty, express or implied, with respect to the contents of the publication. This book should not be relied on apart from the advice of a qualified health care provider.

The authors, editors, and publisher have exerted efforts to ensure that drug selection and dosage set forth in this text are in accordance with current recommendations and practice at the time of publication. However, in view of ongoing research, changes in government regulation, and the constant flow of information relating to drug therapy and drug reactions, the reader is urged to check the package insert for each drug for any change in indications and dosage and for added warnings and precautions. This is particularly important when the recommended agent is a new or infrequently employed drug.

Some drugs and medical devices presented in this publication have Food and Drug Administration (FDA) clearance for limited use in restricted research settings. It is the responsibility of the health care providers to ascertain the FDA status of each drug or device planned for use in their clinical practice.

About the Cover

One of the fun parts of writing this book was dressing it up with a unique cover. We were delighted to learn that Mayo Clinic Scientific Press encouraged our participation in the design of the cover. We wanted the cover not only to represent the contents of the book but also to make a personal statement. Knowing of our interest in abstract art, Karen Barrie, art director for the book, provided several examples of abstract art in a warm color palette. The magnificent paintings by Wassily Kandinsky stood out as the model for our project. Our own abstract line drawings and our favorite Kandinsky paintings were shown to Jim Rownd, a Mayo Clinic illustrator. Jim took our vision and created the cover illustration. We see the cover as analogous to radiographic images—also abstract to many viewers, understood only with a knowledge of anatomy, radiography, and pathology. Our hope is that the interrelated beauty of the components of the gastrointestinal tract is depicted in the illustration. The individual components are placed on the title pages of their respective chapters.

We are most grateful to both Karen Barrie and Jim Rownd for their artistic guidance and talents. We also appreciate the freedom given to our team at Mayo Clinic to create the book of our choice. We hope you enjoy it.

C. Daniel Johnson, M.D.
Grant D. Schmit, M.D.

Preface

The purpose of writing this book was to provide an atlas of common abnormalities that affect the gastrointestinal tract. Emphasis was placed on providing images large enough to study and minimal text including core information about the cases and disease processes. The book is not intended to be an inclusive source of diseases and their many manifestations. Rather, the most important disease processes affecting the gastrointestinal tract and their most common presentations are included. Only a few selected pediatric cases are included to provide a comparison with adult disease processes. Readers are directed to other textbooks for a comprehensive review of pediatric gastrointestinal disorders. The content of the book is directed primarily to residents in training, particularly those studying for board examinations. Practicing radiologists wanting to review the spectrum of abnormalities affecting the gastrointestinal tract will find the book to be an efficient review.

This book should be considered a new book when compared with *Alimentary Tract Imaging: A Teaching File*, authored by me (C.D.J.) more than a decade ago. Although some of the cases used in the earlier book also are used in this text, there are substantial differences. Additions include many new cases and also chapters on the liver, biliary system, pancreas, spleen, and mesentery and peritoneum. The book includes images obtained with state-of-the-art technology, such as computed tomographic colonography and enterography, ultrasonography, and magnetic resonance (including magnetic resonance cholangiopancreatography). The format for case presentation has been standardized to description of the radiographic findings, pertinent differential diagnoses, diagnosis, and discussion. The format is designed to allow the reader to review each case without knowing the diagnosis. Students are urged to commit themselves to the findings, differential diagnoses, and then diagnosis for each case before reading the answer. They can then obtain additional information from the discussion. Numerous summary tables synthesize information and provide key points and case references. The illustrations, drawn by David A. Factor, a medical illustrator at Mayo Clinic, provide a composite of the key diseases discussed in each chapter. We hope these illustrations assist the reader in learning key differential considerations. Selected readings and references are not included—an acknowledgment that readers of this book are likely looking for an efficient single-source review.

C. Daniel Johnson, M.D.
Grant D. Schmit, M.D.

Acknowledgments

I am deeply indebted to the many members of the Department of Radiology at Mayo Clinic who provided cases for the book. I have had many mentors and assistants who made this project possible. My training in radiology was highly influenced by distinguished radiologists, including Harley C. Carlson, David H. Stephens, Robert L. MacCarty, Reed P. Rice, William M. Thompson, and Igor Laufer. I am grateful for the training, mentorship, encouragement, and help from all of them. My colleague, Grant D. Schmit, the coauthor of this book, provided enthusiasm and help with obtaining cases, balancing content, and providing insight into formats and charts and key editorial assistance. He has been delightful to work with, and I hope this experience has cemented our collegial bonds and friendship. Debora L. Shreve performed a herculean job in typing and organizing the contents of the book. Without her dedication and skills, the book could not have been written. The Section of Scientific Publications and Media Support Services at Mayo Clinic worked tirelessly to provide the product that Grant and I envisioned. Roberta Schwartz was the lead project organizer, LeAnn Stee editor, Dianne Kemp editorial assistant, Karen Barrie art director, David Factor medical illustrator, and John Hedlund proofreader. Each one served a critical role in book production. I am grateful to them all.

Most importantly, I thank my dear wife, Therese, for her encouragement to tackle another book. As always, she provided me unselfish support for a project that took me away from family and home activities. I also thank my daughter, Kristina, for her support. Time was not always available to do things together that would have been most fun. I hope that my academic pursuits, such as book writing, will inspire her to activities that are professionally rewarding and enjoyable.

I hope readers find the book an efficient way to learn the myriad and fascinating ways of the gastrointestinal tract.

C. Daniel Johnson, M.D.

In addition to those persons already acknowledged, I thank my wife, Chris, and my sons, Collin and Cameron, for their support and the sacrifice that allowed me to be involved in writing this book. I also thank my friend and mentor, C. Daniel Johnson, for including me in such an educational and rewarding project at this early stage in my academic career.

Grant D. Schmit, M.D.

Author Affiliations

C. Daniel Johnson, M.D.

Consultant, Department of Radiology, Mayo Clinic
Professor of Radiology, Mayo Clinic College of Medicine
Rochester, Minnesota

Grant D. Schmit, M.D.

Senior Associate Consultant, Department of Radiology, Mayo Clinic
Instructor in Radiology, Mayo Clinic College of Medicine
Rochester, Minnesota

Table of Contents

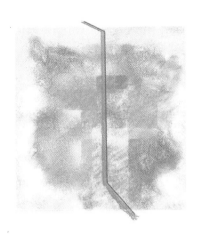

CHAPTER 1

ESOPHAGUS

CASE 1.1

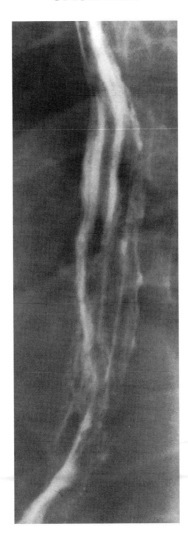

Findings
Double-contrast esophagram. Thickened and somewhat nodular folds are seen in the distal esophagus.

Differential Diagnosis
1. Reflux esophagitis
2. Esophageal varices

Diagnosis
Mild reflux esophagitis

Discussion
Reflux esophagitis is a common indication for and finding at UGI. If fold thickening is the only finding on a triphasic esophagram, mild esophagitis commonly is found endoscopically. Folds are considered abnormal if they exceed 2 to 3 mm in diameter.

Development of reflux esophagitis depends on several factors, including the acidity of the refluxed contents, the efficacy of esophageal clearance, and the frequency of reflux. These factors are particularly important in patients with Zollinger-Ellison syndrome and those with scleroderma, groups commonly affected with reflux esophagitis. Varices (cases 1.38 and 1.39) change shape with fluoroscopic observation and often have a serpentine and nodular configuration.

CASE 1.2

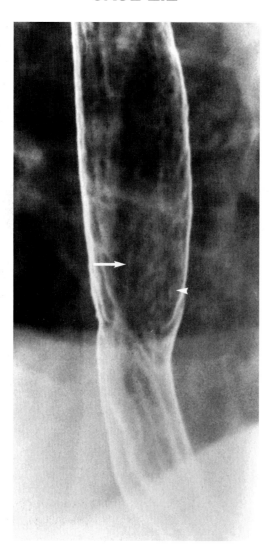

Findings

Double-contrast esophagram. Linear erosions (arrow) and punctate superficial erosions (arrowhead) are present within a mildly nodular mucosal background. The esophagus is shortened, and a small hiatal hernia is present.

Differential Diagnosis

1. Reflux esophagitis
2. Herpes esophagitis
3. *Candida* esophagitis

Diagnosis

Moderate reflux esophagitis

Discussion

Moderate esophagitis usually is characterized by the presence of superficial erosions that may be either punctate or linear. Fold thickening and nodularity also often are findings on the mucosal-relief phase films.

In patients with long-standing disease with esophageal intramural fibrosis, the esophagus shortens and pulls the stomach into an intrathoracic location. This type of "short esophagus" hiatal hernia is present in this case.

Herpes esophagitis (cases 1.12 and 1.13) is usually associated with multiple discrete superficial ulcers that may be located anywhere in the esophagus. *Candida* esophagitis (cases 1.10 and 1.11) most often has multiple plaquelike filling defects throughout the esophagus.

CASE 1.3

CASE 1.4

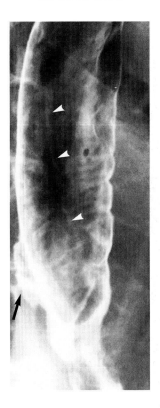

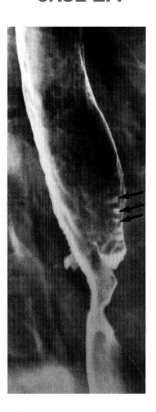

Findings

Case 1.3. Double-contrast esophagram. A large, flat ulcer is present in the distal esophagus (arrow) with associated diminished distensibility of the lower esophageal segment. There is also a long linear ulcer (arrowheads) with a surrounding halo of edema.

Case 1.4. Double-contrast esophagram. Mucosal nodularity, a deep ulcer, and luminal narrowing are present. Transverse folds due to chronic scarring and buckling of the mucosa also are present (arrows). Sharp spiculations are seen just superior to the deep ulcer; these are due to transverse folds seen in profile. Asymmetric scarring causes the distal deformity and narrowing.

Differential Diagnosis

1. Transverse folds and severe reflux esophagitis
2. Feline esophagus
3. Carcinoma of the esophagus

Diagnosis

Severe reflux esophagitis

Discussion

Transverse folds develop as a result of a prior linear ulceration with scar formation within the longitudinal muscle layers of the distal esophagus. They usually do not span the entire esophageal lumen.

Severe esophagitis usually is characterized by the presence of an ulcer crater. Typically, patients with severe esophagitis have superficial erosions and fold thickening in addition to the characteristic ulcer.

Transverse folds from esophagitis should be distinguished from the folds in feline esophagus (case 1.54) because transverse folds are fixed, fewer in number, coarser, and shorter. Changes of both active and chronic disease commonly coexist (as seen in these cases).

CASE 1.5

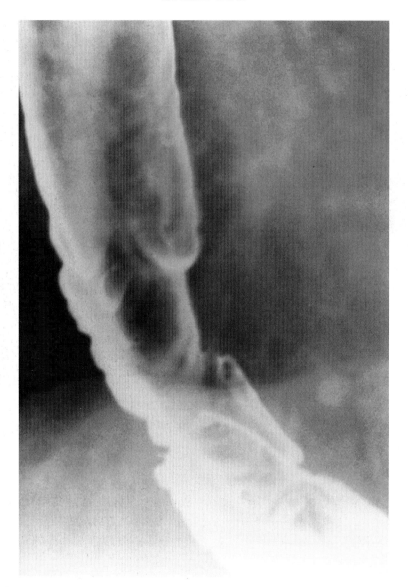

Findings
Double-contrast esophagram. Luminal irregularity and narrowing are present in the distal esophagus with associated asymmetric sacculations.

Differential Diagnosis
1. Active reflux esophagitis
2. Chronic reflux esophagitis
3. Esophageal carcinoma

Diagnosis
Chronic reflux esophagitis

Discussion
Chronic and active changes of reflux esophagitis often coexist. It may be impossible to exclude active ulceration or carcinoma in patients with marked deformity. Endoscopy should be recommended for patients with such problematic findings. Changes of chronic reflux esophagitis can result in scarring and considerable deformity of the esophagus.

CASE 1.6

CASE 1.7

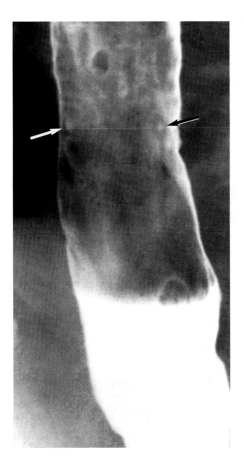

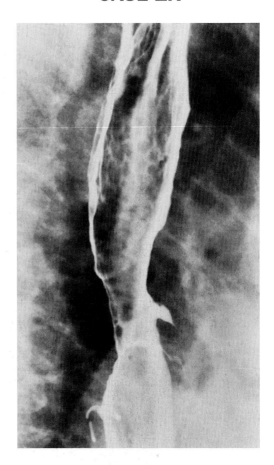

Findings

Case 1.6. Double-contrast esophagram. A featureless distal esophagus is present. Above the featureless zone are findings of active reflux esophagitis (mucosal granularity and superficial erosions [arrows]).

Case 1.7. Double-contrast esophagram. Mucosal reticularity is present in the esophagus. There is a short esophagus-type hiatal hernia. A surgically induced deformity mimics an ulcer crater. A benign-appearing stricture also is present.

Differential Diagnosis

1. Barrett esophagus with active reflux esophagitis
2. Reflux esophagitis
3. *Candida* esophagitis

Diagnosis

Barrett esophagus

Discussion

It is important to recognize Barrett esophagus because the adenomatous tissue is at increased risk for malignant transformation. Some reports suggest adenocarcinoma may develop in up to 10% of affected patients. In fact, 5% to 20% of all esophageal cancers develop in Barrett mucosa.

Reticular changes of Barrett esophagus are often adjacent to an esophageal stricture. The nodularity and crevices may be smaller and more delicate than in case 1.7. The mucosal nodularity associated with usual reflux esophagitis (cases 1.2, 1.3, and 1.4) without adenomatous transformation could have similar radiographic findings. The plaquelike filling defects in patients with candidiasis (cases 1.10 and 1.11) usually involve the entire esophagus and are not associated with other changes of reflux esophagitis.

CASE 1.8

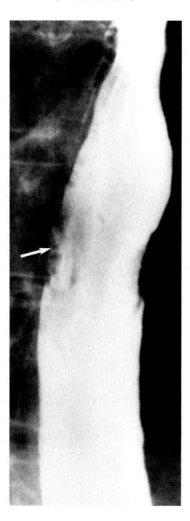

Findings
Single-contrast esophagram. An irregular, linearly oriented ulceration with a surrounding soft tissue mass (arrow) is present in the mid esophagus. There is also a region of reduced distensibility on the opposite wall.

Differential Diagnosis
1. Infectious esophagitis (cytomegalovirus, human immunodeficiency virus)
2. Early esophageal carcinoma
3. Medication-induced esophagitis

Diagnosis
Medication-induced esophagitis

Discussion
Localized inflammation due to medication lodged in the esophagus can lead to focal edema, ulceration, and stricture formation. Pills can lodge anywhere within the esophagus, but usually do so at the arch level or within the distal esophagus. Tetracycline, quinidine, and potassium chloride are the usual offending drugs, but others, including ascorbic acid, digitoxin, digoxin, and iron sulfate, also have been implicated. Patients usually complain of odynophagia, dysphagia, and retrosternal pain.

Radiographic findings are usually single or multiple shallow ulcerations. Associated fold thickening also may be seen. Double-contrast examination of the esophagus is sensitive for detecting these small, subtle ulcers. Endoscopy is required to exclude other differential possibilities unless the patient's history is typical.

CASE 1.9

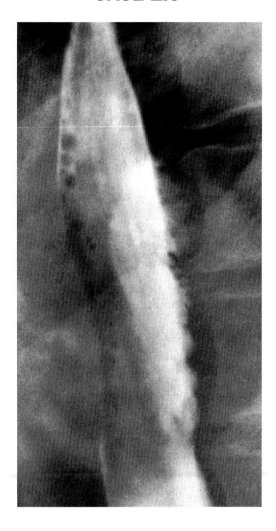

Findings

Double-contrast esophagram. A segmental region of deep ulceration affects a noncircumferential portion of the mid esophagus.

Differential Diagnosis

1. Infectious esophagitis
2. Crohn esophagitis
3. Acute caustic ingestion
4. Esophageal carcinoma

Diagnosis

Crohn esophagitis

Discussion

Crohn disease rarely affects the esophagus; when it does, disease is almost always present in the small bowel and colon. Most patients seek medical attention because of symptoms from disease elsewhere in the alimentary tract or from an esophageal stricture that is causing dysphagia.

The usual radiographic finding is aphthous ulcers (discrete ulcers surrounded by a mound of edema), which usually require double-contrast radiography for detection. Confluent ulcerations and deep ulcers (as seen in this case) can be found in more severe disease. Transmural disease may lead to esophageal perforation and fistula formation. Progressive scarring can lead to stricture formation.

The lack of surrounding mass makes cancer unlikely. A caustic ingestion nearly always involves a larger segment of the esophagus (and ingestion history). The ulceration is larger than that usually found with cytomegalovirus (case 1.14) or human immunodeficiency virus.

CASE 1.10

CASE 1.11

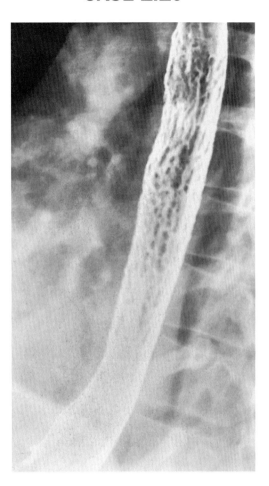

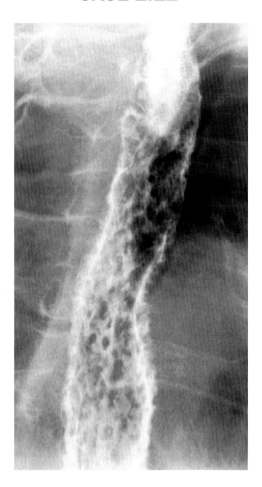

Findings

Case 1.10. Double-contrast esophagram. Multiple plaquelike filling defects are seen throughout the esophagus.

Case 1.11. Double-contrast esophagram. Shaggy, irregular luminal contours due to extensive plaquelike filling defects are present throughout the esophagus.

Differential Diagnosis
1. Candidiasis
2. Reflux esophagitis
3. Glycogenic acanthosis
4. Herpes esophagitis

Diagnosis
Candidiasis

Discussion

There is a spectrum of radiographic findings associated with candidiasis. Patients may present early with findings only of dysmotility (atonicity and tertiary contractions). Discrete plaquelike lesions are the most common finding, ranging from a few to diffuse esophageal involvement. Nodularity, granularity, and fold thickening may occur as a result of mucosal inflammation and edema. More severe disease is manifested as a shaggy, irregular luminal surface. Rarely, large filling defects occur as a result of giant plaques and fungus balls.

Reflux esophagitis usually is confined to the lower esophagus and rarely is associated with well-defined plaques. Patients with glycogenic acanthosis are usually asymptomatic and older but could present with similar radiographic findings. Herpes esophagitis occasionally can present with multiple plaquelike filling defects, but discrete ulcerations are more common.

CASE 1.12

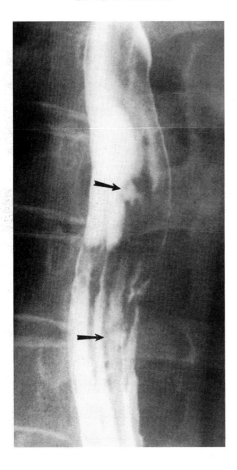

CASE 1.13

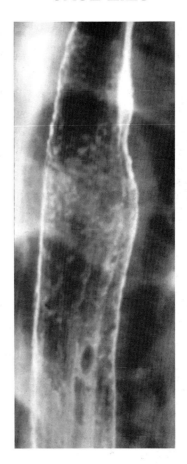

Findings

Case 1.12. Double-contrast esophagram. Multiple discrete ulcerations (arrows) are present on a normal esophageal background. (From Laufer I. Double contrast gastrointestinal radiology. Philadelphia: Saunders. 1979;115-8. By permission of the publisher.)

Case 1.13. Double-contrast esophagram. Multiple discrete ulcerations are clustered within the mid esophagus. (Courtesy of M. Levine, M.D., Philadelphia, Pennsylvania.)

Differential Diagnosis

1. Herpes esophagitis
2. Candidiasis
3. Reflux esophagitis
4. Cytomegalovirus/varicella esophagitis

Diagnosis

Herpes esophagitis

Discussion

Radiographically, discrete ulcerations on an otherwise normal esophageal mucosal background are characteristic findings in herpes esophagitis. Multiple plaquelike filling defects, with or without ulcerations, also can be seen.

Differential considerations include candidiasis, which usually presents with plaquelike filling defects (cases 1.10 and 1.11). Other members of the herpesvirus group, including cytomegalovirus and varicella zoster, can present with identical radiographic findings. Cytomegalovirus infection often presents with a large, solitary, discrete ulcer (case 1.14). Ulcers from reflux esophagitis (cases 1.3 and 1.4) are usually confined to the distal esophagus and associated with hiatal hernia, reflux, and lower esophageal stricture.

CASE 1.14

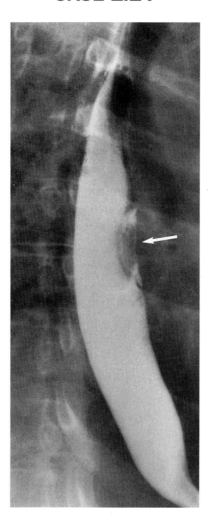

Findings

Double-contrast esophagram. A large, flat ulceration (arrow) is present in the distal esophagus. (Courtesy of Kyunghee C. Cho, M.D., Bronx, New York.)

Differential Diagnosis

1. Cytomegalovirus esophagitis
2. Human immunodeficiency virus esophagitis
3. Herpes esophagitis
4. Crohn esophagitis

Diagnosis

Cytomegalovirus esophagitis

Discussion

Cytomegalovirus infection is a disorder arising from the herpesvirus family. Most patients with this opportunistic infection have acquired immunodeficiency syndrome (AIDS). The small bowel and colon are most frequently affected. Diagnosis is usually made histologically by examining endoscopic brushings and biopsy specimens. Intranuclear inclusions are seen within endothelial cells or fibroblasts.

Radiographically, cytomegalovirus esophagitis may be indistinguishable from herpes esophagitis (cases 1.12 and 1.13) or human immunodeficiency virus (HIV) infection with multiple discrete ulcerations. Advanced disease may be associated with extensive ulceration. Giant ulcers suggest cytomegalovirus or HIV infection rather than herpes esophagitis. These large ulcers are often flat and ovoid. Cytomegalovirus esophagitis should be considered in any patient with AIDS and esophageal ulcerations.

Peptic and Inflammatory Esophagitis

		Case
Mild reflux esophagitis	Thickened folds only	1.1
Moderate reflux esophagitis	Thickened folds and tiny linear ulcerations	1.2
Severe reflux esophagitis	Thickened folds and moderate to large ulcer	1.3 and 1.4
Chronic reflux esophagitis (with or without active disease)	Smooth, tapering stricture immediately above gastroesophageal junction. Scarring with deformity, transverse folds	1.5
Barrett esophagus	Benign stricture at an abnormally high location, transition zone with active esophagitis above normal distal segment, or reticulated mucosal pattern	1.6 and 1.7
Medication-induced esophagitis	Single or multiple shallow ulcers, usually at level of arch or distal esophagus	1.8
Crohn esophagitis	Aphthous ulcers. Confluent ulcers in more severe disease	1.9

Infectious Esophagitis

Candidiasis	Multiple plaquelike filling defects Advanced disease has shaggy appearance	1.10 and 1.11
Herpes esophagitis	Multiple discrete ulcers, normal mucosa between lesions	1.12 and 1.13
Cytomegalovirus and human immunodeficiency virus esophagitis	Large, flat, solitary ulcer. Radiographically indistinguishable	1.14

CASE 1.15

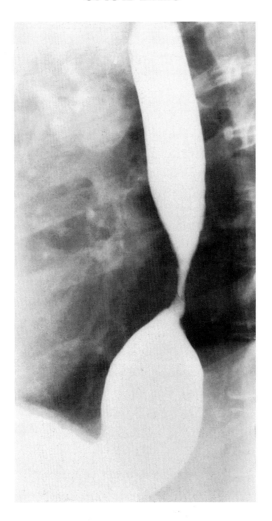

Findings

Single-contrast esophagram. A moderate-sized hiatal hernia is present with esophageal shortening and narrowing beginning at the gastroesophageal junction. The margins of the stricture taper gradually.

Differential Diagnosis

1. Chronic reflux-induced stricture
2. Caustic ingestion-induced stricture

Diagnosis

Chronic reflux esophagitis: focal stricture

Discussion

Stricture formation is the most frequent radiographic manifestation of chronic reflux esophagitis. The classic stricture begins immediately above the gastroesophageal junction and extends proximally a variable distance. Usually the margins are smooth and taper gradually. A mild stricture may present as a subtle region of incomplete esophageal distention. Severe strictures that narrow the lumen to less than 1 cm are nearly always symptomatic—dysphagia is the most frequent complaint. Treatment of symptomatic strictures is usually by either balloon or bougie dilation. Surgical treatment is reserved for patients who do not respond to more conservative therapy. An antireflux operation may be performed in such cases. In many cases, fibrosis causes esophageal shortening, with the development of an esophageal hiatal hernia. Caustic strictures (case 1.21) are usually longer, often involving a longer length of the esophagus.

CASE 1.16

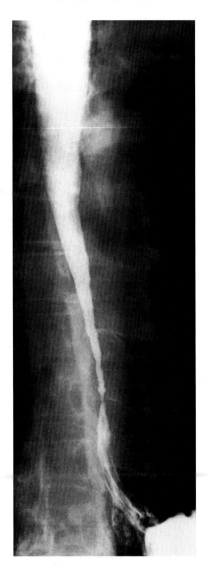

Findings
Single-contrast esophagram. A long distal esophageal stricture, with an associated hiatal hernia, is present.

Differential Diagnosis
1. Caustic ingestion-induced stricture
2. Prolonged nasogastric tube stricture
3. Radiation-induced stricture
4. Blistering skin disorders
5. Chronic reflux-induced stricture

Diagnosis
Chronic reflux esophagitis: long stricture

Discussion
This benign-appearing stricture is due to chronic reflux esophagitis. The smooth, tapered margins usually indicate a benign cause. Long strictures such as this are unusual for peptic esophagitis-induced strictures. Other considerations may have to be excluded after review of the patient's history.

CASE 1.17

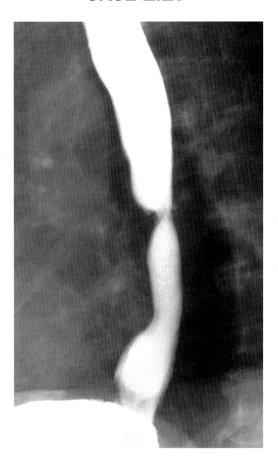

Findings

Single-contrast esophagram. A short stricture is present in the mid esophagus, with some luminal irregularity at the level of the stricture. A short esophagus-type hiatal hernia also is visible.

Differential Diagnosis

1. Barrett esophagus stricture
2. Reflux stricture
3. Medication-induced esophagitis or stricture
4. Caustic ingestion-induced stricture

Diagnosis

Barrett esophagus stricture

Discussion

A focal esophageal stricture above the gastroesophageal junction is suggestive of Barrett esophagus. Barrett esophagus is histologically described as metaplasia and replacement of the normal squamous epithelium with gastric-type adenomatous mucosa. Chronic reflux esophagitis is nearly always the underlying cause of the disease. Some authorities estimate that nearly 10% of patients with reflux esophagitis have some adenomatous transformation in the esophagus.

This case is a typical example of Barrett esophagus. The short-esophagus hiatal hernia indicates long-standing esophagitis. Usual reflux-induced strictures (case 1.15) are located immediately above the gastroesophageal junction. Because adenomatous tissue is acid-resistant, strictures in Barrett esophagus develop near the squamous-adenomatous transition zone. Barrett strictures commonly are seen in the upper and mid esophagus. Medication-induced esophagitis (case 1.8) usually occurs at areas of anatomical narrowing—thoracic inlet, near aortic arch, or left main-stem bronchus. Caustic strictures (case 1.21) are usually long and associated with a typical history of caustic ingestion.

CASE 1.18

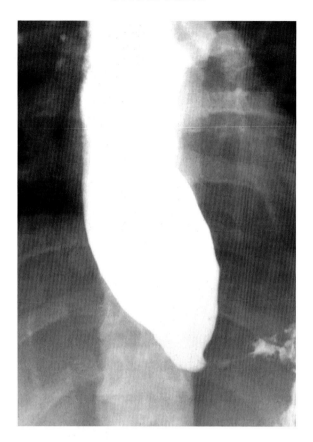

Findings
Single-contrast esophagram. Dilatation of the esophagus with a beaklike deformity near the gastroesophageal junction. Aperistalsis of the smooth muscle portion (distal two-thirds) was observed.

Differential Diagnosis
1. Achalasia
2. Scleroderma
3. Reflux-induced stricture
4. Chagas disease
5. Carcinoma of gastroesophageal junction (pseudoachalasia)

Diagnosis
Achalasia

Discussion
Achalasia is a motor disorder of the esophagus characterized by aperistalsis of the distal two-thirds (smooth muscle portion) of the esophagus and failure of the lower esophageal sphincter to relax. Patients usually complain of dysphagia, recumbent regurgitation, and episodes of aspiration pneumonia.

Radiographically, the esophagus is often dilated and a standing column of contrast material is seen (the height of the column is proportional to the severity of lower esophageal obstruction). Periodic relaxation of the lower esophageal sphincter with continued drinking is a critical observation for distinguishing primary achalasia from pseudoachalasia—carcinoma of the gastroesophageal junction (a fixed, nonrelaxing obstruction) (case 1.20). Manometry is the standard for diagnosing achalasia.

Transesophageal balloon dilation and surgical incision of the lower esophageal muscle fibers (Heller myotomy) are the primary treatment options.

Patients with scleroderma have a patulous gastroesophageal junction, esophagitis, and a lower esophageal stricture. In reflux esophagitis, peristalsis remains normal. Chagas disease may be indistinguishable from achalasia.

CASE 1.19

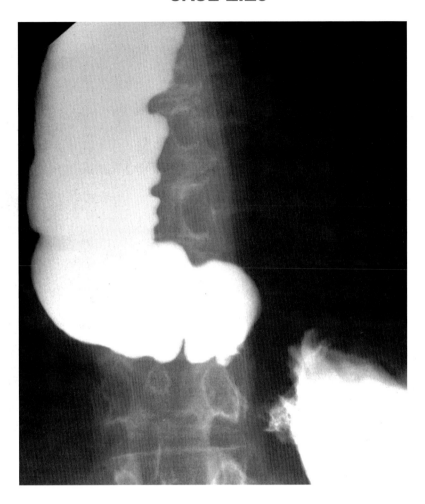

Findings
Single-contrast UGI. The esophagus is dilated to the gastroesophageal junction. The lower esophageal segment has smooth, tapered narrowing and intermittent, transient opening. In addition, multiple nonpropulsive contractions are present in the lower esophageal segment. Normal stripping wave is not observed.

Differential Diagnosis
1. Achalasia
2. Carcinoma gastroesophageal junction (pseudoachalasia)
3. Reflux-induced stricture
4. Scleroderma
5. Chagas disease

Diagnosis
Vigorous achalasia

Discussion
Vigorous achalasia is considered a less severe or early form of achalasia with motor abnormalities similar to those of achalasia seen fluoroscopically, in addition to repetitive, simultaneous, nonpropulsive contractions. Patients may have chest pain and typical dysphagia. Esophageal dilatation may be only minimal.

Complications from achalasia include carcinoma and *Candida* esophagitis. Carcinomas are squamous cell type, developing after 20 years of achalasia. The upper and mid esophagus are common locations for these cancers. Candidiasis (cases 1.10 and 1.11) develops from chronic stasis.

CASE 1.20

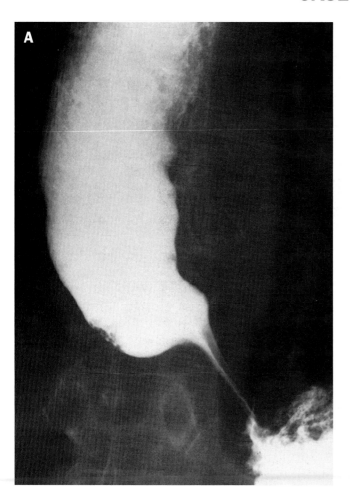

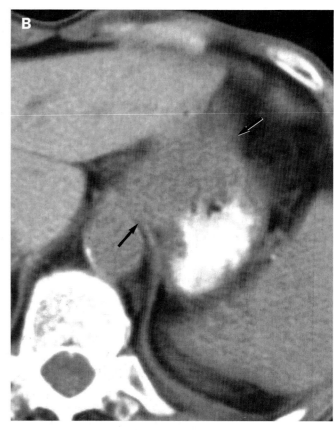

Findings

A. Single-contrast esophagram. Fixed, smooth narrowing is present in distal esophagus. Proximal esophagus is dilated. At fluoroscopy, narrowing remained unchanged, even after esophagus was half filled with contrast material.

B. Abdominal CT with oral contrast. A soft tissue mass (arrows) causing gastric wall thickening is present at the level of the gastroesophageal junction. The mass extends into the distal esophagus.

Differential Diagnosis

1. Carcinoma of gastroesophageal junction (pseudoachalasia)
2. Achalasia

Diagnosis

Carcinoma of the gastroesophageal junction (pseudoachalasia)

Discussion

Tumors such as this have predominantly submucosal growth and often arise from a gastric primary lesion. The radiographic findings can mimic those of achalasia. The terms *pseudoachalasia* and *secondary achalasia* have been used for such cases. On careful fluoroscopic observation of the cancerous esophagogastric junction during swallowing, a fixed, rigid stricture is seen that never distends during esophageal emptying. The esophagogastric junction in achalasia (case 1.18) opens transiently and distends when the hydrostatic barium column in the esophagus exceeds lower esophageal sphincter muscle tone. Peristalsis of the distal esophagus is absent in both conditions. The exact mechanism for this motor abnormality in patients with pseudoachalasia is uncertain.

CT may be helpful when findings are equivocal, because a soft tissue mass may be visible in patients with tumor.

CASE 1.21

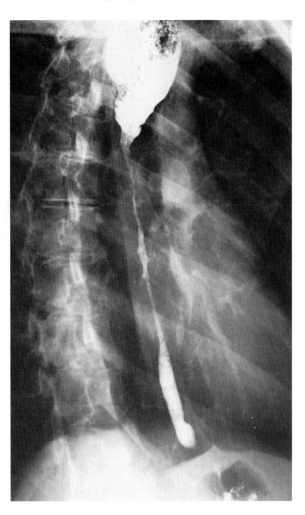

Findings

Single-contrast esophagram. There is a long, narrow stricture involving the mid and distal esophagus.

Differential Diagnosis

1. Caustic stricture
2. Stricture due to bullous skin disease
3. Radiation stricture
4. Prolonged nasogastric tube stricture
5. Chronic reflux stricture

Diagnosis

Caustic (lye-induced) stricture

Discussion

Caustic damage to the esophagus can occur from several agents, including alkali (lye), acid, phenols, ammonium chloride, and silver nitrate. The extent of esophageal damage depends on the concentration of the agent, the amount ingested, and the duration of mucosal contact. Radiographic examinations are helpful for documenting the severity and extent of stricture formation.

Radiographic findings of acute caustic esophagitis include dysmotility, irregular margins, edema, ulcerations, plaques of sloughing mucosa, and occasionally an intramural collection of contrast material. Esophageal strictures usually develop 1 to 3 months after the injury. The strictures may be focal and confined to the upper esophagus, or the esophagus may be diffusely involved with asymmetric regions of narrowing and sacculations. Patients are also at increased risk (1%-4%) of esophageal cancer after 20 years.

CASE 1.22

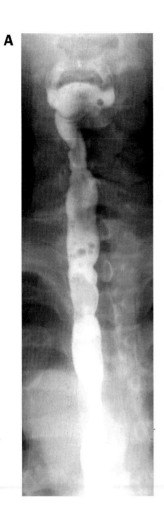

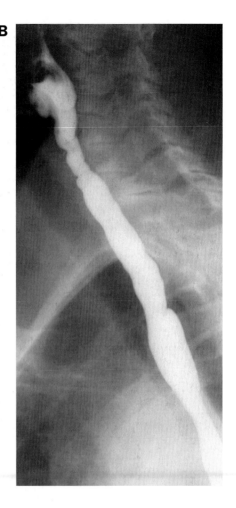

Findings
Single-contrast esophagram. Frontal (**A**) and lateral (**B**) images show persistent multifocal strictures in the cervical and upper thoracic esophagus.

Differential Diagnosis
1. Caustic ingestion strictures
2. Strictures due to medication-induced esophagitis
3. Strictures due to bullous disease

Diagnosis
Cicatricial pemphigoid strictures (benign mucous membrane pemphigoid)

Discussion
This patient had a known history of cicatricial pemphigoid with characteristic blistering lesions of the oral mucosa and face. Bullous diseases of the esophagus include cicatricial pemphigoid and epidermolysis bullosa dystrophica. Cicatricial pemphigoid is a rare (1:20,000), chronic, autoimmune blistering disorder involving the mucous membranes of the mouth, eyes, nose, esophagus, larynx, urethra, and anus. Peak incidence is between 60 and 80 years of age. Transient skin lesions (small blisters and erosions) occur in more than 20% of patients and usually are located on the head and neck. Biopsy often is required for diagnosis. Patients generally are treated with corticosteroids, the results of which are variable. Chronic changes of the disease in the esophagus often result in strictures. Scarring due to other causes of esophagitis also could present as multifocal strictures. Caustic (lye) ingestion (case 1.21) usually results in a long esophageal stricture, but multifocal strictures also could occur with variable areas of mucosal damage and healing.

CASE 1.23

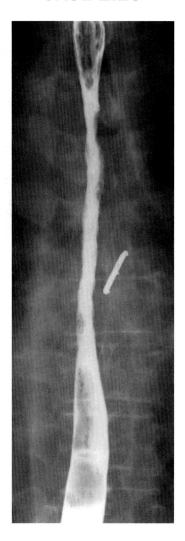

Findings
Double-contrast esophagram. A long, smooth stricture is present in the mid esophagus.

Differential Diagnosis
1. Radiation stricture
2. Caustic stricture
3. Nasogastric tube peptic stricture
4. Zollinger-Ellison reflux stricture

Diagnosis
Radiation stricture

Discussion
This patient had radiation therapy 1 year previously for lung cancer. Severe esophagitis and strictures can occur with high-dose (generally >50 Gy) radiation therapy to the chest. Acute radiation esophagitis usually occurs 1 to 4 weeks after the start of radiation therapy, whereas strictures often develop 4 to 8 months after its completion.

Long-segment esophageal strictures also can be caused by caustic ingestion (case 1.21), peptic stricture due to acid reflux with long-term nasogastric tube placement, or reflux stricture in Zollinger-Ellison syndrome. However, these strictures almost always extend to the gastroesophageal junction. A radiation stricture should be a primary diagnostic consideration for a long, smooth esophageal stricture that spares the distal esophagus.

CASE 1.24

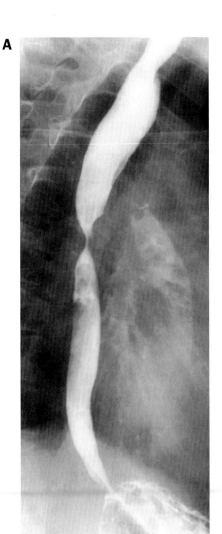

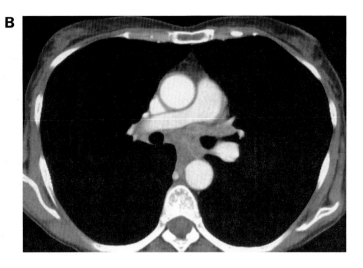

Findings
A. Single-contrast esophagram. Extrinsic compression and narrowing involve the mid esophagus.

B. Contrast-enhanced CT. Bulky mediastinal and hilar lymphadenopathy is present.

Differential Diagnosis
1. Mediastinal adenopathy
2. Esophageal carcinoma

Diagnosis
Extrinsic esophageal compression by lymphomatous mediastinal adenopathy

Discussion
Lymphomatous involvement of the esophagus is unusual. Usually patients have known generalized lymphoma before esophageal disease is discovered. This disease can affect the esophagus by mass effect or by direct spread from enlarged, contiguous lymph nodes. Lymphomatous involvement of the stomach can spread directly to the esophagus, or a lesion can develop in the esophagus simultaneously with disease elsewhere in the body. Benign inflammatory causes of mediastinal adenopathy also can result in extrinsic narrowing of the esophagus.

Esophageal Strictures

		Case
Peptic stricture	Immediately above gastroesophageal junction, often above esophageal hiatal hernia. Smooth, tapered margins	1.15 and 1.16
Barrett esophagus stricture	Usually seen in mid esophagus near squamous-adenomatous transition zone	1.17
Carcinoma	Irregular luminal contour with abrupt, shouldered margins	1.29
Achalasia	2-cm smooth stricture in region of gastroesophageal junction. Transiently relaxes with column of barium in esophagus while patient is standing	1.18 and 1.19
Pseudoachalasia	Carcinoma of the gastroesophageal junction. Fixed obstruction, never relaxes with full column of esophageal barium	1.20
Caustic stricture	Usually long and very narrow. Childhood injury, prolonged nasogastric tube common	1.21
Blistering skin disorders	Strictures, webs, cicatricial deformity. Epidermolysis bullosa dystrophica or benign mucous membrane pemphigoid	1.22
Radiation stricture	Long, narrow, smooth stricture. History of radiation therapy	1.23
Lymphoma	Extrinsic compression by mediastinal adenopathy	1.24

CASE 1.25

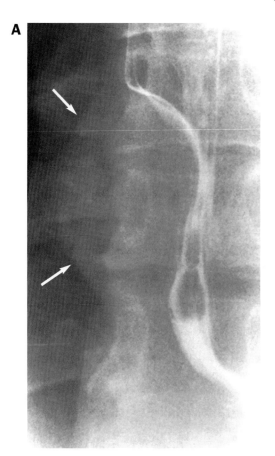

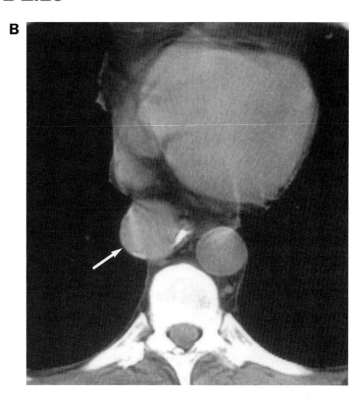

Findings

A. Double-contrast esophagram. There is a smooth impression on the esophageal contour by a well-circumscribed mass. The lateral margins of the mass (arrows) extend to the right of the spine.

B. Contrast-enhanced CT of the chest. A well-circumscribed, exophytic, enhancing tumor (arrow) is seen along the right side of the distal esophagus.

Differential Diagnosis

1. Gastrointestinal stromal tumor
2. Fibroma, neuroma, neurofibroma, lipoma, hemangioma
3. Duplication cyst
4. Lymphoma

Diagnosis

Gastrointestinal stromal tumor

Discussion

The location of the mass in relationship to the esophagus, its smooth surface, and the obtuse angle between the mass and the esophageal lumen suggest a submucosal mass. Gastrointestinal stromal tumors (GISTs) are the most frequently occurring submucosal neoplasm of the esophagus, accounting for more than half of all benign esophageal tumors. They are more common in the mid esophagus and distal esophagus—segments where smooth muscle is most abundant. Approximately 3% to 4% of tumors are multiple. Most GISTs are found incidentally.

Differential considerations include other types of intramural tumors such as fibromas, neuromas, neurofibromas, lipomas, and hemangiomas. Enteric duplication cysts or a lymphomatous mass could have a similar appearance.

A focal and enhancing mass makes a neoplasm most likely at CT. Duplication cysts often show water attenuation and do not enhance with intravenous contrast material.

CASE 1.26

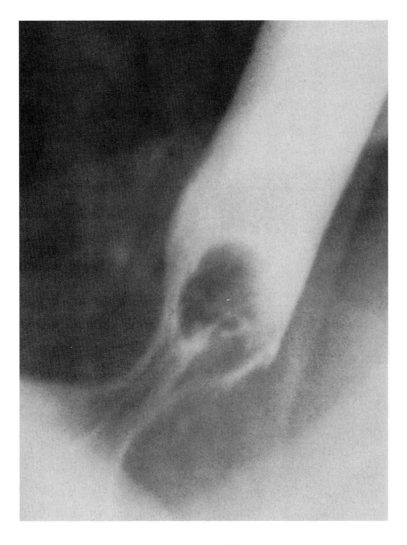

Findings
Single-contrast esophagram. A lobulated filling defect is present in the distal esophagus.

Differential Diagnosis
1. Adenoma
2. Papilloma
3. Inflammatory esophagogastric polyp

Diagnosis
Adenoma

Discussion
Adenomas of the esophagus are rare lesions arising from adenomatous tissue in the distal esophagus, usually within Barrett esophagus. Malignant degeneration has been reported in these lesions; therefore, endoscopic removal is recommended. Large polyps are more likely to be malignant than small polyps.

Esophageal papillomas (fibrovascular excrescences that are covered with squamous epithelium) can have a similar radiographic appearance and are probably more common than previously believed. These polyps are usually removed endoscopically, but no malignant transformation has been reported in humans. Inflammatory esophagogastric polyps (case 1.27) also could be confused with adenomas; however, these polypoid protuberances are enlarged gastric folds that protrude into the lower esophagus.

CASE 1.27

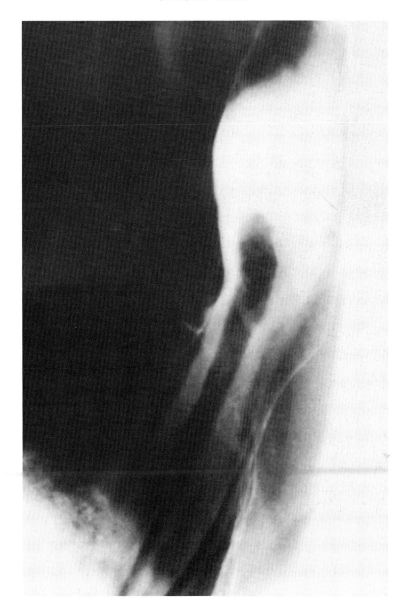

Findings

Double-contrast esophagram. An enlarged polypoid fold extends from the stomach into the esophageal lumen.

Differential Diagnosis

1. Inflammatory esophagogastric polyp
2. Adenoma
3. Papilloma

Diagnosis

Inflammatory esophagogastric polyp

Discussion

The inflammatory esophagogastric polyp is an enlarged gastric fold that projects into the lower esophagus. Inflammation is due to reflux esophagitis in affected patients. These polyps have no malignant potential. Usual radiographic features are a clubbed, bulbous fold that arises from the fundus of the stomach and projects into the lower esophagus. Occasionally, it may be difficult to differentiate an inflammatory esophagogastric polyp from a papilloma or an adenoma. In these cases, endoscopy is recommended to obtain a definitive diagnosis.

CASE 1.28

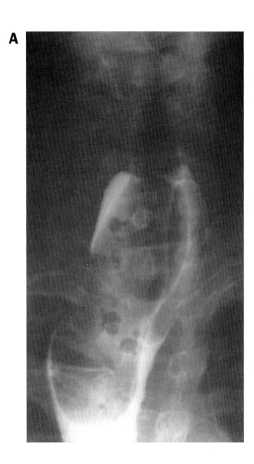

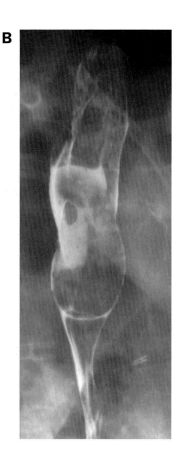

Findings

Double-contrast esophagram. **A** and **B**. A large, smooth, intraluminal mass arising from a thin stalk is present in the cervical esophagus. The esophagus is dilated around the intraluminal mass.

Differential Diagnosis

1. Fibrovascular polyp
2. Adenomatous polyp
3. Spindle cell carcinoma (carcinosarcoma)
4. Intraluminal gastrointestinal stromal tumor

Diagnosis

Fibrovascular polyp

Discussion

Fibrovascular polyps are benign, pedunculated, intraluminal lesions composed of various mesenchymal elements. They are covered by normal squamous esophageal mucosa and usually occur in the cervical esophagus. *Fibrovascular polyp* is the unifying term recommended for these lesions by the World Health Organization in 1990. In the past, they were named according to the predominant histologic component (fibroepithelial polyps, pedunculated lipomas, fibrous lipomas, fibromyxomas, fibrolipomas). Fibrovascular polyps are typically longer than 7 cm and can exceed 20 cm in length. Occasionally, they present dramatically with regurgitation of the polyp into the pharynx. This can result in respiratory compromise or even death. Fibrovascular polyps are not at risk for malignant transformation. Treatment of these lesions is surgical or endoscopic excision. Fibrovascular polyps often have a considerable lipomatous component and have fatty density on CT.

Adenomatous polyps (case 1.26) rarely attain this size. Spindle cell carcinomas (case 1.37) can arise from a stalk, but the site of attachment is usually in the mid or distal esophagus. Gastrointestinal stromal tumor is also a diagnostic consideration, but it rarely has this large an endoluminal component and does not arise from a stalk.

CASE 1.29

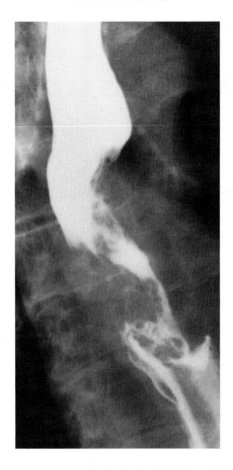

Findings
Single-contrast esophagram. A large, centrally ulcerated mass with an irregular luminal contour and an abrupt inferior edge is present in the mid esophagus.

Differential Diagnosis
1. Primary esophageal carcinoma
2. Metastases
3. Lymphoma

Diagnosis
Ulcerative esophageal carcinoma (squamous cell)

Discussion
Features of a malignant mass include an irregular contour of the barium-filled lumen, abrupt (shouldered) edges, and an ulcer that does not project beyond the expected location of the normal esophageal mucosa. This case illustrates these features of a malignancy. Esophageal carcinoma is a highly lethal disease that usually presents with chest pain or progressive dysphagia. Symptomatic tumors are often large and of advanced stage. Small tumors are usually discovered incidentally. Important risk factors in the development of esophageal cancer include tobacco and alcohol consumption, sex (3- to 4-fold increase in males), race (twice as common in nonwhites), lye ingestion, achalasia, prior head and neck cancer, nontropical sprue, tylosis, Plummer-Vinson syndrome, and exposure to tannins and nitrosamines. Tobacco and alcohol consumption are the most important risk factors in the United States.

Squamous cell carcinomas and adenocarcinomas are the most common histologic types of esophageal cancers. Squamous cell tumors do not usually cross the esophagogastric junction, whereas adenocarcinomas arising in Barrett esophagus frequently extend into the stomach. Most adenocarcinomas arise in Barrett esophagus and, as expected, are usually located in the distal esophagus.

CASE 1.30

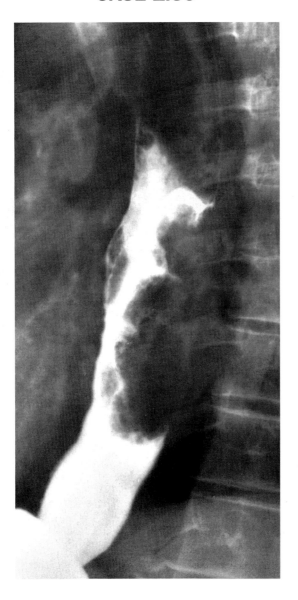

Findings

Double-contrast esophagram. A large polypoid filling defect with irregular borders and abruptly shouldering edges is present within the distal esophagus.

Differential Diagnosis

1. Esophageal carcinoma
2. Spindle cell carcinoma (carcinosarcoma)
3. Lymphoma

Diagnosis

Polypoid esophageal adenocarcinoma

Discussion

An esophageal adenocarcinoma, spindle cell carcinoma (carcinosarcoma) (case 1.37), or lymphoma (case 1.36) should be suspected when a bulky polypoid tumor is identified. Squamous cell carcinomas rarely have this morphologic configuration. Adenocarcinomas nearly always arise within Barrett esophagus and are therefore usually located in the distal esophagus. Esophageal adenocarcinomas are increasing in frequency because of an increase in the number of patients with Barrett esophagus.

CASE 1.31

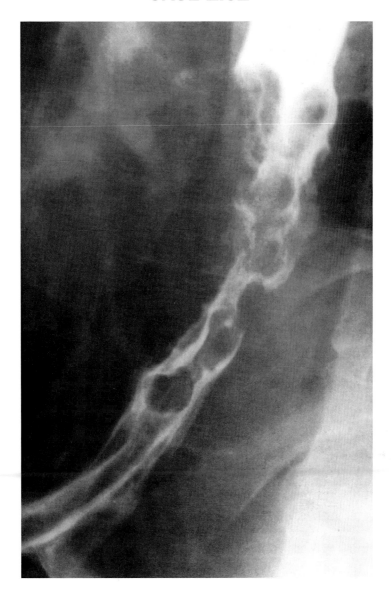

Findings

Single-contrast esophagram. A large mass is present in the distal esophagus with associated thickened and nodular folds. An abrupt edge forms the superior margin of the tumor.

Differential Diagnosis

1. Primary esophageal carcinoma
2. Varices

Diagnosis

Varicoid esophageal adenocarcinoma

Discussion

Most esophageal tumors do not have a varicoid appearance. This type of adenocarcinoma has a substantial proportion of tumor extending within the submucosa, causing the distorted fold appearance. Tumors are fixed and rigid, unchanging with swallowing. Usually a peristaltic wave will not pass through such a diseased esophageal segment. Varices change shape, especially with passage of a peristaltic stripping wave (cases 1.38 and 1.39).

CASE 1.32

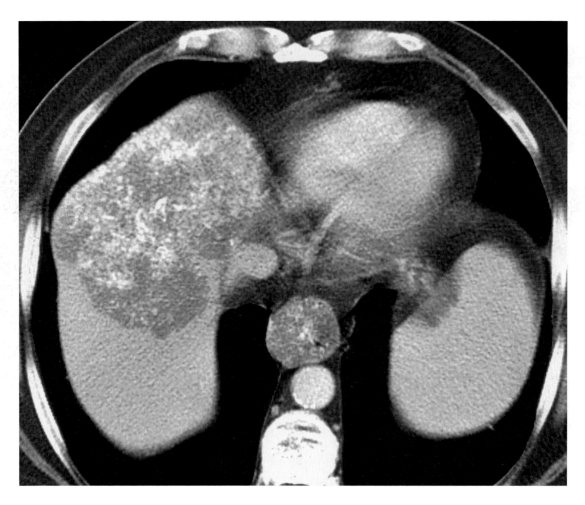

Findings

Contrast-enhanced CT. Marked distal esophageal wall thickening and calcification are present. A large, finely calcified hepatic mass is also visible.

Differential Diagnosis

1. Primary esophageal carcinoma
2. Lymphoma
3. Peptic esophagitis
4. Infectious esophagitis

Diagnosis

Esophageal carcinoma with hepatic metastases

Discussion

The normal esophageal wall is less than 3 mm thick. Wall thickening by itself is a nonspecific finding; both benign and malignant processes can have this appearance. Often, endoscopy is necessary to determine the cause of the wall thickening. Detection of paraesophageal invasion can be difficult, especially if the patient has a paucity of mediastinal fat or the fat planes are obliterated by operative or radiation therapy. Intravenously administered contrast material may help display tissue boundaries better in some patients with questionable findings. The presence of enlarged nodes (1.0–1.5 cm) suggests metastases; however, the absence of adenopathy does not exclude disseminated disease. Metastases to normal-sized lymph nodes (often undetectable at CT) often occur in microscopic quantities. In addition, even enlarged nodes can be due to benign inflammatory disease. Acute inflammatory changes can sometimes be distinguished from tumor infiltration by visualization of water attenuation within the thickened wall.

CASE 1.33

CASE 1.34

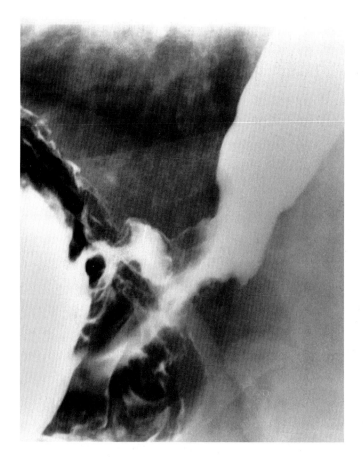

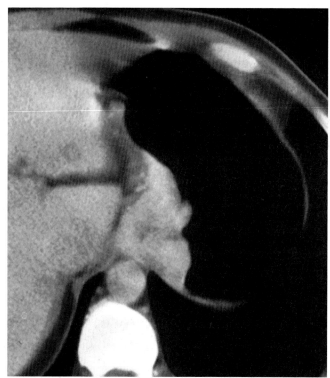

Findings

Case 1.33. Double-contrast barium esophagram. Distal esophagus has irregular luminal narrowing and nodularity.

Case 1.34. Contrast-enhanced CT. A circumferential soft tissue mass encases the esophagogastric junction.

Differential Diagnosis

Primary esophageal carcinoma

Diagnosis

Infiltrative adenocarcinoma of the gastroesophageal junction

Discussion

Esophageal adenocarcinomas nearly all arise from Barrett esophagus or from a fundal carcinoma extending into the esophagus. The spread of adenocarcinoma resembles that of squamous cell carcinoma, except there is a higher likelihood of involvement of the gastric cardia or fundus. Radiographic features that suggest an adenocarcinoma rather than a squamous carcinoma include distal location, gastric invasion, and evidence for chronic reflux esophagitis. CT can be used to identify mediastinal invasion and subdiaphragmatic extent of tumor. If extensive metastases are identified, the patient often receives radiation therapy rather than surgery. CT often understages tumors at the gastroesophageal junction.

CASE 1.35

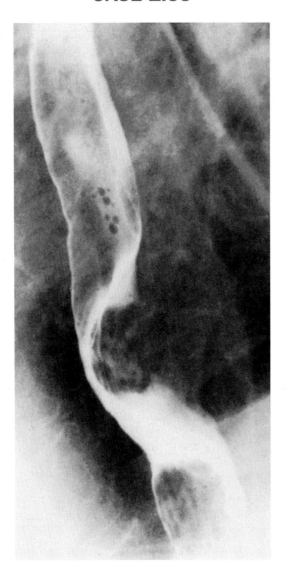

Findings

Double-contrast esophagram. There is a polypoid, lobulated filling defect in the distal esophagus, and an associated extrinsic mass displaces the esophagus posteriorly.

Differential Diagnosis

1. Esophageal carcinoma
2. Metastases

Diagnosis

Lung cancer with metastatic invasion into the esophagus

Discussion

CT (not shown) showed extensive mediastinal lymphadenopathy causing the changes on the esophagram. Metastases to the esophagus usually arise from cancers of the stomach, lung, or breast. Most of these tumors metastasize to mediastinal lymph nodes, and with growth they can displace or directly invade the esophagus. In some patients, the abnormality may resemble a primary esophageal cancer or present as a long, narrow stricture. Displacement of the lumen by a nodal mass is common. The mid esophagus is most commonly affected because mediastinal lymph nodes are most often affected. Hematogenous metastases to the esophagus are unusual.

CASE 1.36

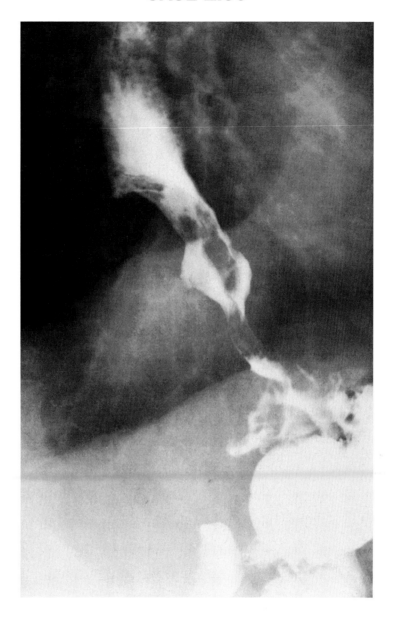

Findings

Esophagram. A large lobulated and ulcerated mass constricts the distal esophagus.

Differential Diagnosis

1. Esophageal carcinoma
2. Lymphoma
3. Varices

Diagnosis

Esophageal lymphoma

Discussion

The appearance of lymphoma can closely resemble that of primary carcinoma. The most common intrinsic manifestation of lymphoma is a polypoid, ulcerative, or infiltrative mass—usually indistinguishable from primary esophageal cancer. Less frequently, submucosal infiltration of lymphoma results in varicoid folds, discrete small submucosal masses, or diffuse nodular changes. Varices are usually more serpentine, and they change shape during fluoroscopic observation (especially from a peristaltic stripping wave).

CASE 1.37

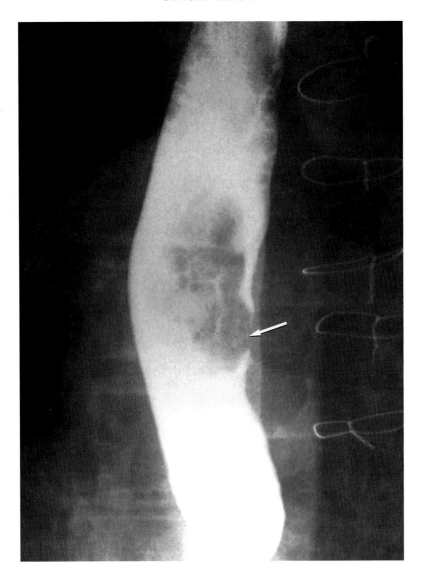

Findings

Single-contrast esophagram. A large, bulky filling defect is seen within the distal esophagus. A pedicle (arrow) is seen attaching the tumor to the left side of the esophagus.

Differential Diagnosis

1. Pedunculated gastrointestinal stromal tumor
2. Fibrovascular polyp
3. Spindle cell carcinoma
4. Adenocarcinoma

Diagnosis

Spindle cell carcinoma (carcinosarcoma)

Discussion

Spindle cell carcinomas are rare malignancies that contain histologic elements of both carcinoma and sarcoma. In the past, these tumors have been called carcinosarcomas. These tumors usually appear as bulky, polypoid, intraluminal tumors in the mid or distal esophagus. The mass may expand the esophageal lumen, but obstruction is rare.

CASE 1.38

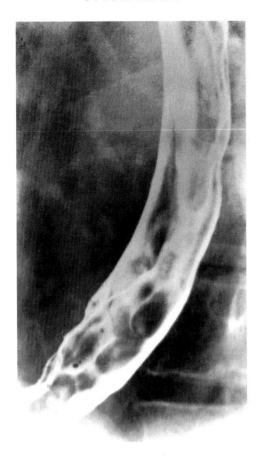

CASE 1.39

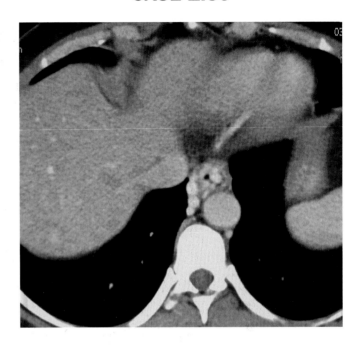

Findings

Case 1.38. Double-contrast esophagram. Multiple serpentine filling defects are seen in the distal esophagus. These defects changed in size and shape.

Case 1.39. Contrast-enhanced CT. Several esophageal varices are present within the distal periesophageal tissues.

Differential Diagnosis

1. Esophageal varices
2. Varicoid esophageal carcinoma

Diagnosis

"Uphill" esophageal varices

Discussion

Esophageal varices are dilated submucosal veins that develop as a result of portal venous hypertension. Hepatic cirrhosis is the most frequent cause of portal venous hypertension.

Increased portal venous pressure reverses normal venous blood flow such that flow occurs "uphill" from the portal vein, to the left gastric (coronary) vein, to the periesophageal venous plexus, and, finally, to the azygous and hemiazygous collaterals that empty into the superior vena cava. Varices almost never cause dysphagia, but they can bleed and cause life-threatening hemorrhage.

The radiographic diagnosis of esophageal varices is most sensitive when the partially collapsed esophagus is examined. Varices can be obliterated by the filled, distended esophagus as well as the collapsed esophagus immediately after a stripping peristaltic wave. Varices appear as linear, often serpentine, filling defects with a scalloped esophageal contour. Uphill varices are more prominent in the distal esophagus. The changing nature of varices with esophageal distention, peristalsis, and respiratory effort is helpful in differentiating varices from varicoid carcinoma (case 1.31) that appears fixed, is noncompliant, and often has shouldered margins.

CASE 1.40

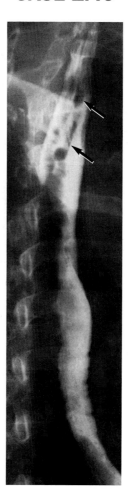

Findings
Single-contrast esophagram. Tubular thickened folds (arrows) are present in the upper thoracic esophagus.

Differential Diagnosis
1. Esophageal varices
2. Varicoid esophageal carcinoma

Diagnosis
"Downhill" esophageal varices

Discussion
"Downhill" varices develop as a result of obstruction of the superior vena cava, most commonly due to bronchogenic carcinoma, lymphoma, or fibrosing mediastinitis. Collaterals of the supreme intercostal vein, bronchial veins, and inferior thyroidal veins and other periesophageal collaterals enlarge and may be visible on an esophagram in the upper one-third of the esophagus. Blood flows "down" (caudally) the azygous-hemiazygous system and reenters the systemic circulation by way of the left gastric and portal veins. Unlike uphill varices, which often cause gastrointestinal bleeding, downhill varices usually are asymptomatic. In fact, in clinical practice, these varices are rare. In the absence of the superior vena cava syndrome, other diagnostic considerations should be entertained, such as varicoid carcinoma (case 1.31).

Rarely, a varix is identified in patients without portal venous hypertension or superior vena cava obstruction. Varices in these patients are considered idiopathic. These varices change size and shape (as do varices of any cause) with esophageal distention and after a peristaltic stripping wave. If the varix is thrombosed, it may be indistinguishable from a submucosal tumor.

CASE 1.41

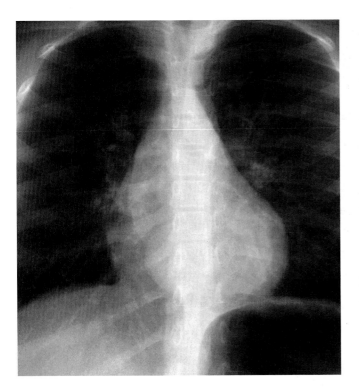

CASE 1.42

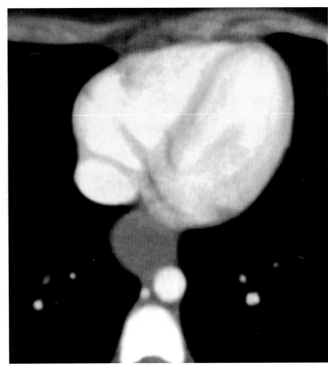

Findings

Case 1.41. Chest radiograph. There is a well-circumscribed mass behind the heart.

Case 1.42. Contrast-enhanced CT. A paraesophageal mass with the attenuation of water is present in the lower mediastinum.

Differential Diagnosis

Bronchopulmonary foregut malformation

Diagnosis

Esophageal (enteric) duplication cyst

Discussion

Esophageal duplication cysts are a type of foregut cyst, as are bronchogenic cysts and neurenteric cysts. Pathologically, esophageal duplication cysts are lined with squamous epithelium and have a smooth muscle wall. Bronchogenic cysts have respiratory epithelium, and neurenteric cysts have associated vertebral body anomalies. Symptoms from these cysts can be caused by compression on the adjacent esophagus or tracheobronchial tree or by infection of the cyst. If acid is secreted by the lining mucosa, peptic ulceration, perforation, and bleeding occur rarely.

Esophageal duplication cysts can be located anywhere in the posterior mediastinum. Contrast esophagraphy usually shows an extramucosal (smooth, well-demarcated) mass, which is often impossible to differentiate from a gastrointestinal stromal tumor (GIST) (case 1.25) or other mass arising from the esophageal wall. CT allows differentiation of an enteric cyst (attenuation of water) from a solid-enhancing GIST.

CASE 1.43

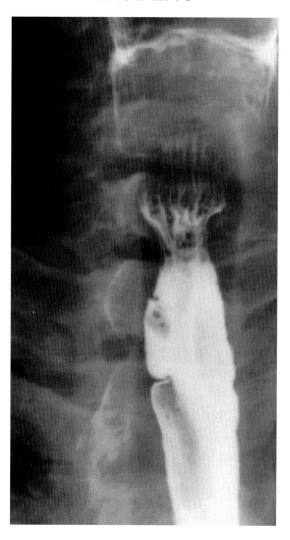

Findings

Double-contrast esophagram. A pair of shallow indentations approximately 2 cm apart are seen along the lateral wall of the cervical esophagus.

Differential Diagnosis

1. Ectopic gastric mucosa
2. Blistering skin disorder

Diagnosis

Ectopic gastric mucosa

Discussion

Ectopic gastric mucosa is thought to be a congenital abnormality, resulting from residue of columnar epithelium not replaced by stratified squamous epithelium during normal embryogenesis. Ectopic gastric mucosa usually is located in the cervical esophagus, which is the last place in the esophagus to undergo replacement with stratified squamous epithelium. Radiographic evidence of ectopic gastric mucosa in the upper esophagus can be found in up to 3% of patients. The patches of ectopic gastric mucosa are usually less than 2 cm in diameter. Recognition of the characteristic radiographic features of this abnormality makes endoscopy and follow-up unnecessary. However, ectopic gastric mucosa occasionally results in dysphagia and appears polypoid or irregular in shape. An atypical appearance should be evaluated endoscopically. A blistering skin disorder could present with similar findings.

CASE 1.44

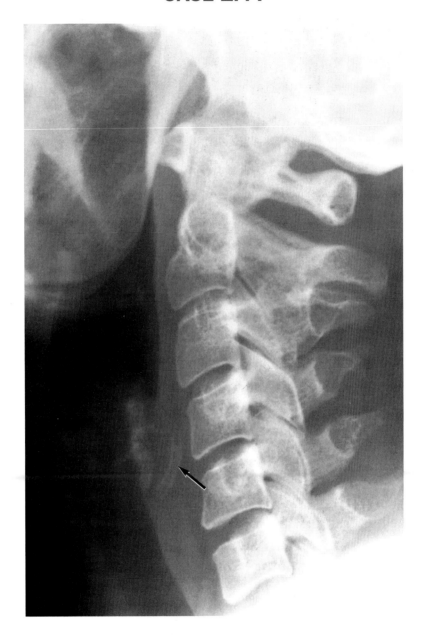

Findings

Lateral radiograph of the neck. There is a bone fragment (arrow) in the region of the esophagus at the level of the C4 interspace.

Differential Diagnosis

Foreign body

Diagnosis

Esophageal foreign body

Discussion

This patient complained of food sticking and pain while eating chicken. A chicken bone was removed endoscopically.

Bony foreign bodies such as chicken or fish bones often lodge in the upper esophagus, whereas meat impactions (case 1.45) most commonly occur at the gastroesophageal junction. Impacted bones often are best visualized on a lateral radiograph of the cervical region or at CT. Contrast material may obscure a small fragment.

CASE 1.45

A
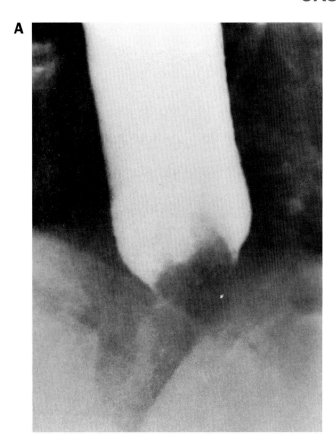

B
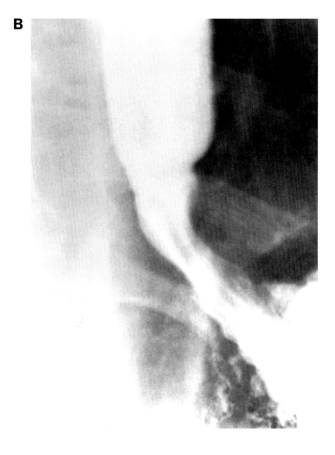

Findings

A. Single-contrast esophagram. An intraluminal filling defect is present in the distal esophagus just above the gastroesophageal junction.

B. Subsequent esophagram shows that the filling defect is no longer present and also shows a lower esophageal ring.

Differential Diagnosis
1. Foreign body
2. Esophageal carcinoma
3. Esophageal adenoma

Diagnosis
Esophageal foreign body

Discussion
This patient had a typical history of swallowing a large piece of meat and immediately experiencing odynophagia. Glucagon (1 mg) was administered intravenously after image

A was obtained, and the meat bolus passed into the stomach.

Impacted food typically lodges above the gastroesophageal junction. Several techniques can be used to remove the food. Intravenously administered glucagon decreases pressure of the lower esophageal sphincter and may facilitate passage of the food bolus into the stomach. Generally, if the bolus reaches the stomach, it will pass through the remainder of the alimentary tract without difficulty. Endoscopic retrieval is the traditional means of treatment. Baskets and balloon catheters also have been used successfully to extract these foreign bodies. Effervescent granules and meat tenderizer have been used successfully by some, but they are not used in our practice because of the possible risk of perforation with these methods. If an impaction has persisted for more than 24 hours, the risk of perforation increases because of possible transmural ischemia. Special care must be taken in these cases. It is important to examine the esophagus after the food bolus has passed or been removed in order to exclude an underlying lesion.

Esophageal Filling Defects

		Case
Benign tumors		
Gastrointestinal stromal tumor	Smooth surface. 90° angle with esophageal lumen. Most common submucosal tumor	1.25
Adenoma	Resembles a polyp. Usually <1.5 cm in diameter	1.26
Inflammatory polyp	Always contiguous with gastric fold. Due to esophagitis	1.27
Fibrovascular polyp	Large polyp in the cervical esophagus on a thin stalk	1.28
Malignant tumors		
Carcinoma	Polypoid, ulcerative, or annular. Squamous cell carcinoma, proximal; adenocarcinoma, distal. Most adenocarcinomas are from Barrett esophagus, usually polypoid	1.29–1.34
Metastases	Can appear mucosal or extramucosal	1.35
Lymphoma	Primary or secondary involvement of esophagus. Associated lymphadenopathy should be sought	1.36
Spindle cell carcinoma (carcinosarcoma)	Polypoid tumor in mid or distal esophagus. May expand the esophageal lumen	1.37
Malignant gastrointestinal stromal tumor	Submucosal, bulky. Can present as intraluminal mass	Not shown
Nonneoplastic		
Varices	Serpentine shape, shape changes. Also can be present in the stomach	1.38–1.40
Duplication cyst	Smooth surface. Oblique angle with esophageal contour, lumen displacement away from mass. Water attenuation at CT	1.41 and 1.42
Ectopic gastric mucosa	Usually a pair of shallow indentations in cervical esophagus. Occasionally polypoid or irregular in shape	1.43
Foreign body	Bones lodge in upper esophagus; meat impactions occur above gastroesophageal junction	1.44 and 1.45

CASE 1.46

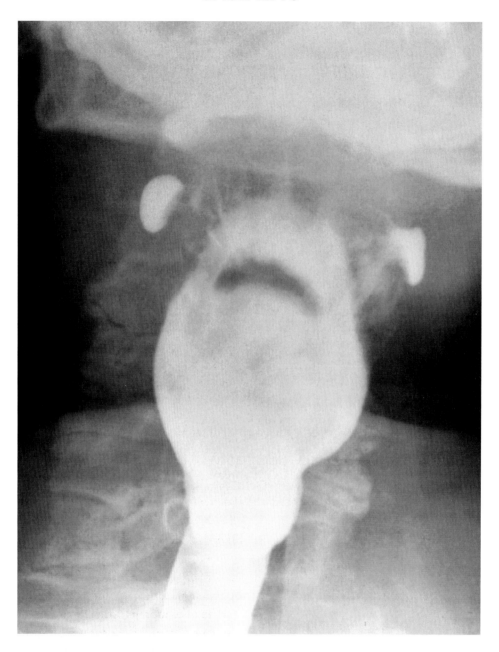

Findings

Single-contrast esophagram. Small outpouchings arise from both sides of the hypopharynx.

Differential Diagnosis

Lateral pharyngeal pouches

Diagnosis

Lateral pharyngeal pouches

Discussion

Lateral pharyngeal pouches arise from an unsupported "weak area" of the thyrohyoid membrane which does not contain a muscular covering. Pouches may be best shown during the pharyngeal phase of swallowing or by asking a patient to blow through closed lips (modified Valsalva maneuver). These pouches are common in asymptomatic patients and can reach a large size in glassblowers, wind instrument players, and the elderly.

CASE 1.47

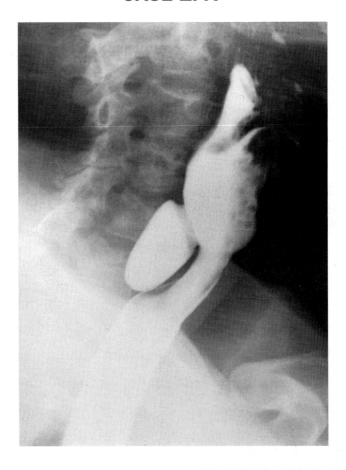

Findings
Double-contrast esophagram. A diverticulum arises from the posterior wall of the cervical esophagus.

Differential Diagnosis
1. Zenker diverticulum
2. Pseudo-Zenker diverticulum

Diagnosis
Zenker diverticulum

Discussion
Zenker diverticulum is a protrusion of the esophageal mucosa through an anatomically weak area in the posterior wall of the cervical esophagus. The site of weakness lies between the oblique and horizontal fibers of the esophageal wall, known as a Killian dehiscence or triangle. The cricopharyngeus muscle is invariably prominent just caudal to the diverticulum.

Zenker diverticula result from abnormally increased pressure generated in the hypopharynx. This high pressure is due to failure of the cricopharyngeus muscle to relax after pharyngeal contraction during swallowing. Many patients with gastroesophageal reflux have a prominent cricopharyngeus muscle.

Retention of food and fluid within the diverticulum can be uncomfortable, cause halitosis, or even lead to aspiration when the patient is recumbent. Cricopharyngeal myotomy and either surgical diverticulopexy or diverticulectomy may be required.

A pseudo-Zenker diverticulum results from barium being trapped between a pharyngeal contraction wave and a prominent cricopharyngeus muscle. This can result in a transient, small, saclike bulge off the posterior pharyngeal wall superior to the cricopharyngeus muscle.

CASE 1.48

A

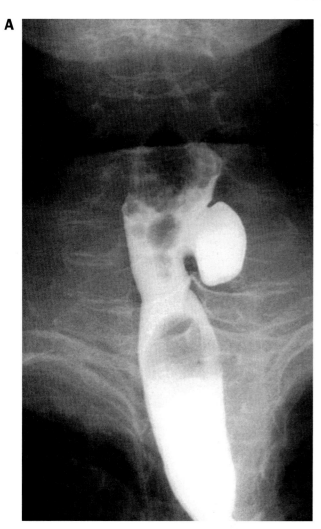

B

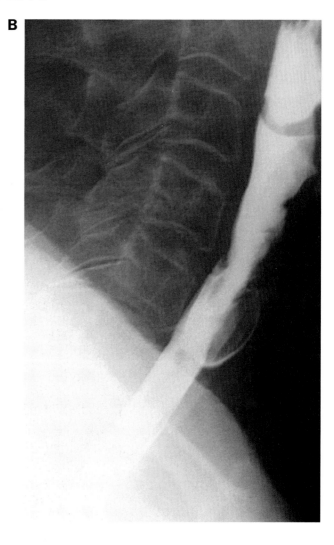

Findings
A. Single-contrast anteroposterior esophagram.

B. Lateral esophagram. A rounded, barium-filled diverticulum protrudes off the lateral wall of the upper cervical esophagus.

Differential Diagnosis
1. Killian-Jamieson diverticulum
2. Zenker diverticulum

Diagnosis
Killian-Jamieson diverticulum

Discussion
A Killian-Jamieson diverticulum protrudes through an area of weakness below the attachment of the cricopharyngeus muscle on the cricoid cartilage and lateral to the suspensory ligaments of the esophagus inserting on the cricoid cartilage, known as the Killian-Jamieson space. It presents radiographically as a diverticulum off the anterolateral wall of the proximal cervical esophagus just below the level of the cricopharyngeus muscle. Killian-Jamieson diverticula are more often bilateral than unilateral. A unilateral diverticulum can sometimes be confused with a Zenker diverticulum. However, on a lateral view, a Killian-Jamieson diverticulum should protrude anteriorly in relation to the cervical esophagus, unlike a Zenker diverticulum, which protrudes posteriorly.

CASE 1.49

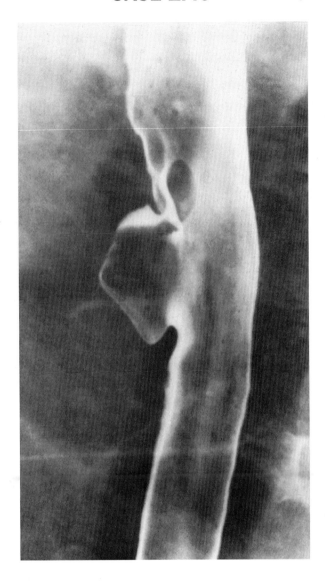

Findings
Double-contrast esophagram. A wide-based outpouching arises from the mid esophagus.

Differential Diagnosis
1. Traction diverticulum
2. Pulsion diverticulum

Diagnosis
Mid-esophageal traction diverticulum

Discussion
The triangular shape of this diverticulum is often found among traction diverticula as a result of fibrosis in the periesophageal tissues. In the past, tuberculosis with inflammatory mediastinal lymph nodes was implicated as an important cause of traction diverticula. Today, most esophageal diverticula are pulsion in origin, developing as a result of esophageal motor disorders. Pulsion diverticula usually are rounded and fail to empty (they contain no muscle in their walls) with a peristaltic contraction.

Most mid-esophageal diverticula are asymptomatic. A large diverticulum can compress the esophagus and lead to dysphagia. If a diverticulum overflows into the esophagus, aspiration can occur. Inflammation and infection can lead to rare complications of perforation or fistulization.

CASE 1.50

CASE 1.51

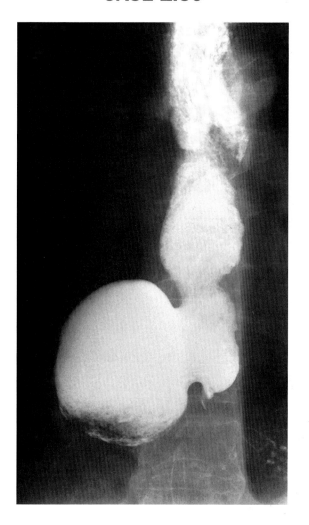

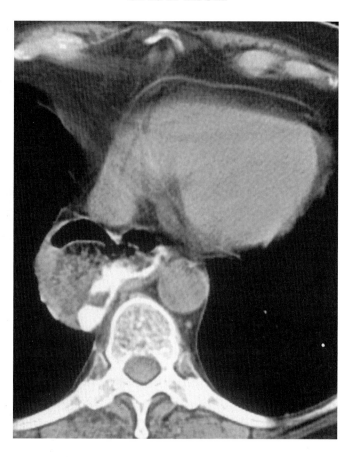

Findings

Case 1.50. Single-contrast esophagram. A large diverticulum is seen in the distal esophagus just above the gastroesophageal junction. Esophageal contractions also are visible.

Case 1.51. Contrast-enhanced CT. A large, thin-walled sac communicates with the esophagus. Orally administered contrast material and food are seen within the diverticulum.

Differential Diagnosis
Pulsion diverticulum

Diagnosis
Epiphrenic pulsion diverticulum

Discussion

Diverticula arising in the distal esophagus just above the gastroesophageal junction are referred to as epiphrenic diverticula. These outpouchings are nearly always pulsion in origin. Achalasia or other motor abnormalities of the esophagus often are associated with this condition. Both of these patients had achalasia. The visible contractions were nonpropulsive and characteristic of vigorous achalasia.

CASE 1.52

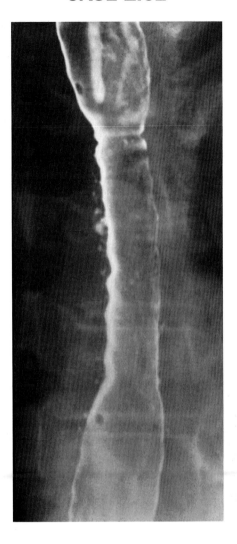

Findings
Double-contrast esophagram. Multiple tiny outpouchings are seen within the mid esophagus around a localized stricture.

Differential Diagnosis
Intramural esophageal pseudodiverticulosis

Diagnosis
Intramural esophageal pseudodiverticulosis

Discussion
Intramural esophageal pseudodiverticulosis is seen as multiple tiny outpouchings that either diffusely or segmentally affect the esophagus. The tiny necks may not fill completely, resulting in an apparent lack of communication with the esophageal lumen. Pathologically, these outpouchings are dilated submucosal glands, most commonly due to chronic reflux esophagitis. Elderly patients are most frequently affected and complain of progressive dysphagia due to the often-associated esophageal strictures. Up to 90% have an associated smooth stricture in the mid or upper esophagus. Dilation of the stricture usually cures the symptoms. The radiographic appearance is analogous to Rokitansky-Aschoff sinuses in the gallbladder and is virtually pathognomonic of this condition. *Candida* is frequently cultured from the esophagus in patients with this condition, but this is believed to be a secondary invader rather than a causative factor.

Esophageal Diverticula

		Case
Pharyngeal	Usually referred to as pouches; due to weakness in region of tonsillar fossa and thyrohyoid membrane. Usually asymptomatic	1.46
Zenker	Posterior, immediately above prominent cricopharyngeus muscle	1.47
Killian-Jamieson	Arise from lateral esophagus just below cricopharyngeus muscle	1.48
Mid-esophageal	In the past, due to traction from granulomatous disease (tuberculosis); today, nearly always pulsion diverticula due to motor abnormalities	1.49
Epiphrenic	Distal esophageal segment due to motor abnormality of esophagus	1.50 and 1.51
Pseudodiverticulosis	Dilated submucosal glands cause multiple small outpouchings. Usually due to chronic reflux esophagitis. *Candida* is often cultured but is not the causative factor	1.52

CASE 1.53

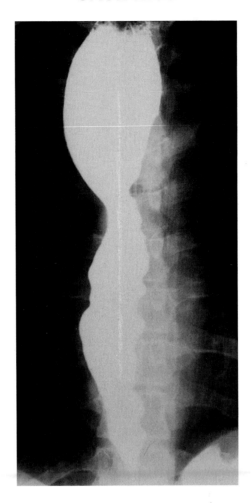

Findings
Single-contrast esophagram. Multiple nonpropulsive contractions are present in the lower esophagus.

Differential Diagnosis
1. Tertiary contractions
2. Vigorous achalasia

Diagnosis
Nonspecific motor incoordination, tertiary esophageal contractions

Discussion
Esophageal contractions can be categorized as three separate types: primary, secondary, or tertiary. Primary esophageal peristalsis is initiated by a swallow and propagates a smooth, continuous contraction the length of the esophagus. Secondary esophageal peristalsis appears fluoroscopically identical to a primary wave, except it is not initiated by a swallow but rather by a bolus within the esophagus or by intraesophageal distention. Tertiary esophageal contractions are nonpropulsive contractions that may be single or multiple, and they do not result in clearing of esophageal contents. These contractions increase in frequency with age. Tertiary contractions also can be associated with many other conditions. Incomplete relaxation of the lower esophageal sphincter also can occur in some patients. The single esophagraphic image shown here could be seen in vigorous achalasia (case 1.19). However, more esophageal dilatation might be expected, and, in this case, barium was seen to flow freely into the stomach across a normal gastroesophageal junction during real-time imaging.

CASE 1.54

A

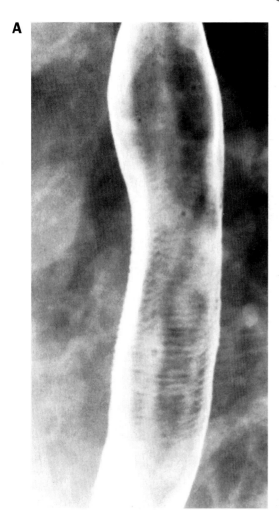

B

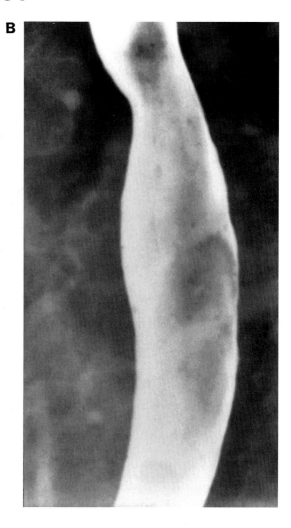

Findings
Double-contrast esophagram. **A.** Multiple thin, transverse folds are present in the lower esophagus. **B.** An exposure taken a few seconds later is normal, without evidence of the previously seen folds.

Differential Diagnosis
1. Feline esophagus
2. Transverse folds of chronic reflux esophagitis

Diagnosis
Feline esophagus

Discussion
Feline esophagus can be recognized by the presence of multiple transverse folds that are present transiently as the esophagus begins to collapse. The folds are fine and delicate, numerous, and symmetric. They usually cross the entire esophageal lumen. Their transient nature distinguishes them from the fixed, larger folds occasionally seen in patients with reflux esophagitis (case 1.4). Transverse folds of esophagitis usually do not cross the esophageal lumen. They also should be distinguished from the broad transverse bands seen in patients with nonpropulsive tertiary contractions (case 1.53).

The name is derived from the similar-appearing esophagraphic findings in cats. Often this finding is a normal variant that is due to contraction of the longitudinally oriented muscularis mucosae. Some investigators have suggested that this finding may be more common in patients with esophagitis.

CASE 1.55

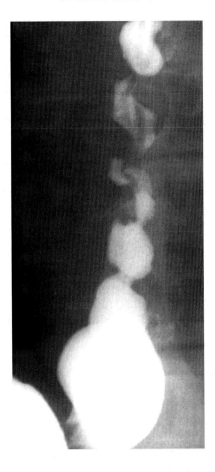

Findings

Single-contrast esophagram. Numerous nonpropulsive contractions are present in the lower esophagus. This appearance has been likened to a corkscrew.

Differential Diagnosis

1. Diffuse esophageal spasm
2. Vigorous achalasia
3. Nonspecific motor incoordination

Diagnosis

Diffuse esophageal spasm (nutcracker esophagus)

Discussion

Diffuse esophageal spasm is characterized by dysphagia or chest pain, and at least 30% of swallows are associated with vigorous, repetitive, nonpropulsive contractions. Careful fluoroscopy eventually shows a normal peristaltic sequence. Lower esophageal sphincter function may be normal; however, nearly a third of patients have impaired relaxation or increased resting pressures. Various terms have been used to describe the radiographic appearance of the nonpropulsive contractions, including corkscrew, curling, rosary bead, and shish kebab esophagus.

The term *nutcracker esophagus* refers to a disorder characterized by the manometric findings of high-amplitude (>180 mm Hg) contractions in conjunction with chest discomfort. Radiographically, peristalsis is normal. Some authorities believe that this disorder is a precursor to diffuse esophageal spasm.

The principal differential consideration is vigorous achalasia (case 1.19). Achalasia can be excluded by a normal stripping wave in response to swallowing. Some patients are symptomatic, and others are not but have identical radiographic findings (nonspecific motor incoordination). It is important to exclude other causes of chest pain, especially coronary artery disease, before attributing it to the esophageal abnormalities.

CASE 1.56

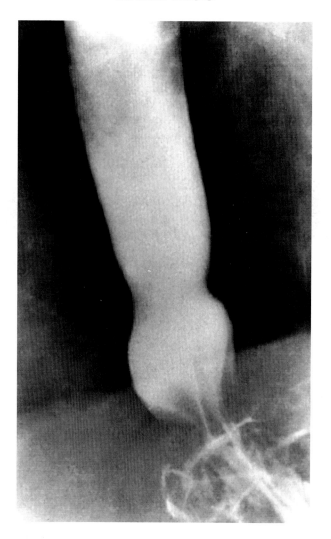

Findings

Single-contrast esophagram. A ring (circumferential impression) is seen within the distal esophagus. At fluoroscopy, the ring was noted to be transient.

Differential Diagnosis

1. Muscular ring (A ring)
2. Mucosal ring (B ring)

Diagnosis

Muscular ring (A ring)

Discussion

A muscular ring appears as a broad, smooth indentation in the lower esophagus, just superior to the esophageal vestibule. It is caused by a muscular thickening and can be observed to change shape and disappear at fluoroscopy. A prominent muscular ring is encountered more often in patients with a hiatal hernia or gastroesophageal reflux and in some esophageal motor disorders. It is not known whether these associations are significant. The esophageal vestibule roughly corresponds in location to the manometrically defined lower esophageal sphincter and should not be confused with a hiatal hernia. At fluoroscopy, a peristaltic wave can be seen to pass through this region. Often a mucosal ring (B ring) also is visible during the examination. The B ring is a thin, fixed ring that does not change appearance and marks the location of the esophagogastric junction.

CASE 1.57

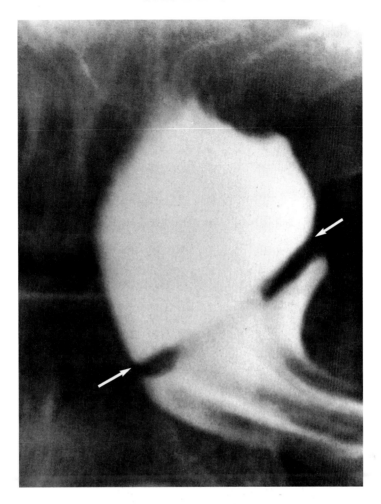

Findings

Single-contrast esophagram. There is a thin, smooth, circumferential filling defect at the gastroesophageal junction (arrows) with a small associated hiatal hernia.

Differential Diagnosis

1. Schatzki ring
2. Chronic reflux stricture

Diagnosis

Schatzki ring

Discussion

A Schatzki ring is a symptomatic, thin constricting ring at the level of the gastroesophageal junction. The pathogenesis of this condition is unknown. Most patients complain of dysphagia with solid foods. Large pieces of meat are often most troublesome. Treatment varies from instructions on chewing more carefully to endoscopic mechanical disruption of the ring with a bougie or pneumatic dilation.

Radiographically, a thin, weblike constriction is present at the gastroesophageal junction. A hiatal hernia is often present. Some patients experience dysphagia if the luminal diameter is between 10 and 15 mm at the level of the ring. Virtually all patients are symptomatic if the ring narrows to 10 mm or less.

The term *lower esophageal ring* denotes a visible B ring that is asymptomatic. A Schatzki ring has a very characteristic appearance, and other conditions are rarely mistaken for it. It was originally defined as a B ring with luminal narrowing of 13 mm or less. A chronic reflux stricture should be longer and of different morphologic appearance.

CASE 1.58

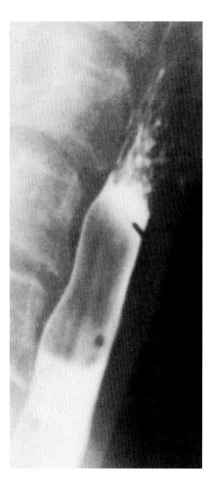

Findings

Double-contrast esophagram. A thin, smooth, shelflike filling defect is present along the anterior wall of the cervical esophagus.

Differential Diagnosis

1. Esophageal web
2. Prominent anterior venous plexus

Diagnosis

Esophageal web

Discussion

Esophageal webs are thin folds composed of mucosa and submucosa which result in a 1- to 2-mm–wide shelflike filling defect along the anterior wall of the lower hypopharynx, pharyngoesophageal segment, or proximal cervical esophagus. Occasionally, webs may be multiple and more masslike in configuration. Esophageal webs are usually asymptomatic. However, dysphagia can develop when the web results in marked luminal narrowing. Clinically significant narrowing may present as a jet phenomenon, in which a thin column of barium jets through the center of a circumferential web. Many investigators have attempted to associate cervical esophageal webs with other conditions. The association between esophageal webs and iron deficiency anemia (Plummer-Vinson syndrome) remains controversial. Reports also have suggested an association between webs and upper esophageal or pharyngeal carcinoma. The great majority of webs remain an isolated finding, often incidentally discovered without an associated disorder.

Distinction of an esophageal web from the anteriorly located venous plexus may be difficult. Careful study of the venous plexus will show variability in its size, whereas a web remains fixed and unchanging from swallow to swallow.

CASE 1.59

A

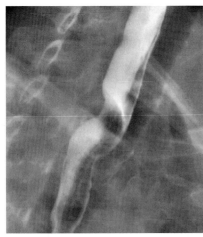

B

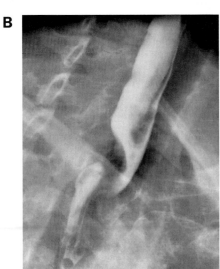

CASE 1.60

A

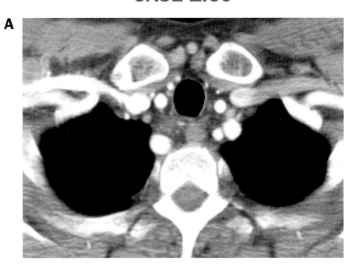

B

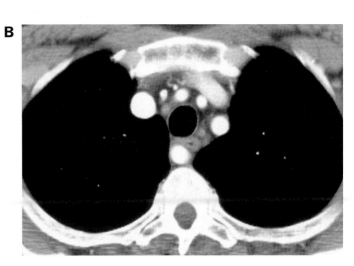

Findings
Case 1.59. Double-contrast esophagram. **A** and **B**. There is a prominent oblique, smooth-surfaced, tubular-shaped filling defect on the posterior aspect of the esophagus.

Case 1.60. Contrast-enhanced CT. **A** and **B**. An aberrant right subclavian artery is present coursing posterior to the esophagus.

Differential Diagnosis
Aberrant right subclavian artery

Diagnosis
Aberrant right subclavian artery

Discussion
An aberrant right subclavian artery is the most common aortic arch anomaly seen as an impression on the esophagus. The aberrant right subclavian artery arises just distal to the normal left subclavian artery and traverses obliquely to the right, posterior to the esophagus. The impression is extramucosal and is so typical of the abnormality that no further studies are needed. The abnormality is rarely symptomatic and needs no treatment.

CASE 1.61

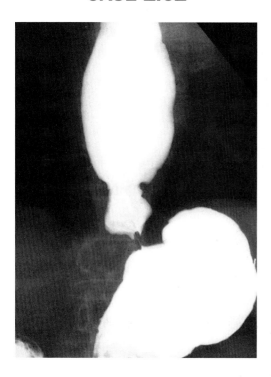

CASE 1.62

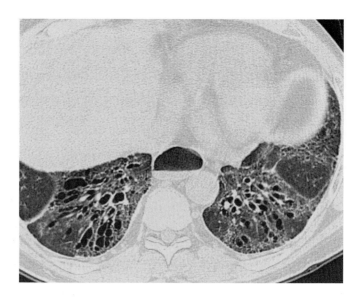

Findings

Case 1.61. Single-contrast esophagram. There is dilatation of the esophagus with a small esophageal hiatal hernia. Real-time imaging showed absent peristalsis in the distal two-thirds of the esophagus and free gastroesophageal reflux of barium in the recumbent position. Slight irregularity is present at the gastroesophageal junction.

Case 1.62. Unenhanced high-resolution CT. Peripheral interstitial fibrotic changes are present in the lung bases with associated ground-glass infiltrates and traction bronchiectasis. Pulmonary findings are consistent with nonspecific interstitial pneumonitis. Dilatation of the distal esophagus also can be seen with an air-fluid level.

Differential Diagnosis
1. Scleroderma
2. Achalasia
3. Pseudoachalasia

Diagnosis
Scleroderma

Discussion

Scleroderma (progressive systemic sclerosis) involves the esophagus in 80% of cases, and the radiographic changes in the esophagus often precede development of the characteristic skin changes. Pathologically, degeneration and atrophy of the smooth muscle and fibrosis are present within the distal two-thirds of the esophagus.

Radiographic changes relate to decreased peristalsis in the distal two-thirds of the esophagus, with an incompetent lower esophageal sphincter. Gastroesophageal reflux and changes of peptic esophagitis often are observed. Chronically, a lower esophageal stricture is often present.

Diminished esophageal clearance results in stasis and the possibility of secondary esophageal candidiasis and aspiration pneumonitis. Chronic reflux esophagitis can be complicated by Barrett esophagus.

The lungs are involved pathologically in nearly 90% of patients with scleroderma. However, radiographic evidence of pulmonary involvement is found in only 25% of patients. The appearance is indistinguishable from other causes of interstitial pulmonary fibrosis. Findings of scleroderma in the small bowel include diminished peristalsis, dilatation, sacculations, and closely spaced valvulae conniventes.

CASE 1.63

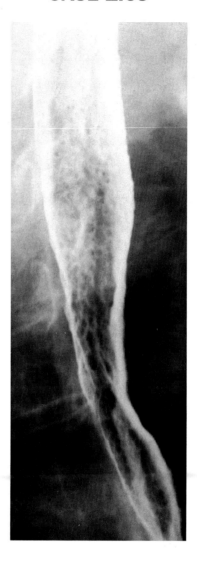

Findings
Double-contrast esophagram. Multiple nodular filling defects throughout the esophagus.

Differential Diagnosis
1. Reflux esophagitis
2. Glycogen acanthosis
3. *Candida* esophagitis

Diagnosis
Glycogen acanthosis

Discussion
Glycogen acanthosis is an occasional incidental finding in older patients, caused by increased cytoplasmic glycogen within the squamous epithelial cells of the esophagus. Radiographically, nodular filling defects are seen, ranging in size from 1 to 15 mm. Rarely, nodules coalesce to form larger plaques. Often, the margins of these lesions are hazy and fade peripherally.

Reflux esophagitis is the main differential consideration. *Candida* esophagitis also may have a nodular mucosal appearance. However, patients with *Candida* esophagitis almost always present with odynophagia, unlike patients with glycogen acanthosis, who are almost always asymptomatic.

CASE 1.64

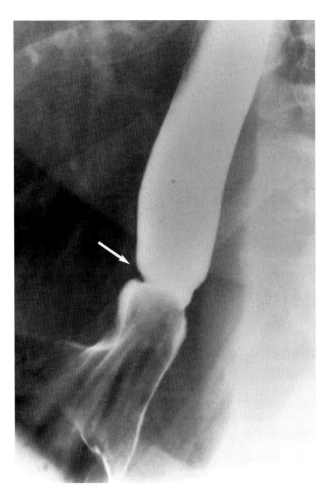

Findings
Double-contrast esophagram. A portion of the gastric cardia protrudes through the esophageal hiatus into the thorax. Gastric rugae are seen within the hernia sac. A lower esophageal mucosal ring (arrow) (B ring) demarcates the gastroesophageal junction.

Differential Diagnosis
1. Sliding hiatal hernia
2. Schatzki ring

Diagnosis
Sliding hiatal hernia

Discussion
Identification of a B ring at least 2 cm above the diaphragm allows hiatal hernia to be diagnosed with confidence. The significance of esophageal hiatal hernias is controversial. Usual symptoms are from gastroesophageal reflux: heartburn, chest pain, and water brash. Occasionally, large hernias can be associated with aspiration, respiratory distress, and compromised lung excursion. A hiatal hernia as a single radiographic finding is a poor predictor of gastroesophageal reflux or reflux esophagitis. Most patients with significant reflux esophagitis, however, have a hiatal hernia.

The main differential consideration in this case is a Schatzki ring (case 1.57). A lower esophageal ring has little clinical relevance unless there is significant compromise of the esophageal lumen. Some patients experience dysphagia if the luminal diameter is between 10 and 15 mm, whereas virtually all patients are symptomatic if the diameter is 10 mm or less. Pneumatic dilation of the mucosal ring is often successful in treating symptomatic patients.

CASE 1.65

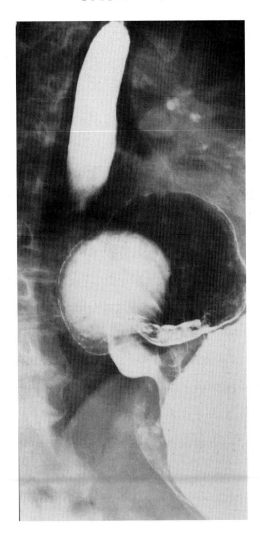

Findings

Double-contrast esophagram. The gastroesophageal junction is normally positioned, and a portion of the stomach herniates into the thorax by way of the esophageal diaphragmatic hiatus.

Differential Diagnosis

1. Paraesophageal hernia
2. Sliding esophageal hiatal hernia

Diagnosis

Paraesophageal hernia

Discussion

Paraesophageal hernias are more prone to complication than sliding esophageal hiatal hernias. Complications include gastritis and bleeding in the hernia (due to edematous and hemorrhagic rugal folds from venous and lymphatic obstruction), gastric ulcers at the level of the diaphragmatic hiatus, and strangulation of the hernia sac.

Radiographic diagnosis is dependent on identifying a normally positioned esophageal junction with the stomach passing through the esophageal hiatus anteriorly. A sliding esophageal hiatal hernia can at times mimic a paraesophageal hernia, but in these cases the esophageal junction is always abnormally located within the thoracic cavity. Most paraesophageal hernias undergo surgical repair because a high mortality is associated with strangulation—a complication that may occur in up to 30% of patients.

CASE 1.66

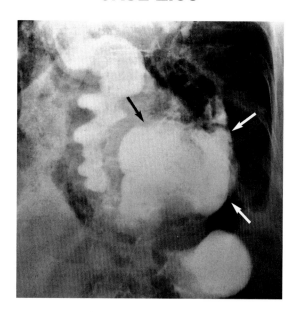

CASE 1.67

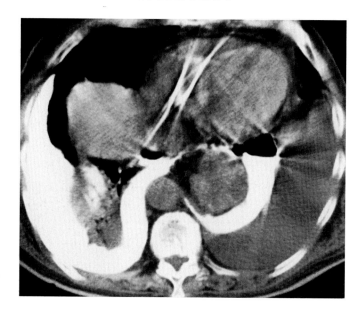

Findings
Case 1.66. Single-contrast esophagram with water-soluble contrast. A large collection of extravasated contrast (arrows) is present in the mediastinum.

Case 1.67. CT with oral contrast. Extravasated oral contrast is seen in the pleural spaces bilaterally. Air also is present within the mediastinum and pleural spaces.

Differential Diagnosis
Esophageal perforation

Diagnosis
Esophageal perforation

Discussion
In case 1.66, the patient had a known history of achalasia, and pain developed after dilation of the lower esophageal sphincter. In case 1.67, the patient also had pain after endoscopy. Surgical repair was necessary in both cases.

Esophageal perforation usually is due to iatrogenic procedures (endoscopic perforations cause 75%-80% of all esophageal leaks and occur in about 1 of 1,000 patients undergoing fiberoptic endoscopy) or spontaneous perforation (Boerhaave syndrome) from violent retching or vomiting. Most endoscopic perforations involve the cervical esophagus near the cricopharyngeus muscle. Spontaneous rupture nearly always occurs just above the gastroesophageal junction on the left. Early detection of these perforations is critical to patient survival. Small cervical esophageal leaks often can be treated conservatively, but large leaks must be surgically repaired to prevent development of a retropharyngeal abscess. Untreated thoracic esophageal perforations have at least a 70% mortality rate (due to mediastinitis) if the leak is undiscovered.

Esophageal perforations can be suspected from the chest radiograph by detection of pneumomediastinum, widening of the mediastinum, hydropneumothorax, pleural effusion, and subcutaneous emphysema. Perforations suspected on the basis of the chest radiograph or on clinical grounds should be confirmed by an esophagram with water-soluble contrast material. Small leaks may be overlooked with water-soluble contrast agents, and negative studies should be followed by barium esophagraphy.

CT is excellent for evaluating patients with suspected or known esophageal perforation. Small amounts of extravasated air (pneumomediastinum) or contrast material and its location within the chest can be identified readily.

Miscellaneous Esophageal Conditions

		Case
Nonspecific motor incoordination	Nonpropulsive contractions. Stripping wave present with observation. Common in the elderly	1.53
Feline esophagus	Transient, numerous fine folds traverse entire lumen. Can be normal; esophagitis should be suspected	1.54
Esophageal spasm	Tertiary contractions with pain	1.55
Muscular ring	Transient, nonobstructing	1.56
Schatzki ring	Fixed, narrows lumen ″13 mm. B ring, esophagogastric junction	1.57
Esophageal web	Membranous, usually cervical esophagus. Association with anemia is controversial	1.58
Aberrant right subclavian artery	Oblique, smooth filling defect in upper thoracic esophagus	1.59 and 1.60
Scleroderma	Aperistalsis of distal two-thirds. Patulous gastroesophageal junction, reflux. Reflux esophagitis, lung fibrosis	1.61 and 1.62
Glycogen acanthosis	Multiple elevated nodules in asymptomatic elderly patients	1.63
Hiatal hernia	Gastroesophageal junction in thorax. Sliding (common) or short (due to chronic reflux esophagitis)	1.64
Paraesophageal hernia	Gastroesophageal junction normally positioned. High incidence of incarceration and strangulation	1.65
Esophageal perforation	Contained within mediastinum or pleural communication. Iatrogenic—usually cervical location; vomiting (Boerhaeve syndrome)— usually distal esophageal tear	1.66 and 1.67

DIFFERENTIAL DIAGNOSES

Esophagitis

Peptic (reflux) esophagitis
Barrett esophagus
Medication-induced esophagitis
Crohn esophagitis
Infectious esophagitis
    Candidiasis
    Herpes esophagitis
    Cytomegalovirus esophagitis
    Human immunodeficiency
       virus esophagitis

Strictures

Benign
    Peptic (reflux) stricture
    Barrett stricture
    Caustic stricture
    Radiation stricture
    Achalasia
    Blistering skin disorders
Malignant
    Annular carcinoma
    Pseudoachalasia
    Lymphoma (extrinsic
      compression by adenopathy)

Diverticula

Pharyngeal
Zenker
Killian-Jamieson
Mid-esophageal
Epiphrenic
Pseudodiverticulosis

Filling Defects

Benign tumors
    Gastrointestinal stromal tumor
    Adenoma
    Inflammatory esophagogastric
      polyp
    Fibrovascular polyp
Malignant tumors
    Carcinoma
    Metastases
    Lymphoma
    Malignant gastrointestinal
      stromal tumor
    Spindle cell carcinoma
Nonneoplastic filling defects
    Varices
    Esophageal duplication cyst
    Ectopic gastric mucosa
    Foreign body

ESOPHAGEAL STRICTURES

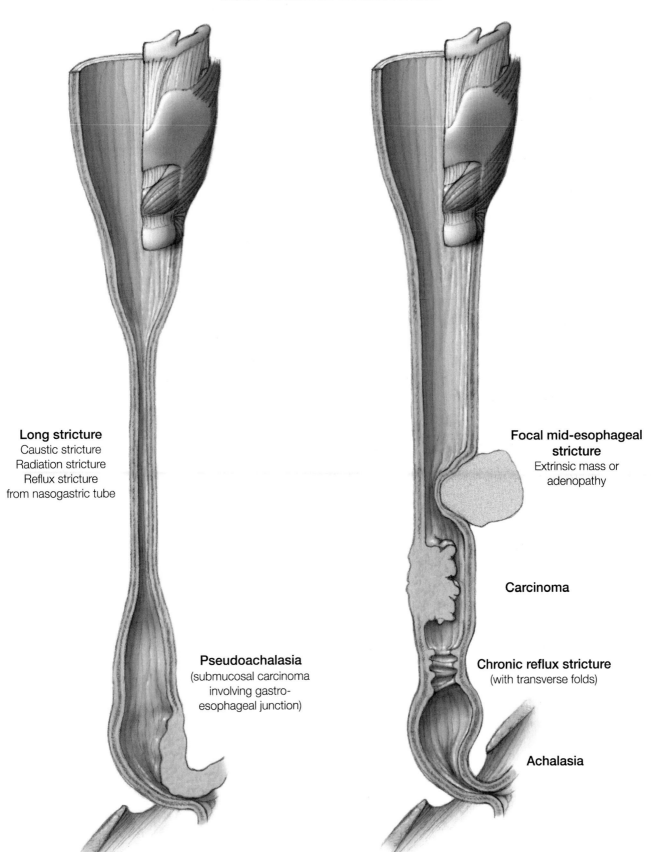

Long stricture
Caustic stricture
Radiation stricture
Reflux stricture
from nasogastric tube

Pseudoachalasia
(submucosal carcinoma
involving gastro-
esophageal junction)

**Focal mid-esophageal
stricture**
Extrinsic mass or
adenopathy

Carcinoma

Chronic reflux stricture
(with transverse folds)

Achalasia

ESOPHAGEAL NARROWINGS

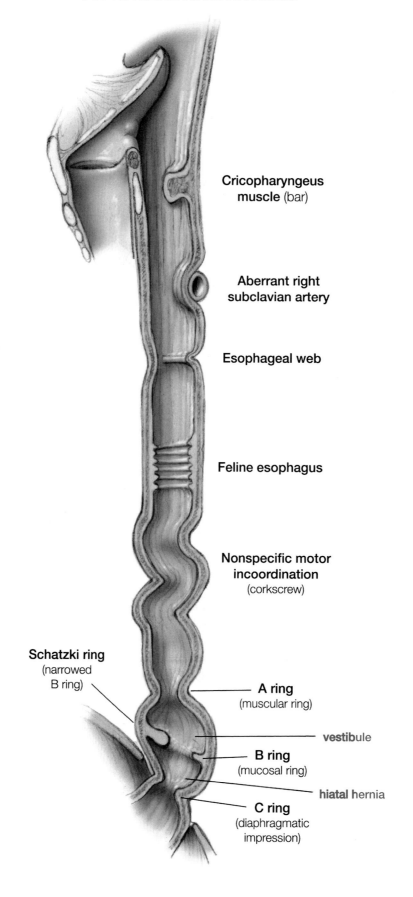

Cricopharyngeus
muscle (bar)

Aberrant right
subclavian artery

Esophageal web

Feline esophagus

Nonspecific motor
incoordination
(corkscrew)

Schatzki ring
(narrowed
B ring)

A ring
(muscular ring)

vestibule

B ring
(mucosal ring)

hiatal hernia

C ring
(diaphragmatic
impression)

ESOPHAGEAL DIVERTICULA

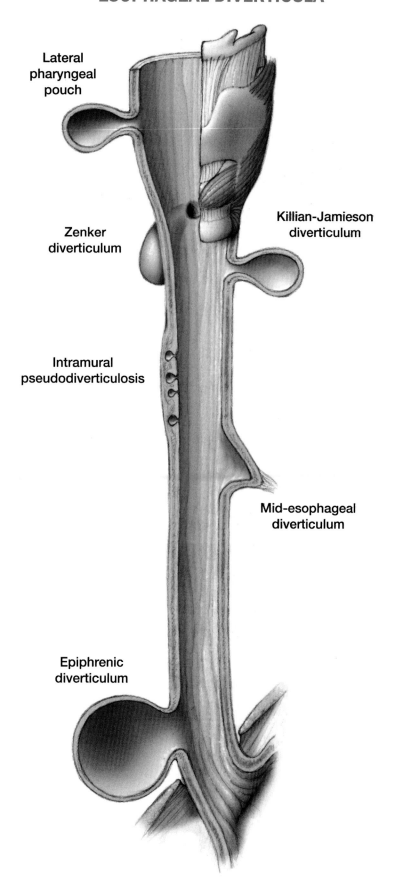

Lateral pharyngeal pouch

Zenker diverticulum

Killian-Jamieson diverticulum

Intramural pseudodiverticulosis

Mid-esophageal diverticulum

Epiphrenic diverticulum

ESOPHAGEAL FILLING DEFECTS

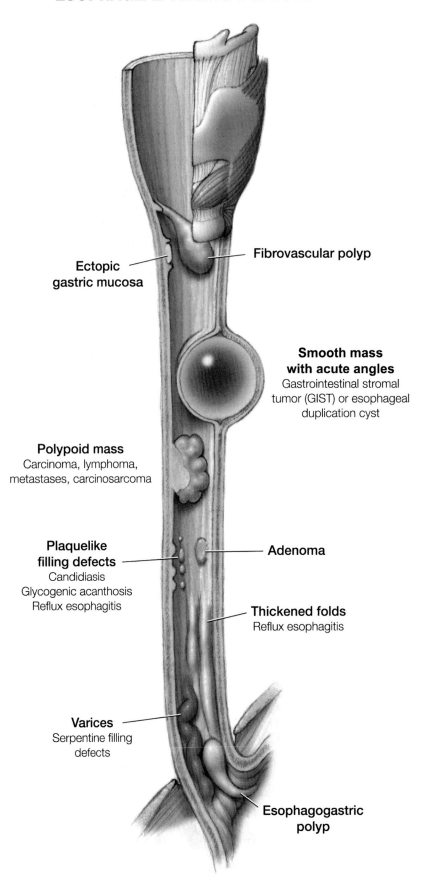

Ectopic
gastric mucosa

Fibrovascular polyp

**Smooth mass
with acute angles**
Gastrointestinal stromal
tumor (GIST) or esophageal
duplication cyst

Polypoid mass
Carcinoma, lymphoma,
metastases, carcinosarcoma

**Plaquelike
filling defects**
Candidiasis
Glycogenic acanthosis
Reflux esophagitis

Adenoma

Thickened folds
Reflux esophagitis

Varices
Serpentine filling
defects

Esophagogastric
polyp

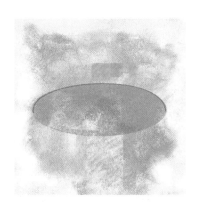

CHAPTER 2
STOMACH

CASE 2.1

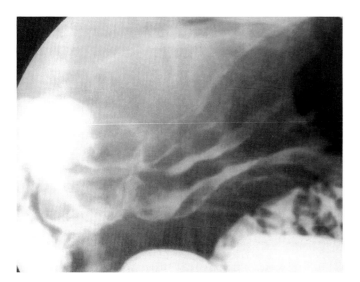

CASE 2.2

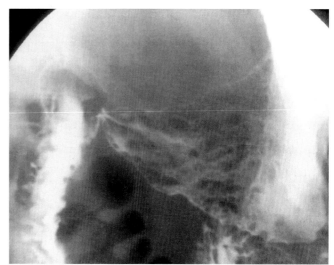

Findings

Case 2.1. Double-contrast UGI. Thickened, lobulated folds are present in the body and antrum of the stomach.

Case 2.2. Double-contrast UGI. Nodular fold thickening is present in the gastric antrum.

Differential Diagnosis
1. Gastritis (e.g., caused by *Helicobacter pylori*, alcohol, medication)
2. Zollinger-Ellison syndrome
3. Lymphoma

Diagnosis
H. pylori gastritis

Discussion
H. pylori infection is the major cause of gastritis (70%), gastric ulcers (70%), and duodenal ulcers (90%). It also has been identified as a significant risk factor for development of gastric adenocarcinoma and lymphoma. *H. pylori* is a gram-negative rod that colonizes the stomachs of a large percentage of the U.S. population (>50% of those older than 60 years), most of whom are asymptomatic. However, eradication of the *H. pylori* infection with antibiotics in addition to acid blockers has been effective for curing gastritis and ulcers in up to 90% of patients. *H. pylori* infection usually is diagnosed with serologic tests or endoscopic biopsy. Treatment of asymptomatic patients currently is not recommended because of the cost and possible side effects of the medical therapy.

H. pylori gastritis usually presents as smooth, nonspecific fold thickening involving the body and antrum of the stomach on barium examinations. Occasionally, *H. pylori* gastritis causes markedly thickened nodular folds indistinguishable from lymphoma or submucosal carcinoma. In these cases, endoscopy is recommended to exclude malignancy. Zollinger-Ellison syndrome (cases 2.11 and 2.12) also can cause gastric fold thickening.

CASE 2.3

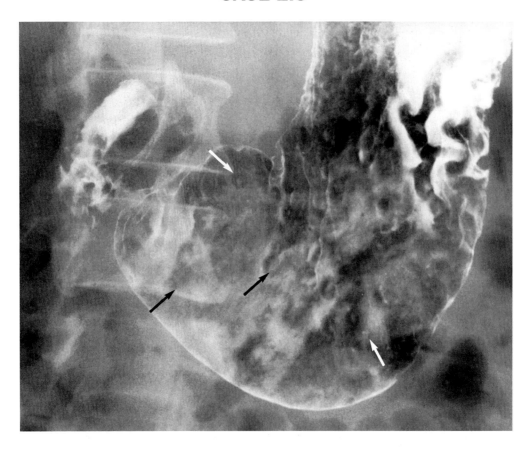

Findings
Double-contrast UGI. Multiple small, round filling defects (mounds of edema) (arrows) containing a small central collection of barium (erosion or tiny ulceration) are present in the gastric antrum and body.

Differential Diagnosis
1. Acute erosive (varioliform) gastritis
2. Barium precipitate
3. Crohn disease
4. Infectious gastritis (viral or fungal)

Diagnosis
Acute erosive gastritis

Discussion
Acute gastritis often presents with symptoms mimicking those of peptic ulcer disease. This disorder has many causes, including stress reactions, *Helicobacter pylori*, alcohol, aspirin, nonsteroidal anti-inflammatory drugs (NSAIDs), chemotherapeutic agents, and several other medications. In our practice, aspirin and NSAIDs are the most common causes.

Typically, multiple small, elevated mounds of edema with central ulcerations are identified, often in line with a rugal fold. These typical erosions are often referred to as varioliform erosions.

It is important not to mistake barium precipitates for punctate erosions. Precipitates never have a surrounding mound of edema and often are randomly oriented—not along the crest of a rugal fold, as often seen with true erosions. The early aphthous ulcerations found in Crohn disease, gastric candidiasis, or viral infections may be indistinguishable from erosive gastritis. Erosions are almost always multiple. Crohn disease usually presents with additional lesions in the small bowel. Single lesions may represent an artifact or a small submucosal process, such as pancreatic rest (case 2.39), gastrointestinal stromal tumor (cases 2.19, 2.20, and 2.21), or metastasis (case 2.37).

CASE 2.4

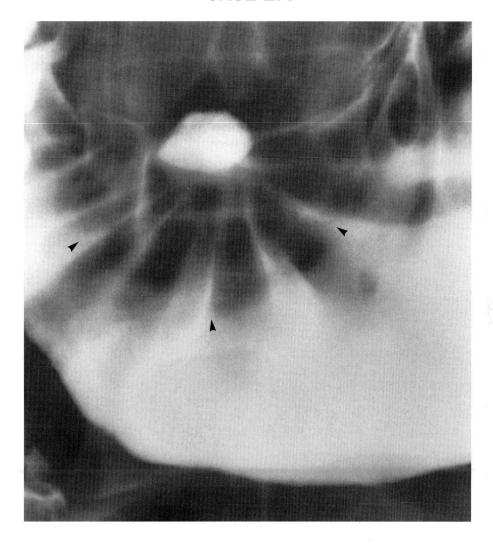

Findings

Single-contrast UGI. An ulcer crater is located along the lesser curvature of the gastric antrum. Symmetric and smoothly contoured folds radiate to the crater. The mound of edema (arrowheads) is smooth in contour, and the crater is located centrally within the mound.

Differential Diagnosis

Benign gastric ulcer

Diagnosis

Benign gastric ulcer

Discussion

This ulcer has some of the typical signs of benignity: a round or oval crater, folds that cross the mound of surrounding edema and extend up to the crater, a symmetric and smooth filling defect (edema) about the crater, extension of the ulcer beyond the normal gastric lumen contour, and radiating gastric folds that are smooth and symmetric (without nodularity or clubbing). Most benign ulcers occur along the lesser curvature or posterior wall of the antrum or body of the stomach. The anterior wall is affected least often. The greater curvature is a somewhat unusual location for benign ulcers. Benign ulcers along the greater curvature of the body and antrum of the stomach are often associated with ingestion of aspirin-containing medication (case 2.7).

CASE 2.5

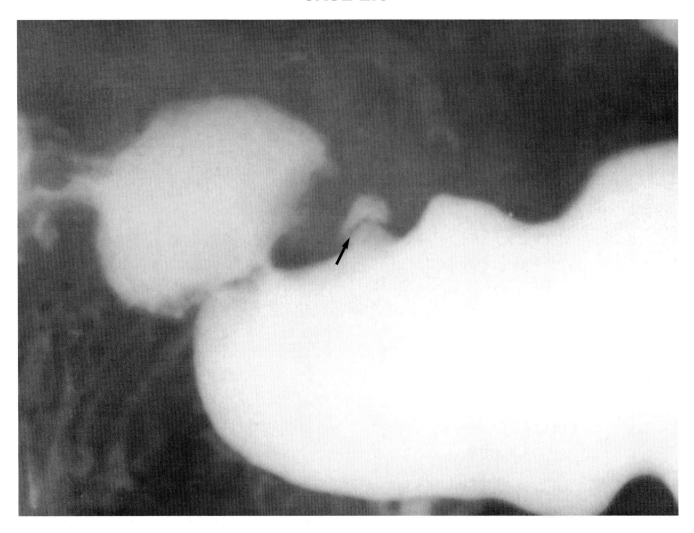

Findings
Single-contrast UGI. An ulcer crater is seen on this tangential view of the gastric antrum. A Hampton line (arrow) is seen at the base of the crater.

Differential Diagnosis
Benign gastric ulcer

Diagnosis
Benign gastric ulcer (Hampton line)

Discussion
Gastric ulcers are common abnormalities, in large part a result of the widespread use of anti-inflammatory agents and *Helicobacter pylori* infection. The radiographic examination is a reliable method for distinguishing benign from malignant ulcers. Characteristics of a benign ulcer on the tangential view include a Hampton line (as seen in this case) or a smooth and symmetric ulcer collar or mound. A Hampton line represents nonulcerated acid-resistant mucosa around the ulcer crater. An ulcer collar represents edematous submucosal tissue surrounding the ulcer cavity. A collar is always wider than the thin, delicate Hampton line. Ulcers with typical radiographic features of benignity are nearly always benign and can be followed radiographically until complete healing has occurred.

CASE 2.6

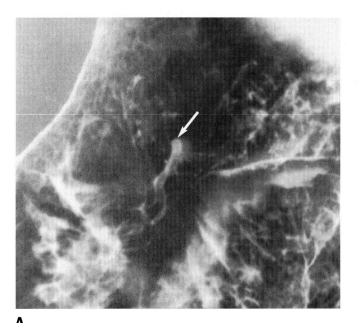

A

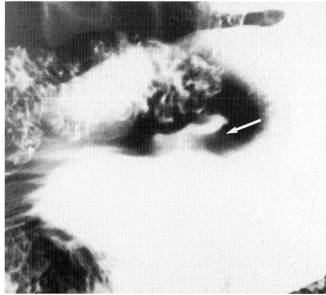

B

Findings

Double-contrast UGI. **A.** A linear collection of barium (arrow) is visible on the en face view of the gastric body. Several folds radiate to the edge of the crater. **B.** The elongated ulcer collection and surrounding collar (arrow) are seen when viewed in profile.

Differential Diagnosis

Benign linear ulcer

Diagnosis

Benign linear ulcer

Discussion

An ulcer collar represents edematous submucosa about the ulcer crater. The crater extends within the submucosa because this tissue is not as acid resistant as the mucosa. A linear configuration of the crater is often seen in patients with healing ulcers. Healing ulcers may be asymmetric or "split" into two smaller craters as reepithelialization occurs. The average time required for healing of an ulcer is 8 weeks. Large ulcers require more time to heal than do smaller ones. For this reason, follow-up studies should probably not be performed less than 6 to 8 weeks after the initial diagnosis. Most ulcers leave a scar after healing has occurred. Scars often appear as a depression or pit on the mucosal surface. Radiating folds often can be seen extending up to the depression. Retraction (as a result of intramural fibrosis) of the adjacent gastric wall is also common. The finding of areae gastricae covering the scarred region confirms ulcer healing; however, this is only rarely identified on double-contrast examinations.

CASE 2.7

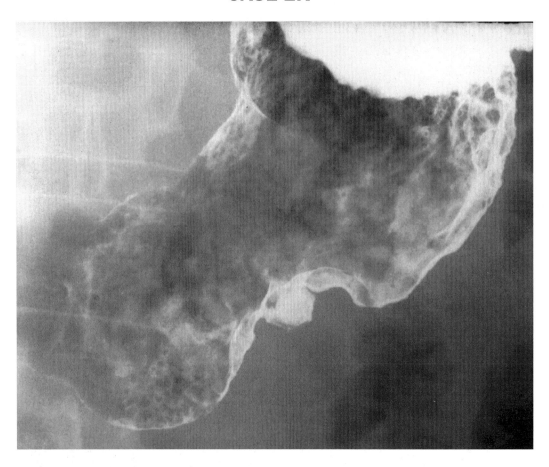

Findings

Double-contrast UGI. An ulcer crater is present on the greater curvature of the stomach. A smooth mound of edema surrounds the centrally located ulcer. The crater does not extend beyond the normal gastric lumen contour.

Differential Diagnosis

1. Benign sump ulcer
2. Gastric adenocarcinoma
3. Intramural diverticulum

Diagnosis

Benign gastric sump ulcer

Discussion

Benign ulcers of the greater curvature may not have all of the usual radiographic features associated with benignity. The location of an ulcer is not a reliable predictor of benignity or malignancy. As a general rule, however, benign ulcers are rarely located in the proximal half of the stomach along the greater curvature. Occasionally, benign gastric ulcers are found in the proximal stomach along the lesser curvature in elderly patients. Many of the ulcers in the distal stomach are benign and medication-induced. Aspirin-induced ulcers often develop along the greater curvature because it is a dependent location where pills collect and directly cause mucosal injury. Sometimes they are referred to as sump ulcers (as in this case). Usually the mound of edema surrounding a benign ulcer is smooth-surfaced and tapers gradually, merging imperceptibly with the normal gastric wall. In this patient, the surrounding mass of edema has rather abrupt margins with the normal gastric wall. Endoscopy is often necessary to exclude malignancy if equivocal or worrisome findings are present. A gastric intramural diverticulum usually does not have significant surrounding mass effect and changes shape with peristaltic contractions.

CASE 2.8

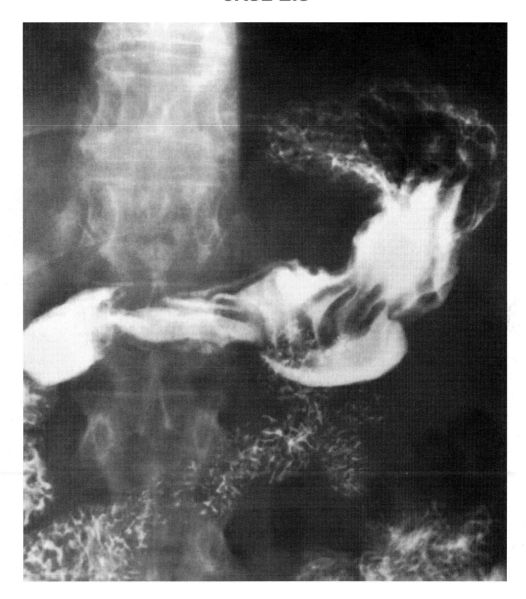

Findings

Single-contrast UGI. A large ulcer is present along the greater curvature of the stomach. Gastric folds extend up to the crater. The crater projects beyond the expected location of the greater curvature mucosa.

Differential Diagnosis

1. Giant gastric ulcer
2. Postoperative deformity

Diagnosis

Benign giant gastric ulcer

Discussion

Giant ulcers are defined as those larger than 3 cm in diameter. The size of the crater has no bearing on their benign or malignant nature. They are commonly associated with contained perforations. Usually, a large mass is visible in patients with giant malignant ulcers (case 2.24). Multiple ulcerations can be seen in 12% to 20% of patients with benign gastric ulcers. Multiplicity favors a benign cause, but each ulcer should be evaluated individually. Concurrent gastric and duodenal ulcers are unusual.

CASE 2.9

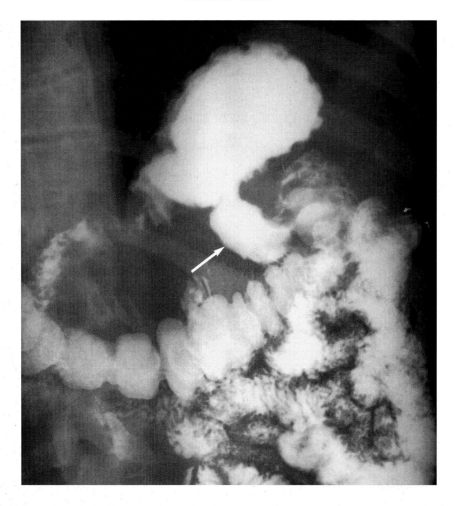

Findings
Single-contrast UGI. A large fistulous communication (arrow) exists between the greater curvature of the stomach and the left transverse colon.

Differential Diagnosis
1. Benign gastric ulcer with fistula
2. Malignant gastric ulcer with fistula
3. Postoperative anastomosis

Diagnosis
Gastrocolic fistula due to a benign gastric ulcer

Discussion
In this patient, a penetrating benign gastric ulcer was found at operation. Major complications of gastric ulcers include bleeding, perforation, obstruction, and penetration. Bleeding is the most frequent complication, occurring in 10% to 24% of patients with peptic ulcer disease. Most actively bleeding ulcers are assessed endoscopically. An ulcer can penetrate into any adjacent organ or tissue. Common sites include the pancreas, omentum, biliary tract, liver, and colon. Most gastrocolic fistulas are due to primary carcinomas or lymphomas arising from either the stomach or the colon. Offending ulcers usually are located along the greater curvature, and offending benign ulcers are usually found in patients receiving aspirin or corticosteroid therapy or both. Penetration of an ulcer into the pancreas may result in pancreatitis or a pancreatic abscess.

An enteric anastomosis is unlikely because the communication does not contain enteric folds (suggesting ulceration or cavity), and intentional anastomosis to the colon is never performed.

CASE 2.10

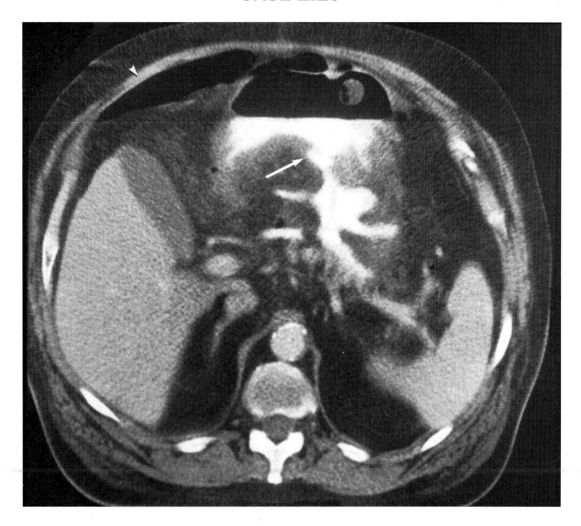

Findings
Enhanced abdominal CT. Orally administered contrast material is seen within the body of the stomach and within an ulcer crater (arrow) in the posterior gastric wall. There is a communication between the stomach (at the site of the ulcer) and into an irregularly shaped cavity within the lesser sac. Pneumoperitoneum (arrowhead) is seen anteriorly within the peritoneal cavity (postoperative in origin).

Differential Diagnosis
1. Perforated benign gastric ulcer
2. Perforated malignant ulcer

Diagnosis
Perforated benign gastric ulcer

Discussion
CT can be helpful for determining the extraluminal extent of disease in a patient with a known or suspected penetrating ulcer. This information can be helpful for preoperative planning and for assessment of possible percutaneous drainage. It may not be possible to distinguish a benign from a malignant ulcer at CT. Endoscopy is often required for further evaluation.

CASE 2.11

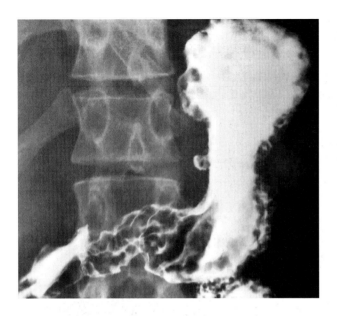

CASE 2.12

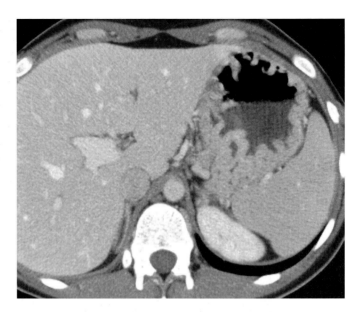

Findings

Case 2.11. Single-contrast UGI. Enlarged rugal folds are present in the gastric antrum. A benign ulcer is present along the lesser curvature.

Case 2.12. Enhanced abdominal CT. The gastric wall and rugal folds are markedly thickened.

Differential Diagnosis

1. Zollinger-Ellison syndrome
2. Lymphoma
3. Primary gastric carcinoma
4. Ménétrier disease

Diagnosis

Zollinger-Ellison syndrome

Discussion

Zollinger-Ellison syndrome is caused by a gastrin-secreting islet cell neoplasm (usually in the pancreas) that results in marked gastric hypersecretion of hydrochloric acid and severe peptic ulcer disease. At least half of these tumors are malignant, metastasizing to regional lymph nodes and liver. Approximately one-fourth of patients have multiple endocrine neoplasia type 1 (parathyroid adenoma, pituitary adenoma, pheochromocytoma). Patients usually are middle-aged and present with intractable peptic ulcer

disease, often with associated malabsorption (due to inactivation of lipase and bile salt precipitation from hyperacidity). Serum gastrin levels are always increased, and paradoxical increase in gastrin levels occurs after an injection of secretin. This result distinguishes Zollinger-Ellison syndrome from other diseases with increased serum gastrin levels (e.g., retained gastric antrum, antral G-cell hyperplasia, short-bowel syndrome, and uremia).

Upper gastrointestinal radiographic findings include enlarged rugal folds, hypersecretion, peptic ulcers, and thickened folds in the proximal small bowel. At CT, gastric and duodenal wall thickening and hypersecretion may be seen. The primary tumor in the pancreas (or nearby organs) and evidence of metastases also may be visible.

Small gastrinomas without evidence of metastases are surgically resected. Advanced lesions are treated with a combination of histamine$_2$-receptor blockers, chemotherapy, and hepatic artery embolization. Multiphase CT and octreotide scintigraphy are most commonly used for identification of the primary tumor. CT and MRI are commonly used for follow-up imaging studies.

Gastric lymphoma produces disorganized, enlarged folds, whereas adenocarcinoma presents as a focal mass or diffusely narrowed stomach (linitis plastica). Neither of these diseases results in inflammatory changes in the duodenum. Thickened folds in Ménétrier disease usually are confined to the proximal stomach.

CASE 2.13

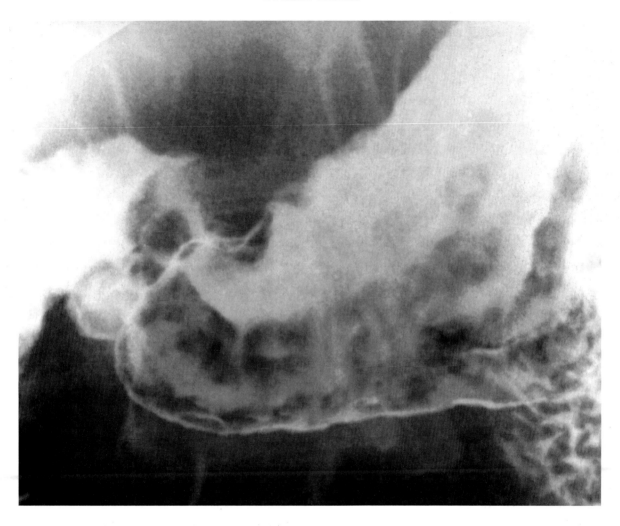

Findings

Single-contrast UGI. Multiple erosions are present in the gastric antrum.

Differential Diagnosis

1. Erosive gastritis
2. Crohn disease

Diagnosis

Crohn disease

Discussion

In this patient, Crohn disease was proved by endoscopic biopsy (chronic inflammation and granulomas). Crohn disease (regional enteritis) of the stomach is uncommon, but when present it usually is associated with disease in the small bowel or colon or both. The earliest changes from Crohn disease include aphthous ulcers and fold thickening (as in this case). Continued inflammation results in confluent ulcers, cobblestoning, denuded mucosa, fibrosis, and strictures. The distal half of the stomach usually is affected, often with concomitant duodenal involvement.

The finding of aphthous ulcerations (superficial erosions) is nonspecific and could be due to peptic ulcer disease or medication-induced gastritis (e.g., aspirin). Endoscopy and histologic examination also are often nonspecific.

CASE 2.14

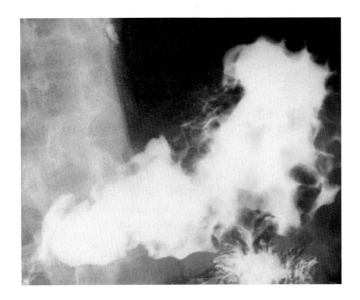

CASE 2.15

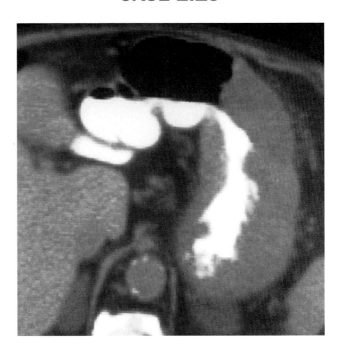

Findings

Case 2.14. Single-contrast UGI. Markedly enlarged gastric folds are present within the proximal half of the stomach.

Case 2.15. Unenhanced abdominal CT. The wall of the gastric fundus and body is markedly thickened, especially along the greater curvature. The antral wall is of normal thickness. Bilateral adrenal masses are present.

Differential Diagnosis

1. Lymphoma
2. Ménétrier disease
3. Zollinger-Ellison syndrome
4. Eosinophilic gastritis

Diagnosis

Ménétrier disease

Discussion

Ménétrier disease is a disorder of unknown cause, sometimes referred to as a hypertrophic gastropathy. Pathologically, hyperplasia of surface epithelial cells is present with abundant mucous cells and mucoid secretions. Parietal cells may be replaced by the epithelial cells, causing achlorhydria.

The process is not primarily inflammatory, but inflammatory cells may be present. Erosions and hemorrhage may cause anemia. Carcinoma has been reported in patients with this disorder, but whether it predisposes to malignancy is unknown. Treatment (antisecretory drugs and occasionally gastrectomy) is often unnecessary unless pain, bleeding, or protein loss is severe.

Radiologic findings are usually those of enlarged rugal folds, often sparing the antrum. The folds are pliable, with a distensible stomach. Folds are enlarged but organized and follow the distribution of normal rugae. Occasionally, segmental rugal enlargement is seen and presents as a polypoid mass.

Gastric folds may be enlarged without any associated clinical disorder. These folds nearly always can be effaced with adequate distention of the gastric fundus. Enlarged folds in patients with lymphoma are usually disorganized and can be nodular and irregular (cases 2.31, 2.32, and 2.33). Zollinger-Ellison syndrome with enlarged gastric folds often is associated with hypersecretion, peptic ulcers, a dilated duodenum, and thickened folds in the proximal small bowel (cases 2.11 and 2.12). Patients with eosinophilic gastritis have thickened folds within the stomach and small bowel as well as a history of allergy.

Thickened Gastric Folds

		Case
H. pylori gastritis	Usually in antrum. Commonest manifestation	2.1 and 2.2
Zollinger-Ellison syndrome	Hypersecretion and ulcerations in stomach and duodenum. Enhancing pancreatic mass	2.11 and 2.12
Crohn disease	Stomach is uncommon location. Aphthous ulcers and fold thickening	2.13
Varices	In patients with portal hypertension, esophageal varices also should be sought. Usually in cardia and fundus	2.41–2.43
Ménétrier disease	May have hypersecretion. Usually in cardia and fundus. Often a diagnosis of exclusion	2.14 and 2.15
Lymphoma	Variable size and nodularity	2.31–2.33

CASE 2.16

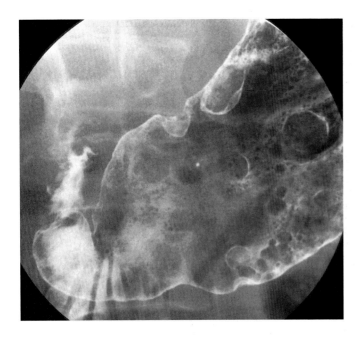

CASE 2.17

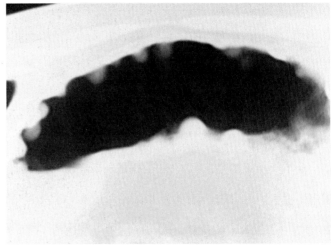

Findings

Case 2.16. Double-contrast UGI. Multiple polypoid filling defects are present in the stomach.

Case 2.17. Unenhanced abdominal CT. Multiple polyps arise from the anterior and posterior walls of the stomach.

Differential Diagnosis

Gastric polyps

Diagnosis

Gastric polyps

Discussion

In this patient, hyperplastic polyps were found at endoscopic biopsy. Gastric polyps occur in about 2% of the population. Most polyps are either hyperplastic or adenomatous histologically. Hyperplastic polyps develop as a reactive change to chronic inflammation with mucosal proliferation and cystic dilatation of gastric glands. Some authors refer to them as regenerative or inflammatory polyps. They are often multiple and usually small (<1 cm in diameter). They have a propensity to develop in the fundus of the stomach, but they may be found anywhere. Hyperplastic polyps are believed to be benign, without malignant potential; however, rare malignant transformation has been reported. Innumerable hyperplastic polyps in the gastric fundus occur in patients with familial adenomatous polyposis syndrome (fundic gland polyposis syndrome).

Adenomatous polyps are infrequent, often solitary lesions, with diameters usually exceeding 1 cm. These polyps can develop into carcinomas, but this is an unusual occurrence, generally among large (>2 cm) lesions. Overall, development of a cancer from gastric polyps is rare, perhaps occurring in 1% to 2% of patients. Endoscopic biopsy and polypectomy are safe and should be considered for solitary large polyps.

CASE 2.18

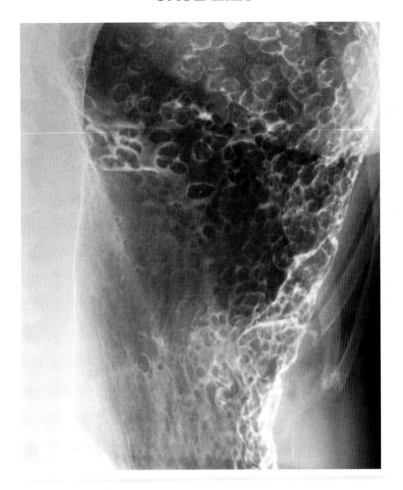

Findings
Double-contrast UGI. Innumerable small polyps are present throughout the stomach. They are most numerous within the fundus.

Differential Diagnosis
1. Gastric polyps
2. Fundic gland polyposis syndrome

Diagnosis
Fundic gland polyposis syndrome

Discussion
This patient had known familial adenomatous polyposis (FAP) syndrome. Gastric polyps in patients with FAP are usually hyperplastic, whereas polyps elsewhere in the intestines are adenomatous. Gardner syndrome and Turcot syndrome are variations of FAP with associated manifestations outside the gastrointestinal tract. In patients with Gardner syndrome, desmoid tumors, osteomas, epidermoid cysts, or papillary thyroid cancer can develop. Patients with Turcot syndrome have development of central nervous system tumors, including gliomas and medulloblastomas. The common association of multiple hyperplastic polyps in the gastric fundus in patients with FAP is known as fundic gland polyposis syndrome. Gastric adenomatous polyps are uncommon, but when they occur in these patients they usually are located in the antrum and may be multiple. Gastric polyps developing in the other polyposis syndromes (Peutz-Jeghers syndrome, juvenile polyposis, and Cronkhite-Canada syndrome) are classified as hamartomas. Patients with FAP also are predisposed to adenomas and adenocarcinomas developing in the periampullary region. Colorectal cancer eventually develops in nearly all patients who have FAP without proctocolectomy.

Polyposis Syndromes

Syndrome	Polyp type	Inheritance	Comment
Familial adenomatous polyposis (FAP)	Hyperplastic: stomach Adenomatous: small bowel, colon	Autosomal dominant	Includes Gardner syndrome and Turcot syndrome
Gardner syndrome	Hyperplastic: stomach Adenomatous: small bowel, colon	Autosomal dominant	FAP and extraintestinal manifestations: desmoid tumors, osteomas, epidermoid cysts, papillary thyroid cancer
Turcot syndrome	Hyperplastic: stomach Adenomatous: small bowel, colon	Autosomal dominant	FAP and central nervous system tumors: gliomas, medulloblastomas
Hereditary nonpolyposis colon cancer syndrome (Lynch syndrome)	Adenomatous	Autosomal dominant	DNA mismatch repair, mutation. 90% of colon cancers associated with microsatellite instability. Associated endometrium, stomach, small bowel, liver, biliary, brain, ovary, ureter, and renal pelvis cancers
Peutz-Jeghers syndrome	Hamartomatous: usually small bowel	Autosomal dominant	Mucocutaneous pigmentation, gastroduodenal and colon malignancy, extraintestinal neoplasms (gynecologic)
Cowden disease	Hamartomatous	Autosomal dominant	Mucocutaneous lesions, thyroid abnormalities, breast abnormalities
Cronkhite-Canada syndrome	Hamartomatous	Sporadic	Stomach, small bowel, colon, ectodermal changes (skin, hair, nails)
Juvenile polyps	Hamartomatous	Familial—autosomal dominant; nonfamilial form	Classification: 1. Isolated juvenile polyps of childhood 2. Juvenile polyposis of gastrointestinal tract 3. Juvenile polyps of infancy

CASE 2.19

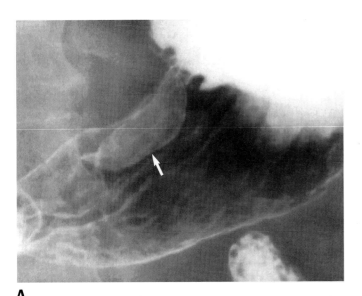

A

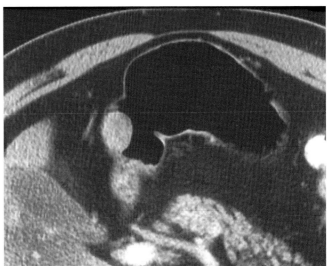

B

Findings
A. Single-contrast UGI. A well-demarcated, smooth-surfaced mass (arrow) is present within the gastric body.

B. Contrast-enhanced CT. A well-defined soft tissue mass arises from the distal stomach.

Differential Diagnosis
1. Gastrointestinal stromal tumor
2. Fibroma
3. Lipoma
4. Carcinoid tumor

Diagnosis
Gastrointestinal stromal tumor

Discussion
Gastrointestinal stromal tumors (GISTs) are the most common submucosal gastric tumor. They can occur anywhere within the stomach. Depending on their growth characteristics, they can occupy an intramural location (as in this case), extend intraluminally (cases 2.20 and 2.21), or extend as an exophytic mass from the stomach (case 2.36). The smooth surface is characteristic of a submucosal tumor. A 90° angle is often formed between the edges of the mass and the normal gastric wall.

GISTs are often asymptomatic lesions that are discovered incidentally. Melena is a common complaint in patients with symptomatic lesions that are ulcerated. Abdominal pain and obstruction also can occur.

Any tumor arising from the cellular elements of the submucosa could have similar radiographic features: fibromas and lipomas (case 2.22), neurogenic tumors, malignant GISTs (case 2.36), vascular tumors, and carcinoids.

CASE 2.20

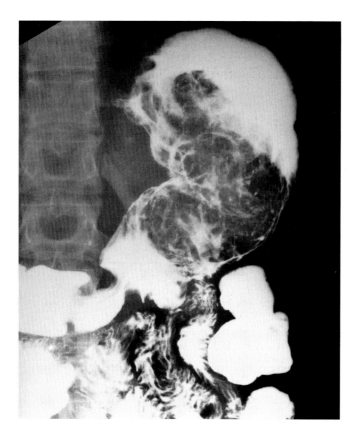

CASE 2.21

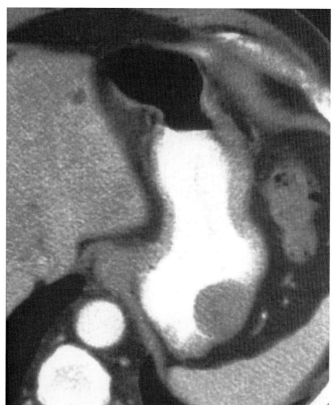

Findings

Case 2.20. Single-contrast UGI. A large intraluminal mass is present within the stomach.

Case 2.21. Enhanced abdominal CT. A mass arising from the gastric wall is present within the fundus.

Differential Diagnosis
1. Gastrointestinal stromal tumor
2. Bezoar

Diagnosis

Intraluminal gastrointestinal stromal tumor

Discussion

In these patients, a large gastrointestinal stromal tumor (GIST) was removed at operation. Some submucosal tumors grow intraluminally and resemble a polypoid neoplasm (carcinoma or lymphoma) (cases 2.25, 2.26, and 2.30) or a foreign body (bezoar) (case 2.38). Large tumors such as this may cause gastric obstruction.

CT may be helpful for determining the origin and extent of exophytic tumors. Malignant GISTs tend to be larger (often >10 cm in diameter) than their benign counterparts, have an irregular shape, and are often inhomogeneous with regions of central necrosis (case 2.36). The presence of distant metastases and adjacent organ invasion also can be assessed at CT.

CASE 2.22

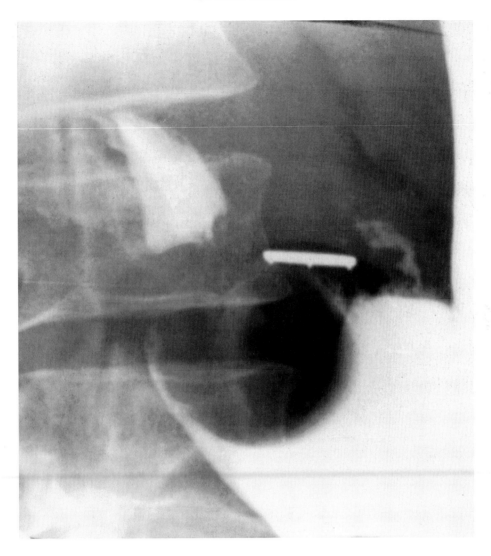

Findings

Single-contrast UGI. A well-circumscribed, round filling defect is visible in the distal gastric antrum. The mass has a smooth surface, indicating intact overlying mucosa. A 2-cm metallic marker attached to a compression device is visible adjacent to the mass.

Differential Diagnosis

1. Gastrointestinal stromal tumor
2. Lipoma
3. Ectopic pancreatic rest

Diagnosis

Gastric lipoma

Discussion

Gastric lipomas may be radiologically indistinguishable from GISTs. Lipomas usually present as solitary intraluminal masses within the antrum and may change shape during peristalsis or compression. These tumors may be pedunculated and can prolapse into the duodenum or, rarely, obstruct the pylorus. The surface of these tumors may ulcerate. CT is diagnostic if the typical fatty density is identified within the tumor. They may be indistinguishable at fluoroscopy from a GIST or an ectopic pancreatic rest (case 2.39). The finding of a small central depression favors the diagnosis of an ectopic pancreatic rest.

CASE 2.23

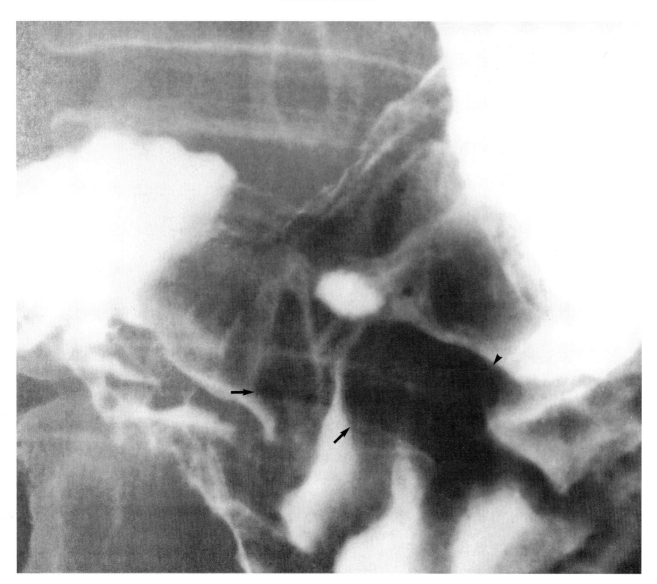

Findings
Single-contrast UGI. A small ulcer crater is present in the gastric antrum. Several abnormal folds are present adjacent to the ulcer crater. The folds have a clubbed (arrows) and fused (arrowhead) appearance.

Differential Diagnosis
1. Gastric adenocarcinoma (malignant ulcer)
2. Benign ulcer

Diagnosis
Gastric adenocarcinoma (malignant ulcer)

Discussion
At operation in this patient, a gastric adenocarcinoma was removed. Early depressed cancers are often recognized by the characteristic changes of the converging folds about the cancer or ulcer. Malignant fold alteration usually includes clubbing, tapering, interruption (amputation), and fusion. When these findings are identified, a cancer should be suspected and an endoscopic biopsy should be performed. Benign ulcers have smooth, tapered folds that radiate to the ulcer crater.

CASE 2.24

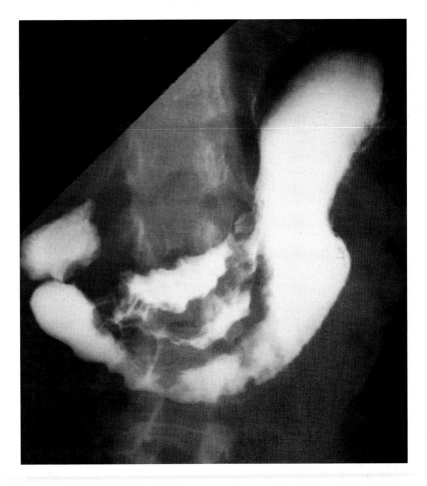

Findings
Single-contrast UGI. A large, ulcerated mass straddles the lesser curvature of the gastric body and antrum. The ulcer does not extend beyond the expected location of the normal gastric wall, and the surrounding mass has a lobulated contour.

Differential Diagnosis
Gastric adenocarcinoma

Diagnosis
Gastric adenocarcinoma: Carman meniscus sign

Discussion
Gastric cancer remains a lethal disease. Most patients in the United States have advanced-stage disease at diagnosis (stage III or IV) and a very low 5-year survival rate (<10% with these advanced-stage lesions).

Radiologic features of malignancy in lesions that are ulcerated include the following: 1) the tissue surrounding the ulcer is nodular—often the orifice and floor of the crater are also nodular, 2) there is abrupt transition between the surrounding tissue and the normal gastric wall (usually forming an acute angle), 3) the crater does not project beyond the expected location of the gastric wall, 4) radiating folds stop at the edge of the surrounding tissue and do not reach the crater itself, 5) the crater is asymmetrically placed within the surrounding tissue, and 6) the crater is often wider than it is deep.

The Carman meniscus sign is seen when the malignant ulcer straddles the lesser curvature and compression is applied apposing both surfaces of the surrounding tumor. The ulcer appears as a crescent (half-moon) on the lesser curvature, with nodular tumor surrounding the periphery of the ulcer. This sign is reported to be pathognomonic of carcinoma.

CASE 2.25

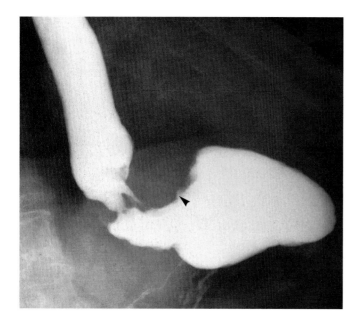

CASE 2.26

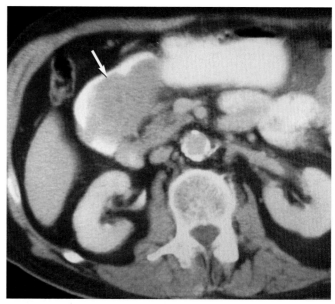

Findings

Case 2.25. Double-contrast UGI. A polypoid irregular-surface filling defect (arrowhead) is present in the gastric fundus and cardia.

Case 2.26. Enhanced abdominal CT. A large polypoid, intraluminal soft tissue mass (arrow) is present in the gastric antrum.

Differential Diagnosis

1. Gastric adenocarcinoma
2. Gastrointestinal stromal tumor
3. Lymphoma
4. Solitary varix
5. Metastases

Diagnosis

Polypoid gastric adenocarcinoma

Discussion

Gastric adenocarcinoma was found at operation in these patients. The incidence of gastric cancer has decreased in the United States. It now is the third most frequent gastrointestinal cancer, after colorectal and pancreatic cancer, and the sixth most frequent cancer overall. A few decades ago, gastric cancer was the most frequent gastrointestinal malignancy. There is considerable geographic variability throughout the world in the incidence of this disease. High cancer rates are found in Japan, Finland, Iceland, and Chile. Several etiologic factors are likely to contribute to the development of this disease, including high-starch diets, polycyclic hydrocarbons (found in home-smoked foods), and nitrosamines (found in processed meats and vegetables). Patients with some gastric conditions, including atrophic gastritis, pernicious anemia, post-subtotal gastrectomy, and adenomatous polyps, also are considered to have a higher risk for development of gastric malignancy.

The use of routine preoperative CT for patients with known gastric cancer is controversial. Some investigators have found CT unreliable for determining the true extent of disease. Nodal metastases can be particularly problematic, because normal-sized lymph nodes can contain metastases and enlarged lymph nodes may be inflammatory.

Gastrointestinal stromal tumors usually have a very smooth surface, whereas lymphomas and metastases usually present with multiple masses. A solitary varix should be considered in patients with portal venous hypertension. Endoscopy is usually required for a definitive diagnosis.

CASE 2.27

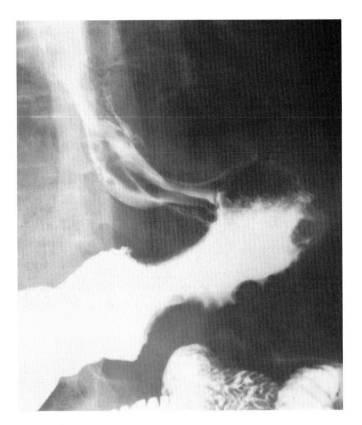

CASE 2.28

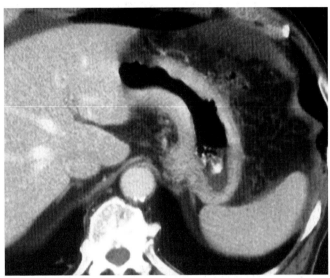

Findings

Case 2.27. Single-contrast UGI. Several filling defects are seen within a nondistensible segment of the gastric body. The mass encases and narrows the stomach. Gastric folds can be seen at the level of the mass along the greater curvature.

Case 2.28. Contrast-enhanced CT. Thickening of the wall of the gastric fundus and body is present. The luminal contour is irregular.

Differential Diagnosis

1. Lymphoma
2. Gastric adenocarcinoma
3. Ménétrier disease
4. Metastases

Diagnosis

Polypoid, infiltrative gastric adenocarcinoma

Discussion

Gastric adenocarcinoma was found at operation. Differential considerations may be indistinguishable radiographically. The stomach often remains distensible in Ménétrier disease. Today, most patients with gastric cancers will have preoperative endoscopy for histologic confirmation. A correct diagnosis of gastric cancer usually can be made endoscopically; however, infiltrative tumors may be detected in only 70% of patients. The presence of intact gastric folds indicates the submucosal location of the infiltrative process.

Resection is the only treatment that can result in cure. Many authorities favor an extensive gastric and lymph node resection. Approximately 40% of patients with gastric cancer have advanced disease that precludes a curative resection. Many patients undergo a palliative bypass procedure to prevent obstruction or to relieve dysphagia.

CASE 2.29

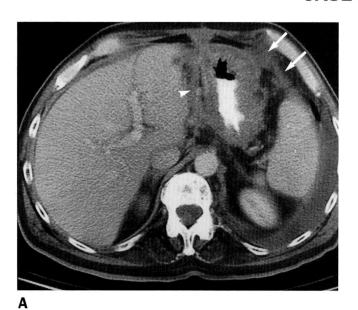

A

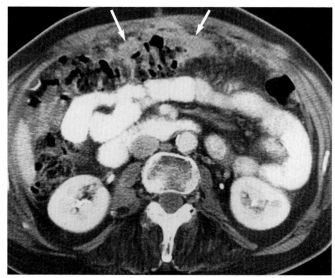

B

Findings

Contrast-enhanced CT. **A.** The stomach is circumferentially thickened. The serosal contours are irregular and poorly defined. Abnormal soft tissue masses are seen about the anterior peritoneal surface (arrows). There is soft tissue thickening (arrowhead) within the gastrohepatic ligament, representing adenopathy. A left pleural effusion is present. **B.** Multiple soft tissue masses (arrows) are seen within the omentum, anterior and adjacent to the transverse colon.

Differential Diagnosis

Metastatic gastric carcinoma

Diagnosis

Metastatic gastric carcinoma

Discussion

The lesser and greater omentum represent tissues that are in direct contiguity with the gastric serosa. Once cancer extends to the serosa, extension to the omentum occurs in most patients. More than 90% of patients have omental involvement if the tumor has reached the serosa, whereas only approximately a third of patients with tumor limited to the muscular layer have omental tumor.

Lymphatic metastases are common within nodes along the lesser curvature (within the gastrohepatic ligament) and greater curvature. Other commonly involved nodal groups include parapancreatic, para-aortic, and nodes around the middle colic artery.

After tumor spreads beyond the serosa, cells may seed the peritoneal cavity. Usual locations for peritoneal metastases include the pouch of Douglas, sigmoid mesocolon, right paracolic gutter, and the small bowel mesentery. Metastatic spread to the ovary is referred to as a Krukenberg tumor. Most liver and lung metastases occur as a result of hematogenous dissemination.

Direct invasion of gastric cancer to the pancreas or liver can be difficult to recognize at CT. Only if there are obvious findings of invasion should the diagnosis be made confidently.

CASE 2.30

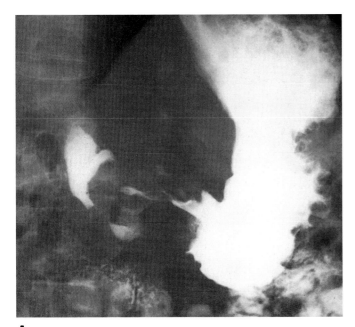

A

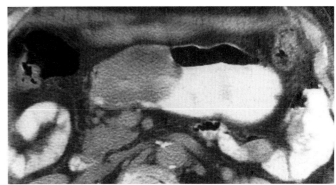

B

Findings

A. Single-contrast UGI. The gastric antrum is markedly narrowed by a large constricting mass.

B. Enhanced abdominal CT. A large polypoid mass is seen arising from the anterior wall of the gastric antrum.

Differential Diagnosis

1. Gastric carcinoma
2. Lymphoma

Diagnosis

Gastric lymphoma (solitary)

Discussion

Solitary lymphoma, as in this case, can mimic gastric adenocarcinoma (cases 2.23 and 2.24). Diagnostic tissue may be difficult to obtain at endoscopic biopsy because the overlying mucosa may be intact and prevent adequate tumor sampling. For this reason, multiple biopsy specimens at sites of possible mucosal involvement need to be obtained at endoscopy.

CASE 2.31

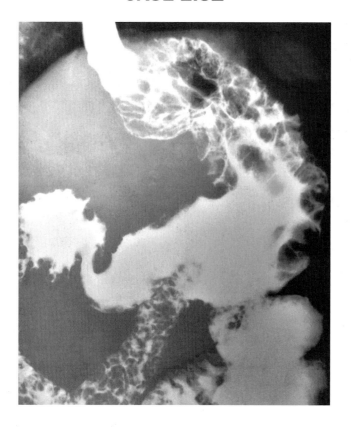

CASE 2.32

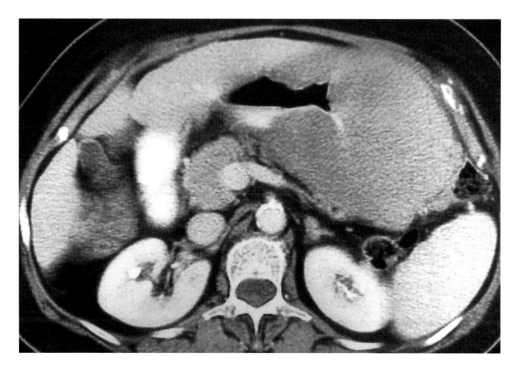

CASE 2.33

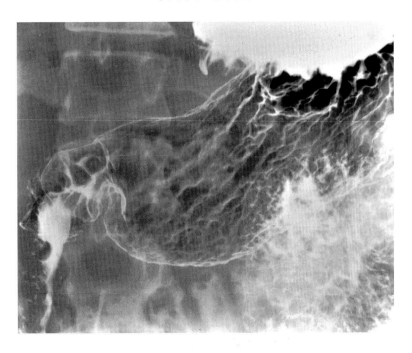

Findings

Case 2.31. Double-contrast UGI. Marked rugal fold thickening is present throughout the stomach. Multiple nodules are also present throughout the duodenum.

Case 2.32. Enhanced abdominal CT. Marked wall thickening is seen throughout the stomach.

Case 2.33. Double-contrast UGI. Diffuse nodularity and fold thickening are present within the gastric body and fundus.

Differential Diagnosis

1. Lymphoma
2. Ménétrier disease
3. Gastric adenocarcinoma
4. Metastases

Diagnosis

Gastric lymphoma (diffuse infiltrating)

Discussion

The amount of wall thickening in this case is characteristic of gastric lymphoma. Infiltrative lymphoma is often confined to the submucosal layer of the stomach.

Ulcerations may be present. Despite extensive disease, there is little restriction in gastric volume.

Lymphoma occasionally crosses the pylorus and affects the adjacent duodenum (as in case 2.31). Lymphoma also can occur within other regions of the alimentary tract. Because treatment and prognosis differ if the disease has spread beyond the stomach, it is often helpful to extend a UGI examination and also study the small bowel.

CT can be helpful in patients with known or suspected gastric lymphoma. The extent of extraluminal disease (usually adenopathy) can be documented and complications such as perforation and fistulization can be detected. Perigastric adenopathy is a common finding in patients with lymphoma, but it also can be found in patients with carcinoma. Lymphadenopathy at or below the level of renal pedicles is uncommon in patients with gastric carcinoma, but it has been reported in at least one-third of patients with lymphoma.

Differential considerations include Ménétrier disease (cases 2.14 and 2.15) and linitis plastica (gastric adenocarcinoma) (cases 2.48 and 2.49). Ménétrier disease usually affects the proximal stomach, and linitis plastica narrows the gastric lumen and produces a noncompliant affected segment.

CASE 2.34

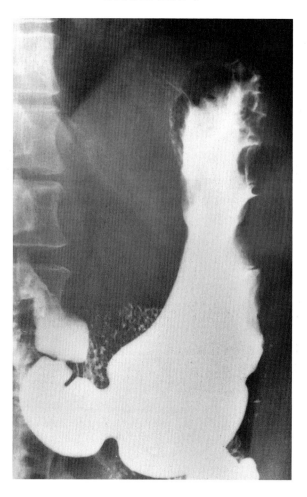

Findings
Single-contrast UGI. Multiple smooth-surfaced filling defects (arrows) are present along the greater curvature of the gastric fundus.

Differential Diagnosis
1. Gastric adenocarcinoma
2. Lymphoma
3. Metastases
4. Varices

Diagnosis
Gastric lymphoma (multiple submucosal masses)

Discussion
The stomach is the most common extranodal site for non-Hodgkin lymphoma. Disease confined to the stomach has a much better prognosis than does disseminated tumor, and it is often treated surgically rather than with chemotherapy.

Several radiographic forms of lymphoma have been identified, including infiltrative, ulcerative, polypoid, and intraluminal-fungating. There is often overlap among the radiographic forms. Radiographic features that are helpful in suggesting lymphoma instead of gastric adenocarcinoma include multiplicity of lesions, involvement of a large extent of stomach, evidence for a submucosal origin of the tumor, extension of the tumor across the pylorus, and less luminal narrowing than expected.

Gastric varices can have a polypoid submucosal appearance (cases 2.41, 2.42, and 2.43) and can change shape during the examination.

CASE 2.35

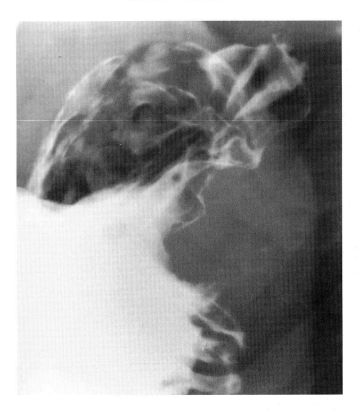

CASE 2.36

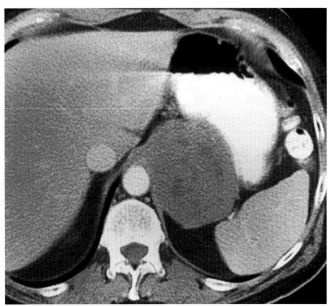

Findings

Case 2.35. Double-contrast UGI. A smooth-surfaced mass is present in the posterior wall of the gastric fundus.

Case 2.36. Contrast-enhanced CT. A large, mixed-density, predominantly exophytic mass lies between the posterior wall of the fundus and the aorta.

Differential Diagnosis

Gastrointestinal stromal tumor

Diagnosis

Malignant gastrointestinal stromal tumor

Discussion

Gastrointestinal stromal tumors (GISTs) are unusual primary gastric tumors of smooth muscle origin. Diagnosis of a GIST is important because it has a much better prognosis than does gastric adenocarcinoma. These intramural tumors often extend exophytically from the stomach, as in these cases. However, they may present with a large endogastric component, depending on the direction of growth.

There are no reliable radiographic criteria to differentiate benign from malignant GISTs, except that the larger the mass, the more likely it is to be malignant. CT can assist in determining the origin and extent of the tumor, as well as evaluating for possible metastases. Metastases from malignant GISTs often spread to the liver and peritoneal cavity, whereas metastases to local lymph nodes are unusual. Most submucosal tumors are removed regardless of size because even small tumors can harbor malignancy.

CASE 2.37

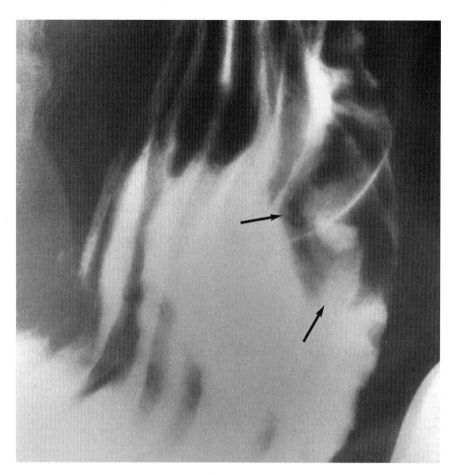

Findings
Double-contrast UGI. A gastric mass (arrows) containing a central ulceration is present in the upper body of the stomach.

Differential Diagnosis
1. Gastric adenocarcinoma
2. Lymphoma
3. Metastasis
4. Gastrointestinal stromal tumor
5. Ectopic pancreatic rest

Diagnosis
Metastatic melanoma

Discussion
Melanoma metastases have a similar radiographic appearance in the stomach and small bowel. They usually present as submucosal masses containing a central ulceration. The appearance has been described as a target or bull's-eye lesion. Although ulcerative metastases can cause gastrointestinal bleeding, other causes of bleeding also should be searched for in symptomatic patients with cancer. Severe gastritis and benign ulcers are more common sources of bleeding in affected patients.

Differential considerations for a solitary ulcerated lesion in the stomach include gastrointestinal stromal tumor (case 2.19), primary gastric adenocarcinoma (case 2.23), lymphoma (case 2.30), or ectopic pancreatic rest (containing a central umbilication) (case 2.39). Multiple lesions favor a diagnosis of metastases or lymphoma. The clinical history of metastatic melanoma in this patient is critical in determining the most likely diagnosis.

CASE 2.38

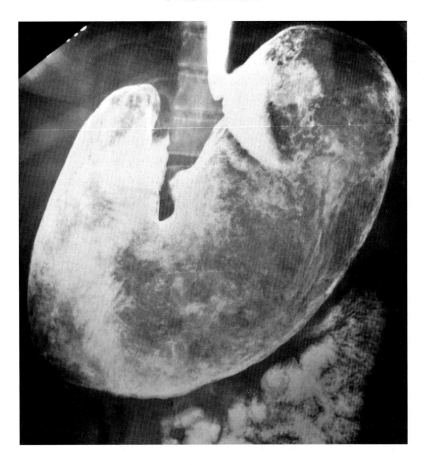

Findings
Single-contrast UGI. A huge filling defect occupies the entire gastric lumen.

Differential Diagnosis
1. Bezoar
2. Adenocarcinoma
3. Gastrointestinal stromal tumor
4. Lymphoma

Diagnosis
Bezoar

Discussion
Bezoars are concretions of ingested material. They are most commonly composed of vegetable material (phytobezoar), hair (trichobezoar), or other substances. Various foods (persimmons, berries, other fruits, vegetables, milk), mucus, pitch, tar, antacids, shellac, and furniture polish have been reported to form bezoars. Delayed gastric emptying, diminished gastric acid and pepsin production, excess or abnormal production of mucus, dietary content, and improper mastication are factors that can contribute to bezoar formation. Patients with prior gastric surgery are particularly prone to bezoar development (case 2.56).

Radiographic features of a bezoar include a mottled soft tissue mass on abdominal plain radiographs. A filling defect is present within the stomach on barium studies. The defect is not attached to the wall, and contrast material often collects within the interstices of the bezoar. Complications are rare but include obstruction, ulceration, hemorrhage, and perforation. Gastric tumor (carcinoma, case 2.26; lymphoma, case 2.30; gastrointestinal stromal tumor, case 2.20) is the most important differential consideration. Free movement of the mass within the stomach and the lack of attachment of the mass to the stomach can usually distinguish it from a true neoplasm.

CASE 2.39

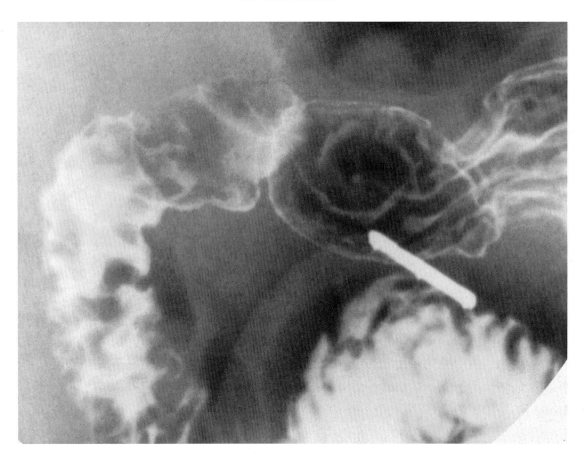

Findings

Double-contrast UGI. A 1.5-cm, round filling defect containing a central umbilication is present within the gastric antrum. The metallic marker is a measuring and compression device scored at 1-cm intervals.

Differential Diagnosis

1. Gastric ulcer (erosion)
2. Ectopic pancreatic rest
3. Gastrointestinal stromal tumor
4. Other submucosal tumors (lipoma, fibroma, neuroma, hemangioma)

Diagnosis

Ectopic pancreatic rest

Discussion

This case shows the typical size, location, and appearance of an ectopic (heterotopic) pancreas. Ectopic rests of pancreatic tissue have been identified in up to 14% of all autopsy specimens. They are more common than gastrointestinal stromal tumors (GISTs). Usually they are found incidentally, but any condition affecting the pancreas also can affect ectopic tissue. Diseases including pancreatitis, pseudocyst formation, carcinoma, and adenoma have been reported.

Although the distal stomach is usually involved, other locations including the duodenum, ileum, and within a Meckel diverticulum are possible. Radiographically, they appear as umbilicated submucosal nodules, although nearly half may not contain the characteristic central depression. The umbilication is not an ulceration; it is covered by normal epithelium. Rudimentary ducts may empty into this depression. These masses are often indistinguishable from a GIST (case 2.19) or other submucosal tumors.

CASE 2.40

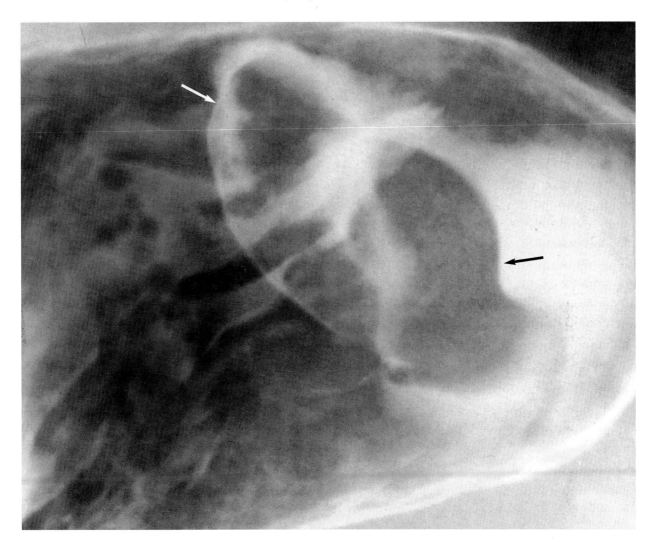

Findings
Double-contrast UGI. A symmetric, smooth filling defect (arrows) surrounds the gastroesophageal junction.

Differential Diagnosis
1. Fundoplication
2. Gastric adenocarcinoma
3. Lymphoma

Diagnosis
Fundal pseudotumor: fundoplication

Discussion
Different fundoplication procedures (Nissen 1, Nissen 2, Hill, Belsey) are performed to correct gastroesophageal reflux. Any of these procedures may give the radiographic appearance of a pseudotumor. The Nissen 2 fundoplication is commonly performed. This procedure involves wrapping a cuff of gastric fundus around the posterior esophagus and then suturing it together anteriorly. The cuff of fundus narrows the distal esophagus to prevent reflux. The main differential consideration is a neoplasm. A history of antireflux operation and the typical radiographic findings (as in this case) usually make the diagnosis straightforward.

CASE 2.41

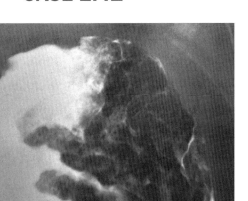

CASE 2.42

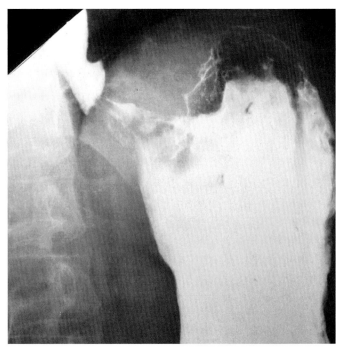

CASE 2.43

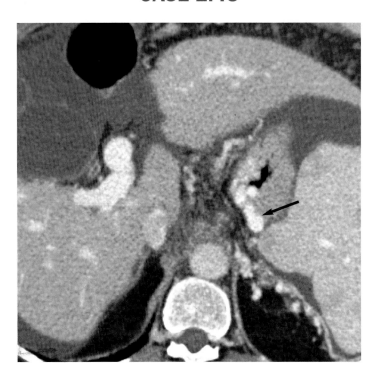

Findings

Case 2.41. Double-contrast UGI. Multiple, serpentine filling defects are present in the gastric fundus. A calcified mass is present in the region of the pancreas, which represents a partially calcified islet cell carcinoma.

Case 2.42. Single-contrast UGI. A lobulated mass is present in the gastric cardia and fundus.

Case 2.43. Contrast-enhanced CT. Enhancing vascular strictures (arrow) are present within the gastric fundus medially. Multiple additional upper abdominal collaterals also are visible.

Differential Diagnosis

Case 2.41

1. Gastric varices
2. Ménétrier disease
3. Lymphoma
4. Zollinger-Ellison syndrome
5. Pancreatitis

Case 2.42

1. Gastric carcinoma
2. Lymphoma
3. Gastric varices

Case 2.43

1. Gastric varices

Diagnosis

Gastric varices

Discussion

Case 2.41 has the typical findings of gastric varices with serpiginous fold thickening in the fundus. The gastric varices in this case were caused by splenic vein occlusion from the islet cell tumor. Case 2.42 shows a rare appearance of gastric varices presenting as a polypoid mass in the gastric fundus, which resembles a carcinoma. The presence of esophageal varices or a history of portal venous hypertension should make the examiner consider a possible gastric pseudotumor. CT (case 2.43) is invaluable for determining the vascular nature of the mass and often allows detection of the underlying disease causing the varices.

Gastric varices develop as a result of portal venous hypertension or splenic vein occlusion. Only one-third to one-half of patients with uphill esophageal varices from portal venous hypertension have gastric varices, but nearly all patients with gastric varices and portal venous hypertension have esophageal varices. This is probably the result of the subserosal location of gastric varices that in many patients cannot be detected at barium examination. Splenic vein occlusion usually is due to pancreatic disease (pancreatitis or pancreatic carcinoma), but it can be idiopathic. Esophageal varices are absent in splenic vein occlusion because blood flow travels from the short gastric veins to the gastric fundus plexus and returns to the portal circulation by way of the left gastric (coronary) vein.

Radiographic findings include serpentine defects, multiple lobulated masses resembling a bunch of grapes, or even a single, polypoid fundal mass (case 2.42). The double-contrast examination may be more sensitive for examining the fundus for varices, because this region is usually not accessible for adequate compression using the single-contrast technique. Examination of the esophagus for varices is important because the combined findings of esophageal and gastric varices indicate portal venous hypertension. A normal esophagus suggests splenic vein occlusion.

Gastric Filling Defects

		Case
Benign tumors		
Polyps	Adenomatous: few and large (>1 cm). Hyperplastic: many and small. Fundic gland polyposis syndrome: hyperplastic in familial adenomatous polyposis	2.16–2.18
Gastrointestinal stromal tumor	Smooth surface. Can ulcerate. Most common gastric submucosal tumor	2.19–2.21
Lipoma	Usually indistinguishable from gastrointestinal stromal tumor without CT. Diagnostic fatty density on CT	2.22
Malignant tumors		
Carcinoma	Can be polypoid, infiltrative, ulcerative, or scirrhous. Usually large with irregular surface	2.23–2.29
Lymphoma	Diverse presentation: solitary or multiple masses, infiltrative. Often has associated adenopathy	2.30–2.34
Malignant gastrointestinal stromal tumor	Smooth surface, but can ulcerate. Can present as intraluminal or exophytic mass	2.35 and 2.36
Metastases	Melanoma, breast, lung are common. Also locally invasive tumors (esophagus, pancreas, and colon)	2.37
Nonneoplastic		
Bezoar, retained food	Moves. Contrast material fills interstices	2.38
Ectopic pancreatic rest	Usually distal stomach. Central umbilication	2.39
Fundoplication defect	Fundus encircles gastroesophageal junction	2.40
Varices	Usually multiple serpentine filling defects in fundus. Splenic vein thrombosis causes isolated gastric varices. Seen with esophageal varices in portal hypertension	2.41–2.43

CASE 2.44

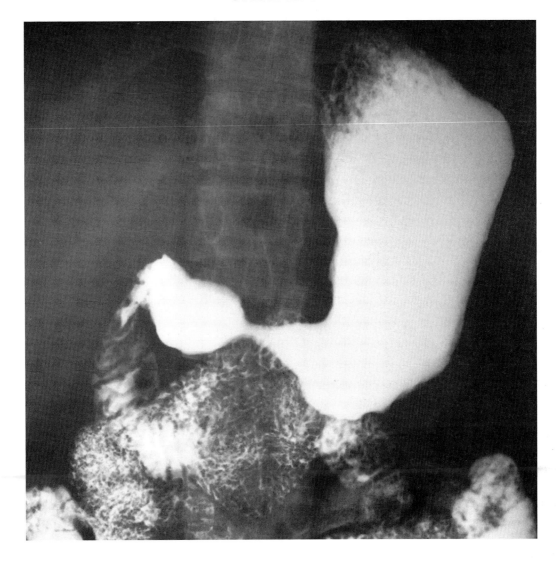

Findings
Single-contrast UGI. Within the gastric antrum, there is symmetric, smooth, tapered narrowing.

Differential Diagnosis
1. Scarring from chronic peptic ulcer disease
2. Granulomatous disease (Crohn disease, sarcoidosis, tuberculosis, syphilis, eosinophilic gastroenteritis)
3. Scirrhous carcinoma

Diagnosis
Crohn disease

Discussion
Chronic changes of Crohn disease are usually due to previous intramural inflammation and subsequent fibrosis. Because the distal stomach is most commonly involved, diffuse narrowing of this region often results in a tubular configuration resembling a ram's horn or pseudo-Billroth I appearance. The scarring may not affect the circumference of the antrum evenly, resulting in irregular deformity of the antrum and proximal duodenum. Fistula formation and mass effect are less frequent in the stomach than in the small bowel or colon. Without a history of peptic ulcers or other evidence of Crohn disease, it may not be possible to narrow the differential possibilities without endoscopic biopsy of this region.

CASE 2.45

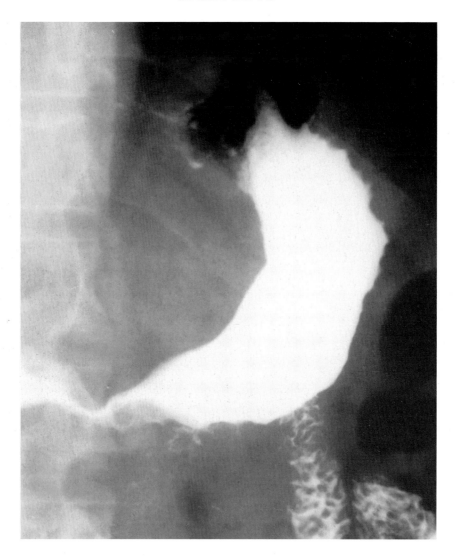

Findings
Single-contrast UGI. The distal third of the stomach is narrowed, tapered, and nondistensible.

Differential Diagnosis
1. Chronic peptic ulcer disease
2. Granulomatous disease (Crohn disease, sarcoidosis, tuberculosis, syphilis, eosinophilic gastroenteritis)
3. Gastric carcinoma
4. Metastatic breast cancer
5. Prior caustic ingestion

Diagnosis
Granulomatous gastritis (sarcoidosis)

Discussion
The most frequent cause of granulomatous gastritis is Crohn disease (case 2.44). Most patients with Crohn disease have concomitant disease in the small bowel. Sarcoidosis involving the stomach nearly always presents in association with disseminated disease. In fact, disease in other organs usually is critical for distinguishing sarcoidosis from the other granulomatous diseases. No specific radiologic findings are helpful for differentiating the various granulomatous diseases. Gastric carcinoma (cases 2.48 and 2.49), metastatic breast cancer (case 2.50), and scarring from corrosive ingestion (case 2.47) could have similar radiographic changes.

CASE 2.46

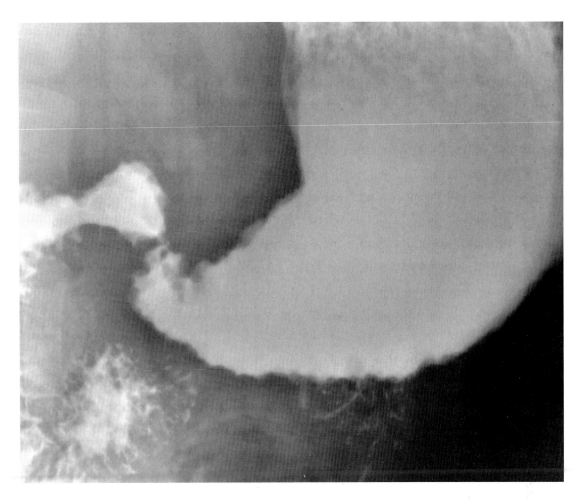

Findings
Single-contrast UGI. Tapered narrowing is present in the antrum of the stomach with nodular fold thickening of the distal stomach and visualized proximal duodenum.

Differential Diagnosis
1. Granulomatous disease (Crohn disease, sarcoidosis, tuberculosis, syphilis, eosinophilic gastroenteritis)
2. Gastric carcinoma
3. Gastric lymphoma

Diagnosis
Eosinophilic gastroenteritis

Discussion
Eosinophilic gastroenteritis is a rare idiopathic disease of the gastrointestinal tract that virtually always affects the gastric antrum, as well as all or part of the small bowel (case 4.51). It is caused by an eosinophilic infiltrate of the mucosa and submucosa and commonly results in mucosal nodularity and narrowing of the distal stomach and diffuse or segmental nodular fold thickening in the small bowel. The disease also may rarely involve the colon.

Patients with eosinophilic gastroenteritis often present with abdominal pain, diarrhea, and occasionally malabsorption. The gastric antrum is usually the best site for diagnostic biopsy. Most patients have peripheral eosinophilia demonstrable on blood smears. In addition, many patients have an allergy history. The clinical course is usually self-limited, and the disease often responds to corticosteroid therapy or resolves spontaneously.

CASE 2.47

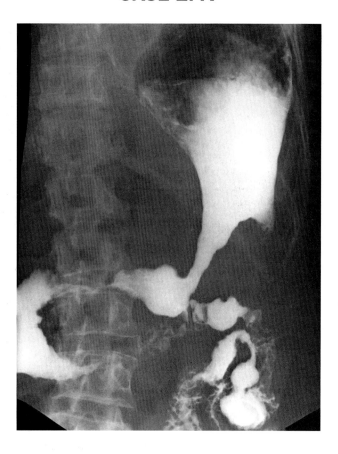

Findings

Double-contrast UGI. The antrum of the stomach is irregularly narrowed. There is an abrupt margin at the junction of the antrum and body along the greater curvature.

Differential Diagnosis

1. Caustic gastric stricture
2. Annular carcinoma
3. Granulomatous infection

Diagnosis

Caustic stricture of the gastric antrum

Discussion

This patient had a history of ammonia ingestion. Caustic injury to the stomach from acid, alkali, or other chemicals usually affects the antrum more severely than the proximal stomach. The amount of gastric damage depends on the depth of the burn. Mucosal damage (first-degree burn) alone heals without sequelae. Second-degree burns involve the submucosa and muscular layers of the stomach. Healing occurs with fibrosis and stricture formation. The secretory and peristaltic functions of the stomach also may be inhibited, depending on the amount of damage. Third-degree burns involve transmural damage, usually resulting in inflammation in the surrounding affected tissues. Hemorrhage, sepsis, and shock can occur.

Ulceration of the stomach and duodenum can be seen 2 to 3 days after caustic ingestion. Subsequent changes include 1) large intraluminal filling defects from hematomas, 2) contraction of the distal stomach with atony, 3) rigidity, and 4) contour irregularity. Late changes include antral stenosis (as seen in this case). Abrupt annular narrowing of the gastric lumen can be confused with a carcinoma (cases 2.48 and 2.49). Associated lesions in the esophagus and duodenum, in addition to a history of caustic ingestion, can help differentiate this lesion from cancer. Granulomatous disease usually results in smooth, tapered narrowing of the antrum.

CASE 2.48

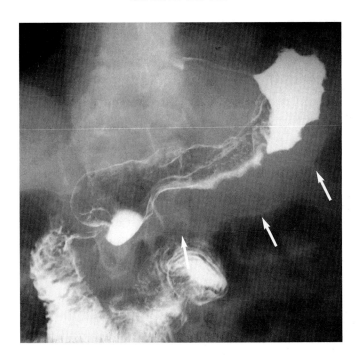

CASE 2.49

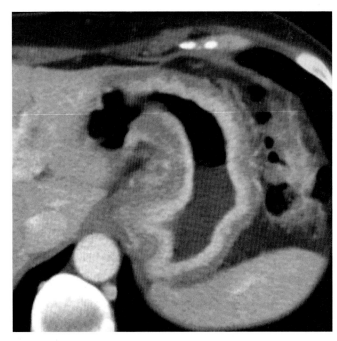

Findings

Case 2.48. Double-contrast UGI. The wall of the stomach is markedly thickened (arrows), with narrowing and scalloping of the gastric contour.

Case 2.49. Contrast-enhanced CT. Marked thickening and enhancement of the gastric wall are visible.

Differential Diagnosis

1. Gastric carcinoma
2. Metastases
3. Lymphoma

Diagnosis

Scirrhous gastric adenocarcinoma

Discussion

Scirrhous carcinomas spread within the submucosa of the gastric wall, often inciting a desmoplastic reaction. Because of the narrowing and rigidity that often accompany these tumors, the radiographic appearance of the stomach has been likened to a leather bottle (linitis plastica). Gastric narrowing is not detectable in all patients. In patients with these lesions, there may be mucosal nodularity, fold thickening, or ulceration. Scirrhous tumors often enhance after intravenous administration of contrast material. These tumors usually involve a large extent of the stomach and often spread to peritoneal surfaces. Polypoid and ulcerative adenocarcinomas usually do not enhance.

Many conditions can present with similar radiographic findings. Breast cancer metastases can resemble scirrhous tumors and often narrow the gastric antrum. Omental metastases, often arising from a primary carcinoma in the transverse colon, can invade and narrow the stomach by way of the gastrocolic ligament.

Histologic confirmation of scirrhous adenocarcinoma of the stomach may be difficult to obtain by endoscopic biopsy. Located in the submucosal tissues, a deep biopsy is often required for diagnosis. In addition, the associated desmoplastic reaction may widely intersperse cancer cells between large areas of fibrosis.

CASE 2.50

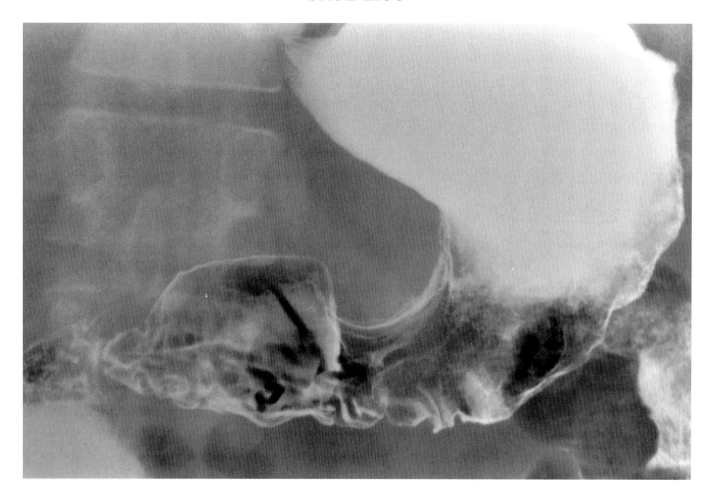

Findings
Double-contrast UGI. The body and antrum of the stomach are deformed and narrowed. Gastric folds are visible in this region of narrowing.

Differential Diagnosis
1. Scirrhous adenocarcinoma
2. Metastatic breast cancer
3. Granulomatous diseases affecting the stomach

Diagnosis
Metastatic breast cancer

Discussion
Metastatic breast cancer involving the stomach may produce a linitis plastica appearance indistinguishable from that of primary scirrhous gastric adenocarcinoma (cases 2.48 and 2.49). Whenever a scirrhous carcinoma is identified in a woman, breast metastases also should be considered. Both scirrhous carcinoma and granulomatous disease can have an identical radiographic appearance. Endoscopic biopsy is usually required for definitive diagnosis.

Gastric Narrowings

		Case
Benign		
Peptic scarring	Nearly always antral with loss of normal antral shoulders. Duodenal changes are commonly associated	Not shown
Granulomatous disease	Ram's horn deformity of antrum. Smooth narrowing, Crohn disease, sarcoidosis, tuberculosis, syphilis, eosinophilic gastroenteritis	2.44–2.46
Corrosive ingestion	Usually acid. Distal stomach	2.47
Malignant		
Carcinoma	Irregular luminal contour. Scirrhous: long segment with intact rugal folds	2.48 and 2.49
Metastases	Linitis plastica. Often seen with metastatic breast cancer. Identical appearance to that of scirrhous adenocarcinoma	2.50
Lymphoma	Infiltrative form can cause gastric narrowing. Thickened, disorganized folds	2.30–2.34

CASE 2.51

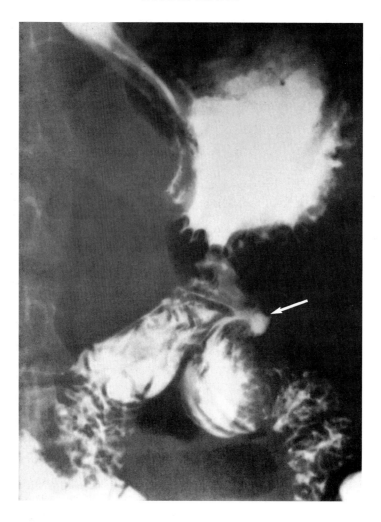

Findings

Single-contrast UGI. An ulcer crater (arrow) is present within the efferent limb, adjacent to the gastrojejunal anastomosis, in this patient with a Billroth II gastroenterostomy.

Differential Diagnosis

Marginal ulcer

Diagnosis

Marginal ulcer

Discussion

A marginal or stomal ulcer is a perianastomotic ulcer developing after a gastroenterostomy. Most ulcers occur in the efferent limb of the jejunum, within 2 cm of the stoma. Marginal ulcers should raise suspicion of several possible conditions: incomplete vagotomy, retained gastric antrum, Zollinger-Ellison syndrome, hypercalcemia, smoking, or ulcerogenic drug abuse.

A spectrum of radiographic findings of peptic disease affecting the postanastomotic jejunum can be seen, including typical ulcer craters, giant craters resembling large diverticula, thickened jejunal folds, and rigidity of the affected jejunal segment. Despite ideal radiographic techniques, some postoperative ulcers are not detected (reports vary between 20% and 50%). Endoscopy should be recommended for symptomatic patients with negative radiologic studies. Delayed diagnosis can lead to perforation, bleeding, or penetration—often into the colon, creating a jejunocolic fistula.

CASE 2.52

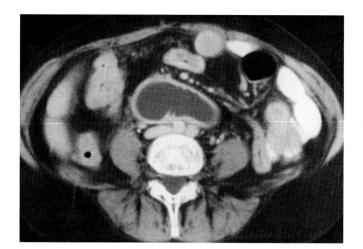

CASE 2.53

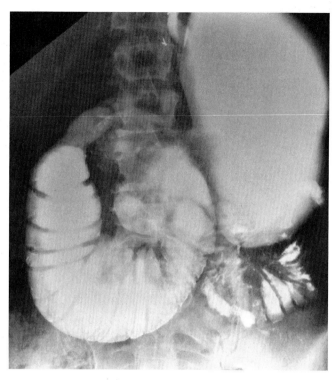

Findings

Case 2.52. Contrast-enhanced CT. A dilated, fluid-filled duodenum is visible in this patient, who had a previous Billroth II gastroenterostomy.

Case 2.53. Single-contrast UGI. The afferent limb of a Billroth II anastomosis is markedly dilated. A cause for the obstruction near the gastroenterostomy is not visible.

Differential Diagnosis
Afferent loop syndrome

Diagnosis
Afferent loop syndrome

Discussion
The usual cause of afferent loop syndrome is obstruction of the afferent loop due to adhesions, recurrent ulcer, recurrent tumor, or internal herniation. Patients with afferent loop syndrome often present with distention, pain, and nausea. Conventional barium studies occasionally identify the site of obstruction and its cause. Often, however, only nonfilling of the afferent limb is detected. CT is helpful for directly imaging the fluid-filled and dilated afferent loop. Fixed obstruction of the loop may lead to blind loop syndrome with bacterial overgrowth, vitamin B_{12} deficiency, and megaloblastic anemia. Perforation of the afferent limb with peritoneal spillage has been reported and may cause death.

Afferent loop syndrome also can be due to a nonphysiologic surgical anastomosis, in which food preferentially empties into the afferent limb. Preferential filling of the afferent loop and delayed emptying often can be appreciated fluoroscopically in patients with nonphysiologic anastomoses. Both of these patients had twisting of the afferent loop around adhesions, which required surgical revision.

CASE 2.54

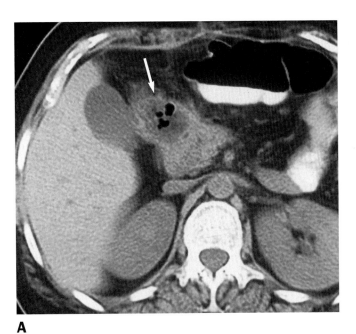

A

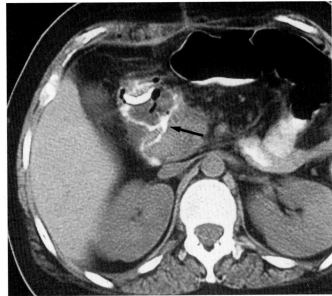

B

Findings

A. Unenhanced abdominal CT. An abscess (arrow) containing fluid and air is located adjacent to the duodenal stump in this patient with a recent Billroth II gastrojejunostomy.

B. Follow-up CT sinogram obtained after placement of a percutaneous locking loop catheter into the abscess cavity shows communication (arrow) between the abscess and the duodenum.

Differential Diagnosis

1. Blown duodenal stump (duodenal anastomotic dehiscence)
2. Intra-abdominal abscess

Diagnosis

Blown duodenal stump

Discussion

Breakdown or leakage of the duodenal stump (blown duodenal stump) is a serious complication after Billroth II anastomosis. Recognition of this condition is important because it has a high mortality. Anastomotic breakdown can occur anytime between the first day and up to 3 weeks after operation. Early intervention and drainage are important for proper management.

The diagnosis may be suggested by the findings on an abdominal plain radiograph, by identifying extraluminal gas, or by abnormal soft tissue in the subhepatic space or about the duodenal stump. CT is excellent for evaluating patients for this complication. The presence and location of abnormal fluid collections can be identified, and in some patients percutaneous drainage can be performed.

CASE 2.55

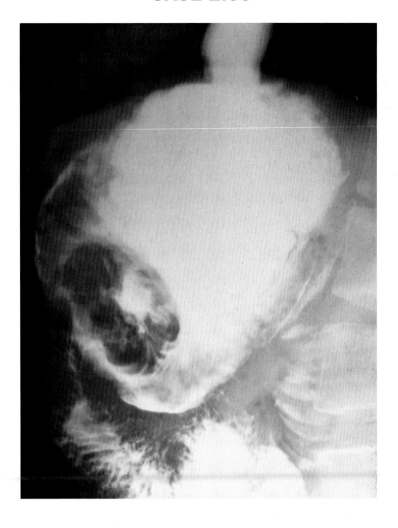

Findings

Single-contrast UGI. A filling defect is present within a gastric remnant. The defect is tubular, and valvulae conniventes are seen within it.

Differential Diagnosis

1. Jejunogastric intussusception
2. Gastric remnant carcinoma

Diagnosis

Jejunogastric intussusception

Discussion

Clinically significant intussusception is an unusual complication after gastroenterostomy. Intussusception can occur antegradely or retrogradely, acutely or chronically. In patients with acute intussusception, clinical signs and symptoms of gastric outlet obstruction can develop, including hematemesis and an upper abdominal mass or fullness. Chronic intussusception is usually intermittent and self-reducing. Symptomatic patients should be regarded as surgical emergencies because of the high mortality associated with untreated patients in whom bowel perforation develops. The efferent limb is most commonly the intussuscipiens, but the afferent or both limbs also can intussuscept. A mass acting as a lead point should be searched for in patients with an antegrade intussusception, when the jejunum is the intussusceptum.

CASE 2.56

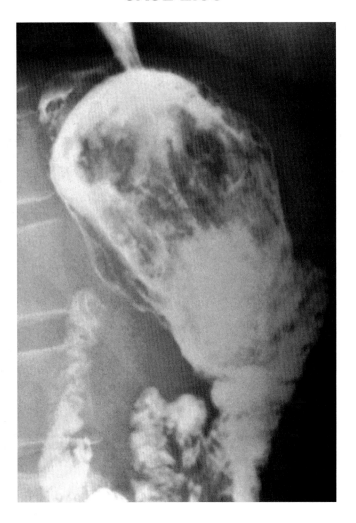

Findings
Single-contrast UGI. There is a large filling defect within the gastric remnant in this patient with a Billroth II gastroenterostomy. Contrast material was seen completely surrounding the filling defect during the examination.

Differential Diagnosis
1. Gastric bezoar
2. Polypoid gastric cancer
3. Gastrointestinal stromal tumor

Diagnosis
Gastric remnant bezoar

Discussion
Bezoar formation, usually from retained vegetable matter (phytobezoar), is a relatively common complication after a gastroenterostomy. Bezoar formation often occurs in patients with a narrowed gastroenterostomy stoma and as a result of surgical vagotomy that slows gastric transit and decreases acid production.

Radiologic diagnosis is based on finding a filling defect within the gastric remnant that is not attached to the gastric wall. Often, interstices within the phytobezoar fill with barium and give it a variegated appearance. Retained food can simulate a bezoar, and it is probably prudent to reexamine the fasting patient several hours later to determine whether the finding is still present. Yeast bezoars due to yeast overgrowth and blood clot bezoars also can occur and cause gastric outlet obstruction.

CASE 2.57

CASE 2.58

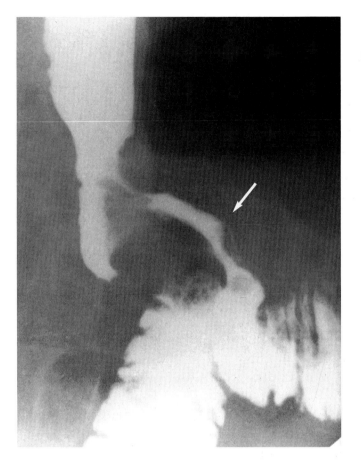

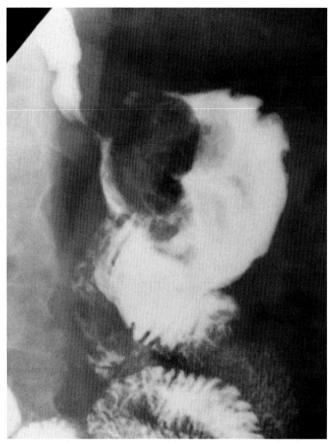

Findings

Case 2.57. Single-contrast UGI. Postoperative changes of a Billroth II gastroenterostomy are visible with a small and stenotic residual gastric remnant (arrow). Mass effect deforms the distal esophagus eccentrically.

Case 2.58. Single-contrast UGI. A polypoid intraluminal mass is present within the gastric remnant in another patient with a Billroth II gastroenterostomy.

Differential Diagnosis

1. Postgastrectomy carcinoma
2. Postoperative deformity
3. Gastric obstruction from adhesions
4. Gastrointestinal stromal tumor

Diagnosis

Postgastrectomy carcinoma

Discussion

These two cases have different appearances of postgastrectomy carcinomas. Case 2.57 illustrates an advanced case of gastric remnant shrinkage due to a constricting, diffuse carcinoma. Detection of this type of gastric remnant cancer can be difficult. Baseline examinations are helpful to assess for subtle changes in the gastric pouch. The polypoid cancer in case 2.58 is much easier to diagnose on the UGI examination. The changes in case 2.57 are too extensive to be attributed to postoperative deformity or adhesions. No mucosal markings (gastric folds) are visible in the narrowed segment. This finding usually indicates ulceration. The filling defect in case 2.58 could be due to a gastrointestinal stromal tumor. Inspection of its contour can be helpful to differentiate submucosal (smooth surface) from mucosal (irregular surface)-based lesions.

CASE 2.59

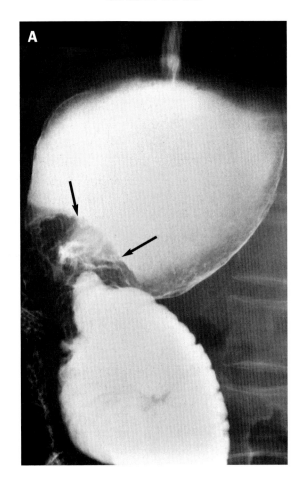

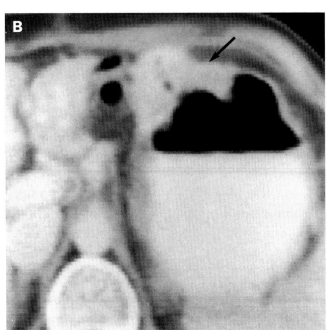

CASE 2.60

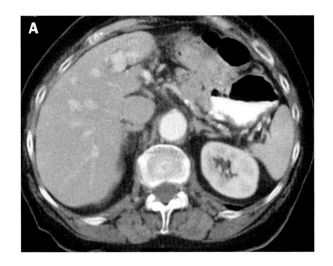

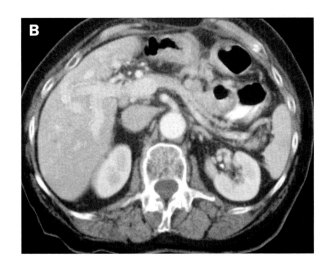

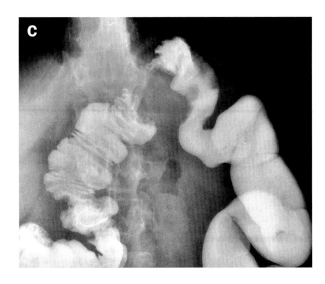

Findings

Case 2.59. A. Single-contrast UGI. A lobulated filling defect (arrows) is present within the gastric remnant near the anastomosis. The stomach is distended because of partial mechanical obstruction from the mass.

B. Contrast-enhanced CT. A soft tissue mass corresponds to the filling defect (arrow).

Case 2.60. A and **B.** Contrast-enhanced CT. A soft tissue mass at the level of the gastrojejunostomy extends anteriorly and abuts the transverse colon.

C. Single-contrast barium enema. Narrowing of the lumen of the transverse colon with mass effect along its inferior margin and tethered mucosal folds.

Differential Diagnosis

1. Postgastrectomy carcinoma
2. Jejunogastric intussusception

Diagnosis

Postgastrectomy carcinoma

Discussion

Gastric carcinoma in a gastric remnant usually occurs either soon (several months) after surgical resection for gastric adenocarcinoma as a result of subtotal tumor removal or as a primary cancer developing 20 to 30 years after gastric surgery for ulcer disease. A 2- to 6-fold increased risk has been reported for development of carcinoma within the gastric remnant in patients with a gastroenterostomy performed for managing gastric ulcer disease. The increased risk is believed to be related to long-standing gastritis as a result of reflux of bile acids and pancreatic secretions into the stomach. Increased cancer risk remains controversial, because some investigators have not confirmed this relationship.

Radiologic detection can be difficult. Filling defects, mucosal ulceration, and stomal or gastric pouch narrowing are the usual findings. Suspicious findings should be evaluated further with endoscopy. Examination of the gastric remnant with the air-contrast technique is recommended because the remaining pouch is rarely accessible for compression.

CASE 2.61

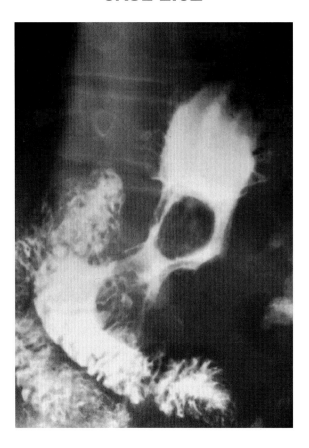

Findings
Single-contrast barium UGI. Postoperative changes of partial gastrectomy with Billroth II gastroenterostomy are present. There is a large filling defect within the gastric remnant. There is also narrowing and deformity of the remaining distal stomach and jejunum about the anastomosis.

Differential Diagnosis
1. Postgastrectomy carcinoma
2. Bile reflux gastritis
3. Gastric polyp

Diagnosis
Bile reflux gastritis with inflammatory polyp

Discussion
The filling defect was identified at endoscopy and found to be an inflammatory polyp. The markedly edematous folds were due to bile reflux gastritis.

Gastritis after operation is common, but usually it resolves within a few weeks. Reflux of bile by way of the afferent loop in a patient with a Billroth II anastomosis also can produce gastritis and can lead to considerable pain. Bile reflux gastritis rarely is diagnosed radiographically, but it may be suggested by identifying enlarged gastric folds (as seen in the distal portion of the gastric remnant in this patient). This patient's inflammatory polyp was probably due to chronic inflammatory changes from bile reflux. Other types of polyps (hyperplastic and adenomatous) also can develop in a gastric remnant. The filling defect in this case cannot be differentiated from a polypoid carcinoma. Endoscopic biopsy was necessary to make the distinction. Roux-en-Y procedures often are performed in patients with complications from a Billroth II gastroenterostomy.

Postoperative Stomach

		Case
Marginal ulcer	Usually distal to gastrojejunal anastomosis. Can be multiple	2.51
Afferent loop syndrome	Dilated duodenum. May not fill at UGI. CT helpful for directly visualizing	2.52 and 2.53
Blown duodenal stump	Fluid or abscess adjacent to proximal duodenum or subhepatic space	2.54
Jejunogastric intussusception	Filling defect in postoperative stomach. Valvulae confirm enteric nature	2.55
Gastric remnant bezoar	Filling defect in postoperative stomach. No wall attachment	2.56
Postgastrectomy carcinoma	Filling defect, luminal irregularity, or shrinkage of gastric pouch	2.57–2.60
Bile reflux gastritis	Usually associated with Billroth I or II gastroenterostomy. Thickened folds, filling defect(s)	2.61

CASE 2.62

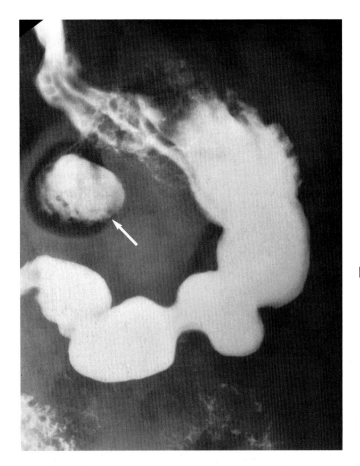

CASE 2.63

A

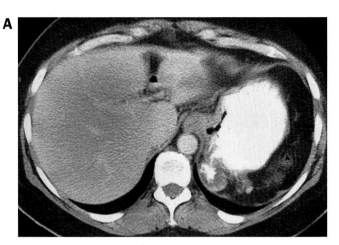

B

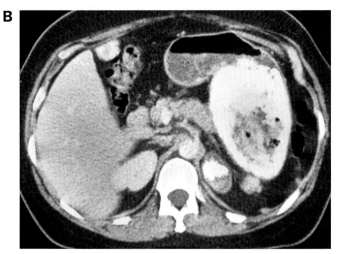

Findings

Case 2.62. Single-contrast UGI. A moderate-sized pouch (arrow) arises from the gastric fundus posteriorly. Its narrow neck arises near the esophagogastric junction. Folds extend from the stomach into the pouch.

Case 2.63. A and **B.** Contrast-enhanced CT. An outpouching arises from the gastric fundus. The most caudal slice does not appear connected to the stomach.

Differential Diagnosis

Gastric diverticulum

Diagnosis

Gastric diverticulum

Discussion

Diverticula of the stomach are unusual congenital entities. Most arise from the posterior surface of the gastric fundus near the esophagogastric junction. Gastric diverticula are rarely symptomatic, but diverticular bleeding has been reported.

Radiologic recognition of these entities depends on identifying mucosal folds within the diverticulum and observing its characteristic changing size and shape. A connecting neck is also a helpful finding. Occasionally, gastric diverticula can simulate an adrenal mass at CT. The use of oral contrast material can be very helpful for establishing the correct diagnosis.

CASE 2.64

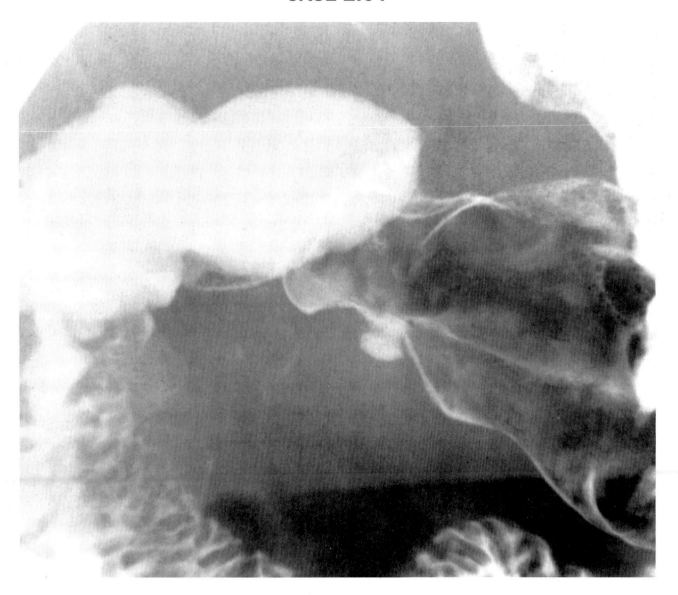

Findings

Double-contrast UGI. An intramural collection of barium is present along the greater curvature of the gastric antrum. This collection was observed fluoroscopically to change in size and shape.

Differential Diagnosis

1. Gastric ulcer
2. Partial gastric diverticulum

Diagnosis

Partial gastric diverticulum

Discussion

A partial gastric diverticulum is a protrusion of mucosa into the muscular wall of the stomach without disturbing the serosa. It is rare (found in approximately 0.05% of the population) and asymptomatic. Its importance lies in differentiating it from a peptic ulcer. Most partial diverticula are located along the greater curvature of the antrum. They often have a narrow neck and change in shape during fluoroscopic visualization. Ectopic pancreatic tissue (case 2.39) in the distal stomach is reported to be a frequent finding. The exact role this aberrant tissue plays in the development of these diverticula is unclear.

CASE 2.65

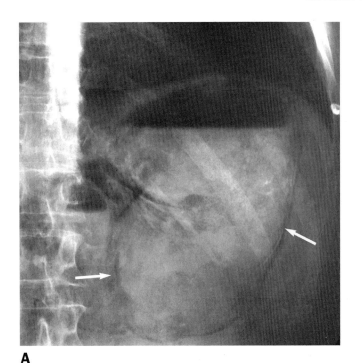

A

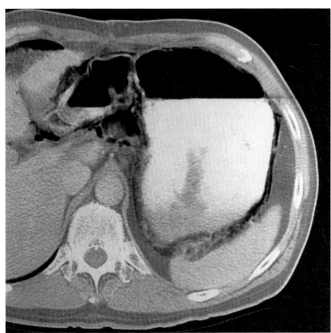

B

Findings

A. Abdominal radiograph. Intramural gas (arrows) is present throughout the fluid- and gas-filled stomach.

B. Contrast-enhanced CT. Intramural gastric air is confirmed at CT. In addition, retroperitoneal gas is seen in the region of the lesser sac.

Differential Diagnosis

Emphysematous gastritis

Diagnosis

Emphysematous gastritis

Discussion

Emphysematous gastritis refers to gas within the stomach wall. Infection with a gas-forming organism (e.g., *Escherichia coli* or *Clostridium perfringens*) is a common cause. Affected patients are usually severely ill and often

die. Other causes of intramural gastric gas include gastric obstruction (due to a pyloric or prepyloric ulcer or tumor) with associated increased intragastric pressure, severe vomiting, and mucosal disruption due to ischemia, infection, or corrosive ingestion. Clinical evaluation of the patient and a brief history are often helpful for excluding many of these causes. Patients receiving corticosteroids are particularly prone to intramural pneumatosis that has no clinical sequelae. Benign pneumatosis usually occurs in either the small bowel or the colon.

Radiologically, a gaslike lucency is identified within the gastric wall. The diagnosis often can be made successfully on the basis of abdominal radiographs, upper gastrointestinal barium studies, or CT. It is impossible to differentiate infectious from noninfectious pneumatosis on the radiograph. The patient in this case was receiving corticosteroid medication and recovered uneventfully without operation.

CASE 2.66

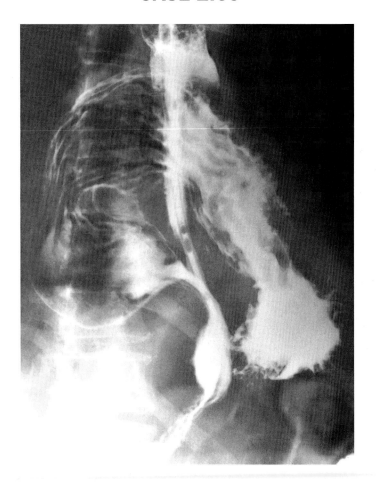

Findings

Double-contrast UGI. An intrathoracic stomach is present and has rotated 180° around the longitudinal axis of the stomach, with the greater curvature cephalad to the lesser curvature.

Differential Diagnosis

Intrathoracic stomach with gastric volvulus

Diagnosis

Intrathoracic stomach with gastric volvulus

Discussion

Gastric volvulus is a rare occurrence defined as 180° torsion either along the longitudinal axis of the stomach (organoaxial) or about the gastric mesentery (mesenteroaxial). Ischemia and gangrene can develop in either type, necessitating emergency surgical repair.

Organoaxial volvulus is the more common type, and it is often associated with a long-standing hiatal hernia, paraesophageal hernia, or eventration of the diaphragm. The intrathoracic stomach rotates so that the greater curvature is located superiorly, with the gastric body cranial to the fundus (as in this case). This type of volvulus often presents as an upside-down stomach. Acute symptoms are those of epigastric pain, retching without vomitus, and an inability to pass a nasogastric tube. Mesenteroaxial volvulus presents with the pylorus and antrum folded anteriorly and superiorly. This type often causes either partial or complete obstruction in the pyloroantral region.

Radiologic examination usually shows an intrathoracic location of the stomach and the anatomical alterations described above. It may not be possible to demonstrate filling or emptying of the stomach if obstruction is present.

CASE 2.67

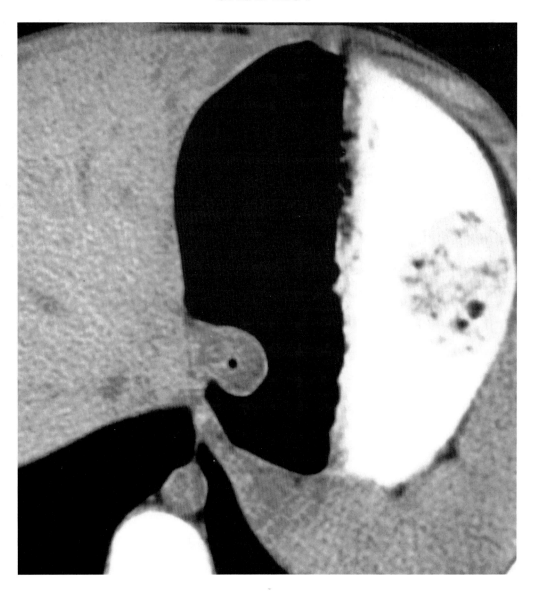

Findings

Unenhanced left decubitus abdominal CT. The distal esophagus at the level of the gastroesophageal junction is protruding into the gastric lumen.

Differential Diagnosis

1. Fundal pseudotumor
2. Gastrointestinal stromal tumor
3. Carcinoma of the gastroesophageal junction

Diagnosis

Fundal pseudotumor

Discussion

This pseudotumor can be shown to be esophageal in origin by its contiguity with the esophagus on more cephalad CT sections. In addition, the air in its lumen and its round shape confirm its esophageal nature. Protrusion of the distal esophagus into the stomach causing a filling defect is a normal variant.

CASE 2.68

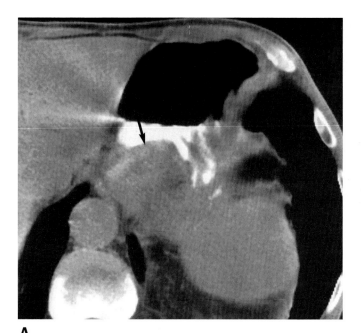

A

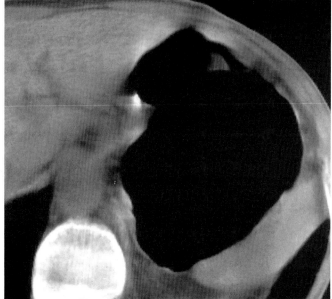

B

Findings

Enhanced abdominal CT. **A.** Mass-like thickening of the gastric fundus (arrow) is present near the esophagogastric junction. **B.** After administration of effervescent granules, the apparent mass is no longer seen.

Differential Diagnosis

1. Pseudothickening of a normal stomach
2. Gastrointestinal stromal tumor
3. Carcinoma of the esophagogastric junction

Diagnosis

Pseudothickening of a normal stomach

Discussion

The gastric fundus near the esophagogastric junction nearly always appears thickened in an incompletely distended stomach. This region is particularly prominent in this patient. Adequate fundal distention with orally administered contrast material, water, or gas usually helps exclude a mass in this region. Scanning the patient in a prone or right posterior oblique position, after administration of effervescent granules, is one of the most effective ways to ensure adequate fundal distention.

Miscellaneous Stomach Conditions

		Case
Diverticulum	Usually posterior fundus. Can simulate adrenal mass on CT without oral contrast material	2.62 and 2.63
Partial diverticulum	Simulates ulcer, usually along greater curvature of antrum, changes shape with peristalsis	2.64
Emphysematous gastritis	Air within stomach wall, often infectious cause	2.65
Volvulus	Upside-down stomach commonest (organoaxial). Can result in obstruction and ischemia	2.66
Pseudotumor	1. Protrusion of esopahgus into stomach, a normal variant. No associated mass	2.67
	2. Collapsed fundus has masslike appearance, distention of stomach makes mass disappear	2.68

DIFFERENTIAL DIAGNOSES

Thickened Folds

Benign
- Gastritis (*Helicobacter pylori*)
- Peptic ulcer disease
- Zollinger-Ellison syndrome
- Ménétrier disease
- Varices

Malignant
- Lymphoma
- Carcinoma
- Metastases

Ulcerative Lesions

Nonneoplastic
- Superficial gastric erosions
- Peptic or medication-induced ulcers

Tumors
- Adenocarcinoma
- Gastrointestinal stromal tumor
- Lymphoma
- Metastases

Filling Defects

Benign tumors
- Polyp(s)
- Gastrointestinal stromal tumor
- Lipoma

Malignant tumors
- Adenocarcinoma
- Malignant gastrointestinal stromal tumor
- Metastases
- Lymphoma

Nonneoplastic
- Ectopic pancreatic rest
- Bezoar
- Fundoplication defect
- Varices

Gastric Narrowings

Benign
- Peptic scarring
- Corrosive ingestion
- Granulomatous disease (Crohn disease, sarcoidosis, tuberculosis, syphilis, eosinophilic gastroenteritis)

Malignant
- Scirrhous adenocarcinoma
- Metastases
- Lymphoma

GASTRIC FILLING DEFECTS

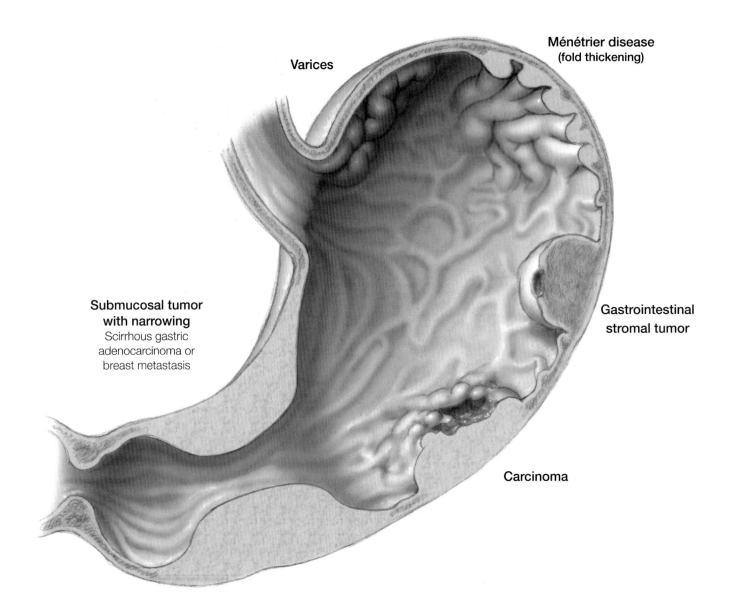

Varices

Ménétrier disease
(fold thickening)

**Submucosal tumor
with narrowing**
Scirrhous gastric
adenocarcinoma or
breast metastasis

Gastrointestinal
stromal tumor

Carcinoma

GASTRIC FILLING DEFECTS

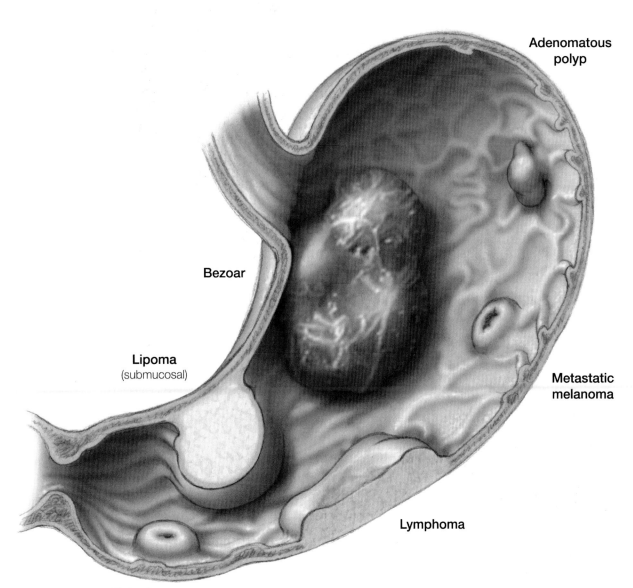

Adenomatous
polyp

Bezoar

Lipoma
(submucosal)

Metastatic
melanoma

Lymphoma

Ectopic pancreas

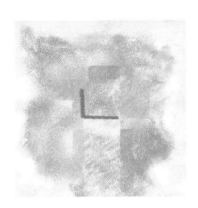

CHAPTER 3

DUODENUM

CASE 3.1

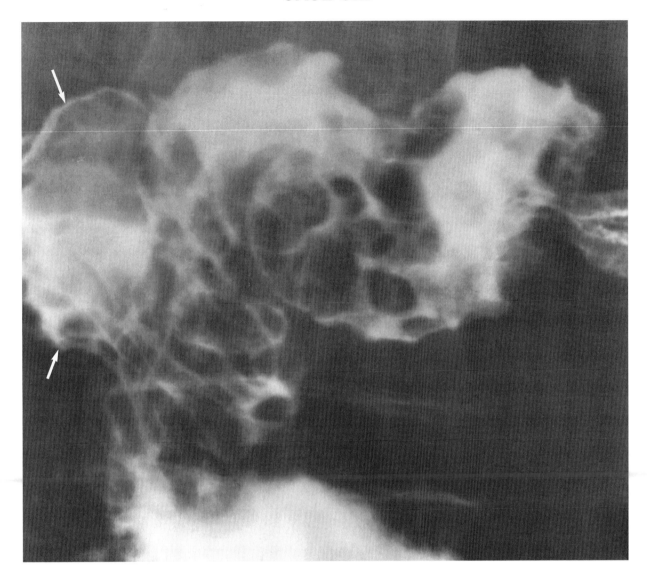

Findings

Single-contrast UGI. Multiple thick and nodular folds are present in the first and second portions of the duodenum. A diverticulum (arrows) is seen lateral to the descending duodenum.

Differential Diagnosis

1. Duodenitis
2. Brunner gland hyperplasia
3. Crohn disease

Diagnosis

Duodenitis

Discussion

The most frequent cause of thickened duodenal folds is peptic ulcer disease. The folds may be enlarged as a result of edema, or Brunner gland hyperplasia (case 3.34) may simulate fold thickening. Usually, multiple enlarged, discrete nodules that form a cobblestone appearance are present in patients with Brunner gland hyperplasia. Most cases of duodenitis are caused by *Helicobacter pylori* infection. Treatment is with antibiotics and acid blockers. Patients with Crohn disease (cases 3.15, 3.16, and 3.17), giardiasis (case 4.48), sprue (case 3.18), Whipple disease (case 4.49), and lymphoma (case 4.55) also can present with thickened duodenal folds.

CASE 3.2

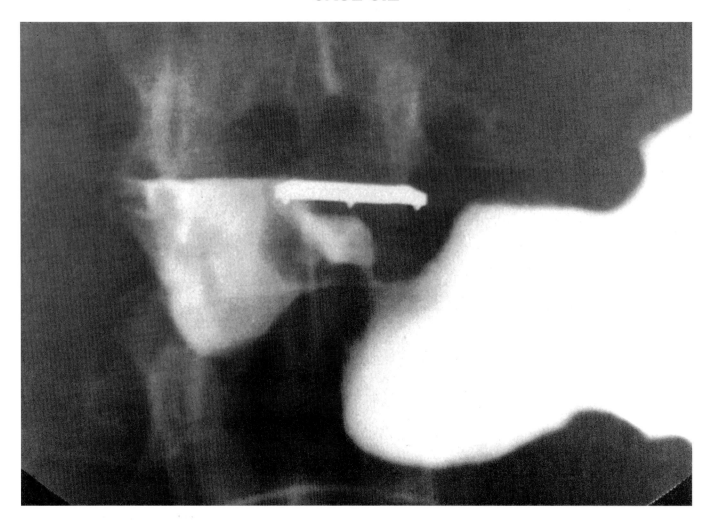

Findings
Single-contrast UGI. A collection of barium is present within the pyloric canal. A metallic compression device is present adjacent to the pylorus.

Differential Diagnosis
1. Pyloric channel ulcer
2. Pyloric torus defect

Diagnosis
Pyloric channel ulcer

Discussion
Ulcers can occur within the pyloric canal. In some cases, they are difficult to visualize because of secondary gastric outlet obstruction. Ulcers can be differentiated from the pyloric torus defect by the unchanging shape of an ulcer. The mid-channel widening of a pyloric torus is often diamond or triangular in shape and changes as the pyloric muscle contracts and relaxes.

CASE 3.3

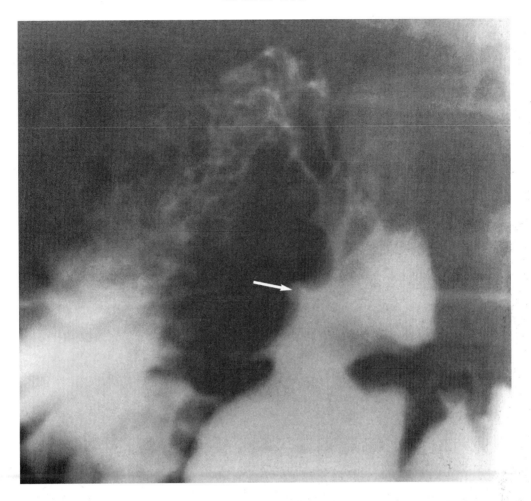

Findings

Single-contrast UGI. The duodenum is deformed along its inferior margin. A small ulcer niche (arrow) with a surrounding mound of edema is present.

Differential Diagnosis

1. Duodenal ulcer
2. Duodenal scarring

Diagnosis

Duodenal ulcer

Discussion

Duodenal ulcers are common problems and are encountered 2 to 3 times more often than gastric ulcers. More males are affected than females. Correlation between clinical symptoms and radiographic findings is often imprecise.

Some patients with relatively large duodenal ulcers remain asymptomatic, whereas other patients have typical symptoms and normal radiologic findings.

Duodenal ulcers are associated with increased secretion of acid and with a high incidence of *Helicobacter pylori* infection. The exact relationship between *H. pylori* infection and duodenal ulcers is uncertain. Other contributing causes include stress, smoking, alcohol, caffeine, and corticosteroid medication.

The key radiologic finding is a persistent collection of barium in the duodenal bulb that does not change shape with compression or peristalsis. Ulcers can vary in shape from pinpoint erosions to linear niches to the commonest round crater. Duodenal deformity is often associated with ulcers but is not present in many cases. Folds usually can be seen to radiate up to an ulcer crater.

CASE 3.4

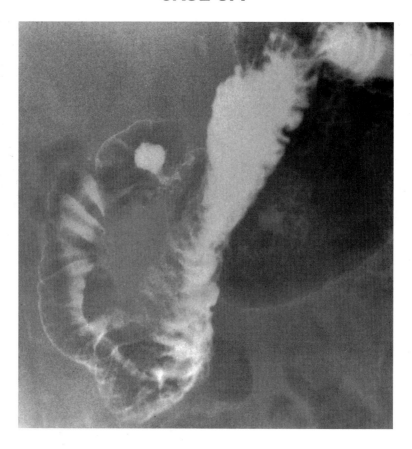

Findings

Double-contrast UGI. A persistent, round ulcer crater is present in the duodenal bulb. Folds radiate up to the crater. This is the classic appearance of a duodenal ulcer.

Differential Diagnosis

Duodenal ulcer

Diagnosis

Duodenal ulcer

Discussion

This radiograph was obtained with the patient in the supine position. Because barium collected within the crater, its location is within the posterior duodenal wall. An anteriorly located ulcer crater could appear as a ring shadow in this position, because barium would empty from the crater, leaving the ulcer edges barium-coated. Anteriorly located ulcers can be difficult to detect with only the double-contrast technique. Compression of the

duodenal bulb is an important part of every UGI. With compression, most anterior wall ulcers can be identified.

Duodenal ulcers are identified less frequently than in the past because of improved medical therapy. Duodenal ulcers alone are rarely malignant. These ulcers tend to follow the same morphologic patterns as benign gastric ulcers. Most are located along the anterior surface of the duodenum within the bulb. Acute ulcers without fibrosis can heal without scarring. Chronic ulcers with submucosal fibrosis usually result in residual duodenal deformity. Complications of duodenal ulcers are similar to those of benign gastric ulcers: bleeding, perforation, obstruction, and penetration. Perforation is more common among duodenal ulcers (case 3.6). The ulcer can penetrate into adjacent structures, such as pancreas, omentum, biliary tract, colon, liver, and mesocolon. Multiple duodenal ulcers can be identified in 10% to 15% of patients. The presence of multiple postbulbar ulcerations should suggest Zollinger-Ellison syndrome (case 3.11).

CASE 3.5

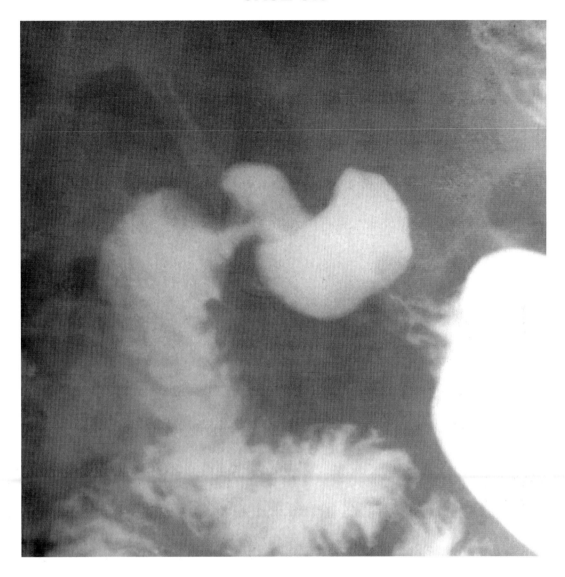

Findings

Single-contrast UGI. A large ulcer crater resides at the junction of the first and second portions of the duodenum. A symmetric mound of edema causes a filling defect around the ulcer base. An ulcer this size is sometimes referred to as a giant ulcer crater.

Differential Diagnosis

1. Duodenal deformity (peptic disease)
2. Duodenal ulcer

Diagnosis

Giant duodenal ulcer

Discussion

Giant ulcers have been described as being larger than 2 to 2.5 cm in diameter or as replacing most of the duodenal bulb. These ulcers may be so large as to mimic a normal duodenal configuration. Recognition depends on observing the fixed shape and size of the ulcer, which contains no normal duodenal folds. Narrowing of the duodenum proximal and distal to the ulcer is common. The complication and mortality rates are higher with this type than with usual duodenal ulcers.

CASE 3.6

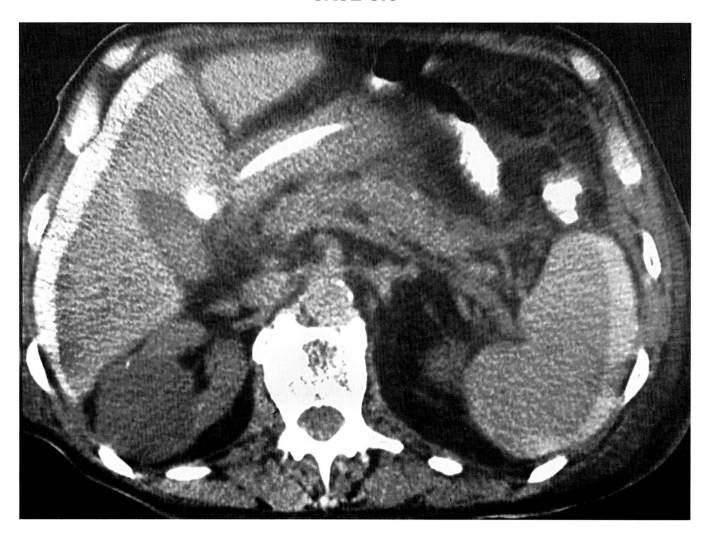

Findings

Unenhanced abdominal CT. High-density contrast material is seen in an extraluminal location (lateral to the duodenum). High-density ascites is visible about the liver and spleen. Benign renal cyst.

Differential Diagnosis

Perforated duodenal bulb ulcer with extravasation of oral contrast material into the peritoneal space

Diagnosis

Perforated duodenal bulb ulcer with extravasation of oral contrast material into the peritoneal space

Discussion

The commonest cause of a perforated viscus in a patient without trauma is a duodenal ulcer. Most duodenal ulcers perforate anteriorly with leakage of air (pneumoperitoneum) or contrast material (as in this case) or both. The presence of high-density contrast material adjacent to the duodenum increases the probability of a perforated duodenal ulcer.

CASE 3.7

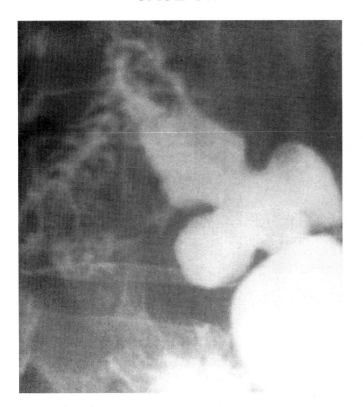

CASE 3.8

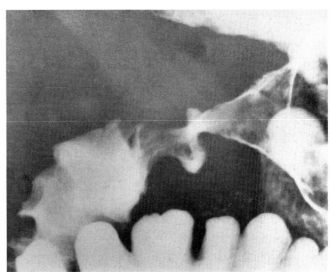

Findings

Case 3.7. Single-contrast UGI. The duodenal bulb is deformed and resembles a cloverleaf. This is the classic appearance of duodenal bulb scarring from a peptic ulcer.

Case 3.8. Double-contrast UGI. Two collections of barium protrude from the pyloric channel. Deformity of the distal gastric antrum and duodenal bulb is present.

Differential Diagnosis

Duodenal bulb scarring from prior ulcer disease

Diagnosis

Duodenal bulb scarring from prior ulcer disease

Discussion

Scarring of the duodenal bulb from previous peptic ulcer disease is a common finding. A centrally located duodenal bulb ulcer characteristically produces this cloverleaf deformity (as seen in case 3.7). The challenge to the radiologist is to exclude an active ulcer in the scarred bulb. Sometimes this is impossible and endoscopy should be recommended to examine the mucosa directly. Active ulcers are fixed abnormalities within the duodenum that do not change shape with peristalsis. Scarred duodenal bulbs change shape as the duodenum fills and empties. Compression should be routinely performed to exclude concomitant ulcers within the deformed bulb.

CASE 3.9

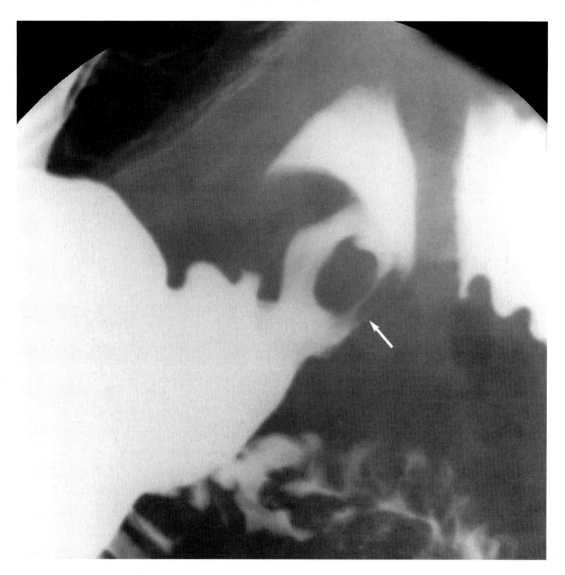

Findings
Single-contrast UGI. Two pyloric channels are present on this radiograph taken with the patient in the prone position. One channel (arrow) connects the greater curvature of the gastric antrum with the apex of the duodenal bulb.

Differential Diagnosis
1. Congenital double pylorus
2. Fistulous channel from peptic ulcer disease

Diagnosis
Fistulous channel from peptic ulcer disease

Discussion
The majority of cases of multichannel pylorus are due to a persistent fistula from peptic ulcer disease or Crohn disease. Rarely, this finding may represent a congenital abnormality. No treatment may be necessary if no active ulcer is present.

CASE 3.10

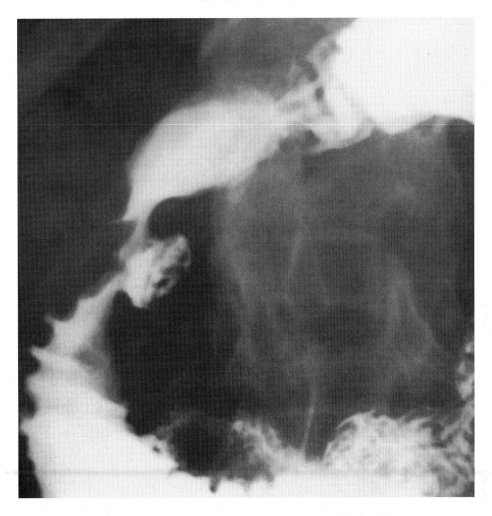

Findings

Single-contrast UGI. A round ulcer crater lies along the medial aspect of the second portion of the duodenum. There is associated duodenal narrowing, concentric edema about the crater, and fold thickening.

Differential Diagnosis

Postbulbar duodenal ulcer

Diagnosis

Postbulbar duodenal ulcer

Discussion

Duodenal ulcers most commonly occur in the duodenal bulb. Postbulbar ulcers are unusual, but when they develop they are usually located proximal to the ampulla and often along the medial wall of the descending duodenum. It has been estimated that 1 in 20 peptic ulcers is located beyond the duodenal bulb. Ulcerations should be considered malignant, or evidence for a gastrin-secreting tumor (Zollinger-Ellison syndrome) should be sought if an ulcer is identified distal to the ampulla of Vater (case 3.11). Healing of these ulcers can result in a ring stricture of the duodenum. Ring strictures can be difficult to diagnose, often necessitating distention of the duodenum with either barium or effervescent gas. Associated ulcer niches also can be easily overlooked and should be suspected if a focal area of narrowing is encountered in the postbulbar duodenum. CT may be useful in assessing for the complications of peptic ulcer disease: abscess, fistula, and pancreatitis. CT has no primary role in the diagnosis of peptic ulcers.

CASE 3.11

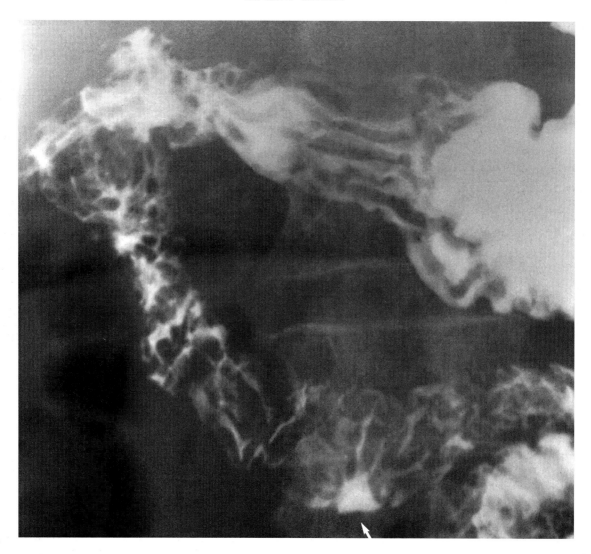

Findings
Single-contrast UGI. An ulceration (arrow) is present within the distal duodenum. The ulcer has benign features radiographically, with no associated mass and folds that radiate to the edge of the crater.

Differential Diagnosis
1. Postbulbar ulcer due to Zollinger-Ellison syndrome
2. Metastases
3. Primary adenocarcinoma

Diagnosis
Postbulbar ulcer due to Zollinger-Ellison syndrome

Discussion
This patient was found to have Zollinger-Ellison syndrome. Peptic ulcers in patients with Zollinger-Ellison syndrome most commonly occur in the pylorus and proximal duodenal region. Ulcers occurring distal to the ampulla are usually malignant, except in patients with Zollinger-Ellison syndrome. Normally, acidic gastric secretions are neutralized by the alkaline pancreatic secretions in the postampullary duodenum. Multiple ulcers occur in about 10% of patients with Zollinger-Ellison syndrome. The stomach and duodenum may appear hypotonic with dilatation of the duodenum ("megaduodenum"). Thickened duodenal folds and Brunner gland hyperplasia (case 3.34) also may be present.

CASE 3.12

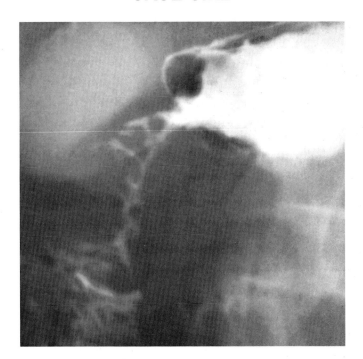

CASE 3.13

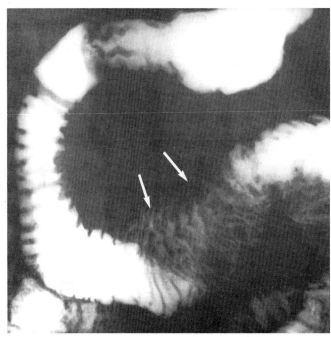

Findings

Case 3.12. Single-contrast UGI. The proximal duodenum is markedly narrowed. The mucosa through this region is intact, and the narrowing ends abruptly.

Case 3.13. Single-contrast UGI. The duodenal C loop is mildly widened. Tethered folds (arrows) are present along the cranial aspect of the transverse duodenum.

Differential Diagnosis

1. Duodenitis
2. Cholecystitis
3. Pancreatitis
4. Annular pancreas
5. Pancreatic carcinoma

Diagnosis

Pancreatitis

Discussion

Occasionally, patients with pancreatitis have a region of focal stenosis in the proximal duodenum. This narrowing is believed to be due to pancreatitis-induced edema and spasm. A persistent stricture can develop. The stenosis may mimic a carcinoma because of the abrupt edges and focal nature of the narrowing. Identifying intact mucosa through the stenosis is a key finding in distinguishing it from a tumor. A history of pancreatitis is also helpful information. Inflammation from cholecystitis or duodenitis could have a presentation similar to that in case 3.12. Annular pancreas should not have associated fold thickening unless superimposed pancreatitis is present.

Tethered folds of the bowel (as seen in case 3.13) usually develop from either an extraluminal inflammatory or neoplastic process. Normally the folds of the bowel are oriented perpendicular to the lumen and meet the edge of the bowel wall with a square, flat appearance. Tethered folds usually appear to be pulled from the normal bowel wall toward a central area extrinsic to the bowel. The folds are usually pointed and elongated.

CASE 3.14

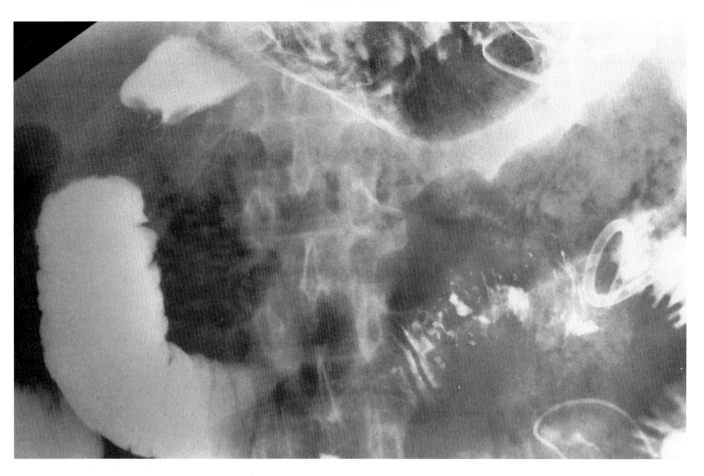

Findings
Double-contrast UGI. A mottled collection of gas is present within the pancreatic bed (the region between the stomach and the duodenum). There is a region of focal narrowing in the proximal duodenum. A drainage catheter is seen in the left upper quadrant.

Differential Diagnosis
Acute pancreatitis with abscess

Diagnosis
Acute pancreatitis with abscess

Discussion
The location and appearance of the extraluminal gas are pathognomonic of a pancreatic abscess. Pancreatic abscess is a dreaded complication of severe acute pancreatitis. High morbidity and mortality are associated with this disease. Pancreatic necrosis is present in many patients with abscess; however, infection of a peripancreatic fluid collection(s) is possible without pancreatic parenchymal necrosis.
If a pancreatic abscess is suspected, CT is the best initial examination. This condition often is diagnosed from plain radiographs in patients with nonspecific abdominal complaints or incidentally when radiographs are obtained for documenting tube position. The key radiographic finding of a pancreatic abscess is a variable amount of extraluminal gas within the pancreatic bed. The gas collection may appear either mottled or homogeneous.

CASE 3.15

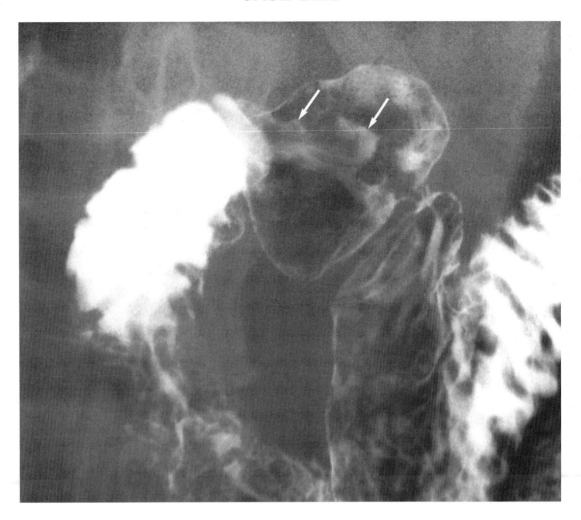

Findings

Double-contrast UGI. Multiple flat ulcerations (arrows) are present within the duodenal bulb and descending duodenum.

Differential Diagnosis

1. Peptic ulcer disease
2. Crohn disease
3. Viral (herpes and cytomegalovirus) ulceration
4. Chemical-induced ulcers (medication, alcohol)
5. Zollinger-Ellison syndrome

Diagnosis

Crohn disease

Discussion

Crohn disease affecting the upper gastrointestinal tract is most common within the proximal duodenum. Aphthous ulcers are probably the earliest radiologic lesion detectable. The ulcers in Crohn disease can vary in appearance from pinpoint ulcers with surrounding halos of edema (aphthous ulcers) to small shallow ulcerations (as seen in this case).

Duodenal erosions are nonspecific lesions. They can be caused by various medications (aspirin and nonsteroidal anti-inflammatory agents), drugs (alcohol), and infectious agents (herpesvirus and cytomegalovirus). The erosions found in patients with Crohn disease are often identical to those due to other conditions. The clinical setting is an important consideration. Usually patients with duodenal Crohn disease also have radiologic findings in the more distal small bowel.

CASE 3.16

CASE 3.17

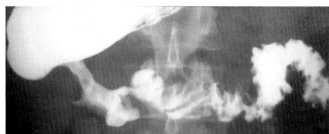

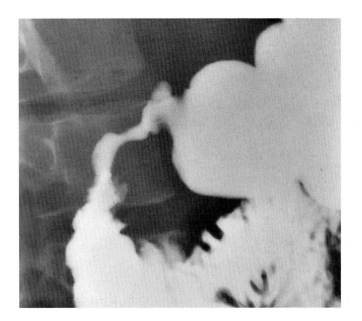

Findings

Case 3.16. Single-contrast UGI. Marked deformity of the pylorus and duodenum is present with asymmetric bowel wall involvement and sacculations.

Case 3.17. Single-contrast UGI. Duodenal narrowing, luminal irregularity, and sacculations (due to asymmetric bowel wall involvement) are visible throughout most of the transverse duodenum.

Differential Diagnosis
1. Scarring from prior peptic ulcer disease
2. Crohn disease
3. Strictures from prior pancreatitis

Diagnosis
Crohn disease

Discussion

Chronic changes of Crohn disease involving the duodenum mimic the findings of Crohn disease found elsewhere in the small bowel. These changes vary from slight luminal narrowing and mucosal thickening to marked narrowing and irregularity causing gastric obstruction. Similar changes can affect the gastric antrum. A differential consideration in this case is scarring from previous peptic ulcer disease. Conceivably, prior severe pancreatitis can leave residual duodenal strictures. If the diagnosis of Crohn disease is not definite, it is often worthwhile extending the examination to include the remainder of the small bowel, because often another characteristic lesion(s) is found (cases 4.64 through 4.69).

CASE 3.18

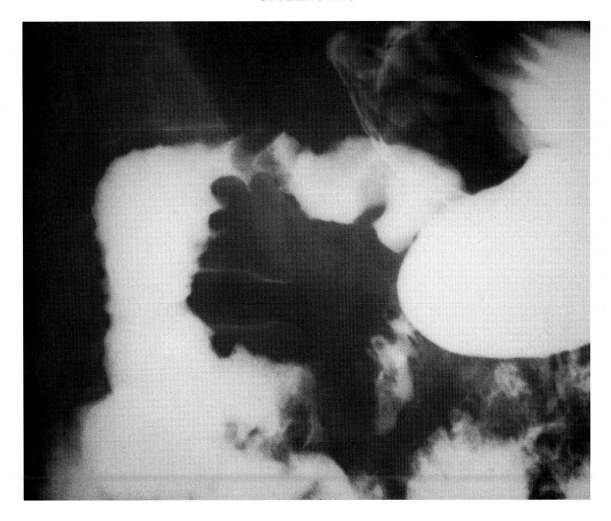

Findings
Single-contrast UGI. The duodenum is mildly dilated, and thickened folds are present in its first and second portions.

Differential Diagnosis
1. Duodenitis
2. Adult celiac disease

Diagnosis
Adult celiac disease

Discussion
Changes of sprue are usually most marked in the jejunum and ileum (cases 4.90, 4.91, and 4.94), but changes in the duodenal mucosa also can be identified both radiographically and endoscopically in a majority of patients. Both villous atrophy and inflammatory changes are usually found histologically. Celiac disease probably impairs the protective effects of the duodenal mucosa against peptic damage.

The radiographic findings of sprue in the duodenum include thickened and often nodular duodenal folds. Duodenal erosions and luminal dilatation may be seen. Brunner gland hyperplasia is often present. Small (1-4 mm), angular filling defects have been reported, resulting in a mosaic or "bubbly" appearance of the duodenal bulb. Patients with long-standing disease may have an atrophic, featureless duodenal mucosal pattern.

Inflammatory and Ulcerative Diseases of the Duodenum

		Case
Peptic disease	Most frequent cause of thickened duodenal folds. Often results in duodenal bulb ulcers	3.1–3.10
Zollinger-Ellison syndrome	Multiple and postbulbar ulcers. Thick gastric folds. Hypersecretion	3.11
Pancreatitis	Narrowing and tethered folds along duodenal C loop	3.12–3.14
Crohn disease	Usually erosions in proximal duodenum. Most patients also have ileal disease	3.15–3.17
Adult celiac disease	Thickened nodular duodenal folds. Classic findings are usually seen in jejunum and ileum. Chronic changes include featureless mucosal pattern	3.18

CASE 3.19

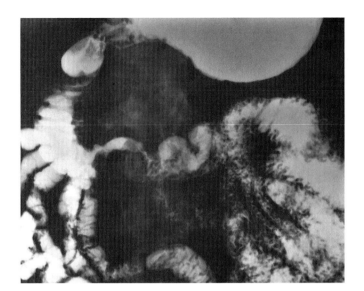

CASE 3.20

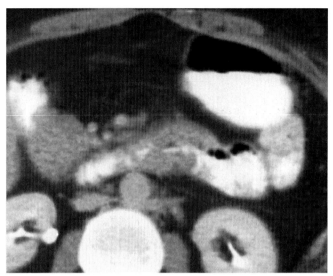

Findings

Case 3.19. Single-contrast UGI. Focal, eccentric narrowing is present within the third portion of the duodenum. The intraluminal characteristics of the lesion are featureless and devoid of any normal mucosal markings (ulcerated surface).

Case 3.20. Contrast-enhanced abdominal CT. Short, segmental bowel-wall thickening is present within the fourth portion of the duodenum. (From Dudiak KM, Johnson CD, Stephens DH. Primary tumors of the small intestine: CT evaluation. AJR. 1989;152:995-8. By permission of the American Roentgen Ray Society.)

Differential Diagnosis
1. Adenocarcinoma
2. Lymphoma

Diagnosis
Duodenal adenocarcinoma

Discussion

Adenocarcinoma was removed surgically. Adenocarcinoma is the primary malignant tumor that most frequently affects the duodenum. It is most commonly distal to the ampulla. Short segmental regions of narrowing (apple core) with abrupt edges or polypoid masses are most common (case 3.19). Lymphoma in the duodenum (cases 3.22 and 3.23) is unusual but can present as a bulky solitary mass.

CT commonly is used to evaluate patients for nonspecific complaints and possible obstruction. Small bowel masses can be detected and staged at CT. Adenocarcinomas characteristically cause short, segmental wall thickening of the duodenum. Luminal narrowing is often present.

CASE 3.21

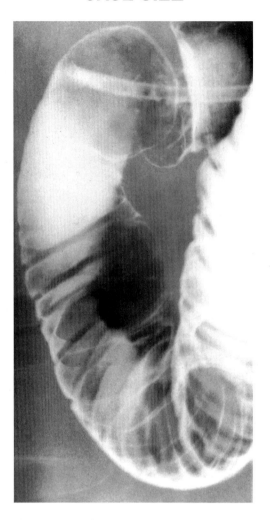

Findings
Double-contrast UGI. A lobulated filling defect occupies the medial wall of the second portion of the duodenum.

Differential Diagnosis
1. Ampullary neoplasm
2. Edematous papilla (recent stone passage or impacted stone)
3. Duodenal polyp

Diagnosis
Ampullary adenocarcinoma

Discussion
Carcinomas involving the ampulla of Vater are nearly always adenocarcinomas arising from the duodenum, distal common bile duct, or distal pancreatic duct. They may present as a polypoid mass or as an annular constricting lesion. Obstruction of the biliary tree is common. Malignant lesions usually have an irregular surface contour. Duodenal (periampullary) adenomas and adenocarcinomas may present as a manifestation of familial adenomatous polyposis syndrome (cases 2.18 and 3.29).

Differential considerations include an edematous papilla, usually due to an impacted distal common bile stone or a large duodenal polyp. Edematous changes nearly always present with the enlarged papilla having a smooth surface.

Endoscopic retrograde cholangiopancreatography is usually indicated in any patient with a suspected ampullary lesion. The tumor is often directly visible, and a biopsy specimen can be obtained. Surgical treatment is usually pancreatoduodenectomy (Whipple procedure).

CASE 3.22

CASE 3.23

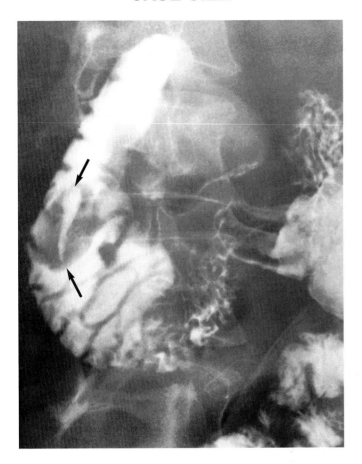

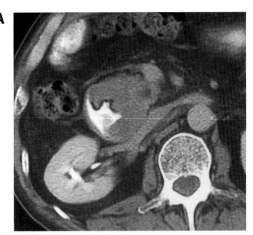

A

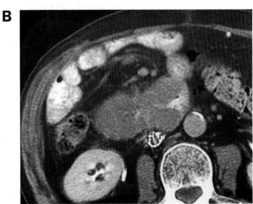

B

Findings

Case 3.22. Single-contrast UGI. A well-defined mass (arrows) with smooth borders is present within the second portion of the duodenum. The mass contains a linear ulcer crater.

Case 3.23. Contrast-enhanced CT. **A** and **B.** A long segment of circumferential bowel-wall thickening involves the second portion of the duodenum. A large ulceration is present within the lesion (best seen in **A**).

Differential Diagnosis

1. Metastases
2. Lymphoma
3. Adenocarcinoma
4. Gastrointestinal stromal tumor

Diagnosis

Lymphoma

Discussion

Any of the primary duodenal tumors and metastases to the duodenum could have the appearance of case 3.22 on the UGI, including adenocarcinoma (cases 3.19 and 3.20), gastrointestinal stromal tumors (case 3.24), and lymphoma. Lymphoma was removed surgically. Notice the well-defined minor and major papillae located medial to the tumor in case 3.22.

Lymphoma involving the duodenum is unusual. It may present as a solitary mass, as one of many lesions within the alimentary tract, or as an ulcerated mass. Occasionally, the ulcer crater is larger than the associated unaffected bowel lumen (aneurysmal ulceration). Characteristic findings of lymphoma on CT include a long segment of marked bowel-wall thickening (as seen in case 3.23). Regional or diffuse adenopathy may be associated with the mass.

CASE 3.24

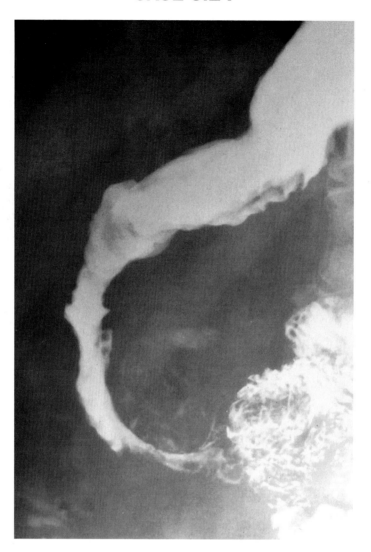

Findings

Single-contrast UGI. An extramucosal mass narrows and deforms the duodenum at the junction of its second and third portions. The smooth surface of the lesion indicates its extramucosal location. Calcification is present within the mass.

Differential Diagnosis

1. Acute and chronic pancreatitis
2. Gastrointestinal stromal tumor
3. Crohn disease

Diagnosis

Malignant gastrointestinal stromal tumor

Discussion

Malignant gastrointestinal stromal tumors are often impossible to differentiate radiologically from those that are benign. They are intramural tumors with a smooth surface. Tumoral calcification (as seen in this case) is usually specific for smooth muscle tumors. Large lesions and ulcerative lesions are more likely malignant. Bulky lesions with areas of central necrosis are typically found on CT. Often the tumor appears larger at CT than anticipated from the barium study. A history and symptoms of pancreatitis are helpful to consider this possibility. Although Crohn disease can alter the duodenal contour, a focal mass is rarely present in this location.

CASE 3.25

CASE 3.26

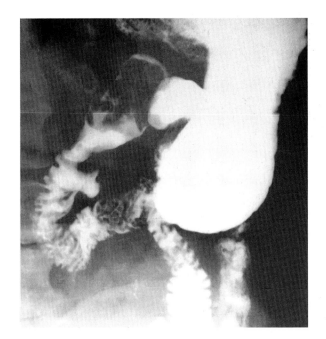

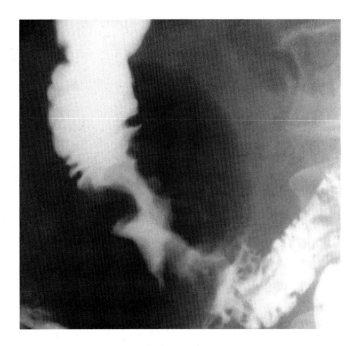

Findings

Case 3.25. Single-contrast UGI. A large polypoid mass fills most of the duodenal bulb. A diverticulum is present along the medial aspect of the second portion of the duodenum.

Case 3.26. Single-contrast UGI. An ulcerated, annular constricting mass is present within the second portion of the duodenum.

Differential Diagnosis

1. Duodenal adenocarcinoma
2. Metastases
3. Lymphoma

Diagnosis

Duodenal metastases

Discussion

Case 3.25. The mass was metastatic renal adenocarcinoma. Renal adenocarcinomas can directly invade or metastasize hematogenously to the alimentary tract. Either route of spread can lead to bulky polypoid filling defects, as seen in this case.

Case 3.26. This mass was a metastatic large cell carcinoma from a primary lesion in the lung. The tumor is radiographically indistinguishable from a primary duodenal adenocarcinoma (cases 3.19 and 3.20). Statistically, a metastasis to the duodenum is more likely than is a primary adenocarcinoma.

CASE 3.27

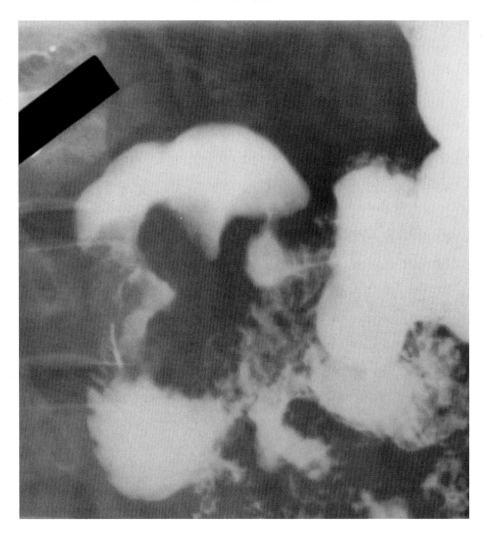

Findings

Single-contrast UGI. The second portion of the duodenum is narrowed and distorted, with ulceration along its medial border. (From Stephens DH. Neoplastic lesions. In: Margulis AR, Burhenne HJ, editors. Alimentary tract radiology. Vol 2. 4th ed. St. Louis: CV Mosby Company; 1989. p. 1167-94. By permission of the publisher.)

Differential Diagnosis

Pancreatic adenocarcinoma

Diagnosis

Pancreatic adenocarcinoma

Discussion

This is a typical example of the reverse 3, or epsilon, sign, described by Frostberg. Barium examination is no longer the method of choice for examination of the pancreas. Direct pancreatic imaging with CT or sonography is preferable. Many intraluminal contrast examinations in patients with pancreatic cancer are negative. Radiographic findings vary depending on the size of the tumor or its location within the pancreas. Tumors in the pancreatic head can compress, invade, and ulcerate the medial border of the duodenal sweep and inferior aspect of the gastric antrum. Masses in the pancreatic body and tail can cause mass effect and tethering of the gastric body and fundus. Tumor also can extend along the normal tissue planes and ligaments of the transverse colon and duodenojejunal flexure.

CASE 3.28

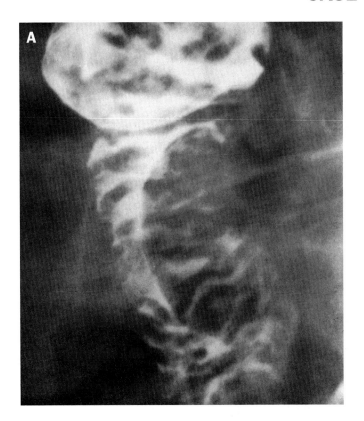

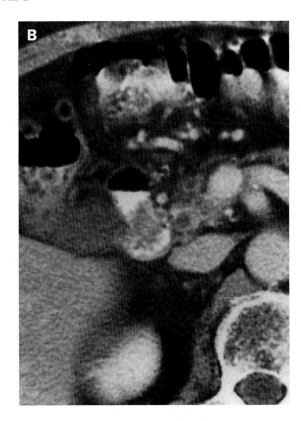

Findings

A. Single-contrast UGI. A well-defined mass is located in the region of the ampulla.

B. Contrast-enhanced CT. A soft tissue mass causes focal wall thickening of the medial wall of the second portion of the duodenum.

Differential Diagnosis

1. Ampullary neoplasm
2. Duodenal polyp
3. Edematous major papilla

Diagnosis

Villous adenoma (duodenal polyp)

Discussion

A villous adenoma was removed at operation. Benign tumors of the duodenum are unusual. Villous adenomas often have a raspberry- or cauliflower-like surface, although the surface of the tumor in this case does not appear villous. These tumors can be suggested radiographically when barium fills the many tiny surface interstices. The incidence of malignant transformation within villous adenomas is higher than in usual tubular adenomatous polyps.

Polyps can be detected at CT with optimal technique. CT is also helpful for determining the extraluminal extent of disease. Local tumor invasion, regional lymphadenopathy, and liver and lung metastases can be assessed preoperatively with CT. Follow-up of these findings with endoscopy is indicated.

CASE 3.29

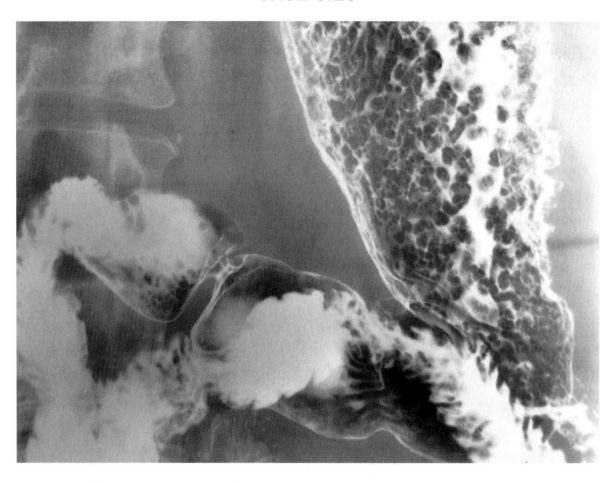

Findings
Double-contrast UGI. Multiple tiny filling defects are present within the duodenal bulb. Larger and more numerous polyps are also present in the stomach in this patient with Gardner syndrome.

Differential Diagnosis
Fundic gland polyposis syndrome (familial adenomatous polyposis syndrome)

Diagnosis
Fundic gland polyposis syndrome (familial adenomatous polyposis syndrome)

Discussion
Duodenal polyps are rare; when present, they are usually adenomas, gastrointestinal stromal tumors, or lipomas. Multiple polyps in the duodenum can be present in patients with a polyposis syndrome. Gastric polyps in familial polyposis (and Gardner syndrome) are most commonly hyperplastic, although adenomas also can be found. Duodenal polyps are usually adenomatous. Because patients with familial polyposis have an increased incidence of ampullary carcinoma, the duodenum should be assessed carefully in all patients with familial polyposis. Hamartomas are usually present in Peutz-Jeghers syndrome.

Other causes of multiple filling defects in the duodenal bulb include heterotopic gastric mucosa (case 3.33), benign lymphoid hyperplasia, and Brunner gland hyperplasia (case 3.34). Heterotopic gastric mucosa usually appears as multiple tiny, angular filling defects. Nodular lymphoid hyperplasia consists of tiny, round, uniform filling defects that usually diffusely involve the entire small bowel (case 4.54). Brunner gland hyperplasia is often larger and involves fewer filling defects that vary in size.

CASE 3.30

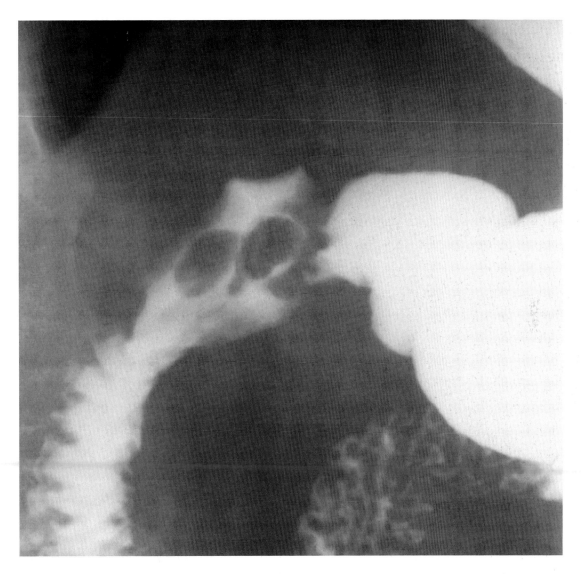

Findings

Single-contrast UGI. Two polypoid filling defects are present within the duodenal bulb. At fluoroscopy, these were observed to traverse the pylorus and return to the stomach.

Differential Diagnosis

1. Prolapsing gastric polyps
2. Brunner gland adenomas
3. Foreign bodies in duodenum

Diagnosis

Prolapsing gastric polyps

Discussion

These lesions were found to be hyperplastic gastric polyps and were removed with endoscopic polypectomy. Gastric polyps are more common than duodenal polyps. In fact, most duodenal bulb polyps are actually gastric polyps that have prolapsed through the pylorus into the duodenum. Fluoroscopic observation can be helpful for watching the polyps move between stomach and duodenum and for identifying the pedicle. Duodenal polyps are attached and do not prolapse into the stomach. Foreign bodies (usually food) will move, during fluoroscopic observation, into the descending duodenum and beyond.

CASE 3.31

CASE 3.32

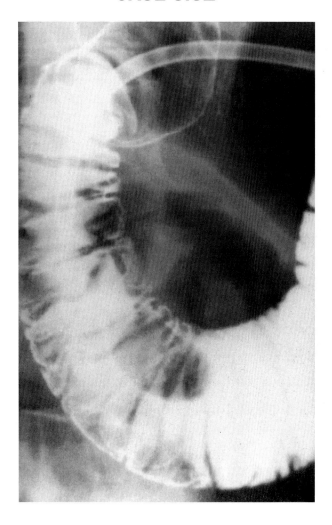

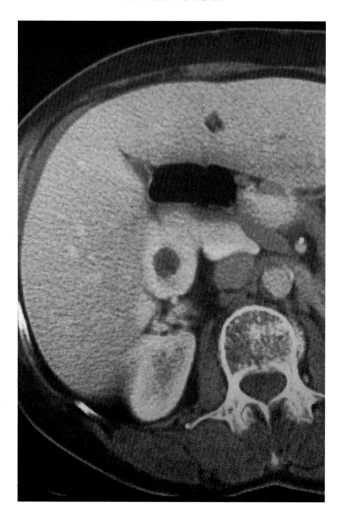

Findings

Case 3.31. Double-contrast UGI. A well-circumscribed mass is located at the junction of the second and third portions of the duodenum. Its smooth surface suggests a submucosal origin of the tumor. The sausage shape of the mass suggests it is soft and pliable.

Case 3.32. Contrast-enhanced CT. A mass the density of fat is present within the duodenum. The mass is well circumscribed.

Differential Diagnosis
Duodenal lipoma

Diagnosis
Duodenal lipoma

Discussion

This radiographic appearance is typical for a lipoma. No further diagnostic tests should be necessary.

Lipomas are submucosal tumors that nearly always have a smooth surface and are compressible at fluoroscopy. These tumors may change shape during a peristaltic contraction. They may grow to be large. The fat attenuation at CT is pathognomonic.

CASE 3.33

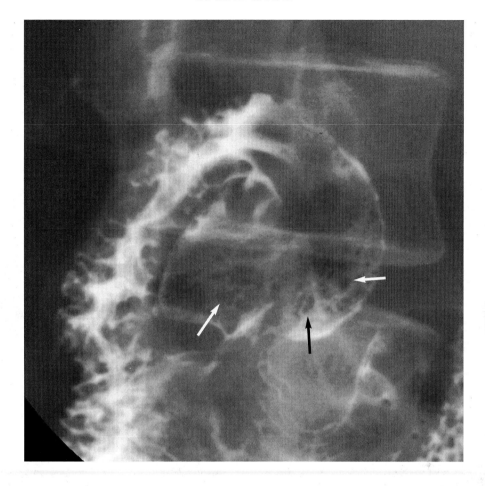

Findings

Double-contrast UGI. Multiple tiny filling defects of variable size (arrows) are present within the duodenal bulb.

Differential Diagnosis

1. Brunner gland hyperplasia
2. Lymphoid pattern
3. Heterotopic gastric mucosa
4. Effervescent granules

Diagnosis

Heterotopic gastric mucosa

Discussion

The normal duodenal mucosa can vary in appearance, but it is often either featureless or a fine nodular pattern. Heterotopic gastric mucosa is a congenital, benign, and asymptomatic condition consisting of islands of gastric mucosa within the duodenal bulb. This type of mucosa may have a protective effect against peptic ulcer disease. Radiographically, raised nodules, often with an angular configuration, that measure one to several millimeters in diameter are seen about the pylorus either diffusely or in clusters. Differential considerations include effervescent granules, Brunner gland hyperplasia, and nodular lymphoid hyperplasia. Brunner glands are usually larger, less numerous, and more uniform in size (case 3.34). Lymphoid nodules (case 4.54) are small and uniform in size, usually evenly distributed throughout the duodenum. Effervescent granules change size and shape on different views as they dissolve. Gastric metaplasia of duodenal epithelium also can occur, analogous to Barrett metaplasia in the esophagus. This condition is commonly associated with peptic ulcer disease. The mucosal changes in metaplasia cannot be appreciated radiologically because the lesions are flat.

CASE 3.34

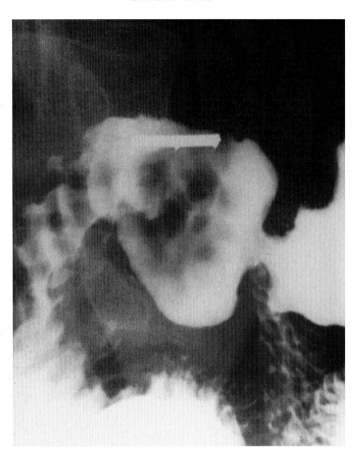

Findings

Single-contrast UGI. Multiple filling defects of various sizes are present within the duodenal bulb. A metallic marker embedded on a radiolucent compression paddle is projected over the bulb.

Differential Diagnosis

1. Duodenitis
2. Brunner gland hyperplasia
3. Nodular lymphoid hyperplasia
4. Heterotopic gastric mucosa
5. Crohn disease

Diagnosis

Brunner gland hyperplasia

Discussion

Brunner glands are normal glandular elements located predominantly in the proximal portion of the duodenum. Glandular secretions are rich in mucus and bicarbonate, substances that protect the duodenum against acid. Hyperplasia of these glands occurs mainly in response to peptic ulcer disease. Radiographically, nodular filling defects are seen in the duodenal bulb and the second portion of the duodenum.

Differential considerations include thickened folds from duodenitis (case 3.1), which often can be obliterated with compression. Crohn disease often involves a more extensive portion of the duodenum and often is associated with changes in the distal stomach and small bowel (cases 3.15, 3.16, and 3.17). Nodular lymphoid hyperplasia usually presents with smaller, uniform-size, and diffusely and evenly distributed nodular filling defects (case 4.54). Heterotopic gastric mucosa is usually smaller and confined to the duodenal bulb (case 3.33).

CASE 3.35

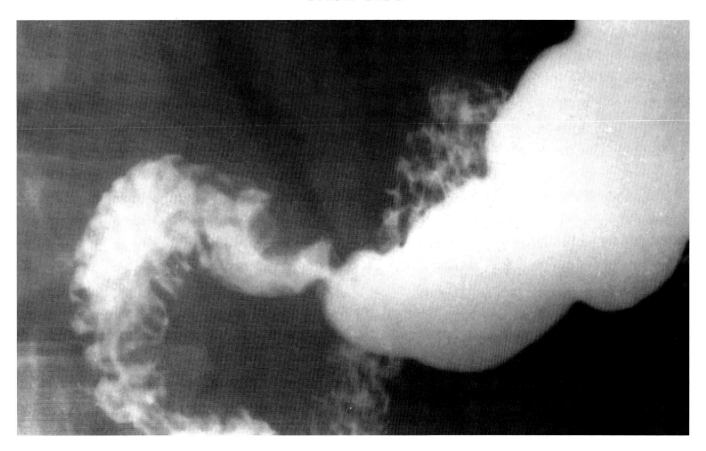

Findings
Single-contrast UGI. An extramucosal (smooth-surfaced) mass indents the superior aspect of the duodenal bulb.

Differential Diagnosis
1. Lipoma
2. Enteric duplication cyst
3. Ectopic pancreatic rest
4. Gastrointestinal stromal tumor

Diagnosis
Enteric duplication cyst

Discussion
Intestinal duplication occurs as a result of abnormal recanalization of the intestinal tract. Duplications can occur anywhere in the alimentary tract, but they usually are found in the esophagus or ileum. With cysts in the small bowel, patients usually present with symptoms of obstruction during late infancy or early childhood. Peptic ulceration and bleeding can occur when ectopic gastric mucosa is present.

Barium studies usually show an extrinsic mass causing narrowing and obstruction of the affected bowel loop. Rarely, communication with the adjacent bowel is seen. Compressibility and pliable shape with palpation and peristalsis are helpful findings that can suggest the diagnosis of either duplication cyst or lipoma. CT often is helpful in a suspected duplication cyst by identifying a well-defined cylindrical or spherical cystic mass the density of water adjacent to the bowel (cases 1.41 and 1.42). Treatment is operative resection.

CASE 3.36

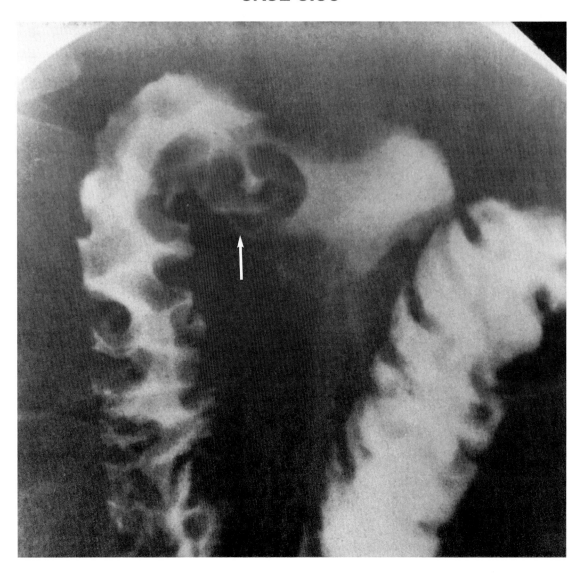

Findings
Single-contrast UGI. A polypoid filling defect (arrow) is present near the junction of the first and second portions of the duodenum.

Differential Diagnosis
1. Duodenal flexural pseudopolyp
2. Polyp
3. Ectopic pancreatic rest
4. Duodenal ulcer

Diagnosis
Flexural pseudopolyp

Discussion
This is the typical appearance of a flexural pseudopolyp. Redundant mucosa is often present at the junction of the first and second portions of the duodenum. This extra mucosa in combination with some buckling medially as the duodenum curves can resemble a polyp (case 3.30), a small ulcer (case 3.3), or ectopic pancreatic tissue (case 2.39). The changing size and configuration of a pseudopolyp can be visualized at fluoroscopy during duodenal filling and emptying.

CASE 3.37

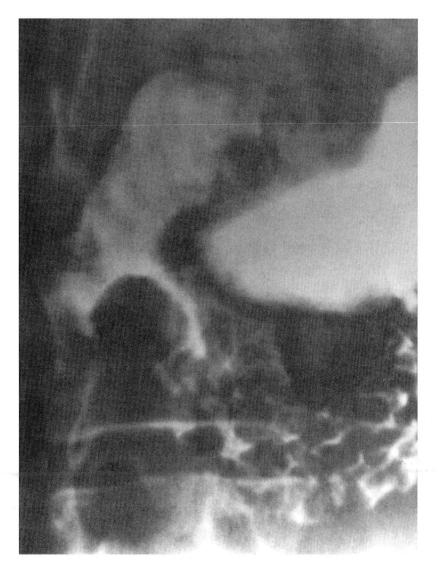

Findings
Single-contrast UGI. A well-defined filling defect with associated narrowing of the descending duodenum is present.

Differential Diagnosis
1. Pancreatitis
2. Duodenal neoplasm (primary or metastatic)
3. Annular pancreas

Diagnosis
Annular pancreas

Discussion
Annular pancreas is a congenital abnormality in which the dorsal and ventral pancreatic tissues encircle and narrow the duodenum at or above the level of the ampulla. Complete duodenal obstruction often occurs in the neonatal period. In patients with duodenal obstruction, the classic "double bubble" is present with gas in the distended stomach and proximal duodenum. Less severe narrowing may be asymptomatic or lead to symptoms that are delayed until adulthood. Endoscopic retrograde cholangiopancreatography or magnetic resonance cholangiopancreatography is diagnostic of this condition when the ventral pancreatic duct encircles the duodenum.

Duodenal Masses and Filling Defects

Malignant tumors		Case
Adenocarcinoma	Most common primary malignant tumor of duodenum. "Apple-core" or polypoid mass	3.19 and 3.20
Ampullary carcinoma	Polypoid mass at ampulla or annular constricting lesion. Usually causes biliary and pancreatic duct obstruction	3.21
Lymphoma	Often long-segment bowel-wall thickening. Aneurysmal ulceration and associated adenopathy should be sought	3.22 and 3.23
Malignant gastro-intestinal stromal tumor	Smooth-surfaced submucosal tumor. Can calcify and ulcerate	3.24
Metastases	Direct extension (pancreatic cancer) or hematogenous spread (e.g., melanoma, lung carcinoma)	3.25–3.27
Benign tumors		
Villous adenoma	Cauliflower-like surface. Higher incidence of malignant transformation than in usual tubular adenomatous polyps	3.28
Polyps	Small sessile or pedunculated lesions	3.29 and 3.30
Gastrointestinal stromal tumor	Submucosal tumor. Can ulcerate	3.24
Lipoma	Smooth submucosal tumor. Fat density on CT	3.31 and 3.32
Nonneoplastic		
Heterotopic gastric mucosa	Often nodules with angular configuration clustered about pylorus	3.33
Brunner gland hyperplasia	Nodular filling defects of varying size in proximal duodenum. Results from gland hyperplasia in response to peptic ulcer disease	3.34
Enteric duplication cyst	Abnormal recanalization of intestinal tract. Fluid density on CT. Extrinsic mass	3.35
Flexural pseudopolyp	Redundant mucosa at junction of first and second portions of duodenum medially	3.36
Annular pancreas	Dorsal and ventral pancreatic tissue encircle and narrow second portion of duodenum	3.37

CASE 3.38

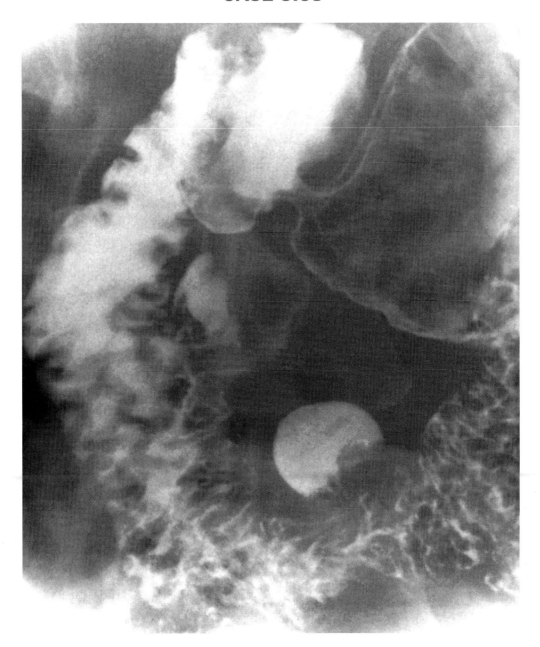

Findings
Double-contrast UGI. Two outpouchings arise from the second and third portions of the duodenum.

Differential Diagnosis
Duodenal diverticula

Diagnosis
Duodenal diverticula

Discussion
Diverticula can occur at any location in the duodenum, but they most commonly arise from the medial wall of its second portion. Usually these are of little clinical significance; however, rarely hemorrhage and perforation have been reported. Diverticula often can be differentiated from ulcers by observing duodenal folds entering the diverticula and the diverticula changing shape and size.

CASE 3.39

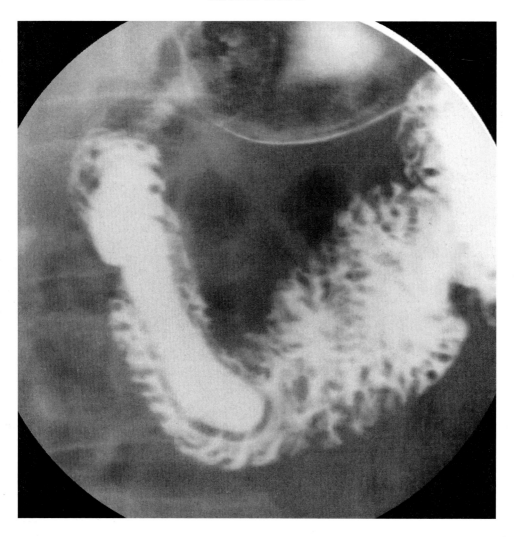

Findings

Double-contrast UGI. A barium-filled, polypoid, intraluminal mass is present within the descending duodenum.

Differential Diagnosis

Intraluminal duodenal diverticulum

Diagnosis

Intraluminal duodenal diverticulum

Discussion

An intraluminal duodenal diverticulum is believed to develop as a result of an intraluminal duodenal diaphragm. The diaphragm usually arises at or near the papilla of Vater. The diaphragm balloons within the duodenum, eventually developing into a sac. Most patients present with intermittent obstructive symptoms and abdominal pain. An obstructive diverticulum near the papilla of Vater may be associated with pancreatitis.

The radiologic appearance of intraluminal duodenal diverticula has been likened to that of a wind sock. Usually a radiolucent band, representing the diverticular wall, surrounds the diverticulum. If the diverticulum is not filled with barium, it resembles a pedunculated polyp (case 3.30).

CASE 3.40

CASE 3.41

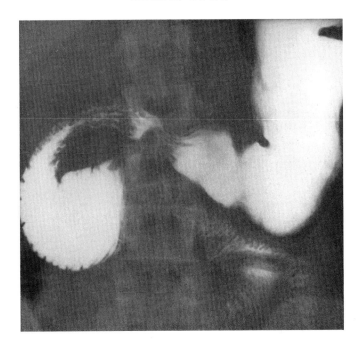

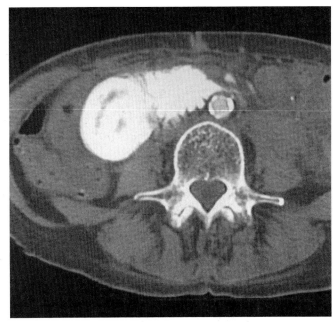

Findings

Case 3.40. Single-contrast UGI. The proximal transverse duodenum is dilated to the level of the spine. The bowel abruptly narrows and appears to be pinched closed by a linear extrinsic mass. The underlying duodenal mucosa is intact.

Case 3.41. Contrast-enhanced CT. The proximal duodenum is dilated and tapers to a region of high-grade narrowing at the level of the superior mesenteric artery. No mass is present at the level of the duodenal stenosis.

Differential Diagnosis

1. Superior mesenteric artery syndrome
2. Duodenal neoplasm
3. Abdominal aortic aneurysm

Diagnosis

Superior mesenteric artery syndrome

Discussion

Findings are characteristic of the superior mesenteric artery syndrome. Narrowing of the third portion of the duodenum can occur as a result of compression by the anteriorly located superior mesenteric artery and posteriorly positioned spine and aorta. This finding often can be observed in asymptomatic persons, but in certain patients a critical narrowing occurs and results in partial duodenal obstruction. Patients who lose weight rapidly or very asthenic persons are most often affected. Patients immobilized for long periods (body casts, hyperextension fixation for spinal injuries, extensive burns) are also at risk.

Radiologically, the first and second portions of the duodenum are dilated to the level of the extramucosal linear obstruction (superior mesenteric artery). Vigorous peristalsis of the proximal duodenum often is observed fluoroscopically as these segments attempt to propel duodenal contents beyond the obstruction. Turning the patient to the left decubitus or prone position may reduce the compression on the duodenum, and contrast material is observed to pass easily into the distal duodenum.

Other conditions causing dilatation of the proximal small bowel include primary or metastatic duodenal tumors (cases 3.25 and 3.26), pancreatitis (cases 3.12 and 3.13), and abdominal aortic aneurysms.

CASE 3.42

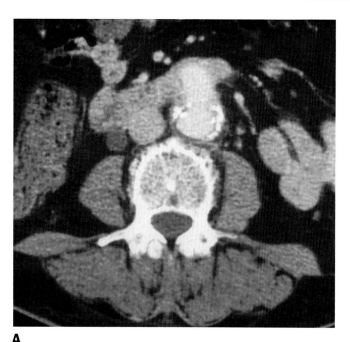

A

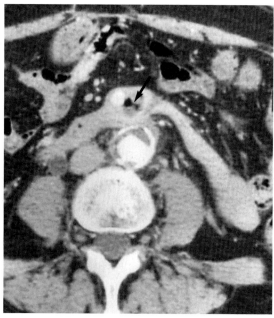

B

Findings
Contrast-enhanced CT. **A.** An end-to-side abdominal aortic graft is in place. **B.** The normally visible fat plane between the aorta/graft and duodenum is absent. Fluid and gas (arrow) are present within the left limb of the graft.

Differential Diagnosis
1. Aortoenteric fistula
2. Aortic graft infection

Diagnosis
Aortoenteric fistula

Discussion
This patient was experiencing gastrointestinal bleeding. Findings are compatible with an aortoenteric fistula. At operation, a 3×3-cm defect was present in the fourth portion of the duodenum. The graft was bile-stained and leaking blood into the duodenum.

An aortoenteric fistula is usually a complication of reconstructive aortic surgery after the placement of a prosthetic graft. Perigraft infection is nearly always present, and fistulization is a potentially catastrophic complication of the infection. The clinical signs and symptoms of this disorder can be subtle; gastrointestinal bleeding is the most obvious manifestation. The commonest CT findings of aortoenteric fistula include an ectopic gas collection and focal bowel-wall thickening. The fat plane is usually lost between the aorta and the duodenum. The finding of perigraft soft tissue, fluid, or ectopic gas is worrisome for perigraft infection. CT is most helpful for excluding this diagnosis by identification of an intact fat plane between the duodenum and the aortic graft. Arteriography is often necessary to confirm the diagnosis.

CASE 3.43

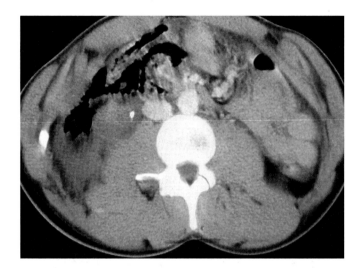

CASE 3.44

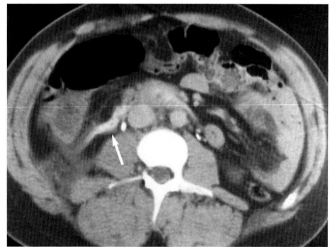

Findings

Case 3.43. Contrast-enhanced CT. Extraluminal gas is present in the subhepatic space, adjacent and anterior to the duodenum. Patient had sustained abdominal trauma in a motor vehicle accident.

Case 3.44. Extravasated orally administered contrast material (arrow) is tracking from the region of the retroperitoneal duodenum into the right anterior pararenal space. Hazy soft tissue stranding is also present in the right flank. This patient had sustained a blow to the abdomen in a motor vehicle accident.

Differential Diagnosis

1. Perforated duodenal ulcer
2. Posttraumatic duodenal rupture
3. Gas-producing retroperitoneal infection

Diagnosis

Posttraumatic duodenal rupture

Discussion

The location of the extraluminal air and the history of abdominal trauma are consistent with duodenal perforation, which was surgically confirmed and repaired.

The diagnosis of duodenal perforation often is not apparent clinically. If the diagnosis is delayed beyond 24 hours, reports suggest that mortality may reach 65%. Repair within 24 hours has only a 5% mortality. For traumatic duodenal perforation, the most important finding on plain radiography is retroperitoneal air. Other nonspecific findings include psoas obliteration, segmental ileus near the duodenum, and scoliosis. Plain radiographic findings of duodenal perforation are present in only one-third of patients. Free intraperitoneal air is unusual in traumatic duodenal perforations, and it is more common in patients with a perforated peptic ulcer. CT can directly visualize the duodenum and adjacent tissues. CT findings of a traumatic duodenal perforation include extravasated gas or orally administered contrast material, fluid collection in the anterior pararenal space, and considerable soft tissue stranding in the retroperitoneum. Retroperitoneal gas and fluid also can occur from traumatic injuries to the thorax, bladder, or pancreas.

CASE 3.45

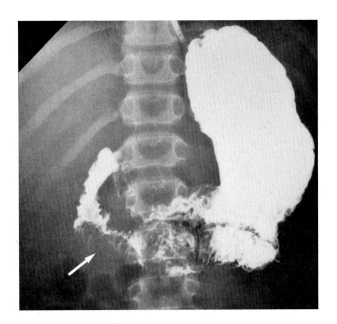

CASE 3.46

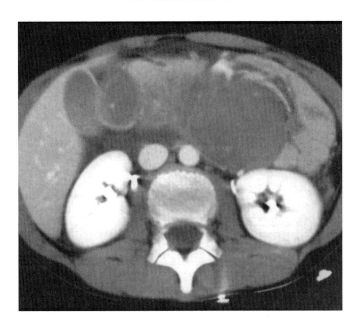

Findings

Case 3.45. Single-contrast UGI. A localized mass (arrow) indents and narrows the duodenum at the junction of its second and third portions. This child was brought to the emergency room after falling from playground equipment onto the abdomen.

Case 3.46. Contrast-enhanced CT. A large, mixed attenuation mass is present in the location of the transverse duodenum. Duodenal folds are thickened and splayed by the mass. This patient was brought to the emergency room after a motor vehicle accident.

Differential Diagnosis

1. Duodenal hematoma
2. Retroperitoneal neoplasm or abscess
3. Pancreatitis
4. Gastrointestinal stromal tumor
5. Metastases

Diagnosis

Duodenal hematoma

Discussion

A duodenal hematoma is most likely, considering the history of trauma. Hemorrhage can affect any portion of the gastrointestinal tract, but the small bowel is most frequently affected. Anticoagulants, trauma, and bleeding diatheses are the usual causes. Patients who sustain blunt abdominal trauma usually have masslike changes involving the duodenum because of its lack of mobility and retroperitoneal fixation. Clearing of the hematoma usually can be appreciated within 1 week, with complete resolution in 2 to 3 weeks.

Radiographic findings include a segmental region of fold thickening where the folds are straight and have been likened to a stack of coins. Smooth or scalloped narrowing of the duodenum with effacement of the folds also can be seen, as in case 3.45. It is important to assess for a duodenal leak (extravasated contrast material or extraluminal gas), an important complication of a severe injury (cases 3.42 and 3.44).

Differential considerations on the barium examination include any process causing localized fold thickening. Generally, the diagnosis is obvious if recent trauma has occurred.

CASE 3.47

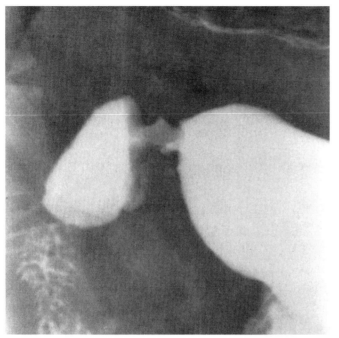

A

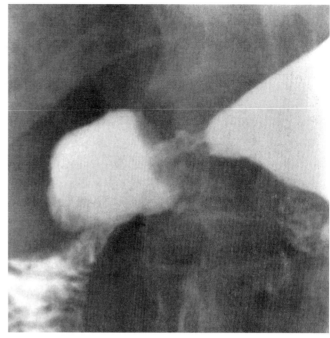

B

Findings
Single-contrast UGI. **A** and **B.** An angular-shaped collection of barium is seen in an elongated pyloric canal. The triangular collection was observed to change shape at fluoroscopy.

Differential Diagnosis
1. Pyloric channel ulcer
2. Pylorus torus defect
3. Adult hypertrophic pyloric stenosis
4. Annular carcinoma

Diagnosis
Pyloric torus defect with hypertrophic pyloric stenosis

Discussion
The normal pylorus is composed of two prominent muscle bundles that converge toward the lesser curvature, known as the torus. In some patients, these muscular bundles diverge far enough to allow mucosa to prolapse between them. This prolapse creates an annulus-shaped niche within the pyloric canal that can simulate a pyloric channel crater. A pyloric torus niche is transient and changes shape and possibly disappears with fluoroscopic observation or serial radiography. It has been reported in 14% of normal patients and is also prominent in patients with hypertrophic pyloric stenosis.

Adult hypertrophic stenosis is rare. Patients frequently complain of nausea, postprandial upset, intermittent vomiting, and heartburn. Radiologically, the pyloric canal is narrowed and elongated. The torus defect is often identified and the pyloric muscle mass indents the base of the duodenal bulb. Nearly half of all patients have concomitant gastric ulceration.

Differential considerations include a pyloric ulcer, carcinoma, and antral gastritis. A fixed pyloric channel should be viewed with suspicion, and endoscopy with biopsy should be recommended to exclude neoplasm.

Miscellaneous Duodenal Conditions

		Case
Diverticula	Often periampullary, but can occur anywhere. Folds radiate into outpouching	3.38
	Intraluminal diverticula have windsock deformity due to prior web	3.39
Superior mesenteric artery syndrome	Dilation of duodenum to superior mesenteric artery. Usually active peristalsis proximally. Asthenic patients	3.40 and 3.41
Aortoenteric fistula	Exclude with fat between aorta and duodenum on all CT slices. Usually due to graft infection	3.42
Rupture	Blunt trauma to abdomen is commonest cause. Retroperitoneal air, soft tissue stranding, oral contrast leakage	3.43 and 3.44
Hematoma	Blunt trauma commonest. Soft tissue mass (often mixed attenuation at CT) involving duodenum	3.45 and 3.46
Pylorus torus	Triangular collection of contrast centered in pylorus. Changes shape with observation	3.47

DIFFERENTIAL DIAGNOSES

Thickened Folds

Benign
- Peptic disease
- Zollinger-Ellison syndrome
- Brunner gland hyperplasia
- Pancreatitis
- Crohn disease
- Adult celiac disease
- Whipple disease
- Hematoma
- Cystic fibrosis

Malignant
- Lymphoma

Filling Defects

Benign tumors
- Polyp
- Gastrointestinal stromal tumor
- Lipoma
- Villous adenoma

Malignant tumors
- Adenocarcinoma
- Lymphoma
- Malignant gastrointestinal stromal tumor
- Metastases
- Ampullary carcinoma

Nonneoplastic
- Pseudotumor
- Hamartoma
- Intraluminal duodenal diverticulum
- Brunner gland hyperplasia
- Enteric duplication cyst
- Ectopic gastric mucosa
- Annular pancreas

Narrowing

Benign
- Peptic ulcer disease
- Pancreatitis
- Crohn disease
- Hematoma
- Superior mesenteric artery syndrome
- Annular pancreas

Malignant
- Adenocarcinoma
- Lymphoma
- Malignant gastrointestinal stromal tumor
- Metastases

DUODENAL FILLING DEFECTS

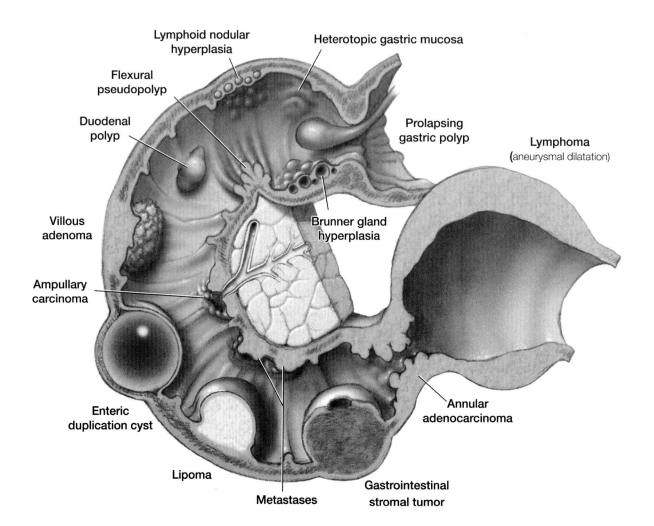

Lymphoid nodular hyperplasia

Heterotopic gastric mucosa

Flexural pseudopolyp

Prolapsing gastric polyp

Lymphoma (aneurysmal dilatation)

Duodenal polyp

Villous adenoma

Brunner gland hyperplasia

Ampullary carcinoma

Enteric duplication cyst

Annular adenocarcinoma

Lipoma

Metastases

Gastrointestinal stromal tumor

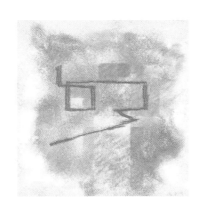

CHAPTER 4

SMALL BOWEL

CASE 4.1

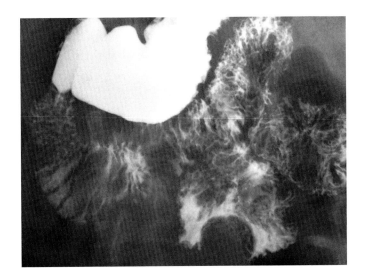

CASE 4.2

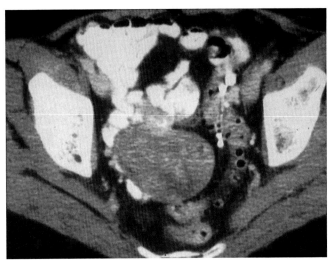

Findings

Case 4.1. Small bowel follow-through. A well-marginated, smooth-surfaced filling defect is present in the jejunum.

Case 4.2. Contrast-enhanced CT. A large, solid soft tissue mass is present in the pelvis, intimately associated with the small bowel.

Differential Diagnosis

1. Gastrointestinal stromal tumor
2. Hemangioma
3. Lipoma
4. Metastasis
5. Lymphoma

Diagnosis

Gastrointestinal stromal tumor

Discussion

Gastrointestinal stromal tumors (GISTs) of the small bowel are most frequent within the jejunum. They are found less often than GISTs of the esophagus or stomach. The radiographic appearance of these tumors depends on their location within the bowel wall. Subserosal GISTs (seen on the CT) may be undetected unless adjacent small bowel loops are displaced by the mass. Submucosal tumors appear as typical intramural lesions elsewhere in the gastrointestinal tract. Some may grow intraluminally and appear as a polypoid mass. Gastrointestinal bleeding is the usual symptom. The bleeding usually occurs as short, repeated episodes of melena or dark-red stool. Even in the absence of active bleeding, these tumors may be detectable at CT or angiography because of their hypervascularity.

CASE 4.3

A
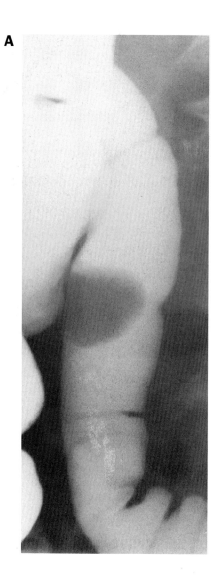

B
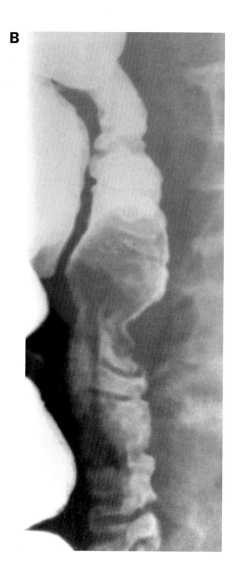

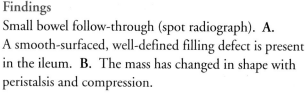

Findings

Small bowel follow-through (spot radiograph). **A.** A smooth-surfaced, well-defined filling defect is present in the ileum. **B.** The mass has changed in shape with peristalsis and compression.

Differential Diagnosis

1. Gastrointestinal stromal tumor
2. Lipoma
3. Hemangioma
4. Metastasis

Diagnosis

Lipoma

Discussion

Lipomas are the third most frequently occurring benign small bowel tumor. They can occur anywhere in the alimentary tract. In the small bowel, they are usually distal. Most are asymptomatic. Symptoms, when present, are often due to an intussusception. Occasionally, obstruction or bleeding can develop. These tumors have no malignant potential.

Radiographically, the smooth surface and compressible nature of these masses suggest the diagnosis. The fatty attenuation of these tumors is diagnostic at CT (case 4.4).

CASE 4.4

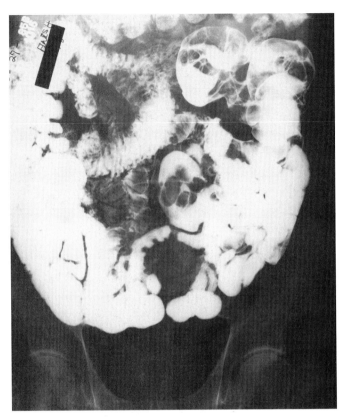

A

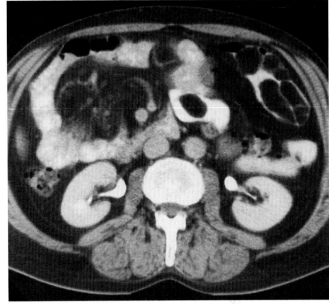

B

Findings

A. Small bowel follow-through. Multiple well-defined, smooth-surfaced filling defects are present within several small bowel loops.

B. Contrast-enhanced CT. Multiple masses the attenuation of fat are present within several loops of small intestine. (From Ormson MJ, Stephens DH, Carlson HC. CT recognition of intestinal lipomatosis. AJR. 1985;144:313-4. By permission of the American Roentgen Ray Society.)

Differential Diagnosis

1. Multiple lipomas
2. Intestinal liposarcoma
3. Metastases

Diagnosis

Multiple intestinal lipomas

Discussion

Multiple small bowel lesions can be found in patients with lymphoma, a polyposis syndrome, hemangiomas, neurofibromas, and metastases. At CT, the tumors in all these other conditions are the attenuation of soft tissue. CT is especially helpful for confirming the diagnosis if a lesion that resembles a lipoma is found on a conventional barium study. If the typical fat density of these tumors is identified at CT, the diagnosis of a lipoma can be made unequivocally. Rarely, multiple lipomas are present (as in this case). No surgical therapy is necessary if patients are asymptomatic. Intestinal lipomatosis can be distinguished from a liposarcoma by the homogeneous fat density and absence of intratumoral soft tissue density in lipomas.

CASE 4.5

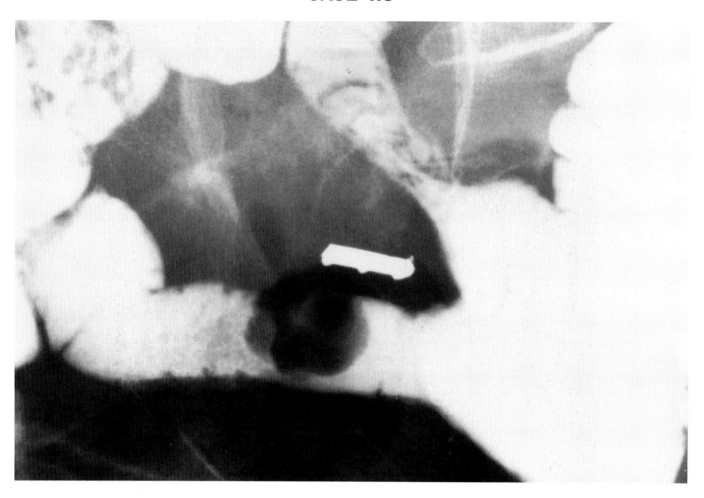

Findings
Small bowel follow-through (spot radiograph). A smooth-surfaced filling defect is present in the small bowel. This is likely due to an intramural tumor. A compression device containing a metallic marker is present.

Differential Diagnosis
1. Gastrointestinal stromal tumor
2. Lipoma
3. Hemangioma
4. Metastasis

Diagnosis
Hemangioma

Discussion
Hemangiomas are rare tumors of the small bowel that usually affect the jejunum. Bleeding, intussusception, and, rarely, obstruction are the most frequently associated complications. Pathologically, multiple thin-walled vessels are seen either intraluminally or within the wall of the small bowel. Patients with Turner syndrome, tuberous sclerosis, blue rubber bleb nevus syndrome, and Rendu-Osler-Weber syndrome have an increased incidence of this disorder.

Radiologically, hemangiomas usually present as focal masses but occasionally can be a diffuse malformation. Many are multiple, small compressible lesions and can be easily overlooked during a small bowel examination. Larger malformations may contain multiple calcified phleboliths that are detectable on a plain film radiograph or at CT.

CASE 4.6

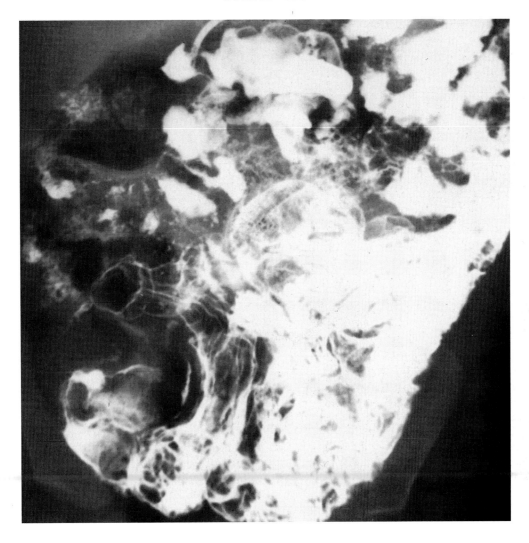

Findings

Small bowel follow-through. Multiple submucosal and intraluminal filling defects are present within the distal small bowel.

Differential Diagnosis

1. Metastases
2. Lymphoma
3. Hemangiomatosis
4. Multiple lipomas

Diagnosis

Diffuse hemangiomatosis

Discussion

Diffuse hemangiomatosis is a rare cause of gastrointestinal bleeding; it usually occurs in infants. Intussusception, obstruction, and malabsorption also can cause symptoms. This condition may be associated with other syndromes, including Klippel-Trénaunay-Weber syndrome (varicose veins, cutaneous hemangiomas, soft tissue and bone hypertrophy), Maffucci syndrome (enchondromas, subcutaneous cavernous hemangiomas), and diffuse hemangiomatosis. There is a spectrum of disease ranging from small submucosal nodules to diffuse intestinal wall involvement with associated extension into the mesentery, retroperitoneum, and other adjacent tissues. Bowel wall phleboliths may suggest a diagnosis but are an unusual radiographic finding.

CASE 4.7

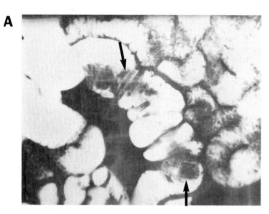

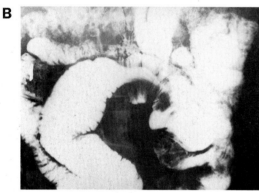

CASE 4.8

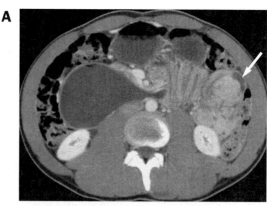

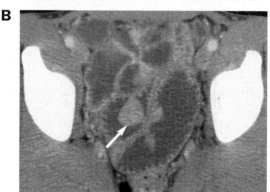

Findings

Case 4.7. Small bowel follow-through. **A.** Two large lobulated polyps (arrows) are present in the mid small bowel. **B.** Transient intussusception with the typical coiled-spring appearance was observed. A polyp was the lead point.

Case 4.8. Contrast-enhanced CT. **A.** The proximal transverse duodenum is dilated and fluid-filled. The distal duodenum has an accordion appearance, and an enhancing mass (arrow) is visible within the small bowel lumen. **B.** Multiple dilated and fluid-filled small bowel loops are visible in the pelvis. An enhancing intraluminal polypoid mass is visible (arrow).

Differential Diagnosis
1. Hamartomas (Peutz-Jeghers syndrome)
2. Lymphoma
3. Metastases

Diagnosis
Hamartomas (Peutz-Jeghers syndrome)

Discussion

Hamartomas were surgically removed in these patients with Peutz-Jeghers syndrome. Hamartomatous polyps are most often found in the small bowel in patients younger than 30 years—the majority of these patients have Peutz-Jeghers syndrome. The small bowel polyps are often cauliflower-like, found in groups, and located within the jejunum. Patients may present with bleeding, pain, or obstruction from intussusception. Usually these lesions are benign, but adenocarcinomas have been reported in the gastrointestinal tract (usually stomach, duodenum, or colon). Ovarian cysts and tumors are found in a minority (5%) of female patients with Peutz-Jeghers syndrome.

Peutz-Jeghers syndrome is inherited as an autosomal dominant disease. Hamartomas most often affect the small bowel, but approximately a fourth of patients have similar polyps in the stomach. Colonic polyps in these patients are adenomatous. Brown pigmented spots on the perioral mucous surfaces are typical.

CASE 4.9

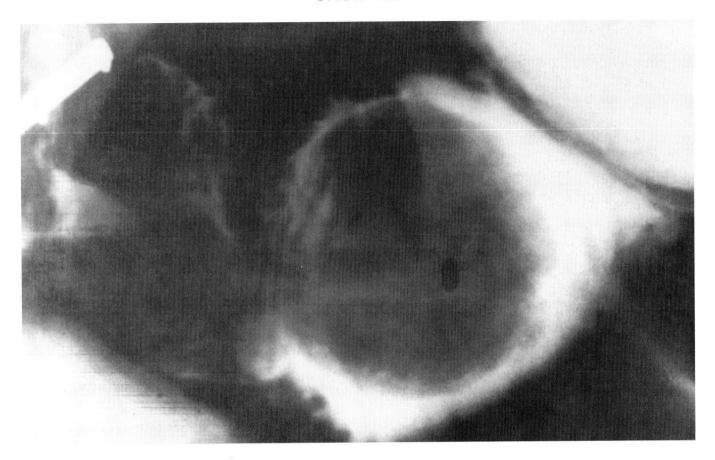

Findings
Small bowel follow-through (spot radiograph). A round, smooth-surfaced filling defect is present in the ileum.

Differential Diagnosis
1. Gastrointestinal stromal tumor
2. Lipoma
3. Hemangioma

Diagnosis
Inflammatory fibroid polyp

Discussion
These polyps are rare and are not true neoplasms histologically. They have been called by various names: infective granuloma, fibroma, hemangiopericytoma, neurinoma, plasma cell granuloma, and Vanek tumor. Histologically, many cell types are found, including fibroblasts, endothelial cells, histiocytes, leukocytes, and small blood vessels. This mixture of cells resembles reparative tissue. The cause of these tumors is unknown, but they can lead to intussusception and obstruction. Radiologically, they are indistinguishable from other polypoid small bowel tumors.

CASE 4.10

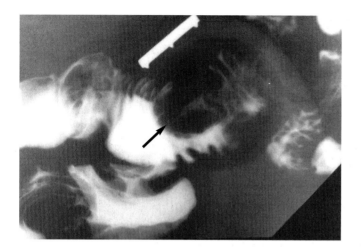

CASE 4.11

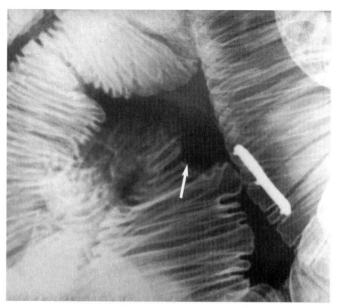

Findings

Case 4.10. Small bowel follow-through (spot radiograph). An ulcerated submucosal mass (arrow) is present in the distal ileum.

Case 4.11. Enteroclysis (spot radiograph). Kinking of a small bowel loop and a submucosal mass (arrow) are present on this examination. A compression device with metallic marker is present.

Differential Diagnosis

1. Gastrointestinal stromal tumor
2. Metastasis
3. Lymphoma
4. Carcinoid

Diagnosis

Carcinoid tumor

Discussion

Carcinoid tumors are neuroendocrine neoplasms derived from Kulchitsky cells that can be found throughout the intestinal tract. Their neural crest origin and biochemical behavior have led to their classification as an amine precursor uptake and decarboxylation tumor. These tumors usually produce 5-hydroxytryptamine (serotonin).

5-Hydroxyindoleacetic acid is a useful biologic marker produced by the degradation of serotonin; it can be measured in the serum or urine of patients with these tumors. Malignant transformation usually occurs in tumors 1 cm or more in diameter. Carcinoids usually are found in the distal small bowel; nearly 40% are within 2 feet of the ileocecal valve. About 30% of patients have more than one tumor.

Small bowel radiographic features of the primary tumor are usually those of an intramural neoplasm, usually 2 to 3 cm in diameter. Ulceration may be present. Often the primary neoplasm is not detected radiographically, and evidence of mesenteric metastases is generally found (case 4.12).

Carcinoid tumors initially spread by direct invasion through the bowel wall into the mesentery. A fibrotic reaction ensues within the mesentery, with kinking and obstruction of the bowel. Usually, obstruction is only partial, and patients may complain of symptoms attributable to partial mechanical obstruction for many years. Advanced disease with mesenteric metastases may result in separation of small bowel loops, tethering of small bowel folds, encasement, and luminal narrowing. The radiographic findings of mesenteric metastases are not specific for carcinoid tumors, and findings can be similar in other malignancies. Kinking and tethered folds also can be caused by adhesions or a localized inflammatory process.

CASE 4.12

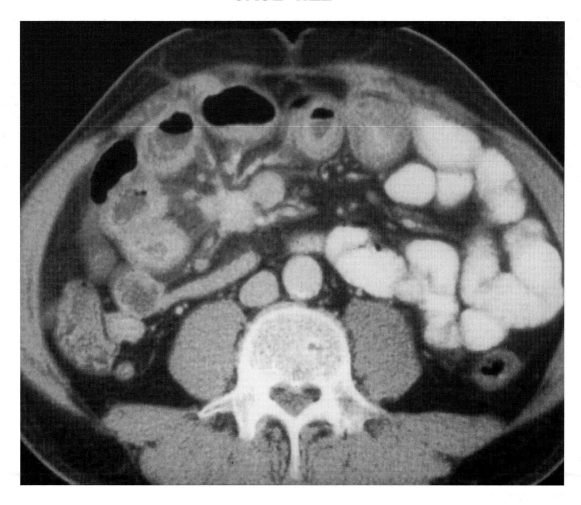

Findings

Contrast-enhanced CT. A soft tissue mesenteric mass is present with associated marked thickening and stranding of mesenteric tissues.

Differential Diagnosis

1. Carcinoid tumor
2. Retractile mesenteritis
3. Mesenteric metastases

Diagnosis

Carcinoid tumor

Discussion

The combination of mesenteric and desmoplastic stranding in this case is typical of a carcinoid tumor. CT evaluation of patients with known or suspected carcinoid tumors can be helpful. The primary tumor is often not detected, but the extent of mesenteric disease, retroperitoneal adenopathy, and hepatic metastases can be assessed. The metastases in the small bowel mesentery often have a typical starburst appearance of linear stranding radiating from a central mesenteric mass and calcification. Liver metastases are hypervascular, often containing regions of central necrosis. Retroperitoneal adenopathy is frequent but rarely is found without hepatic or mesenteric metastases.

Evidence of metastases or a known tumor is helpful for eliminating retractile mesenteritis as a consideration. Although possible, discrete hyperenhancing masses are less common with retractile mesenteritis.

CASE 4.13

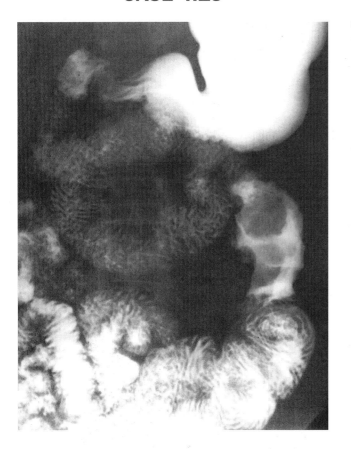

CASE 4.14

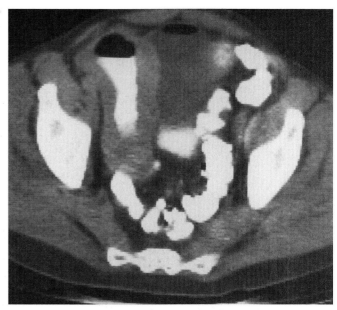

Findings

Case 4.13. Small bowel follow-through. A circumferential ulcerated mass involves a relatively long segment of proximal small bowel. The lumen is larger than the adjacent normal small bowel lumen, exemplifying aneurysmal dilatation.

Case 4.14. Contrast-enhanced CT. A large lesion encases a distal small bowel loop. Marked bowel wall thickening is present. The lumen is dilated. (From Dudiak KM, Johnson CD, Stephens DH. Primary tumors of the small intestine: CT evaluation. AJR. 1989;152:995-8. By permission of the American Roentgen Ray Society.)

Differential Diagnosis

1. Lymphoma
2. Malignant gastrointestinal stromal tumor
3. Metastases

Diagnosis

Lymphoma

Discussion

Small bowel lymphoma constitutes 20% of all malignant small bowel tumors. The vast majority of tumors are of the non-Hodgkin type. Usual symptoms include nausea, vomiting, weight loss, and abdominal pain. Although there are no known predisposing factors, patients with conditions such as acquired immunodeficiency syndrome, celiac sprue, Crohn disease, and systemic lupus erythematosus have a higher risk of the disease.

There are several radiologic classifications for lymphoma. The traditional classification includes multiple nodules (case 4.17), infiltrating form (case 4.15), polypoid (case 4.16), and endo-exoenteric (case 4.19) with excavation and fistula formation. An abbreviated classification includes primary form, lymphoma complicating sprue, and mesenteric nodal form. The traditional classification describes only primary small bowel lymphoma, whereas the abbreviated classification emphasizes secondary forms of the disease.

CASE 4.15

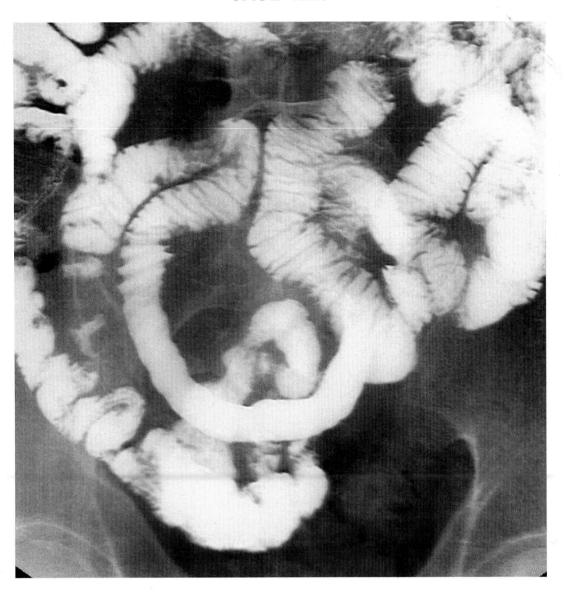

Findings

Small bowel follow-through. A focal segment of small bowel is denuded of folds. The caliber of the small bowel remains normal throughout the length of the abnormality.

Differential Diagnosis

1. Ischemia
2. Amyloidosis
3. Lymphoma

Diagnosis

Lymphoma

Discussion

Focal infiltrative lymphoma may ulcerate the mucosa (with secondary loss of bowel markings). Luminal narrowing occurs when a fibrotic reaction is present. The absence of fibrosis leads to dilatation. The pathologic process is analogous to aneurysmal ulceration, except the lumen through the lymphomatous mass is the same diameter as that of normal small bowel. Chronic changes from ischemia usually result in a narrowed small bowel lumen with loss of folds. Amyloidosis usually causes fold thickening or secondary ischemic changes.

CASE 4.16

CASE 4.17

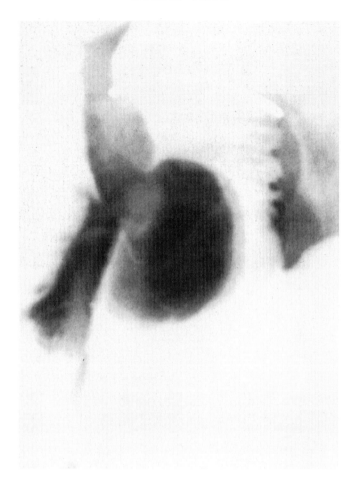

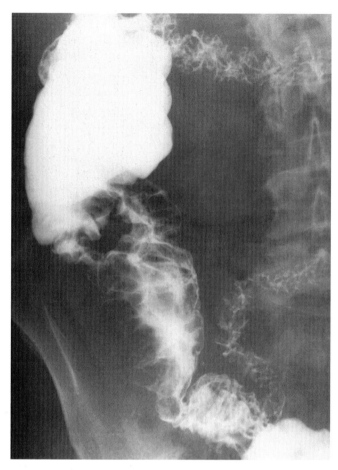

Findings

Case 4.16. Small bowel follow-through (spot radiograph). An intraluminal polypoid mass is present within the small bowel.

Case 4.17. Small bowel follow-through. A long segment of terminal ileum is involved with multiple submucosal, polypoid filling defects. The lumen is increased in diameter.

Differential Diagnosis
1. Metastases
2. Lymphoma
3. Polyposis syndrome (Peutz-Jeghers syndrome)

Diagnosis
Lymphoma

Discussion

A solitary intraluminal mass (as in case 4.16) is an unusual manifestation of lymphoma. The mass is believed to arise within the submucosa of the bowel wall and, as a result of peristalsis, to form a predominantly intraluminal mass, sometimes attached to the bowel wall by a pseudopedicle. The mass could become the lead point for an intussusception.

Multiple masses (as in case 4.17) are a more common presentation for lymphoma. Lymphoma often involves the distal ileum and can cross the ileocecal valve and affect the cecum.

CASE 4.18

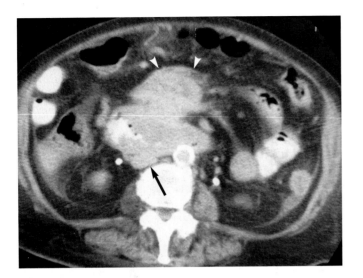

CASE 4.19

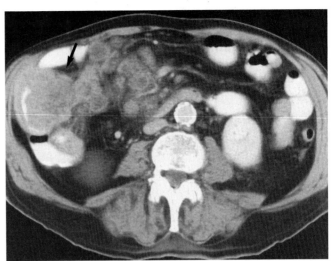

Findings

Case 4.18. Contrast-enhanced CT. Marked wall thickening (arrow) affects a small bowel loop. In addition, adjacent adenopathy (arrowheads) encases mesenteric vessels. (From Dudiak KM, Johnson CD, Stephens DH. Primary tumors of the small intestine: CT evaluation. AJR. 1989;152:995-8. By permission of the American Roentgen Ray Society.)

Case 4.19. Contrast-enhanced CT. Centrally necrotic mesenteric lymphadenopathy is seen in the right side of the abdomen. These lymph nodes coalesce and form a mass (arrow) that displaces and narrows the terminal ileum.

Differential Diagnosis

1. Lymphoma
2. Metastases

Diagnosis

Lymphoma

Discussion

Mesenteric or, less often, retroperitoneal adenopathy, or both, may be present in any form of primary small bowel lymphoma. In case 4.18, lymphoma within the bowel wall appears to be the site of origin of the tumor, and there is secondary spread to mesenteric lymph nodes.

In some patients, the bulk of the tumor is extraluminal, within mesenteric lymph nodes. These nodal masses can become large and cause narrowing, displacement, angulation, and local bowel invasion. Case 4.19 is an example of the mesenteric-nodal form of non-Hodgkin lymphoma.

CASE 4.20

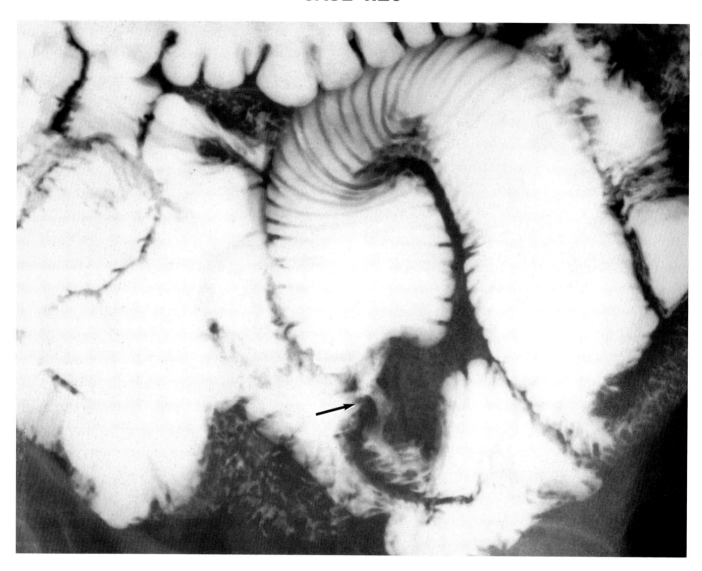

Findings

Small bowel follow-through. A focal region of ulcerative constriction (arrow) is present in the mid small bowel. The loop proximal to the stenosis is dilated, indicating partial mechanical obstruction.

Differential Diagnosis

1. Adenocarcinoma
2. Metastasis
3. Lymphoma

Diagnosis

Lymphoma (Hodgkin type)

Discussion

Hodgkin lymphoma of the small bowel is less common than non-Hodgkin lymphoma. Unlike non-Hodgkin lymphoma, these tumors can incite a desmoplastic reaction, producing luminal narrowing and at times obstruction. Other patterns of Hodgkin lymphoma also can be seen: diffuse fold thickening and irregularity, long segmental regions of involvement, and ulceration. Aneurysmal ulceration, perforation, and fistulization are distinctly uncommon. A primary carcinoma (cases 4.22 and 4.23) could have an identical radiographic appearance.

CASE 4.21

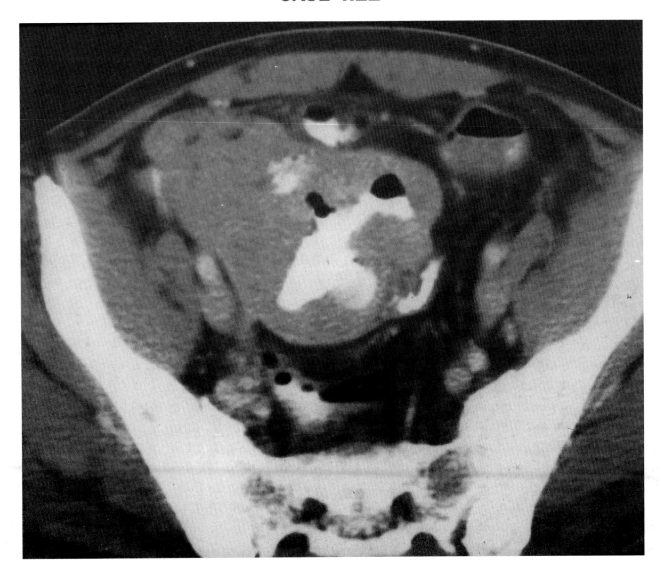

Findings

Contrast-enhanced CT. A bulky soft tissue mass is present in the pelvis. Oral contrast material within its central portion indicates communication of the bowel lumen with its central cavity.

Differential Diagnosis

1. Malignant gastrointestinal stromal tumor
2. Lymphoma
3. Metastases

Diagnosis

Acquired immunodeficiency syndrome–related lymphoma

Discussion

Lymphomas arising from the alimentary tract can present as large bulky tumors. The presence of adenopathy can be very helpful to distinguish it from a malignant gastrointestinal stromal tumor. Patients who are severely immunocompromised are at increased risk for the development of malignancies. Patients with acquired immunodeficiency syndrome (AIDS) have an increased risk for development of opportunistic neoplasms, including Kaposi sarcoma, AIDS-related lymphoma, and several opportunistic infections. Most lymphomas in patients with AIDS are B-cell lymphomas and are aggressive.

CASE 4.22

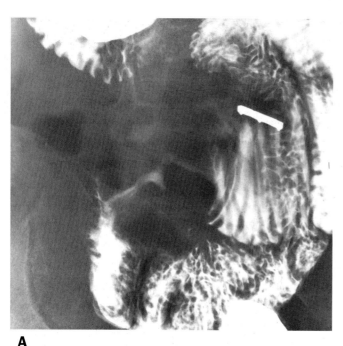

A

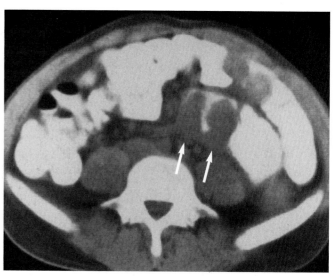

B

Findings

A. Small bowel follow-through (spot radiograph). An ulcerative, annular, constrictive lesion is present in the mid small bowel. The lesion is partially obstructive with mild dilatation of the proximal bowel. A compression device with a metallic marker is present.

B. Unenhanced CT. A lobulated soft tissue mass (arrows) narrows the small bowel lumen and thickens its wall.

(From Dudiak KM, Johnson CD, Stephens DH. Primary tumors of the small intestine: CT evaluation. AJR. 1989;152:995-8. By permission of the American Roentgen Ray Society.)

Differential Diagnosis

1. Primary adenocarcinoma
2. Metastasis
3. Hodgkin-type lymphoma

Diagnosis

Primary adenocarcinoma

Discussion

Primary small bowel adenocarcinoma is most commonly found in the proximal small bowel, usually the duodenum. Patients are often symptomatic: abdominal pain, obstruction, bleeding, or anemia.

There is an increased incidence of this tumor in patients with adult celiac disease and a small increased risk with regional enteritis. Radiographically, a focal region of narrowing with mucosal ulceration is usually seen on barium studies. Detection of these lesions can be challenging at CT if the tumor is less than 2 cm in diameter. Focal circumferential bowel wall thickening in the proximal small bowel is characteristic of an adenocarcinoma at CT.

CASE 4.23

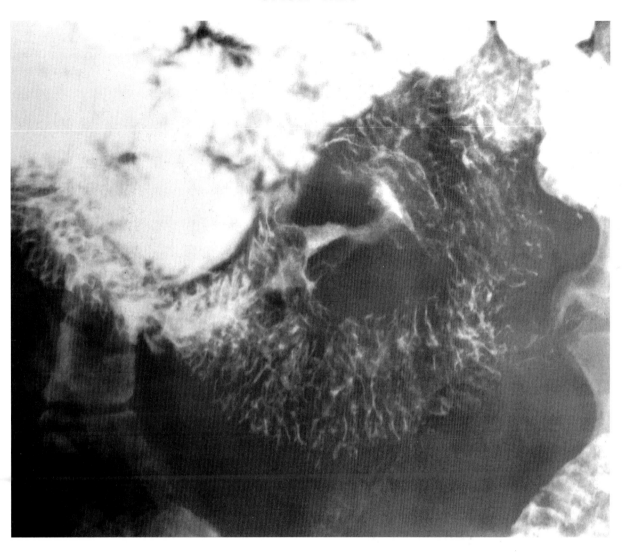

Findings

Small bowel follow-through. An apple-core lesion is present in the jejunum. Notice the absence of normal mucosal markings throughout this lesion. The contour of the lesion is irregular, and the mucosal surface has a smudged appearance due to ulceration.

Differential Diagnosis

1. Primary adenocarcinoma
2. Metastasis
3. Hodgkin lymphoma

Diagnosis

Primary adenocarcinoma

Discussion

The short annular nature of the lesion is characteristic of an adenocarcinoma.

CASE 4.24

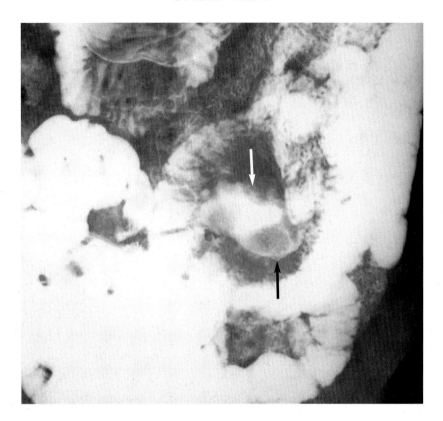

CASE 4.25

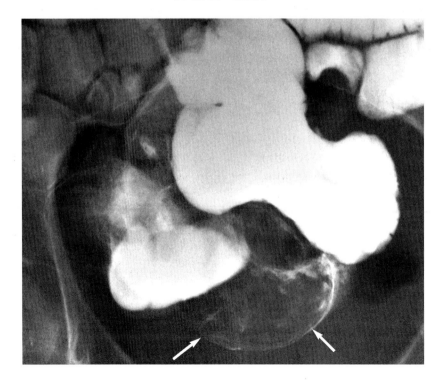

CASE 4.26

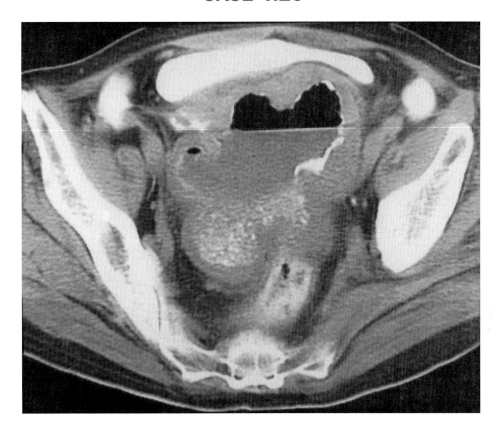

Findings

Case 4.24. Small bowel follow-through. An ulcerated mass (arrows) is present in the proximal small bowel. Ulcerated lumen is expanded compared with adjacent small bowel loops.

Case 4.25. Small bowel follow-through. A large intraluminal filling defect (arrows) is present within the small bowel.

Case 4.26. Contrast-enhanced CT. A large cavitated mass containing air and oral contrast material is present in the pelvis.

Differential Diagnosis

1. Lymphoma
2. Gastrointestinal stromal tumor
3. Metastasis

Diagnosis

Malignant gastrointestinal stromal tumor

Discussion

Gastrointestinal stromal tumors can be divided according to their gross pathologic features into intramural, exoenteric (case 4.24), endoenteric (case 4.25), and dumbbell growths. The exoenteric growths are most common and can incorporate bowel lumen (as in case 4.24). Ulceration, necrosis, degeneration, hemorrhage, fistula, and infection often can be found in these tumors. These tumors metastasize by hematogenous and peritoneal seeding. Nodal metastases are distinctly uncommon. In the absence of metastases, the size of the primary tumor is the most important predictor of malignancy.

CT is particularly helpful in case 4.26 because the nature of the mass can be suggested and hepatic metastases can be identified if present. Surgical removal of smooth muscle tumors is a preferred treatment option because these tumors are radioresistant and unresponsive to current chemotherapeutic agents.

CASE 4.27

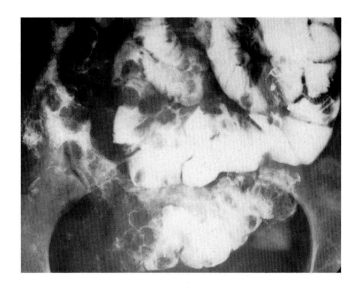

CASE 4.28

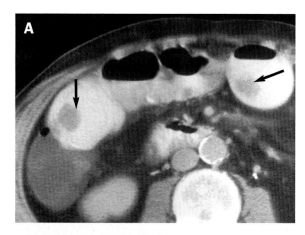

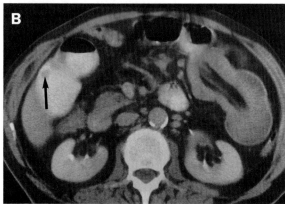

Findings

Case 4.27. Small bowel follow-through. Multiple filling defects are present throughout the small bowel. They are smooth-surfaced and of uniform size.

Case 4.28. Contrast-enhanced CT. **A.** Multiple intraluminal filling defects (arrows) are seen in several bowel loops. **B.** An intussusception is present on the left side of the abdomen. Intraluminal mesenteric fat and vessels are diagnostic of this condition. There is also a small soft tissue nodule (arrow) in another bowel loop.

Differential Diagnosis

1. Metastases
2. Polyposis syndrome
3. Lymphoma

Diagnosis

Metastases, melanoma

Discussion

Metastatic melanoma metastasizes widely and usually spreads hematogenously to the gastrointestinal tract. The small bowel is involved in 50% of cases at autopsy, followed by the colon and stomach. Hematogenous seeding of the small bowel most often occurs in patients with melanoma, breast or lung cancer, and Kaposi sarcoma. If a hematogenous metastasis grows to circumferentially engulf the bowel, it can resemble a primary adenocarcinoma (cases 4.22 and 4.23). Melanoma metastases can present as multiple masses (as in these cases), a solitary large mass (case 4.29), or a bulky ulcerated lesion(s). Intraluminal masses can act as a lead point for an intussusception (case 4.28), causing pain, obstruction, bleeding, ischemia, or even perforation.

CASE 4.29

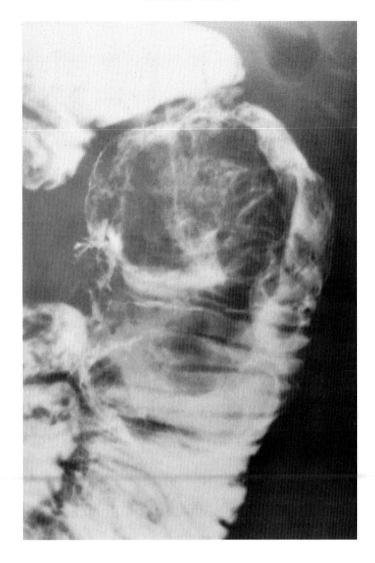

Findings

Small bowel follow-through. A large intraluminal, polypoid mass is present within the dilated proximal small bowel.

Differential Diagnosis

1. Metastasis
2. Gastrointestinal stromal tumor
3. Hamartomatous polyp
4. Lipoma
5. Lymphoma

Diagnosis

Metastasis, melanoma

Discussion

Intraluminal (as in this case) or ulcerated (case 4.30) submucosal metastases can bleed, obstruct, or intussuscept (case 4.28). Renal adenocarcinomas have a propensity to directly invade adjacent organs and present as bulky intraluminal masses. Often, the retroperitoneal duodenum is involved. Any submucosal tumor can extrude in the lumen as a polypoid mass. Lipomas (cases 4.3 and 4.4) and gastrointestinal stromal tumors (cases 4.1 and 4.2) are the commonest primary small bowel tumors to protrude intraluminally as polypoid masses. The history of melanoma in this patient is helpful for making the correct diagnosis.

CASE 4.30

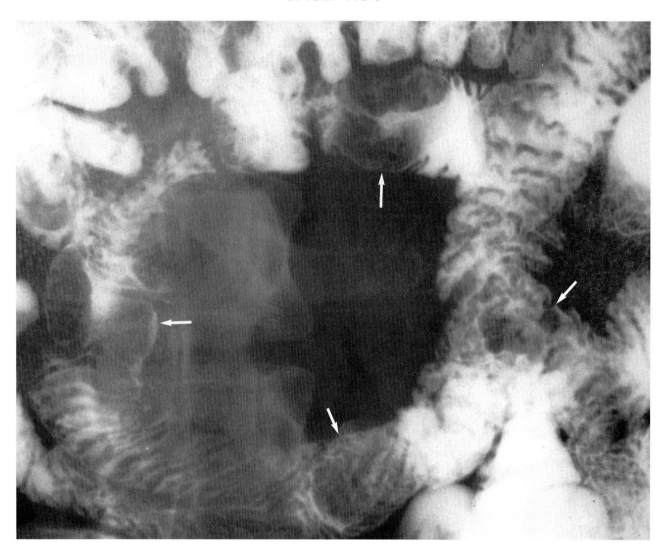

Findings

Small bowel follow-through (spot radiograph). Multiple masses (arrows) are present within a small bowel loop. The central portion of some of these masses appears ulcerated. A large mesenteric mass displaces the small bowel loop around it. Tethered folds adjacent to the mesenteric mass also are present.

Differential Diagnosis

1. Metastases
2. Lymphoma

Diagnosis

Small bowel metastases

Discussion

Multiplicity of lesions should make metastases and lymphoma the main considerations.

CASE 4.31

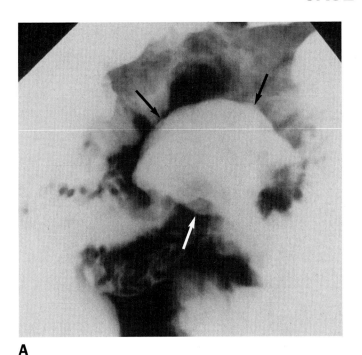

A

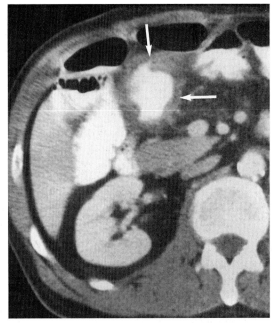

B

Findings

A. Small bowel follow-through (spot radiograph). A large ulcerated mass (arrows) is present within the small bowel. The ulceration has an aneurysmal appearance.

B. Contrast-enhanced CT. The mass (arrows) described above is seen. A rind of soft tissue surrounds the ulcer.

Differential Diagnosis

1. Lymphoma
2. Malignant gastrointestinal stromal tumor
3. Metastases

Diagnosis

Metastases, colon carcinoma

Discussion

Some metastases arise in the bowel wall and grow into the mesentery. Some authors refer to this as exoenteric growth, in which the tumor grows and destroys the bowel wall, forming a large cavitated mass devoid of mucosal markings. Tumors most likely to present in this manner include lymphoma (cases 4.13, 4.14, 4.15, and 4.19), malignant gastrointestinal stromal tumor (case 4.26), and occasionally colon cancer metastases.

CASE 4.32

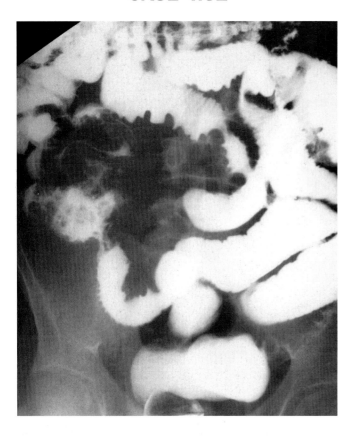

CASE 4.33

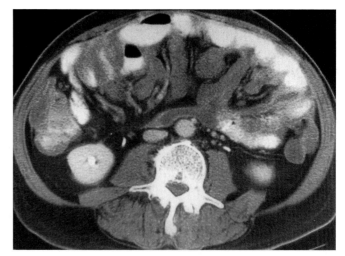

Findings

Case 4.32. Small bowel follow-through. The small bowel loops in the ileocecal region are displaced by a mesenteric mass. Many of the small bowel folds appear tethered and thickened in response to a mesenteric abnormality.

Case 4.33. Contrast-enhanced CT. Soft tissue encasement throughout the leaves of the small bowel. Small bowel loops are displaced by the masses.

Differential Diagnosis
1. Serosal metastases
2. Peritoneal mesothelioma

Diagnosis
Serosal metastases, appendiceal adenocarcinoma

Discussion

Tumors that spread by intraperitoneal seeding often implant and grow in three regions: the pouch of Douglas (the most dependent position in the pelvis), the ileocecal region, and the superior aspect of the sigmoid colon. Meyers described the anatomical regions and usual locations of metastatic implants. Serosal implants displace adjacent bowel loops, narrow bowel lumen(s), cause angulation and kinking of loops, thicken small bowel folds, and result in fold tethering (from direct invasion and mesenteric retraction). Primary tumors arising from the gastrointestinal tract or ovaries often spread by intraperitoneal seeding.

CASE 4.34

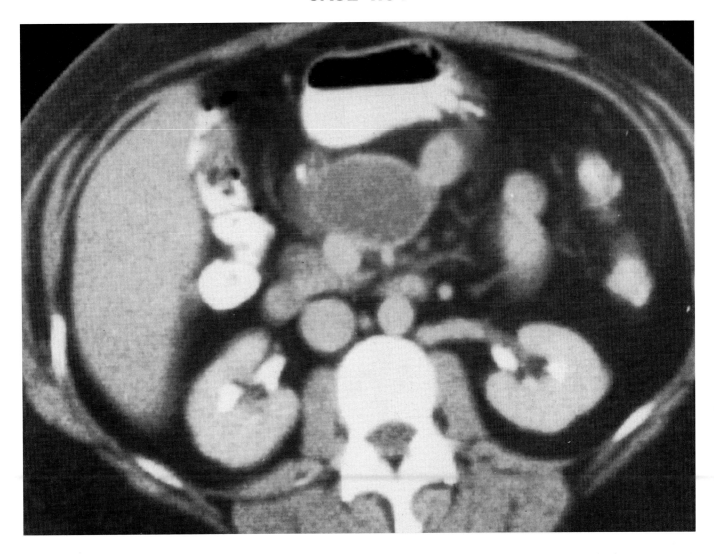

Findings

Contrast-enhanced CT. A well-circumscribed mass the attenuation of water is located within the mesentery.

Differential Diagnosis

1. Duplication cyst
2. Mesenteric cyst
3. Blind loop obstruction
4. Diverticulum
5. Cystic neoplasm
6. Intramural hematoma

Diagnosis

Duplication cyst

Discussion

Duplication cysts can occur anywhere in the gastrointestinal tract, but the terminal ileum is the commonest location. They are usually in proximity to another bowel loop and may communicate with the lumen. The duplication may contain the mucosa of any bowel segment, and up to 25% contain heterotopic gastric mucosa. Most are detected early in life. Treatment is simple excision.

CASE 4.35

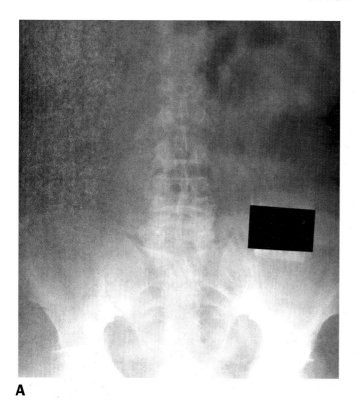

A

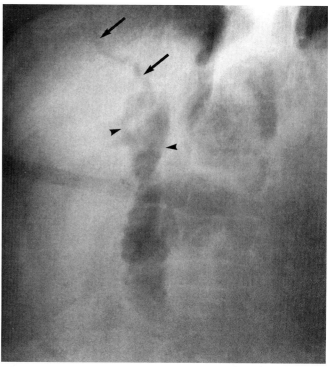

B

Findings
Abdominal radiograph. **A.** Multiple, dilated small bowel loops are present with little visible colonic gas. **B.** A few linear gas lucencies representing the biliary tree (arrows) and gallbladder (arrowheads) are visible in the right upper quadrant.

Differential Diagnosis
1. Gallstone ileus
2. Postoperative biliary-enteric anastomosis with mechanical small bowel obstruction

Diagnosis
Gallstone ileus

Discussion
The combination of biliary gas and mechanical small bowel obstruction is highly suggestive of gallstone ileus if no prior biliary operation has been performed. In this case, an obstructing radiolucent gallstone causing ileal obstruction was removed at laparotomy. Gallstone ileus is a syndrome of mechanical small bowel obstruction by gallstone(s). Classically, elderly women without prior biliary or abdominal disease present with acute intestinal obstruction. Symptoms of acute cholecystitis are unusual, but many patients have a history of gallstones and recurrent cholecystitis. Gallstones can erode into the stomach, small bowel, or colon. Stones in the small bowel most often cause obstruction at the ileocecal valve (the narrowest point). Obstructing stones usually are not spontaneously passed and require surgical lithotomy. Cholecystectomy and fistula repairs are usually performed, but not acutely.

Radiographically, the triad of air within the biliary tree, ectopic calcified gallstone, and mechanical small bowel obstruction is considered characteristic of this entity. Even the findings of biliary air and small bowel obstruction should be regarded as consistent with gallstone ileus.

CASE 4.36

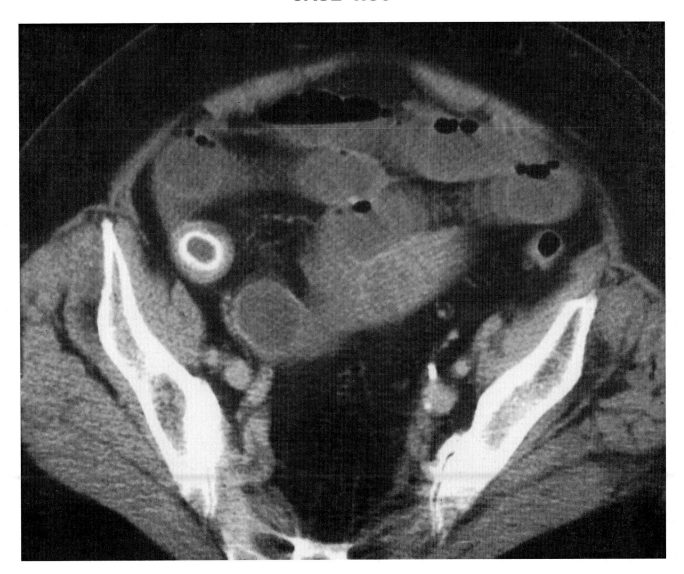

Findings
Contrast-enhanced CT. Multiple dilated small bowel loops are present in the pelvis. A peripherally calcified stone is present within the lumen of a small bowel loop. (This was the site of a transition to normal-caliber loops on other CT sections).

Differential Diagnosis
1. Gallstone ileus
2. Calcified enterolith with small bowel obstruction

Diagnosis
Gallstone ileus

Discussion
CT is a sensitive technique for the detection of calcium-containing gallstones, small bowel obstruction, and biliary air. If gallstone ileus is suspected, CT can be very helpful for confirming the diagnosis. The finding of a stone at the transition point between dilated and normal-caliber small bowel is diagnostic of gallstone ileus.

CASE 4.37

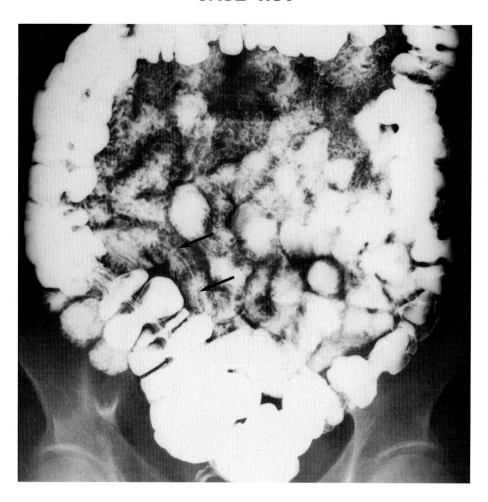

Findings

Small bowel follow-through. An elongated filling defect (arrows) is present in the distal small bowel. A thin white line traverses the length of the filling defect.

Differential Diagnosis

Ascariasis

Diagnosis

Ascariasis

Discussion

The thin white line traversing the length of the worm represents ingested barium in the worm's enteric tract. Ascariasis is a common roundworm infection that most frequently occurs in tropical climates. Infection is acquired by ingesting contaminated water, food, or soil. Ingested eggs hatch in the small bowel, penetrate the intestinal mucosa, and are carried to the lungs by the portal system or intestinal lymphatics. The worms perforate the alveoli, travel up the bronchi, and are swallowed. Worms grow, reproduce, and shed infectious eggs, usually within the distal small bowel. Involved organ systems include respiratory (pneumonia, bronchitis, hemoptysis, and asthma), gastrointestinal (nausea, vomiting, distention, tenderness), and biliary (jaundice, cholecystitis, cholangitis, pancreatitis, and hepatic abscess).

Radiographically, identification of the typical elongated filling defect is characteristic. Mucosal folds may be thickened. Occasionally, the mass of worms can be large enough to cause partial or complete intestinal obstruction. A worm may be identified at sonography or endoscopic retrograde cholangiopancreatography in the biliary tree or pancreatic duct.

Filling Defects of the Small Bowel

		Case
Benign tumors		
Gastrointestinal stromal tumor	Submucosal tumor with smooth contours, most frequent in jejunum	4.1 and 4.2
Lipoma	Pliable submucosal tumor with smooth borders, fat density at CT	4.3 and 4.4
Hemangioma	Focal mass or diffuse malformation (hemangiomatosis), compressible, can contain calcified phleboliths	4.5 and 4.6
Polyp	Solitary or multiple, can occur in patients with polyposis syndromes	4.7–4.9
Malignant tumors		
Carcinoid	Usually distal small bowel, usually 2-3 cm in diameter, mesenteric metastases elicit desmoplastic reaction and can calcify	4.10–4.12
Lymphoma	Mostly non-Hodgkin variety, can present as focal mass, multiple nodules, infiltrative mass, or excavated mass	4.13–4.21
Adenocarcinoma	Usually found in proximal small bowel, often an apple-core lesion	4.22 and 4.23
Malignant gastro-intestinal stromal tumor	Usually large submucosal mass, often exophytic growth, liver metastases should be sought	4.24–4.26
Metastases	Usually present as multiple masses, but may be solitary	4.27–4.33
Nonneoplastic		
Gastrointestinal duplication cyst	Terminal ileum is most common location, fluid density at CT	4.34
Gallstone ileus	Small bowel filling defect, small bowel obstruction, and biliary air. Most common site of obstruction is at ileocecal valve	4.35 and 4.36
Ascariasis	Tubular filling defect with linear barium in worm's gastrointestinal tract	4.37

APPROACH TO DIFFUSE AND SEGMENTAL SMALL BOWEL DISEASE

Diffuse or segmental disease of the small bowel is often confusing, probably because of the infrequency with which many of these rare disorders are encountered and the relatively nonspecific radiographic appearance of many of these diseases.

If a disease diffusely or segmentally affects the small bowel, changes often occur within the wall of the bowel and alter the normal fold pattern. Analysis of, first, the fold pattern and, second, the diffuse or segmental involvement of the small bowel can be helpful for understanding the underlying pathologic condition and for developing a reasonable differential diagnosis. Unfortunately, this classification is somewhat arbitrary, because some diseases may have findings that overlap between designated fold types or a disease may present with different fold patterns in different patients. Despite its limitations, this approach may be helpful as a starting point in the analysis of diffuse and segmental small bowel disease.

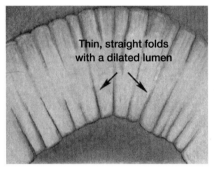

Type I (thin, straight folds)

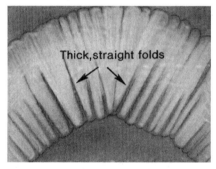

Type II (thick, straight folds)
  Segmental
  Diffuse

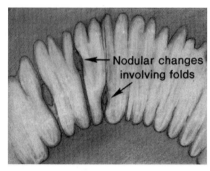

Type III (thick, nodular folds)
  Segmental
  Diffuse

TYPE I FOLDS: THIN (<3 mm), STRAIGHT FOLDS WITH A DILATED LUMEN
(cases 4.38–4.41)

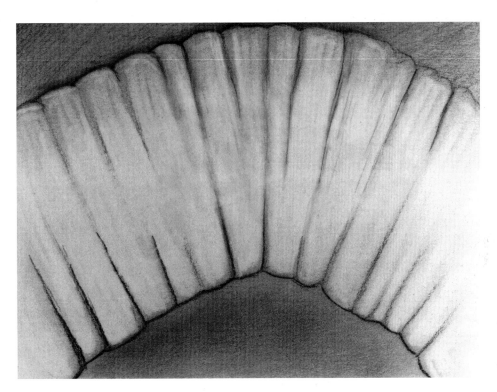

1. Mechanical obstruction
2. Paralytic ileus
3. Scleroderma
4. Sprue

CASE 4.38

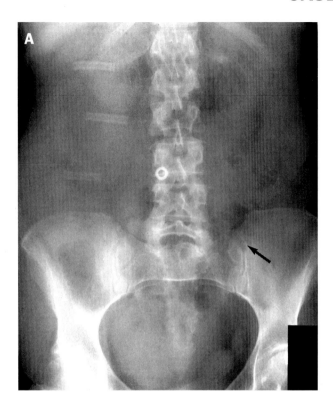

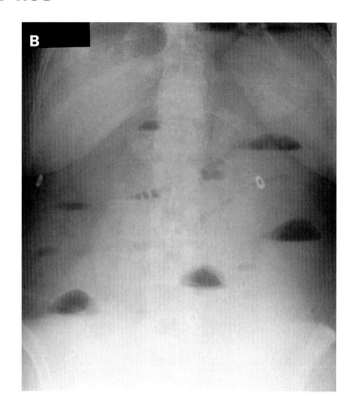

Findings

A. Supine abdominal radiograph. Multiple dilated, partially gas-filled small bowel loops are present with no visible gas in the colon. The valvulae conniventes (arrow) are thin and straight (type I fold pattern).

B. Upright abdominal radiograph. Multiple air-fluid levels are seen throughout the small bowel. Many small collections of gas line up within a small bowel loop and resemble a string of beads.

Differential Diagnosis
1. Mechanical small bowel obstruction
2. Paralytic ileus

Diagnosis
Mechanical small bowel obstruction

Discussion
Partial or complete mechanical small bowel obstruction is a common disease that usually manifests clinically with nausea, vomiting, cramping abdominal pain, and distention.

The common causes of mechanical obstruction of the small bowel are adhesions (from a prior abdominal surgical procedure or severe intraperitoneal inflammation) (case 4.85) or hernias (cases 4.86 and 4.87). Other, less frequent causes include an obstructing neoplasm (cases 4.20 and 4.22), intussusception (cases 4.7 and 4.8), stricture (from Crohn disease, prior ischemia, or idiopathic), or volvulus (case 4.84).

Radiologic evaluation often begins with either an abdominal plain film examination or abdominal CT. Dilated small bowel loops (>3 cm in diameter) are often seen containing air-fluid levels on the film taken with the patient in the upright position. It may be difficult to judge the level of obstruction on an abdominal plain film examination; in fact, a proximal colonic obstruction can masquerade as a mechanical small bowel obstruction on plain films. The lack of gas within the colon makes mechanical small bowel destruction more likely than paralytic ileus in this case. Several additional cases of small bowel obstruction are included in this chapter (cases 4.85, 4.86, and 4.87).

CASE 4.39

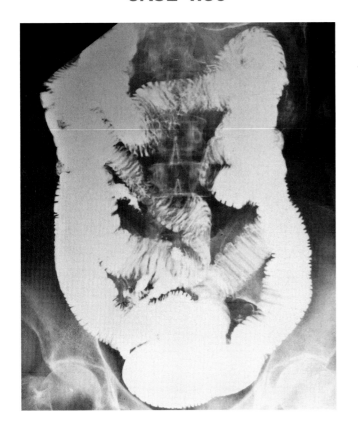

CASE 4.40

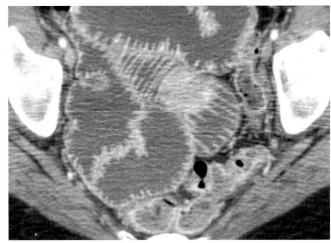

Findings

Case 4.39. Small bowel follow-through. Multiple dilated small bowel loops are present. The valvulae conniventes are thin and straight (type I folds) and closely stacked together.

Case 4.40. Magnified contrast-enhanced CT enterography. Mildly dilated loops of small bowel with crowded thin folds are present in the pelvis.

Differential Diagnosis

1. Scleroderma
2. Celiac disease
3. Mechanical obstruction

Diagnosis

Scleroderma

Discussion

This case has the typical hidebound appearance of scleroderma involving the small bowel, with dilatation and crowding of the straight and thin mucosal folds. Delayed transit time, sacculations on the antimesenteric border of the bowel, and even pneumatosis cystoides intestinalis also can be seen radiographically. Pneumatosis cystoides intestinalis may be related to the frequent use of corticosteroids among patients with scleroderma.

Small bowel changes of scleroderma often occur relatively late in the course of disease, usually after the typical skin changes, Raynaud phenomenon, or arthropathy. Pathologically, atrophy of the mucosa and submucosa, submucosal fibrosis, and round cell infiltration are seen. Mesenteric vascular arteritis may be present.

Distinguishing scleroderma from sprue is usually easy because there is no hypersecretion in scleroderma and patients with sprue usually have normal small bowel motility. In mechanical obstruction, the small bowel usually has more peristaltic activity, the folds are displaced from one another, and there is a considerable amount of retained fluid proximal to the obstruction. Esophageal changes also can be observed in patients with scleroderma (cases 1.61 and 1.62).

CASE 4.41

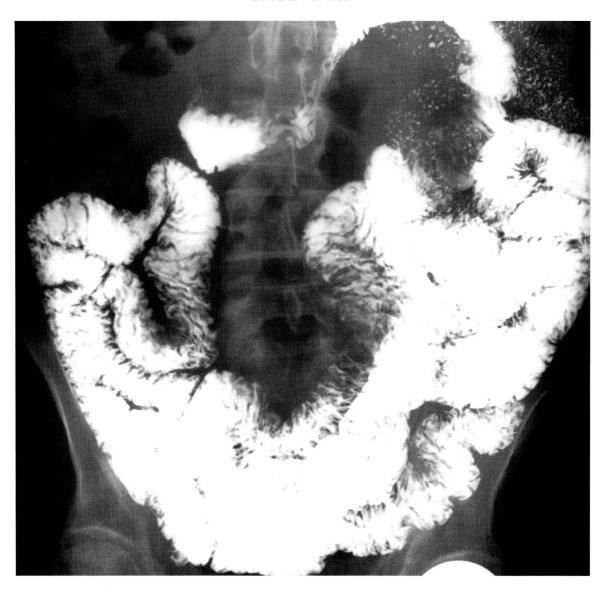

Findings

Small bowel follow-through. Mild dilatation of bowel loops with increased number of thin, straight (type I) folds in the ileum. Reversal of the normal jejunal and ileal fold patterns is seen in this case.

Differential Diagnosis

Celiac disease (sprue)

Diagnosis

Celiac disease (sprue)

Discussion

This typical example of the reversed fold pattern generally is found in patients with celiac disease. The "jejunization" of the ileum is believed to be an adaptive response to the loss of absorptive surface in the proximal small bowel caused by villous atrophy. The jejunal folds have been shown to decrease in number ("ilealization" of the jejunum), a feature particularly evident on enteroclysis examinations. Three folds or less per inch in the jejunum on an enteroclysis examination is strong evidence for this disease. Additional cases of celiac disease are included in this chapter (cases 4.88 through 4.96).

Diffuse and Segmental Small Bowel Diseases: Type I Folds

		Case
Mechanical obstruction	Dilated loops with transition to decompressed loops of small bowel, usually caused by adhesions or hernia	4.38
Paralytic ileus	Diffusely dilated small bowel loops and colon, often due to surgery or narcotic medications	Not shown
Scleroderma	Thin, straight folds stacked together (hidebound appearance), sacculations on antimesenteric border of small bowel	4.39 and 4.40
Celiac disease (sprue)	Fold pattern reversal, hypersecretion, dilatation	4.41

TYPE II FOLDS: THICK (>3 mm), STRAIGHT FOLDS, caused by intramural edema or hemorrhage (cases 4.42–4.46)

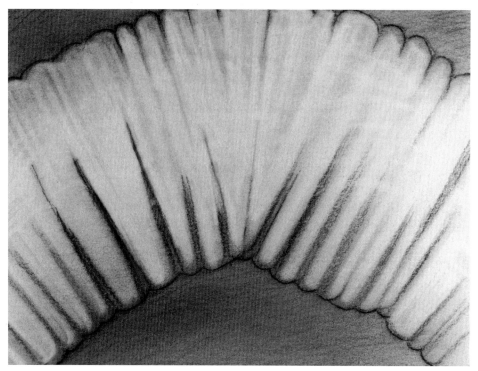

Segmental

1. Ischemia
2. Radiation enteritis
3. Intramural hemorrhage
4. Adjacent inflammatory process

Diffuse

1. Venous congestion
2. Hypoproteinemia
3. Cirrhosis

CASE 4.42

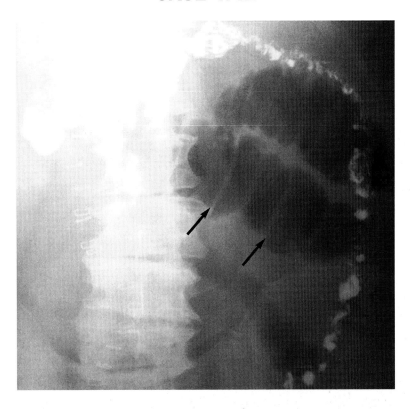

Findings

Supine abdominal radiograph. Two small bowel loops in the left upper abdomen are dilated and contain straight, thickened folds (arrows), characteristic of a segmental type II fold pattern. Residual barium is seen in the colon.

Differential Diagnosis

1. Ischemic bowel
2. Proximal small bowel obstruction
3. Radiation enteritis

Diagnosis

Ischemic bowel

Discussion

Ischemia of the small bowel and colon remains a difficult diagnosis because of the variable and nonspecific clinical findings. Patients may complain of bloating, gas, nausea, or vomiting. Peritoneal signs usually indicate transmural necrosis and possibly perforation. However, this is generally a late and infrequent finding. Gastrointestinal blood loss may be present.

The pathologic findings depend on the extent and duration of ischemia. Ischemia may be due to arterial embolization, hypoperfusion, or venous thrombosis. Arterial hypoperfusion is believed to be the most frequent cause, often due to either congestive heart failure or prolonged hypotension in association with mesenteric atherosclerotic disease. Histologic findings of bowel ischemia within the first 24 hours include initial submucosal edema and intramural hemorrhage, followed by transmural ischemia and eventually necrosis. Depending on the severity and depth of bowel wall injury from the ischemic insult, the three possible results of bowel ischemia are complete healing, stricture formation, and perforation.

Radiologic findings depend on the timing of the examination in relation to the vascular insult. Many abdominal radiographs (up to half) may be normal or have findings of only adynamic ileus. Suggestive findings include an isolated, rigid, often dilated, and unchanging small bowel loop with thickened mucosal folds. Additional cases of small bowel ischemia are included in this chapter (cases 4.72 through 4.83).

CASE 4.43

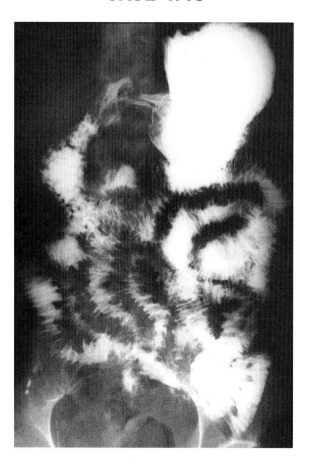

Findings

Small bowel follow-through. Several loops of small bowel in the mid abdomen have straight, thickened folds with separation of the loops, consistent with a segmental type II fold pattern.

Differential Diagnosis

1. Segmental type II folds (ischemia, hemorrhage, radiation)
2. Diffuse type II folds (venous congestion, hypoproteinemia, cirrhosis)

Diagnosis

Radiation enteritis

Discussion

A recent history of abdominal radiation therapy is critical for determining the correct cause of the abnormal, straight, thickened folds in this patient. The small bowel is the portion of the alimentary tract most sensitive to radiation. Usually doses greater than 40 Gy (4,000 rad) are required before radiographic changes occur. Endarteritis obliterans is the underlying pathologic process responsible for the bowel changes. Acute changes can be found several weeks to a few months after treatment. Fold thickening and serration due to edema are frequent. The affected folds may appear fixed and angulated.

Chronic changes can be found 6 months after therapy and may develop many years later. These changes are usually due to bowel ischemia from arteriolar damage. Intestinal loops are often narrowed, separated, and straightened and the bowel wall is thickened. Nodularity and thumbprinting may be observed. These changes may become progressively more severe with stenosis, obstruction, perforation, and fistulization. The majority of patients with chronic radiation changes in the small bowel present with obstruction from adhesion or stenosis rather than with acute ischemia.

CASE 4.44

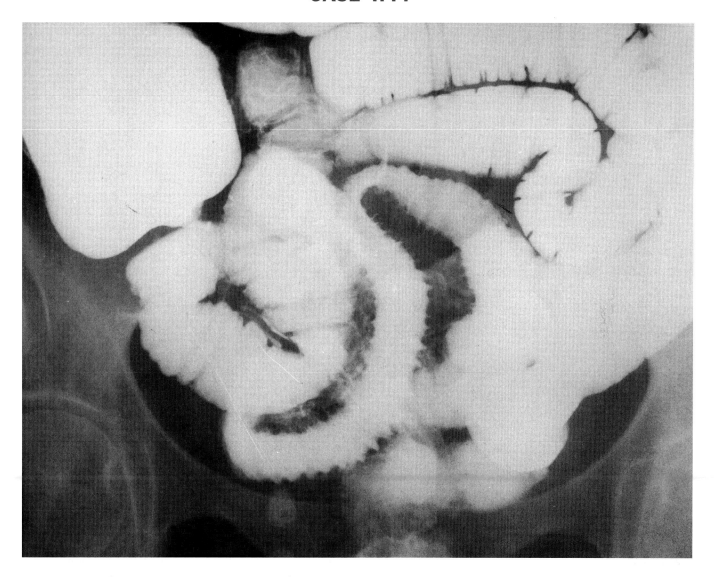

Findings

Small bowel follow-through. A loop of abnormal small bowel is seen in the pelvis. The lumen is slightly narrowed with thick, straight folds (segmental type II pattern).

Differential Diagnosis

1. Ischemia
2. Intramural hemorrhage
3. Adjacent inflammatory process (appendiceal or pelvic abscess)

Diagnosis

Intramural hemorrhage

Discussion

This patient was receiving anticoagulant therapy and had a spontaneous intramural hemorrhage. The small bowel is the most common site for intramural hemorrhage, which can be caused by anticoagulation, bleeding, diathesis, or trauma. Spontaneous bleeds such as this one often result in thick, straight folds with a stack-of-coins appearance. Ischemic bowel or reactive small bowel edema due to an adjacent inflammatory process in the pelvis also could result in similar findings on a barium small bowel examination.

CASE 4.45

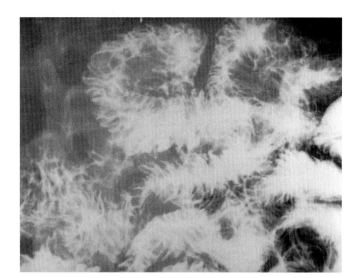

CASE 4.46

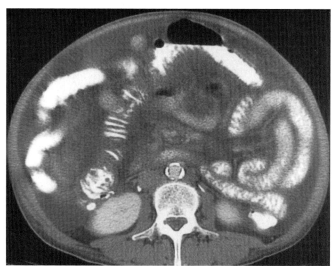

Findings

Case 4.45. Small bowel follow-through. The folds of the small bowel are diffusely thickened. Classification of the fold type is difficult, but it is best classified as diffuse type II folds.

Case 4.46. Contrast-enhanced CT. Diffuse ascites is present in the abdominal cavity. Small bowel fold thickening and increased mesenteric markings are present.

Differential Diagnosis
1. Hypoproteinemia
2. Venous congestion
3. Cirrhosis

Diagnosis
Hypoproteinemia

Discussion

This patient had chronic active hepatitis and secondary hypoalbuminemia. Intestinal edema due to hypoproteinemia (usually the serum albumin level is ″2 g/dL) can be idiopathic or due to various diseases. Cirrhosis of the liver is the most frequent underlying disease.

Various radiographic changes also can be seen with diffusely thickened folds (type II), including haustral thickening and ascites. Venous congestion due to congestive heart failure could give a similar appearance.

CT findings in patients with hypoalbuminemia include not only edematous changes within the bowel and mesentery but also edema within other body tissues. These edematous changes include soft tissue stranding and a generalized increased density within the subcutaneous and mesenteric fat.

Diffuse and Segmental Small Bowel Diseases: Type II Folds

	Segmental Folds	Case
Ischemia (arterial or venous occlusion)	Acute abdomen, pneumatosis and portal venous gas should be sought	4.42
Radiation enteritis	Confined to radiation port	4.43
Intramural hemorrhage (trauma or bleeding diathesis)	History of trauma or anticoagulation	4.44
Adjacent inflammatory process	Appendicitis, diverticulitis, pancreatitis	Not shown
	Diffuse Folds	
Venous congestion	History of congestive heart failure	Not shown
Hypoproteinemia	History of nephrotic syndrome, liver disease	4.45 and 4.46
Cirrhosis	Changes of portal venous hypertension should be sought	Not shown

TYPE III FOLDS: THICK, NODULAR FOLDS,
caused by infiltrative disease of the bowel wall (cases 4.47–4.59)

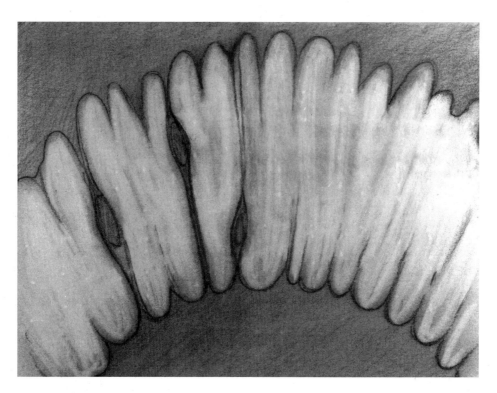

Segmental

1. Crohn disease
2. Infection
3. Lymphoma
4. Metastases

Diffuse

1. Whipple disease
2. Intestinal lymphangiectasia
3. Nodular lymphoid hyperplasia
4. Polyposis syndromes
5. Eosinophilic gastroenteritis
6. Amyloidosis
7. Mastocytosis
8. Lymphoma
9. Metastases

CASE 4.47

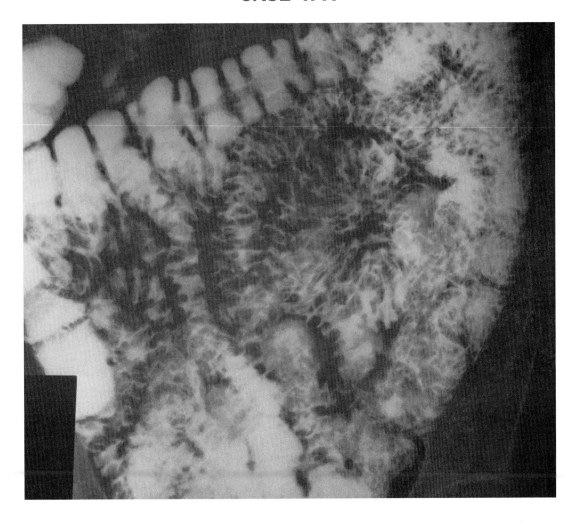

Findings

Small bowel follow-through. Thickened, somewhat nodular (type III) folds are present in the majority of the visualized small bowel loops.

Differential Diagnosis

Segmental and diffuse type III fold differentials

Diagnosis

Crohn disease

Discussion

Crohn disease is a chronic disorder of unknown origin. The disease involves the small bowel in at least 80% of patients. The clinical activity of the disease (abdominal pain, diarrhea, fever, weight loss, anemia) correlates poorly with radiologic changes. The location of the involved small bowel segment does affect prognosis. Crohn disease confined to the distal small bowel has the best long-term prognosis, whereas ileocolic involvement has the highest incidence of complications (abscess, fistula). The terminal ileum is usually involved (spared in only 5% of all patients). Recurrent disease after resection of a diseased small bowel segment invariably occurs about the anastomosis. Recurrences are usually detectable radiographically within 2 years after operation. Additional cases of Crohn disease are included in this chapter (cases 4.60 through 4.71).

CASE 4.48

A

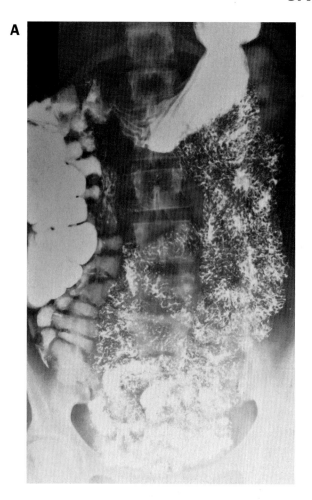

B

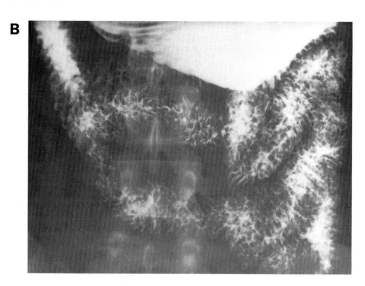

Findings
Small bowel follow-through. **A** and **B.** The folds of the proximal small bowel are thickened; some fold nodularity or contour irregularity (segmental type III folds) is present.

Differential Diagnosis
Segmental and diffuse type III fold differentials

Diagnosis
Giardiasis

Discussion
These findings are nonspecific and could be due to any disease causing a type III fold pattern. Localization of the findings within the proximal small bowel suggests giardiasis. Giardiasis is a disease caused by infection with the protozoan *Giardia lamblia*. Ingested trophozoites attach to the duodenal mucosa and reproduce. Cysts are shed and passed in the stool. The host response to the protozoan varies from the asymptomatic carrier state to severe symptoms of diarrhea and malabsorption. Patients with hypogammaglobulinemia or agammaglobulinemia are believed to be more prone to infection, and often these patients have changes of nodular lymphoid hyperplasia (case 4.54) in the small bowel. The majority of people infected with *G. lamblia* have no clinical or radiographic manifestations of their infection.

Radiographically, the proximal small bowel usually shows inflammatory changes, including fold thickening, increased secretions, irritability, and spasm or rapid transit. Tiny nodular lesions are frequent and result from hypertrophied lymphoid follicles. A spruelike pattern may occur in the distal jejunum and ileum, with reversal of the normal fold pattern. These changes revert to normal after treatment.

CASE 4.49

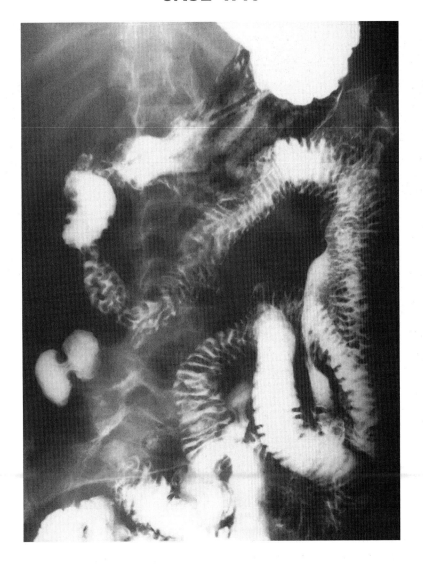

Findings

Small bowel follow-through. Somewhat nodular, thickened folds (type III) are present throughout the proximal small bowel.

Differential Diagnosis

Segmental and diffuse type III fold differentials

Diagnosis

Whipple disease

Discussion

Whipple disease is caused by the bacillus *Tropheryma whippelii*. It is characterized clinically by malabsorption, arthritis or arthralgias, lymphadenopathy, abdominal tenderness, and increased skin pigmentation. Histologically, a periodic acid-Schiff–positive glycoprotein is deposited within macrophages in the lamina propria and lymph nodes of the small bowel. Treatment usually consists of a long-term course of antibiotics.

Radiographically, fold thickening and nodularity are common in the proximal small bowel. Hypersecretion, dilatation, and diffuse small bowel involvement are usually absent, which helps to differentiate this disease from sprue. In the immunocompromised patient, infection with *Mycobacterium avium-intracellulare*, *Giardia*, or *Cryptosporidium* can produce identical radiographic findings and should be considered.

CASE 4.50

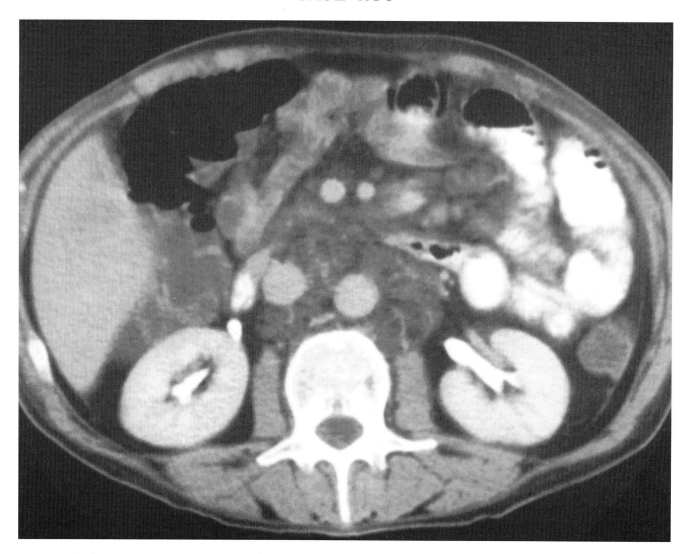

Findings
Contrast-enhanced CT. Multiple low-density lymph nodes are present within the retroperitoneum and small bowel mesentery.

Differential Diagnosis
1. Whipple disease
2. *Mycobacterium avium-intracellulare*
3. Testicular metastases
4. Lymphoma
5. Epidermoid carcinoma

Diagnosis
Whipple disease

Discussion
Whipple disease often is associated with abdominal lymphadenopathy, but this finding is rarely appreciated on small bowel examinations. The lymph nodes usually have a low attenuation on CT because of the deposition of fat and fatty acids within the nodes. Occasionally, only mesenteric lymphadenopathy is present. Sacroiliitis, a component of this systemic illness, also may be detectable on CT of the abdomen. The sacroiliac joints may be affected either unilaterally or bilaterally, and the articular symptoms may precede the gastrointestinal symptoms (usually diarrhea) by 5 years or more.

CASE 4.51

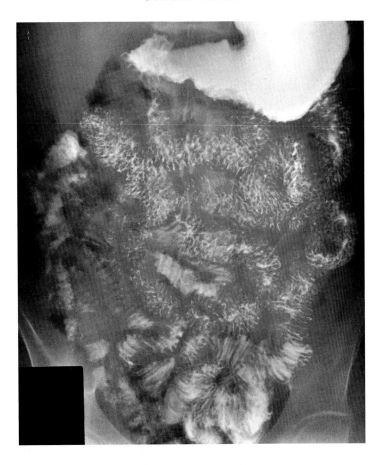

Findings

Small bowel follow-through. Nodular fold thickening is present diffusely throughout the visualized dilated loops of small bowel. There is also nodular deformity of the distal stomach.

Differential Diagnosis

Diffuse type III fold differentials

Diagnosis

Eosinophilic gastroenteritis

Discussion

Although this small bowel pattern is nonspecific, the patient was found to have eosinophilic gastroenteritis. Eosinophilic gastroenteritis is a disease of unknown origin, in which the patient presents with abdominal pain, diarrhea, vomiting, and occasionally malabsorption. Usually eosinophilia is present on the peripheral blood smear.

Often the clinical course is benign and self-limited, responding to corticosteroid treatments. Some patients have a history of allergy.

Pathologically, eosinophils and chronic inflammatory cells are present in the bowel wall. Localized and diffuse bowel involvement occur. Localized eosinophilic granuloma is usually confined to the stomach. Various clinical syndromes have been attributed to the portion of the bowel wall infiltrated by eosinophils. Predominantly mucosal infiltration results in protein loss and malabsorption, intramural disease presents with obstructive symptoms or diarrhea, and serosal eosinophilia results in ascites.

The radiographic findings are similar to those of any other infiltrative small bowel disease. Marked bowel wall infiltration can result in luminal narrowing and rigidity of the affected segment(s). Any portion of the alimentary tract may be affected, but the stomach and small bowel are the usual sites.

CASE 4.52

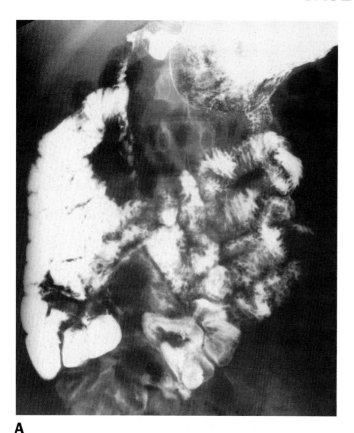

A

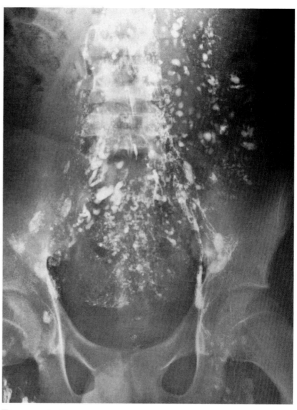

B

Findings

A. Small bowel follow-through. Thickened folds and tiny nodules (type III folds) are present within the proximal small bowel. Dilution of barium as a result of excess intraluminal fluid is seen in the distal small bowel.

B. Lymphangiogram. Multiple dilated and bulbous lymphatic channels are present within the small bowel mesentery.

Differential Diagnosis

Intestinal lymphangiectasia

Diagnosis

Intestinal lymphangiectasia

Discussion

Intestinal lymphangiectasia is a disorder of abnormal lymph flow, with loss of lymphatic fluid (most importantly protein) into the alimentary tract. Patients often present with hypoalbuminemia, hypoproteinemia, and occasionally malabsorptive symptoms. Diarrhea, vomiting, and abdominal pain are often present. Lymphangiectasia is often a congenital condition, or it may be acquired later in life from inflammatory or neoplastic lymphatic obstruction.

Pathologically, lymph channels are dilated in the lamina propria and submucosa of the bowel wall with associated enlarged and distorted villi. These lymph channels rupture into the gut lumen and are responsible for the protein loss. Treatment may be difficult, but some patients respond to a low-fat diet with medium-chain triglycerides, which do not require lymphatic transport for absorption. Lymphatic abnormalities elsewhere in the body are often found.

CASE 4.53

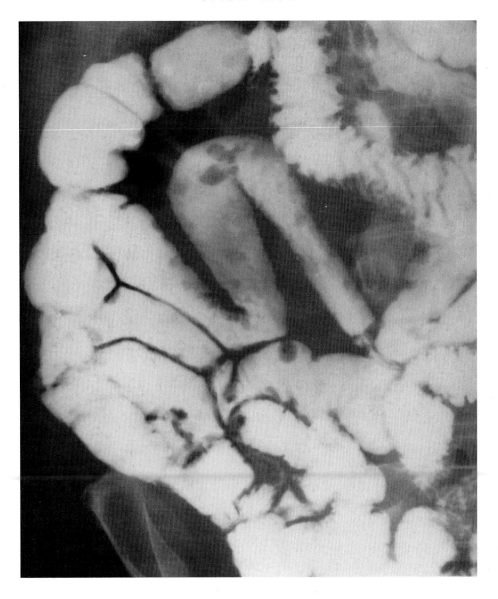

Findings
Small bowel follow-through. Multiple polypoid filling defects are present throughout the small bowel.

Differential Diagnosis
1. Polyposis syndrome
2. Metastases
3. Lymphoma
4. Lymphangiectasia

Diagnosis
Intestinal lymphangiectasia

Discussion
The nodular filling defects that may occur in lymphangiectasia can vary considerably in size. Large filling defects (as seen in this case) can be several millimeters in diameter, whereas tiny defects may appear as sandlike lucencies.

CASE 4.54

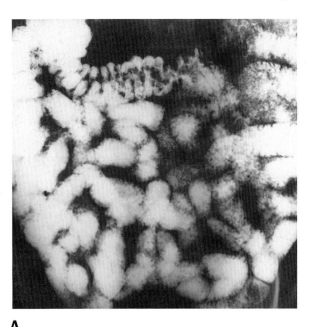

A

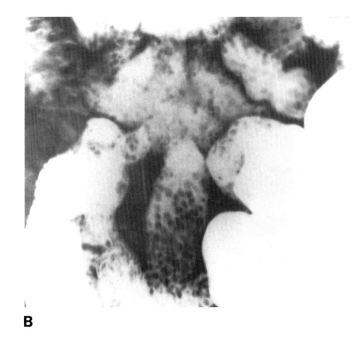

B

Findings
Small bowel follow-through. **A** and **B.** Multiple tiny
nodular filling defects are present throughout the small
bowel (diffuse type III pattern). All the nodules are
uniform in size and shape.

Differential Diagnosis
1. Nodular lymphoid hyperplasia
2. Lymphoma
3. Normal lymphoid nodules

Diagnosis
Nodular lymphoid hyperplasia

Discussion
Nodular lymphoid hyperplasia usually is associated with
an immunologic disorder, primarily a deficiency of IgA
and IgM. Occasionally, this disease may be present without
an immunologic disorder. Malabsorption and an intestinal
infection (*Giardia lamblia*, *Strongyloides*, or *Monilia*) are
often associated conditions. The incidence of gastric and
colonic cancers is increased in all patients with enteropathic
immunoglobulin deficiencies, especially children.

Innumerable tiny nodules are seen in the involved
portions of the small bowel. The nodules are usually less
than 4 mm in diameter and of uniform size. They may be
centrally umbilicated and resemble an aphthous ulcer.
The main differential consideration is lymphoma; however,
lymphomatous nodules are large, vary in size, and may
ulcerate (cases 4.55 and 4.56). Normal lymphoid nodules
can regularly be seen in patients of any age but are usually
found in children and young adults. These nodules are
uniform in size, nearly always less than 4 mm in diameter,
and primarily involve the distal small bowel and proximal
colon.

CASE 4.55

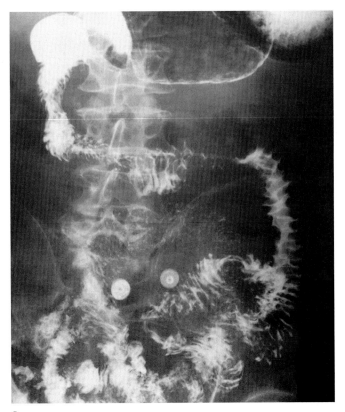

A

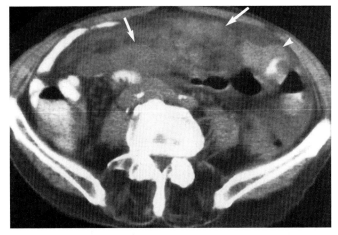

B

Findings

A. Small bowel follow-through. Diffuse nodular fold thickening (type III) is present throughout the small bowel. This appearance is nonspecific.

B. Contrast-enhanced CT. Adenopathy (arrows) is present within the small bowel mesentery. A small bowel loop with thickened wall is visible (arrowhead).

Differential Diagnosis

1. Lymphoma
2. Crohn disease

Diagnosis

Lymphoma

Discussion

CT is often included in the evaluation of patients with nonspecific complaints. In patients with lymphoma affecting the small bowel, CT can be helpful in suggesting the diagnosis. Bowel abnormalities vary from thickened folds (as in this case) to circumferential, long segments of bowel wall thickening (cases 4.14, 4.17, and 4.19). Mesenteric adenopathy is displayed well at CT, and, although nonspecific, it is a supportive finding of lymphoma. Other type III fold differential possibilities are unlikely with the focal bowel wall thickening and mesenteric lymphadenopathy. Both lymphoma and Crohn disease can present with these two findings, although the extensive lymphadenopathy favors lymphoma.

CASE 4.56

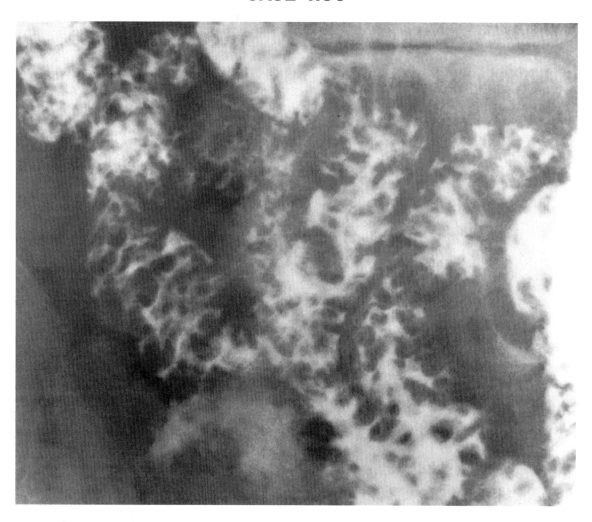

Findings
Small bowel follow-through. Diffuse nodular fold thickening (type III) is present throughout these small bowel loops. The smooth surface of these nodules suggests their submucosal location.

Differential Diagnosis
Diffuse type III fold differentials

Diagnosis
Lymphoma

Discussion
Multiple nodules of varying size and fold thickening are manifestations of lymphoma diffusely involving the small bowel. In addition to the diffuse form, 10% to 20% of patients with gastrointestinal lymphoma have multiple focal lesions. These lesions may appear to be of submucosal origin and their surface may be ulcerated. The polyposis syndromes (cases 2.18, 4.7, 4.8, 5.63, 5.64, and 5.65) are a differential consideration, but usually they are diagnosed before a small bowel examination is performed. A prior history of malignancy (e.g., melanoma) is often known in patients with metastatic tumors of the small bowel (cases 4.27 through 4.31). Metastases are usually not as numerous as the diffuse nodularity in this case. Nodular lymphoid hyperplasia has small (<4 mm) nodules of uniform size (case 4.54). Lymphangiectasia (cases 4.52 and 4.53) usually is diagnosed by early adulthood, whereas non-Hodgkin lymphoma generally occurs during the fifth and sixth decades of life.

CASE 4.57

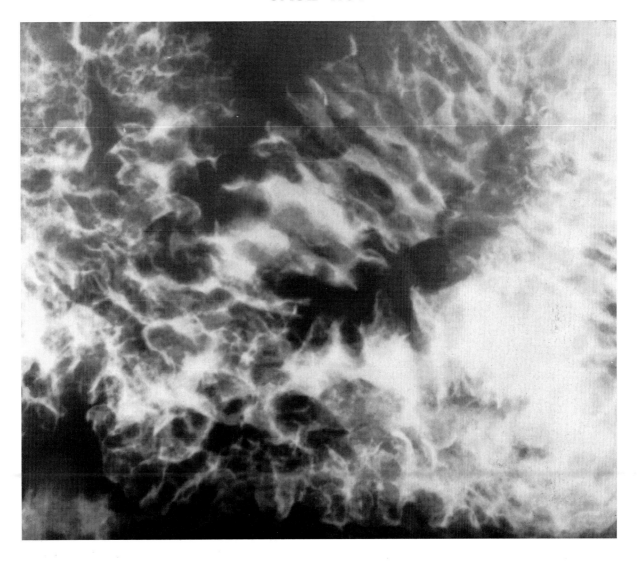

Findings
Small bowel follow-through. The small bowel is involved with diffusely nodular folds (type III fold pattern).

Differential Diagnosis
Diffuse type III fold differentials

Diagnosis
Metastatic melanoma

Discussion
Diffuse hematogenous seeding of the gastrointestinal tract with metastatic tumor can result in nodular changes within the bowel wall. A history of melanoma would make this radiographic appearance nearly diagnostic of metastases. Nodular lymphoid hyperplasia (case 4.54) has smaller nodules (usually <4 mm diameter) of uniform size. Whipple disease affects the proximal small bowel most severely. Patients with Crohn disease usually have segmental areas of intervening normal small bowel, often with luminal stenosis and fistulas. Polyps developing in patients with Peutz-Jeghers syndrome are usually fewer and larger. Lymphoma and lymphangiectasia could present with these findings.

CASE 4.58

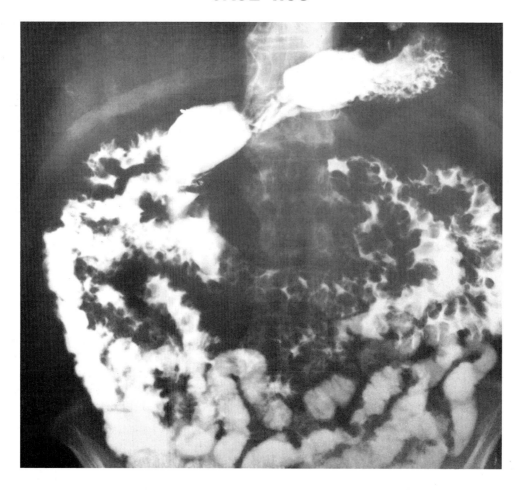

Findings
Small bowel follow-through. Multiple thickened and nodular (type III) folds are present throughout the small bowel.

Differential Diagnosis
Segmental and diffuse type III fold differentials

Diagnosis
Systemic amyloidosis

Discussion
The small bowel is that portion of the alimentary tract most often affected with amyloid. Vascular compromise can result in bowel ischemia, infarction, and bleeding. Submucosal amyloid deposition causes polypoid protrusions, fold thickening, and irregular, fine filling defects.

Amyloidosis is caused by deposition of an insoluble fibrillar protein within the extracellular space of various organs. Deposition within arterial walls is often present, resulting in possible ischemia or infarction of the end organ. Several classifications have been devised for this disease. Generally, systemic and localized forms exist. Systemic amyloidosis is most common and can result from a wide variety of causes; it can be idiopathic, related to a plasma cell dyscrasia (multiple myeloma, light-chain and heavy-chain disease, Waldenström macroglobulinemia), due to chronic infections or inflammatory conditions, or familial. Amyloid can be deposited throughout the gastrointestinal tract. Patients often complain of weight loss, fatigue, and abdominal pain.

Radiographic findings may be normal, even in patients with debilitating gastrointestinal symptoms. Diminished motor activity, thickened or atrophic folds, dilatation, and an obstructive pattern may be seen. Changes identical to those of ulcerative colitis can be seen in the colon.

CASE 4.59

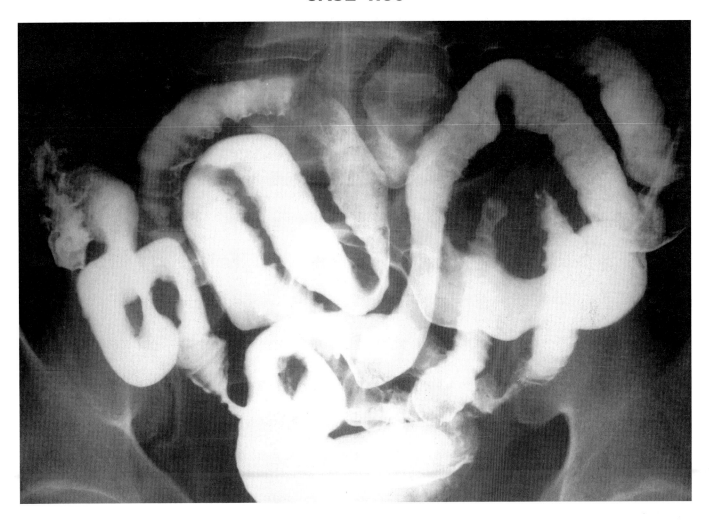

Findings

Small bowel follow-through. Multiple small bowel loops have a featureless, atrophic appearance. Thickened folds are present diffusely.

Differential Diagnosis

1. Ischemic small bowel
2. Infectious enteritis
3. Celiac disease
4. Acute radiation enteritis
5. Graft-versus-host disease
6. Amyloidosis

Diagnosis

Systemic amyloidosis

Discussion

See discussion of case 4.58.

Diffuse and Segmental Small Bowel Diseases: Type III Folds

	Segmental Folds	Case
Crohn disease	Nodules associated with ulcers, usually distal ileum, asymmetric bowel involvement, skip lesions	4.47
Infection	Giardiasis (proximal), *Yersinia* and tuberculosis (distal)	4.48
Lymphoma	Nodules of differing sizes	4.55 and 4.56
Metastases	Multiple nodules with or without ulcers	4.57
	Diffuse Folds	
Whipple disease	Proximal small bowel affected more than distal small bowel, weight loss, arthralgias, lymphadenopathy	4.49 and 4.50
Intestinal lymphangiectasia	May require lymphangiography for diagnosis	4.52 and 4.53
Nodular lymphoid hyperplasia	Diffuse <4-mm monotonous nodules	4.54
Polyposis syndromes	Peutz-Jeghers most common, any type can have small bowel polyps	Not shown
Eosinophilic gastroenteritis	Peripheral eosinophilia	4.51
Amyloidosis	Irregular fine filling defects and fold thickening	4.58 and 4.59
Mastocytosis	Deposits of mass cells in skin and bowel wall, skeletal sclerosis should be sought	Not shown
Lymphoma	Nodules of different sizes, adenopathy	4.55 and 4.56
Metastases	Multiple nodules, history of primary tumor	4.57

CASE 4.60

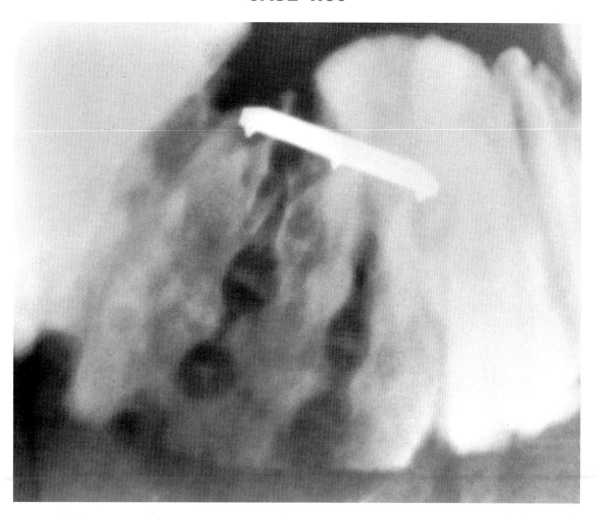

Findings

Small bowel follow-through (spot radiograph). Multiple discrete ulcerations are present in the distal small bowel. The central barium collections (ulcer crater) and mounds of edema are characteristic of aphthous ulcers. A compression device with metallic marker is seen.

Differential Diagnosis

1. Crohn disease
2. Infectious disorders of the ileum
      Yersiniosis
      Amebiasis
      Tuberculosis

Diagnosis

Crohn disease

Discussion

These tiny mucosal ulcers are believed to be the first mucosal lesions of Crohn disease. These lesions may coalesce and form longitudinal and transverse ulcerations that are typical of more advanced disease (case 4.61). Discrete ulcers are not specific for Crohn disease and can be seen in various infectious disorders that affect the terminal ileum.

CASE 4.61

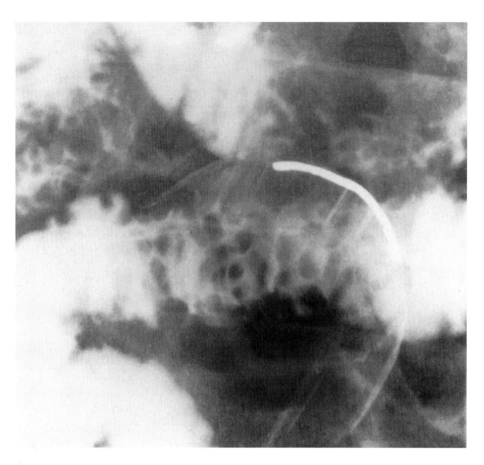

Findings

Small bowel follow-through (spot radiograph). A cobblestone mucosal pattern affects a nonstenotic segment of small bowel. Longitudinal and transverse ulcerations, in conjunction with bowel wall edema, produce a cobblestone mucosal pattern. A metallic marker on a compression device is present.

Differential Diagnosis

1. Crohn disease
2. Small bowel polyps
3. Infectious enteritis

Diagnosis

Crohn disease

Discussion

Patients with Crohn disease often have the insidious onset of abdominal cramping, diarrhea, weight loss, low-grade fever, anorexia, and anemia. Patients usually are treated conservatively with rest, dietary changes, and antidiarrheal and anti-inflammatory agents. In approximately a third to half of patients, the disease can be managed successfully without operation. Surgical treatment is usually reserved for complications of the disease that do not respond to medical therapy—fistulas, obstruction, and abscess.

Extraintestinal manifestations of Crohn disease include arthritis (and ankylosing spondylitis), erythema nodosum, pyoderma gangrenosum, and, rarely, primary sclerosing cholangitis. The incidence of cholesterol gallstones and oxalate renal stones can be increased in patients with ileal disease as a result of abnormalities in the enterohepatic bile acid circulation.

Small bowel polyps usually do not focally involve the bowel and are not associated with ulcerations. Infection can simulate Crohn disease and must be excluded. Yersiniosis and tuberculosis can often mimic Crohn disease.

CASE 4.62

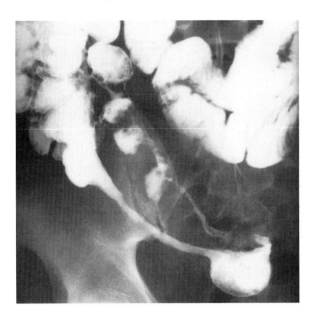

CASE 4.63

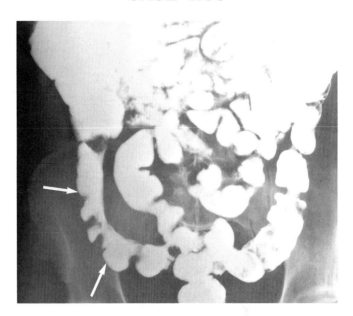

Findings

Case 4.62. Small bowel follow-through. A long segment of narrowed ileum (string sign) is present with areas of bowel wall asymmetry.

Case 4.63. Small bowel follow-through. An abnormal loop of distal small bowel is present in the right lower quadrant (arrows). The loop is separate from others, and the medial wall is flattened and featureless. Pseudodiverticula are present along the lateral wall. These findings are due to circumferential asymmetric bowel wall involvement.

Differential Diagnosis

1. Crohn disease
2. Segmental ischemia
3. Small bowel infection

Diagnosis

Crohn disease

Discussion

The string sign of Crohn disease may or may not represent a fixed stricture. This region of narrowing may be inconstant because of marked spasm, and proximal small bowel dilatation may be lacking. Fixed narrowing from transmural fibrosis usually is associated with a short segmental stricture and dilatation of proximal loops. The terminal ileum often is affected.

Circumferential asymmetry of the bowel lumen can be a helpful radiographic finding in Crohn disease. This finding may be due to skip areas of fibrosis or ulceration with folding and sometimes dilatation of the opposite wall.

Small bowel ischemia can cause featureless strictures; however, multiple skip areas usually are absent. A patient's age and history also can be helpful. Patients with ischemia often are older and have an acute onset of abdominal pain and adynamic ileus. Patients with Crohn disease are usually young adults with a chronic history of abdominal pain and diarrhea. Infectious disorders such as tuberculosis, actinomycosis, histoplasmosis, and blastomycosis can present with findings that are indistinguishable from those of Crohn disease. *Yersinia* and *Salmonella* can produce superficial erosions and fold thickening, but strictures are uncommon.

CASE 4.64

CASE 4.65

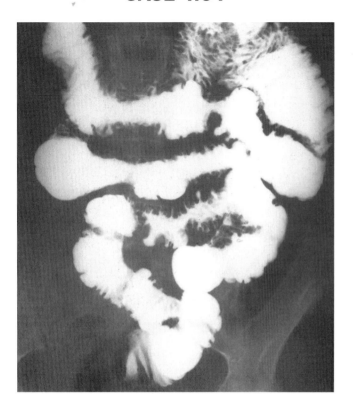

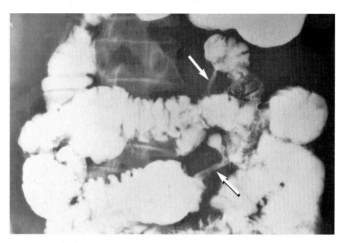

Findings

Case 4.64. Small bowel follow-through. Mucosal fold thickening, ulceration, nodularity, asymmetric bowel wall involvement, regions of narrowing, and separation of small bowel loops are present.

Case 4.65. Small bowel follow-through. Two regions of high-grade stenosis (arrows) are present in the proximal small bowel.

Differential Diagnosis

Case 4.66
1. Crohn disease
2. Acute gastroenteritis
3. Small bowel hemorrhage

Case 4.67
1. Crohn disease
2. Small bowel tumor

Diagnosis

Crohn disease

Discussion

Advanced changes of Crohn disease are often due to transmural inflammation and fibrosis. Transmural inflammation leads to bowel wall thickening and bowel loop separation (as seen in case 4.52). Fistulas and abscesses also result from transmural disease. Fibrosis nearly always accompanies the healing phase of the disease. Patchy discontinuous regions of fibrosis result in circumferential asymmetry of the bowel wall.

Stenotic Crohn disease can affect both long and short segments of the bowel. Proximal dilatation of the small bowel usually indicates significant obstruction by the lesion. Complete obstruction from Crohn disease is rare. In some patients, particularly those with a solitary short stenosis, it may be impossible to exclude neoplasm radiologically. These patients usually require resection of the diseased bowel.

CASE 4.66

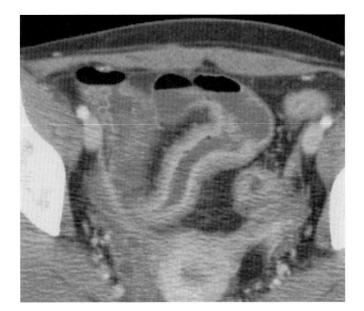

CASE 4.67

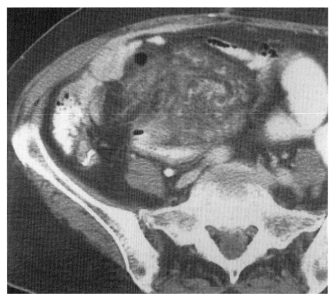

Findings

Case 4.66. Contrast-enhanced CT. Marked homogeneous segmental bowel wall thickening is present in the distal small bowel.

Case 4.67. Contrast-enhanced CT. A mass composed of fat and soft tissue stranding is present in the right lower quadrant. A loop of distal small bowel has mildly thickened walls just posterior to the mass.

Differential Diagnosis

1. Crohn disease
2. Small bowel primary tumor
3. Metastases

Diagnosis

Crohn disease

Discussion

Bowel wall thickening and mesenteric soft tissue stranding are the commonest CT findings of Crohn disease. The location of the bowel wall involvement in the ileum is often helpful for suggesting the diagnosis.

The fibrofatty changes in the mesentery of patients with Crohn disease are referred to as "creeping fat" by surgeons and pathologists. Enlarged and normal-sized lymph nodes are often visible. The mass may be of homogeneous fat density or may contain streaks and poorly defined soft tissue changes within it. Soft tissue changes within the mass are often associated with acute inflammation. This fibrofatty proliferation has been reported to cause ureteral compression and obstruction when the retroperitoneum is affected.

CASE 4.68

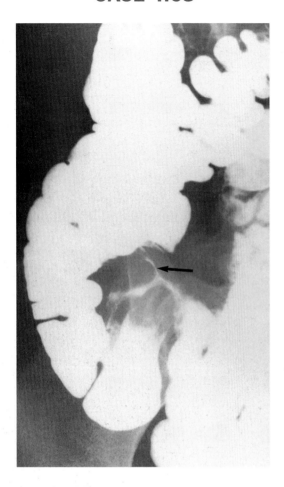

CASE 4.69

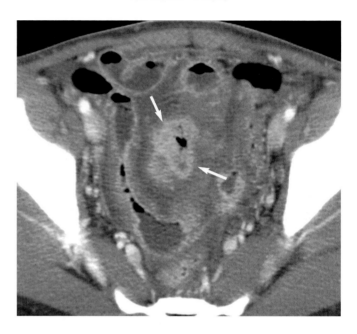

Findings

Case 4.68. Small bowel follow-through. The terminal ileum is narrowed, and a fistulous communication (arrow) exists between the distal ileum and colon. Inflammatory changes with tethered folds are present along the medial aspect of the cecum.

Case 4.69. Contrast-enhanced CT. A segmental loop of small bowel is thick-walled, and the lumen is narrowed. A gas-containing cavity is located within the small bowel mesentery, medial to the affected small bowel loop (arrows). This has the appearance of an interloop abscess.

Differential Diagnosis
Crohn disease

Diagnosis
Crohn disease

Discussion

Fistula formation (case 4.68) is a common finding in patients with transmural disease. Fistulas can communicate with other small bowel loops, colon, genitourinary tract, retroperitoneum, mesentery, and skin. Occasionally they are multiple, and often they are incorporated within an inflammatory mass of bowel and mesentery. Abscess formation (case 4.69) often accompanies fistulization and sinus tracts. CT has the advantage of direct visualization of the entire small bowel, mesentery, and adjacent organs.

CASE 4.70

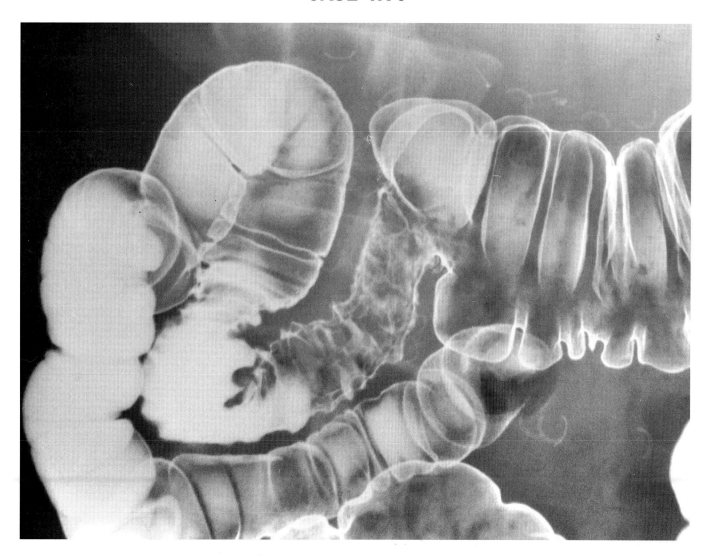

Findings

Double-contrast barium enema. Freely functioning ileotransverse colostomy. The neoterminal ileum is irregular in contour, and the mucosa appears ulcerated and nodular.

Differential Diagnosis

1. Recurrent Crohn disease
2. Infectious ileitis

Diagnosis

Recurrent Crohn disease

Discussion

Recurrent Crohn disease is common after operation. Recurrence almost always involves the neoterminal ileum. The features of recurrent disease are the same as those preoperatively. This is a typical case of nonstenotic recurrent Crohn disease.

CASE 4.71

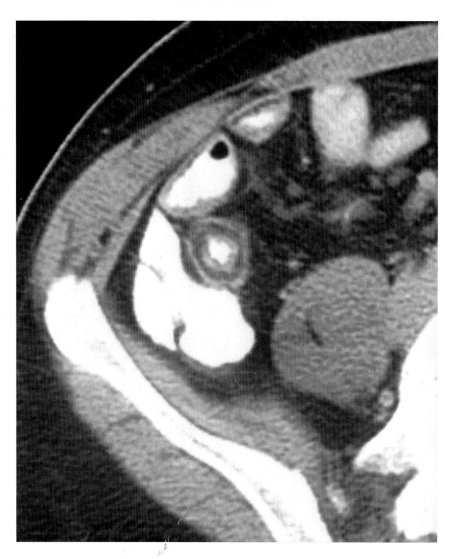

Findings
Contrast-enhanced CT. The terminal ileum has a markedly thickened wall that contains a central ring the attenuation of fat.

Differential Diagnosis
Inactive Crohn disease

Diagnosis
Inactive Crohn disease

Discussion
CT findings of Crohn disease include bowel wall thickening, mesenteric fibrofatty proliferation, abscess, mesenteric inflammation, and lymphadenopathy. In Crohn disease, bowel wall thickening is usually greater than 1 cm and is the commonest CT finding. The wall thickening in active disease may be the density of soft tissue or contain a central water-density ring. Fat within the bowel wall has been shown to accumulate in the submucosa of patients with either ulcerative colitis or Crohn disease. Active inflammation is not present when this finding is identified. The cause of the fat deposition is unknown, although long-term corticosteroid treatment may be responsible.

CASE 4.72

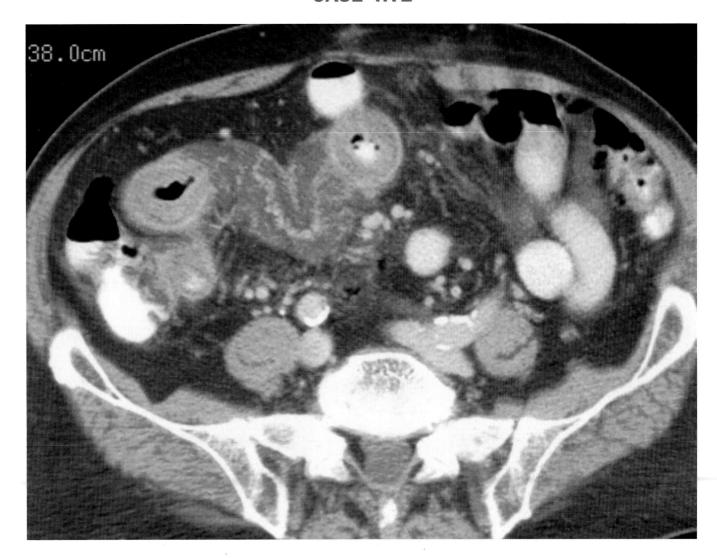

Findings

Contrast-enhanced CT. A thick-walled and dilated small bowel loop is present in the abdomen. A portion of the thickened wall is of low density, near that of water, indicating submucosal edema.

Differential Diagnosis

1. Ischemia
2. Crohn disease
3. Lymphoma
4. Radiation enteritis

Diagnosis

Ischemic small bowel

Discussion

CT findings in patients with bowel infarction include diffuse or focal bowel wall thickening, segmental dilatation, mesenteric edema, ascites, intramural gas, and mesenteric or portal venous gas. Only intramural and venous gases are considered specific for ischemia, but even these findings occasionally are seen in patients without bowel infarction. Edema within the bowel wall is nonspecific and could be due to any inflammatory disease within the bowel or adjacent mesentery or to hypoalbuminemia. Despite its nonspecific nature, bowel dilatation with a thickened and edematous wall without apparent cause in a patient with abdominal pain should be regarded as highly suggestive of ischemia.

CASE 4.73

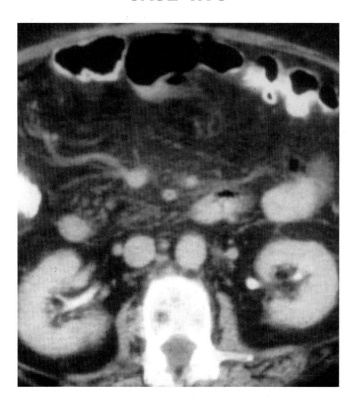

CASE 4.74

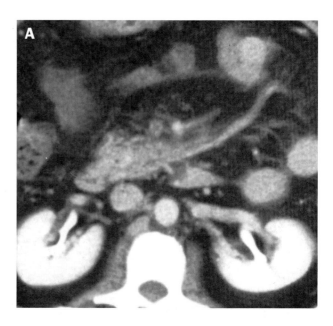

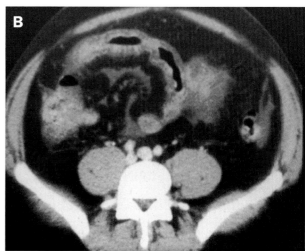

Findings

Case 4.73. Contrast-enhanced CT. A tiny filling defect is present within the superior mesenteric artery. (Courtesy of S. Kriegshauser, M.D., Scottsdale, Arizona.)

Case 4.74. Contrast-enhanced CT. **A.** A filling defect is present within the superior mesenteric vein. **B.** Edematous bowel wall thickening involves several small bowel loops and the right colon.

Differential Diagnosis

Ischemic small bowel

Diagnosis

Ischemic small bowel (superior mesenteric artery embolus in case 4.73, superior mesenteric vein thrombosis in case 4.74)

Discussion

Small bowel ischemia can be due to low flow states (usually from prolonged hypotension), an arterial embolus (case 4.73), or superior mesenteric vein thrombosis (case 4.74). CT often can identify filling defects within the main branches of the superior mesenteric artery or vein.

CASE 4.75

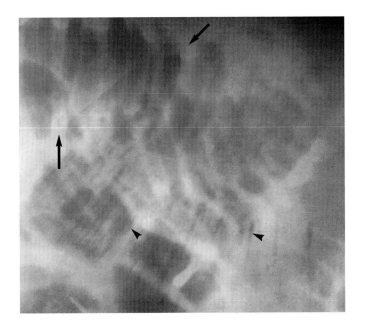

CASE 4.76

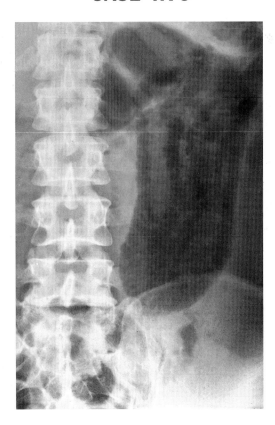

Findings

Case 4.75. Supine abdominal radiograph (close-up). Multiple small bowel folds (arrows) are straight and thickened. In addition, linear intramural pneumatosis (arrowheads) is present.

Case 4.76. Supine abdominal radiograph. Extensive cystic pneumatosis is present within the jejunum.

Differential Diagnosis

1. Small bowel ischemia
2. Benign pneumatosis
3. Mechanical small bowel obstruction

Diagnosis

Small bowel ischemia

Discussion

The finding of intramural pneumatosis in a patient with ischemic bowel disease suggests severe ischemia. Urgent operation usually is required to prevent perforation and to decrease the high morbidity and mortality associated with such a complication.

Pneumatosis intestinalis due to ischemic or infarcted bowel can have either a cystic or a linear appearance. Large cystic collections are unusual and more commonly associated with nonischemic disease. Clinical correlation is always necessary when pneumatosis intestinalis is found so as not to delay treatment or overlook the diagnosis of bowel ischemia.

CASE 4.77

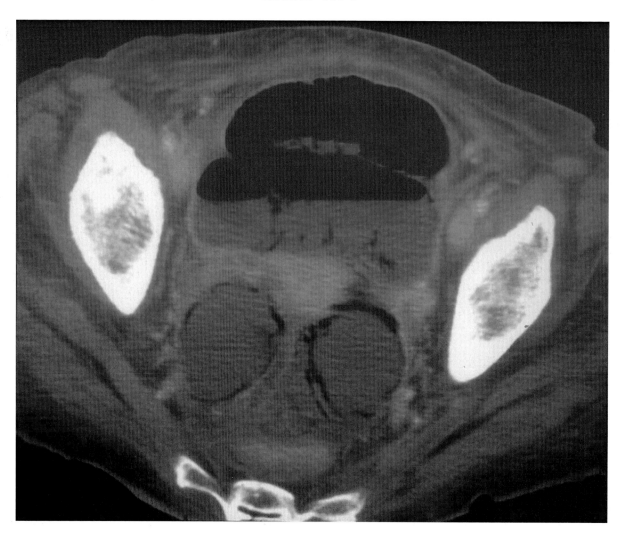

Findings
Contrast-enhanced CT. Linear collections of intramural gas are present within dilated, fluid-filled small bowel loops.

Differential Diagnosis
1. Pneumatosis intestinalis due to small bowel ischemia
2. Benign pneumatosis

Diagnosis
Small bowel ischemia (with pneumatosis intestinalis)

Discussion
The appearance of intramural gas on CT can be either cystic (case 4.78) or linear-curvilinear (case 4.75 and this case). CT is more sensitive than abdominal plain radiography for detecting pneumatosis intestinalis. In addition, other signs of ischemic bowel can be searched for, including portal venous gas (cases 4.81 and 4.82), bowel wall thickening (case 4.72), and thrombi or occlusion of the superior mesenteric artery and vein. If a patient with abdominal pain has pneumatosis, it is most important to review the radiologic and clinical findings with the referring physician because benign pneumatosis and pneumatosis due to bowel ischemia can have a similar radiographic appearance. In some patients, lung window settings are helpful for detecting intramural air at CT.

CASE 4.78

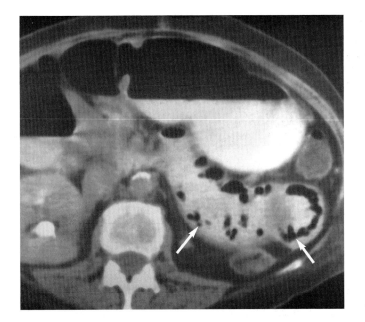

CASE 4.79

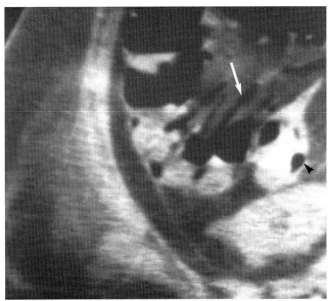

Findings

Case 4.78. Contrast-enhanced CT. A dilated, contrast-filled small bowel loop contains multiple tiny intramural collections of gas (arrows).

Case 4.79. Contrast-enhanced CT. Gas-filled ileocolic veins (arrow) are seen within the mid abdomen. Pneumatosis intestinalis also is present (arrowhead).
(From Smerud MJ, Johnson CD, Stephens DH. Diagnosis of bowel infarction: a comparison of plain films and CT scans in 23 cases. AJR. 1990;154:99-103. By permission of the American Roentgen Ray Society.)

Differential Diagnosis

1. Intestinal ischemia, pneumatosis intestinalis
2. Benign pneumatosis

Diagnosis

Intestinal ischemia, pneumatosis intestinalis

Discussion

Intramural gas is most easily identified within the bowel wall by its posterior, dependent location. Pneumatosis is also usually present within the nondependent wall, but it is often more difficult to distinguish from intraluminal gas. Clinical correlation is necessary to distinguish pneumatosis intestinalis due to intestinal ischemia from other conditions causing pneumatosis, generally referred to as benign pneumatosis. The presence of mesenteric and portal venous gas is usually a sign of advanced ischemia and often is associated with a grave prognosis.

CASE 4.80

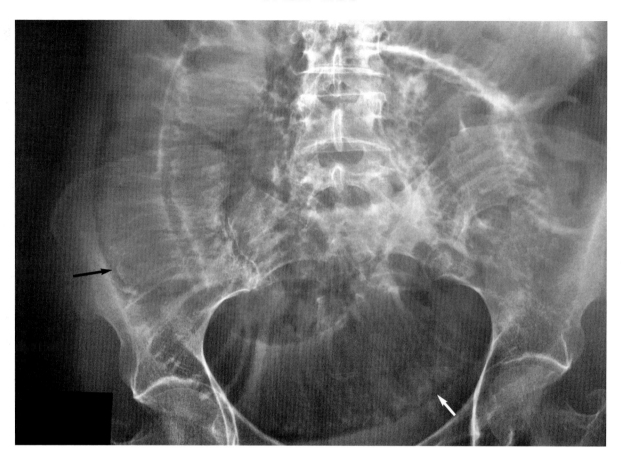

Findings
Abdominal radiograph. Extensive intramural gas (arrows) is present within the small bowel.

Differential Diagnosis
1. Mesenteric ischemia or infarction
2. Benign pneumatosis intestinalis

Diagnosis
Benign pneumatosis intestinalis

Discussion
This patient with scleroderma had been hospitalized several times for intestinal pseudo-obstruction. She recovered uneventfully. The pneumatosis was considered benign, due to her scleroderma and corticosteroid medication.

Pneumatosis intestinalis, or air within the wall of the small bowel, can result from several causes. Commonly associated conditions include corticosteroid medications, scleroderma, chronic obstructive lung disease, and ischemic bowel. The exact cause is often not known, but many theories suggest that a slow-healing mucosal ulceration develops, followed by dissection of gas into the bowel wall. Alternatively, some authors have suggested that in patients with obstructive lung disease, air can dissect from the alveoli into the mediastinum, to retroperitoneum, and eventually to small bowel mesentery and bowel wall. Patients are usually asymptomatic and do not require treatment for this condition unless they have ischemic bowel disease. Patients with ischemic bowel may have associated portal venous gas and bowel wall thickening, and usually they require urgent surgical exploration.

Radiologically, a lucent rim that follows the contours of the bowel wall (as in this case) is pathognomonic. The air collections may appear cystlike or linear. Occasionally, the intramural air collections escape into the peritoneal cavity and cause asymptomatic pneumoperitoneum.

CASE 4.81

CASE 4.82

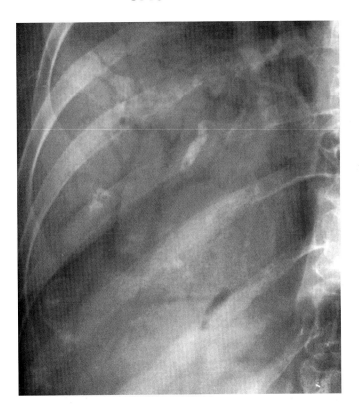

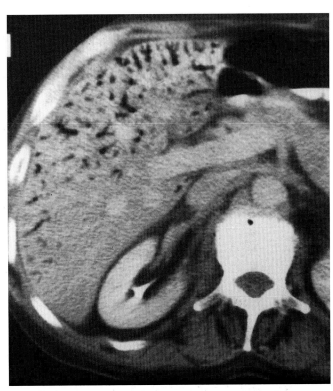

Findings

Case 4.81. Supine abdominal radiograph. Gas-containing tubular structures are visible within the liver. The peripheral distribution of the gas is typical of portal venous gas.

Case 4.82. Contrast-enhanced CT. Multiple gas-filled portal venous branches are visible throughout the periphery of the liver. The nondependent portal veins contain more gas than those in the dependent, posterior right lobe.

Differential Diagnosis

1. Portal venous gas, ischemic bowel
2. Portal venous gas, benign cause

Diagnosis

Portal venous gas, ischemic bowel

Discussion

Portal venous gas is often a late finding in patients with intestinal ischemia. The mucosa is the bowel layer most sensitive to ischemia. As the mucosa breaks down, gas can enter the bowel wall (pneumatosis intestinalis, cases 4.78 and 4.79) and eventually enter the mesenteric and portal venous system. Although nonischemic benign causes of portal venous gas have been reported, portal venous gas is unusual, and urgent clinical assessment of the patient is recommended.

CASE 4.83

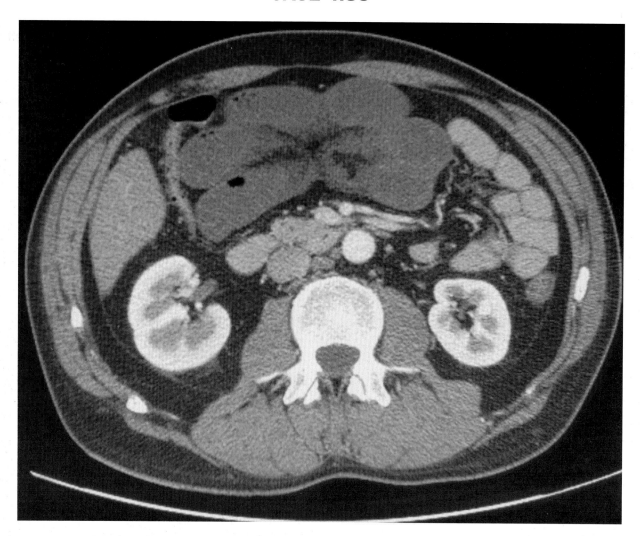

Findings
Contrast-enhanced CT. Several dilated small bowel loops have little or no bowel wall enhancement. The bowel loops appear to be grouped together and pulled toward a central point. Soft tissue stranding is present within the mesentery.

Differential Diagnosis
1. Closed loop small bowel obstruction with secondary ischemia
2. Focal small bowel ischemia (arterial embolus or mesenteric venous thrombosis)

Diagnosis
Closed loop obstruction with secondary ischemia

Discussion
Closed loop obstruction most often is caused by entrapment of a bowel loop(s) by an adhesive band. External and internal hernias also can lead to closed loop obstruction. CT often is helpful for demonstrating the dilated small bowel loop and the site of the compressed adjacent bowel loops. Evidence of vascular compromise by delayed, partial, or absent bowel wall perfusion can be detected at CT.

CASE 4.84

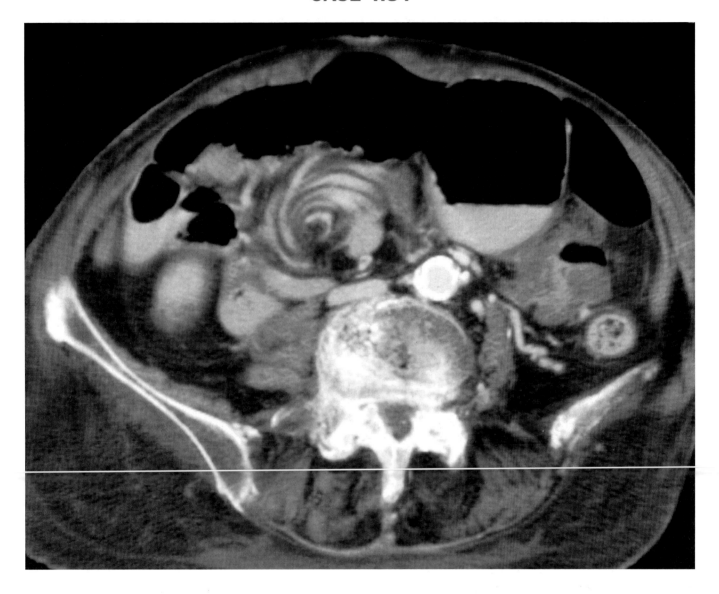

Findings
Contrast-enhanced CT. Small bowel and mesentery encircle the superior mesenteric artery in a whorl-like pattern.

Differential Diagnosis
Midgut volvulus

Diagnosis
Midgut volvulus

Discussion
Patients with rotational anomalies of the gut lack normal posterior peritoneal attachments. Normal peritoneal attachments prevent the small bowel and colon from moving or twisting into an abnormal location or position. In the absence of sufficient fixation, the small bowel can twist about the superior mesenteric artery, leading to bowel obstruction and ischemia. Symptoms of obstruction usually develop. Urgent surgical repair often is required to prevent ischemia or to resect infarcted bowel loops. Intermittent or partial obstruction can lead to bowel congestion, edema, or symptoms of malabsorption.

CASE 4.85

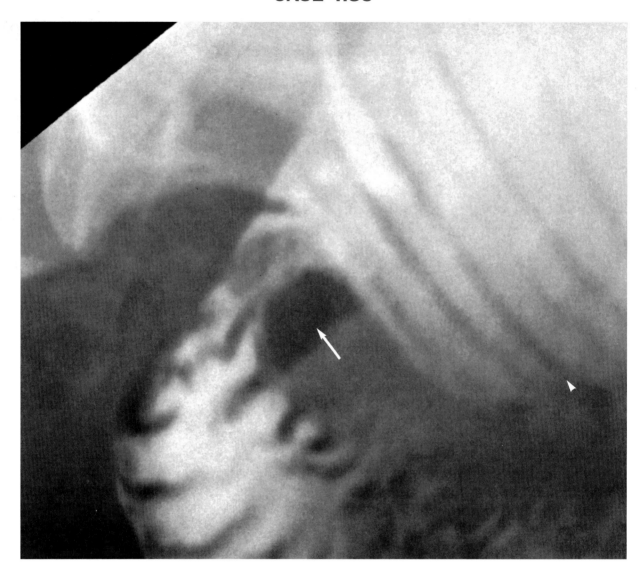

Findings
Small bowel follow-through. The proximal small bowel is dilated and abruptly narrows from a smooth rounded defect (arrow) that eccentrically compresses the lumen and causes partial obstruction. Notice the straight thin folds in the dilated loop (arrowhead).

Differential Diagnosis
1. Mechanical small bowel obstruction due to adhesions
2. Medication-induced focal ulceration and scar

Diagnosis
Mechanical small bowel obstruction due to adhesions

Discussion
Defining the site and cause of obstruction is more commonly done at CT than with a small bowel follow-through or enteroclysis examination. This case illustrates the typical appearance at small bowel follow-through of an obstructing adhesion with the smooth, focal, abrupt transition between dilated and nondistended small bowel.

CASE 4.86

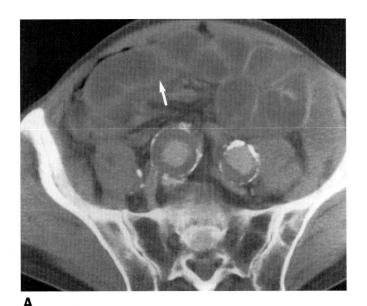

A

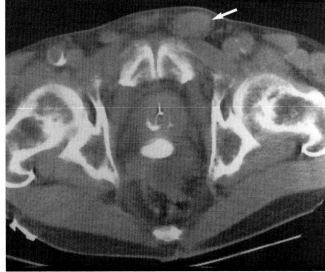

B

Findings

Enhanced abdominal CT. **A.** Multiple dilated fluid-filled small bowel loops are present in the abdomen. Aneurysmal dilatation of both iliac arteries is seen, as are thin, straight small bowel folds (arrow). **B.** A loop of small bowel could be traced into the enlarged inguinal canal (arrow).

Differential Diagnosis

Mechanical small bowel obstruction

Diagnosis

Mechanical small bowel obstruction due to an incarcerated inguinal hernia

Discussion

CT is now widely used as a primary imaging method for evaluating patients with a suspected small bowel obstruction. In nearly three-quarters of the patients, the cause of the obstruction can be identified at CT. The diagnosis of mechanical intestinal obstruction should be suspected when a discrepancy in the caliber of the proximal and distal bowel is identified.

CASE 4.87

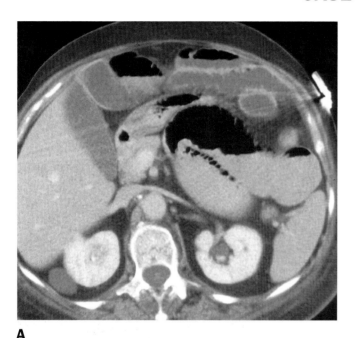

A

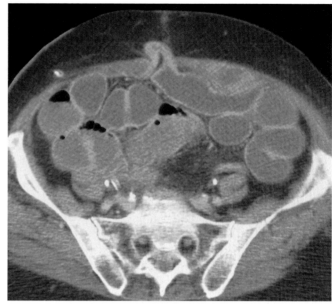

B

Findings
Contrast-enhanced CT. **A** and **B.** Multiple dilated small bowel loops are present throughout the abdomen. A loop of small bowel enters a ventral abdominal wall hernia. At this site, there is an abrupt transition in the caliber of the small bowel.

Differential Diagnosis
Mechanical small bowel obstruction, ventral hernia

Diagnosis
Mechanical small bowel obstruction, ventral hernia

Discussion
Adhesions and hernias are the commonest causes of mechanical small bowel obstruction. In this case, the transition between dilated and collapsed small bowel is visualized as the small bowel loop enters the ventral hernia sac. Operative repair was required.

CASE 4.88

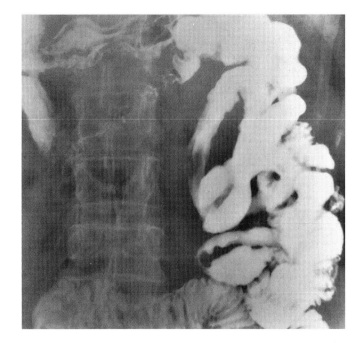

CASE 4.89

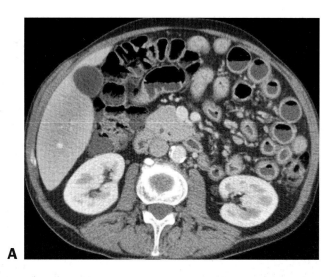

A

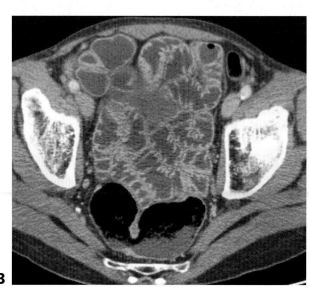

B

Findings

Case 4.88. Small bowel follow-through. The jejunum is devoid of most of its normal mucosal markings. The tubular, featureless appearance of these loops has been referred to as the moulage sign.

Case 4.89. Contrast-enhanced CT. **A.** The jejunum lacks the normal fold pattern. Several loops are fluid-filled and dilated. **B.** Ileal loops in the pelvis have a prominent fold pattern. Many loops are fluid-filled and dilated.

Differential Diagnosis
Celiac disease

Diagnosis
Celiac disease

Discussion
Excessive intraluminal fluid obscures and prevents adequate mucosal coating of the proximal small bowel and results in the moulage sign. Moulage refers to a molded or casted structure. The jejunum in this patient resembles a tubular cast of small bowel because of its paucity of mucosal folds.

CASE 4.90

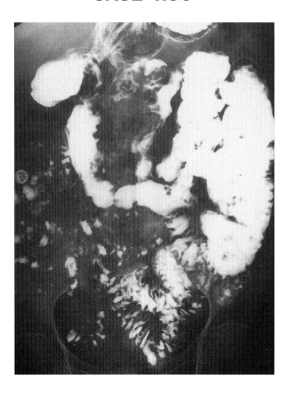

Findings

Small bowel follow-through. Flocculation and segmentation of barium indicate the presence of excessive fluid in the distal small bowel. The normal jejunal fold pattern also is absent. These loops appear featureless. A few small bowel loops in the pelvis have thickened folds.

Differential Diagnosis

1. Celiac disease
2. Zollinger-Ellison syndrome
3. Mechanical small bowel obstruction
4. Acute caustic ingestion

Diagnosis

Celiac disease

Discussion

The term "sprue" is given to three diseases with common radiographic and pathologic manifestations. Childhood and adult (nontropical) sprue are probably the same disease, due to a gluten (a water-insoluble protein found in various cereals and grains, including wheat, rye, oats, and barley) sensitivity. The cause of tropical sprue is unknown, but patients do not respond to dietary gluten restrictions. These patients often respond to folate therapy or antibiotic (usually tetracycline) therapy or both.

Pathologically, villous atrophy is usually seen with elongation of the crypts of Lieberkühn and infiltration of the lamina propria with inflammatory cells. Changes are often more marked in the proximal small bowel.

This case demonstrates many of the radiologic features of excess intraluminal fluid (hypersecretion) that commonly are encountered in patients with sprue. Barium may become radiolucent and separated into clumps (segmentation) or tiny pieces (flocculation) as a result of dilution. This is most common in the distal small bowel. Small bowel folds in patients with sprue may remain normally thin or they may become thickened. Thickened folds usually are due to intramural edema from hypoalbuminemia. The gastrointestinal loss of albumin is the result of the malabsorption that is typically present in these patients. Patients with Zollinger-Ellison syndrome usually have thickened folds in the proximal small bowel. In patients with a mechanical obstruction, a transition to normal-caliber small bowel usually can be shown.

CASE 4.91

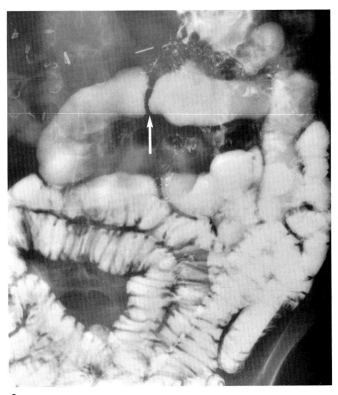

A

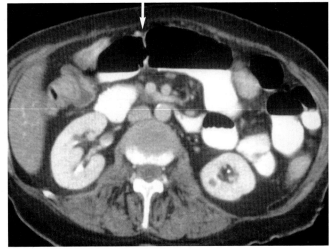

B

Findings

A. Small bowel follow-through. The jejunum has a tubular, featureless appearance without the normal jejunal fold pattern. In addition, there is a focal smooth stricture in the proximal jejunum (arrow) with two or three additional focal strictures in the proximal small bowel which are not well shown on this single image. Extensive postoperative changes also are visible in the abdomen.

B. Contrast-enhanced CT. This corresponding CT image also shows the tubular, featureless appearance of the small bowel with the focal stricture in the proximal jejunum (arrow).

Differential Diagnosis

Celiac disease (sprue) with a benign stricture due to prior ulcerative jejunoileitis

Diagnosis

Celiac disease (sprue) with a benign stricture

Discussion

This patient has the classic moulage sign in the proximal small bowel associated with celiac disease. Patients with long-standing celiac disease occasionally present with benign focal strictures, probably as a result of prior ulcerative jejunoileitis.

CASES 4.92–4.96

Case 4.92

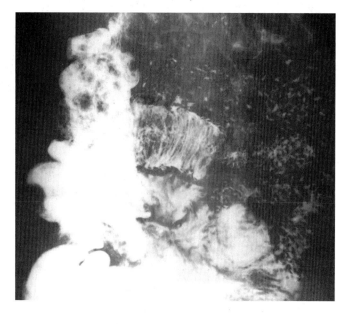

Case 4.94

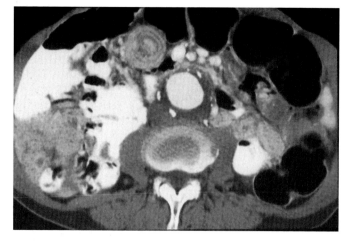

Case 4.95

Case 4.93

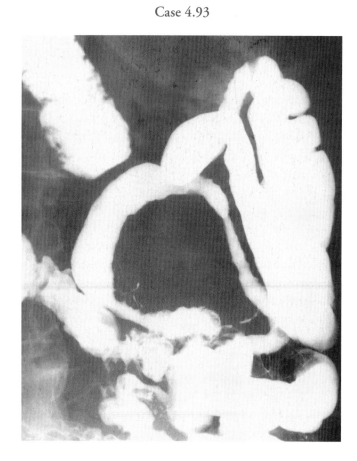

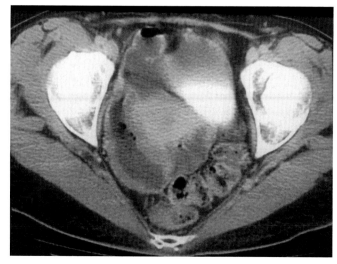

Case 4.96

Findings

Case 4.92. Small bowel follow-through. The typical coiled-spring appearance of a jejunal intussusception is present in the upper abdomen.

Case 4.93. Small bowel follow-through. Several small bowel loops appear featureless, and other loops are narrowed with nodular and thickened folds. The narrowed segments may be ulcerated.

Case 4.94. Contrast-enhanced CT. A small bowel intussusception is present in the central abdomen.

Case 4.95. Contrast-enhanced CT. Multiple low-density lymph nodes are present within the mesentery.

Case 4.96. Contrast-enhanced CT. A dilated, focally thick-walled loop of small bowel is present in the right side of the pelvis.

Differential Diagnosis

Cases 4.92 and 4.94
1. Intussusception
2. Lead point mass
3. Celiac disease

Case 4.93
1. Crohn disease
2. Segmental ischemia
3. Celiac disease with segmental ulceration

Case 4.95
1. *Mycobacterium avium-intracellulare* (tuberculosis)
2. Lymphoma (treated)
3. Celiac disease

Case 4.96
1. Lymphoma
2. Crohn disease
3. Celiac disease with lymphoma

Diagnosis

Complications of celiac disease

Celiac disease with intussusception: cases 4.92 and 4.94
Celiac disease with ulcerating jejunoileitis: case 4.93
Celiac disease with cavitary lymph node syndrome: case 4.95
Celiac disease with small bowel lymphoma: case 4.96

Discussion

Intussusceptions occur often in patients with celiac disease. One report noted this disorder in 20% of patients. Intussusceptions are usually asymptomatic, transient, and self-reducing. As with any intussusception, careful fluoroscopy should be performed to exclude a small bowel mass as a lead point for the intussusception.

Segmental ulceration in patients with sprue is an unusual complication of the disease. Patients often present with worsening of their malabsorptive symptoms and abdominal pain. Bleeding and perforation can occur as a result of the nonspecific ulcers. The ulcers are morphologically nonspecific, are often multiple, and usually involve the jejunum. They can be difficult to detect radiologically. Spasm, irritability, and persistent areas of narrowing can make it difficult to differentiate these changes from lymphoma. As a result, the involved loops are usually resected. In some patients, the nonspecific ulcers may precede the development of strictures or recognition of intestinal lymphoma.

Several disorders are associated with celiac disease, including hyposplenism and cavitary lymph node syndrome (case 4.95). Sometimes the enlarged nodes can have lipid-fluid layers within them. Lymphoma and carcinoma are the best known complications. In addition, dermatitis herpetiformis, immunoglobulin A deficiency, and adenopathy can occur.

Common Small Bowel Diseases

		Case
Crohn disease	Usually distal ileum involved, aphthous ulcers, short-segment strictures, skip lesions, cobblestone pattern	4.60–4.71
Ischemia	Segmental straight, thickened folds, pneumatosis, portal venous gas, mesenteric artery or venous thrombosis or emboli should be sought	4.72–4.83
Small bowel obstruction	Dilated small bowel with transition point, most commonly caused by adhesions or hernias	4.84–4.87
Celiac disease	Reversal of jejunal and ileal fold pattern, hypersecretion, dilatation, transient intussusceptions. Complications: ulcerating jejunoileitis, lymphoma, carcinoma, cavitating lymph node syndrome	4.88–4.96

CASE 4.97

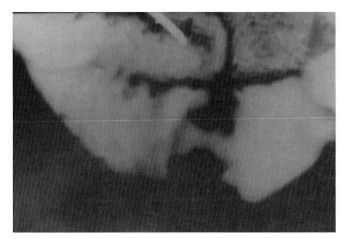

A

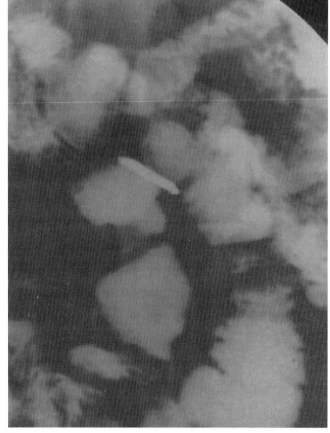

B

Findings

Small bowel follow-through (spot radiograph). **A.** Short focal narrowing of a small bowel loop with an irregular luminal contour and abrupt, shouldered margins. **B.** An eccentric ulceration involves another small bowel loop.

Differential Diagnosis

1. Metastases
2. Lymphoma
3. Crohn disease
4. Nonspecific ulcerations

Diagnosis

Nonspecific ulcerations

Discussion

In the past, intestinal ulcerations frequently were due to enteric-coated potassium chloride. Because this is no longer used, these ulcerations are rarely encountered. Similar-appearing ulcers can occur in patients taking nonsteroidal anti-inflammatory drugs (indomethacin and ibuprofen). The ulcers may be solitary or multiple and can heal with stenosis or diaphragm-like strictures. The ulcers have a sharp demarcation with normal bowel, without surrounding inflammatory change. Other causes of isolated small bowel ulcers include tuberculosis, Crohn disease, Behçet syndrome, celiac disease, ischemia, trauma, heterotopic gastric mucosa, and arsenic poisoning.

CASE 4.98

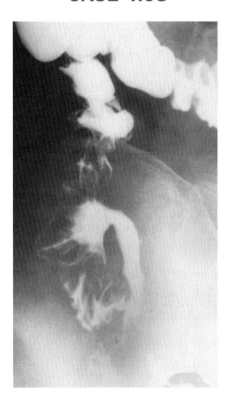

CASE 4.99

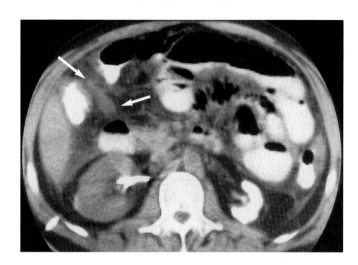

Findings

Case 4.98. Single-contrast barium enema examination. The terminal ileum is narrowed with fine contour irregularities. The cecum is contracted. The ileocecal valve is widely patent.

Case 4.99. Unenhanced CT. The mesenteric fat is of increased attenuation. The anterior pararenal fascia is thickened. The wall of the right colon is thickened (arrows). The left kidney is shrunken and homogeneously hyperdense, consistent with tuberculous nephropathy (putty kidney). A nephrostomy tube is present within the right kidney.

Differential Diagnosis
1. Crohn disease
2. Mycobacterial infection
3. Amebiasis
4. Peritoneal metastases

Diagnosis
Mycobacterial tuberculosis

Discussion

Tuberculosis involving the gastrointestinal tract remains common in parts of the world. Many patients with gastrointestinal tuberculosis have a normal chest radiograph. Tuberculosis most often affects the distal small bowel and cecum. Pathologically, granulomas in the bowel wall ulcerate or form a localized mass. Nodal and peritoneal involvement are common. Chronic infection leads to fibrosis and luminal narrowing.

Radiographically, findings can mimic those of Crohn disease. Ulcerations, luminal narrowing, multiple segmental regions of involvement, bowel wall thickening, fistulas, and a localized mass are typical. The cecum may be shrunken and deformed (acutely as a result of spasm and chronically from fibrosis). The ileocecal valve may be patulous and incompetent.

Tuberculous peritonitis is relatively rare. Ascites, mesenteric soft tissue stranding, and mesenteric adenopathy are usual radiographic findings. Adenopathy involves predominantly the upper abdomen. Low-density centers within the nodes occasionally are identified.

CASE 4.100

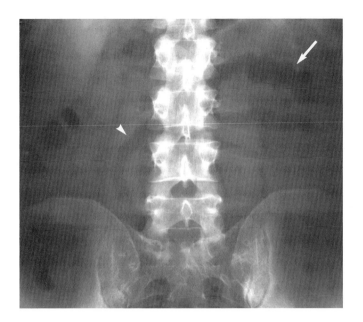

CASE 4.101

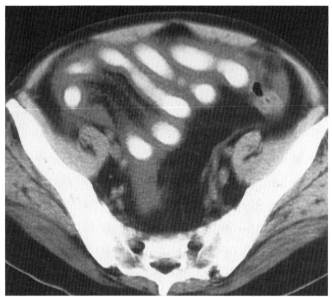

Findings

Case 4.100. Plain abdominal radiograph. Several abnormal small bowel loops are present on this plain film radiograph. The mucosal folds are markedly thickened (arrow) or nearly absent (arrowhead). Separation of small bowel loops suggests bowel-wall thickening.

Case 4.101. Contrast-enhanced CT. Diffuse wall thickening is seen throughout the small bowel. Normal mucosal folds were not visible. The small bowel has a ribbon-bowel appearance.

Differential Diagnosis
1. Ischemic small bowel
2. Infectious enteritis
3. Celiac disease
4. Acute radiation enteritis
5. Graft-versus-host disease
6. Amyloidosis

Diagnosis
Graft-versus-host disease

Discussion

Graft-versus-host disease occurs commonly in patients receiving a bone marrow transplant. New antirejection drugs have reduced this problem such that it develops in only 25% to 35% of patients. The skin, liver, and gastrointestinal tract are affected most often. Severe mucosal inflammation, destruction, and atrophy occur, resulting in a profuse secretory diarrhea. Graft-versus-host disease can affect the stomach, small bowel, and colon; the small bowel usually is affected most severely.

Radiographic changes include fold thickening, effacement, and featureless (atrophic) loops that have been referred to as ribbon bowel. A feature unique to patients who have had bone marrow transplantation is prolonged coating of the affected bowel segments with barium for several days after the examination. The cause of this finding is unknown. Knowledge that the patient has had bone marrow transplantation makes this diagnosis straightforward.

CASE 4.102

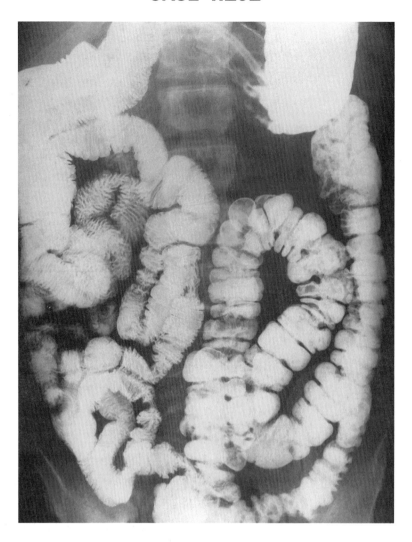

Findings
Small bowel follow-through. All of the small bowel occupies the right side of the abdomen. The colon resides on the left side of the abdomen.

Differential Diagnosis
Intestinal nonrotation

Diagnosis
Intestinal nonrotation

Discussion
Normally, the intestines undergo a rotation of 270° during fetal life. Rotation involves two major segments of intestine: the duodenal-jejunal region, which migrates to its normal position early in fetal life, and the cecocolic segments, which enter the abdominal cavity and rotate into their normal positions later. Abnormalities of rotation can interrupt this sequence of events at any stage of development, resulting in a nonrotation (small bowel resides in the right portion of the abdomen, colon on the left), incomplete rotation (normal small bowel rotation but the cecum is located in the left portion of the abdomen, in the epigastrium, or high on the right side), and incomplete mesenteric fixation (mobile cecum). Midgut volvulus or small bowel obstruction from mesenteric bands is an important complication of malrotation (case 4.84). Congenital diaphragmatic hernias and omphaloceles are also sequelae of nonrotation.

CASE 4.103

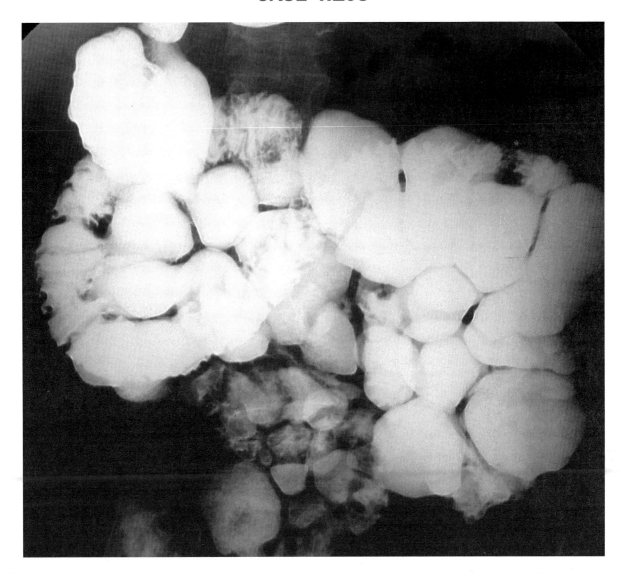

Findings
Small bowel follow-through. Multiple large saclike structures project from multiple small bowel loops.

Differential Diagnosis
Intestinal diverticulosis

Diagnosis
Intestinal diverticulosis

Discussion
Small bowel diverticula are often found incidentally during a small bowel examination. The majority are single or few in number, and most affect the proximal small bowel, especially the duodenum. Tiny diverticula also frequently can be seen arising from the terminal ileum. In our experience, most diverticula are incidental findings and rarely cause clinical symptoms. Occasionally, significant stasis occurs in one or more diverticula, resulting in bacterial overgrowth, vitamin B_{12} deficiency, and macrocytic anemia. Malabsorption can be problematic as a result of bile acid deconjugation by the abundant bacteria and subsequent fat malabsorption. Bacterial exotoxins also can damage the intestinal lining and impair absorption. Bleeding, perforation, diverticulitis, enterolith formation, and pneumoperitoneum are other rarely reported complications.

CASE 4.104

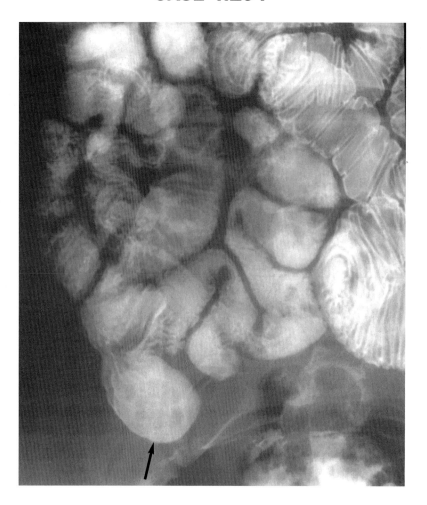

Findings

Enteroclysis. A diverticulum (arrow) arising from the distal small bowel is present in the right lower portion of the abdomen. This location is typical of Meckel diverticulum.

Differential Diagnosis

1. Meckel diverticulum
2. Postoperative deformity

Diagnosis

Meckel diverticulum

Discussion

Meckel diverticulum is an outpouching of the small bowel representing the remnant of the omphalomesenteric duct (a connection between the yolk sac and the midgut). Meckel diverticula usually are located within the distal 3 feet of the small bowel, and approximately two-thirds contain heterotopic gastric mucosa. Symptoms can develop at any age, but most patients seek medical attention before age 3 years. Signs and symptoms usually include melena and abdominal pain. Ulceration, perforation, intussusception, or enterolith formation have all been reported to occur in Meckel diverticulum.

Radiographic evaluation may include an abdominal plain film. Calcified enteroliths and free air or a mechanical small bowel obstruction may be found. Barium examination of the small bowel may reveal the diverticulum; however, this entity is identified less frequently than the expected incidence (3%) for the general population. Some investigators believe an enteroclysis small bowel examination is more sensitive for detecting this entity.

CASE 4.105

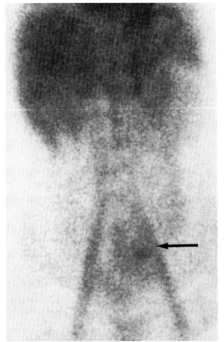

1 minute

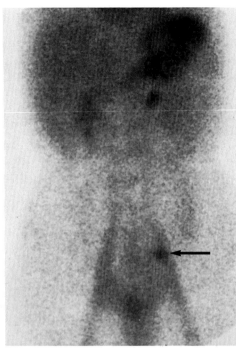

10 minutes

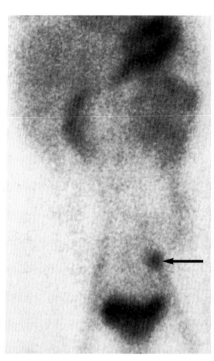

30 minutes

Findings
Technetium pertechnetate radionuclide examination.
A region of abnormally increased tracer (arrows) is visible in the left lower portion of the abdomen.

Differential Diagnosis
1. Duplication cyst
2. Ectopic island of gastric mucosa
3. Meckel diverticulum

Diagnosis
Meckel diverticulum

Discussion
This finding is consistent with a Meckel diverticulum containing ectopic gastric mucosa; however, usually tracer is identified in the right lower quadrant in this condition. Technetium pertechnetate scans are useful for identifying a Meckel diverticulum because the tracer is taken up and secreted by gastric mucosa. Some controversy exists as to which cell type specifically accumulates the tracer. Because many Meckel diverticula contain ectopic gastric mucosa, they can be identified with this examination. Organs that normally take up pertechnetate include stomach, salivary glands, and urinary tract (because a small amount of tracer is cleared by the kidneys). Uptake also can occur in other organs with gastric mucosa, including Barrett esophagus, duplication cysts, and ectopic islands of gastric mucosa in the small bowel.

CASE 4.106

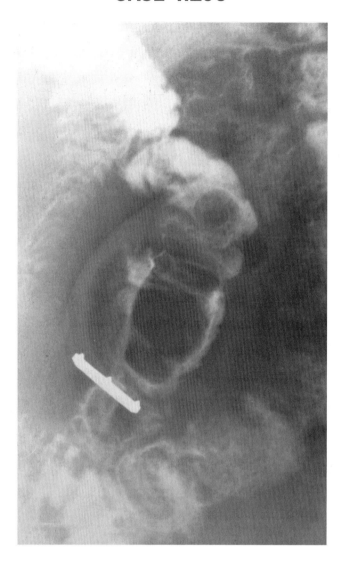

Findings

Small bowel follow-through (spot radiograph). An oblong, sausage-shaped filling defect is present within the lumen of the distal small bowel. A compression device with a metallic marker is present.

Differential Diagnosis

1. Large polyp
2. Gastrointestinal stromal tumor
3. Foreign body
4. Inverted Meckel diverticulum

Diagnosis

Inverted Meckel diverticulum

Discussion

Complications that can occur from Meckel diverticulum include ulceration, bleeding, perforation, obstruction, intussusception, and enterolith formation. Occasional inversion of a diverticulum can present as an intraluminal filling defect and simulate a polypoid tumor.

CASE 4.107

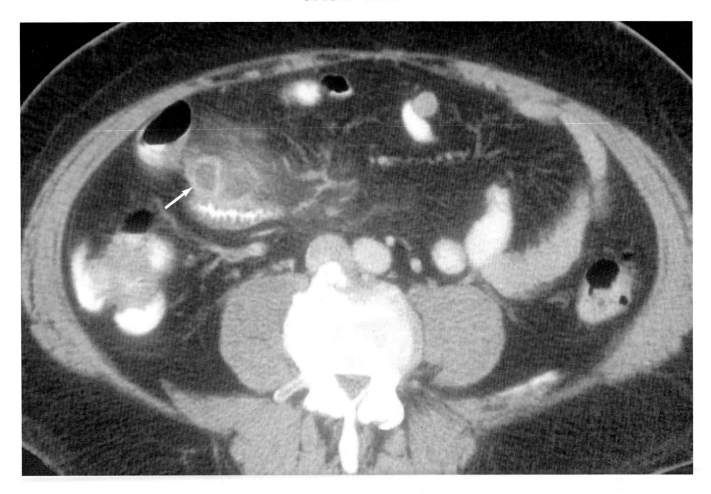

Findings

Contrast-enhanced CT. A blind-ending tubular structure arises from the ileum. The wall of this structure is thickened (arrow), and there is considerable soft tissue stranding in the adjacent fat.

Differential Diagnosis

1. Meckel diverticulitis
2. Crohn disease
3. Mesenteric panniculitis

Diagnosis

Meckel diverticulitis

Discussion

The presence of a blind-ending tubular structure arising from the ileum is typical of a Meckel diverticulum. The wall thickening and mesenteric soft tissue stranding indicate acute inflammation of this structure. The ileum is not thickened, thereby excluding Crohn disease. Panniculitis can be excluded because the process is not centered in the mesentery.

Miscellaneous Small Bowel Conditions

		Case
Nonspecific ulcerations	Potassium chloride, nonsteroidal and anti-inflammatory drugs. Ulcers can be solitary or multiple. Can heal with bandlike narrowing	4.97
Tuberculosis	Resembles Crohn disease, peritoneal nodules, masses, adenopathy may be low-attenuation	4.98 and 4.99
Graft-versus-host disease	Ribbon bowel (thickened, featureless loops). Usually occurs after bone marrow transplantation	4.100 and 4.101
Nonrotation	Abnormal duodenal-jejunal flexure or colon location or both. Predisposes to midgut volvulus and cecal ileus	4.102
Diverticulosis	Usually asymptomatic, bacterial overgrowth and malabsorption occasionally	4.103
Meckel diverticulum	Within 3 feet of distal ileum, ectopic gastric mucosa bleeds, infection, inversion possible	4.104–4.107

DIFFERENTIAL DIAGNOSES

Solitary Filling Defects

Benign tumors
    Lipoma
    Hemangioma
    Adenoma
    Hamartoma
Malignant tumors
    Carcinoid
    Lymphoma
    Adenocarcinoma
    Malignant GIST
    Metastasis
Nonneoplastic
    Duplication cyst
    Gallstone ileus
    Ascariasis

Type I Folds (Thin, Straight, Dilated Lumen)

Mechanical obstruction
Paralytic ileus
Scleroderma
Celiac disease (sprue)

Type II Folds (Thick, Straight)

Segmental
    Ischemia
    Intramural hemorrhage
    Radiation enteritis
    Adjacent inflammatory process
Diffuse
    Venous congestion
    Hypoproteinemia
    Cirrhosis

Type III Folds (Thick, Nodular)

Segmental
    Crohn disease

    Infection
    Lymphoma
    Metastases
Diffuse
    Whipple disease
    Intestinal lymphangiectasia
    Nodular lymphoid hyperplasia
    Polyposis syndromes
    Eosinophilic gastroenteritis
    Amyloidosis
    Mastocytosis
    Lymphoma
    Metastases

Atrophic (Featureless) Folds

Graft-versus-host disease
Ischemic small bowel (chronic)
Celiac disease (sprue)
Radiation enteritis (chronic)
Amyloidosis
Infectious enteritis

Excessive Fluid in Lumen

Proximal to mechanical obstruction
Celiac disease (sprue)
Zollinger-Ellison syndrome

Luminal Narrowing

Adhesions or bands
Crohn disease
Adenocarcinoma
Lymphoma
Metastases
Intramural hemorrhage
Tuberculosis
Ischemia
Radiation enteritis

SMALL BOWEL FILLING DEFECTS AND MASSES

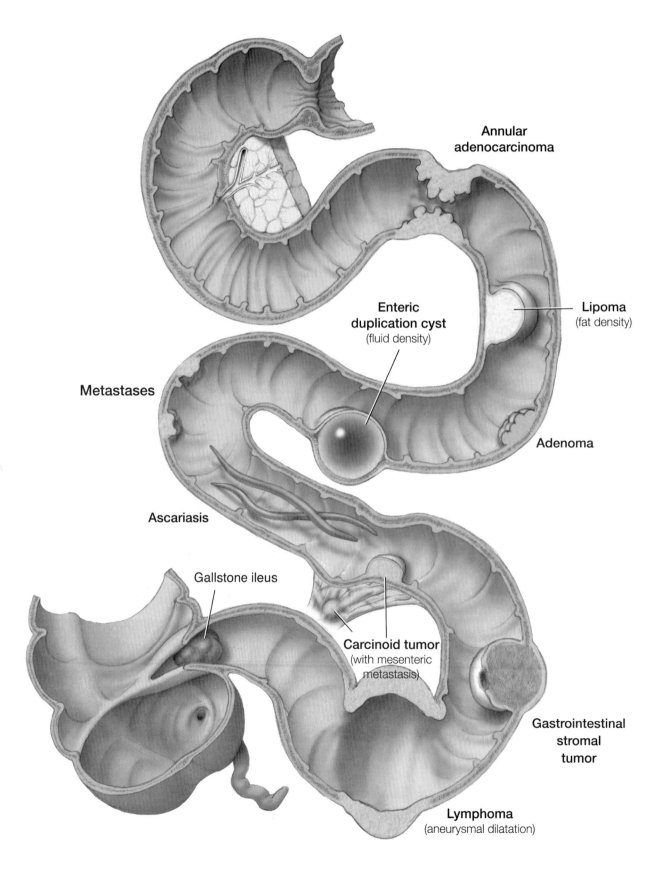

Annular
adenocarcinoma

Enteric
duplication cyst
(fluid density)

Lipoma
(fat density)

Metastases

Adenoma

Ascariasis

Gallstone ileus

Carcinoid tumor
(with mesenteric
metastasis)

Gastrointestinal
stromal
tumor

Lymphoma
(aneurysmal dilatation)

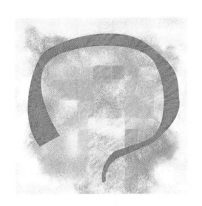

CHAPTER 5
COLON

275

CASE 5.1

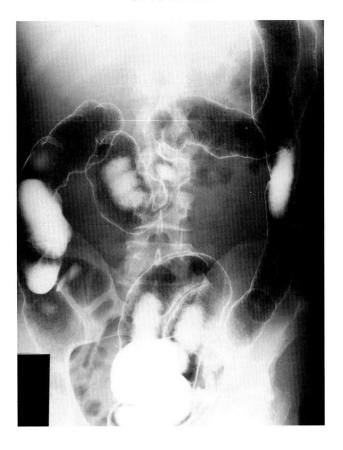

Findings

Double-contrast barium enema. The entire colon is ahaustral, with a diffuse granular-appearing mucosa. The air-filled terminal ileum is dilated.

Differential Diagnosis

1. Ulcerative colitis
2. Infectious colitis

Diagnosis

Ulcerative colitis

Discussion

Ulcerative colitis is a disease of unknown origin. Granulomas are conspicuously absent. Ulceration of the mucosa is nearly always present in patients with active inflammation.

Clinically, many patients initially experience the sudden onset of bloody diarrhea, abdominal cramping, and fever. The initial diagnosis often can be suggested at proctosigmoidoscopy. Extraintestinal manifestations of this disease include erythema nodosum, pyoderma gangrenosum, primary sclerosing cholangitis, cholangiocarcinoma, arthritis, sacroiliitis, spondylitis, and iritis. Spondylitis activity has no relationship to the activity of the colon inflammation. Patients with HLA-B27 histocompatibility antigen are more likely to have spondylitis and iritis develop than patients without the marker.

Radiologically, the following are critical for diagnosis:

1. The involved mucosa on an air-contrast barium enema has a granular (sandpaper-like) or stippled appearance.
2. The distribution of the disease is usually one of rectal involvement with disease affecting the more proximal colon in a continuous manner, without skip areas.
3. Circumferential bowel wall symmetry is maintained. Mucosal ulcerations affect both sides of the bowel with equal severity.

Infectious colitides can present with similar radiographic features. Stool cultures are always required at initial evaluation.

CASE 5.2

CASE 5.3

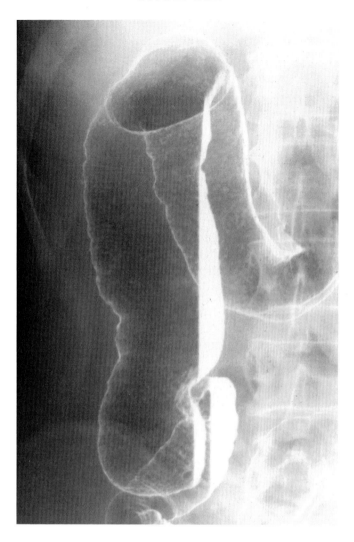

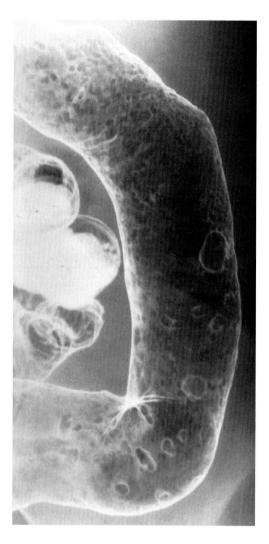

Findings

Case 5.2. Double-contrast barium enema. Coarsely granular mucosal ulcerations are visible in the right colon.

Case 5.3. Double-contrast barium enema. The colon is affected with a coarsely granular mucosal pattern. Numerous polypoid filling defects also are present.

Differential Diagnosis
Ulcerative colitis

Diagnosis
Ulcerative colitis

Discussion
Polypoid changes may develop in any stage of ulcerative colitis. In patients with severe, acute inflammation, pseudopolyps are likely to be present. Pseudopolyps refer to islands of normal colonic mucosa surrounded by denuded ulcerative mucosa. Inflammatory polyps refer to regions of inflamed, elevated mucosa surrounded by granular mucosa. Inflammatory polyps may be sessile or pedunculated, and they more often are found in patients with less severe inflammation than in those with pseudopolyps.

CASE 5.4

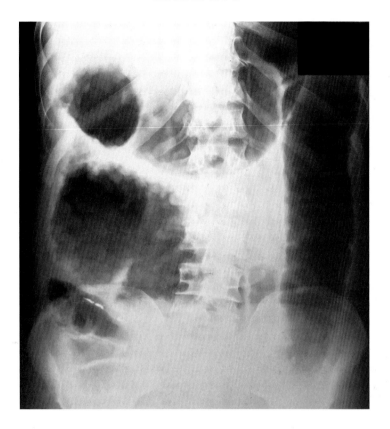

Findings

Abdominal radiograph. The colon is distended with gas (adynamic ileus pattern), and multiple polypoid masses protrude into the colonic lumen.

Differential Diagnosis

1. Adynamic ileus
2. Colonic obstruction
3. Toxic megacolon

Diagnosis

Toxic megacolon

Discussion

Toxic megacolon is a serious complication that can occur in either ulcerative colitis or Crohn colitis (although it is most frequent in patients with ulcerative colitis). This condition occurs during a severe episode of acute inflammation. Dilatation (>6 cm) and adynamic ileus often occur because the inflammatory changes have extended into the muscular layers and usually to the serosa of the colon. Extensive mucosal disease can be visualized by identifying nodularity and polypoid changes within the colonic lumen. These polyps usually represent pseudopolyps. Bowel wall and haustral thickening are due to intramural edema and congestion.

Colonic perforation can occur in toxic megacolon, and it is associated with a high morbidity and mortality. Perforation may be suggested by identifying either intramural pneumatosis or pneumoperitoneum. Iatrogenic intervention is a common cause of perforation. In patients with this condition, a contrast enema or colonoscopy should be avoided. Even inflation of a rectal balloon in patients with a fragile, narrowed, and inflamed rectum can easily result in perforation.

Toxic megacolon always occurs with adynamic ileus. Patients usually have fever, leukocytosis, and a tender abdomen. A single supine radiograph in adynamic ileus can simulate a distal colonic obstruction because of the posterior location of the rectosigmoid. If clinical symptoms suggest an obstruction, a supine or decubitus view is often helpful for demonstrating air filling of the rectosigmoid.

CASE 5.5

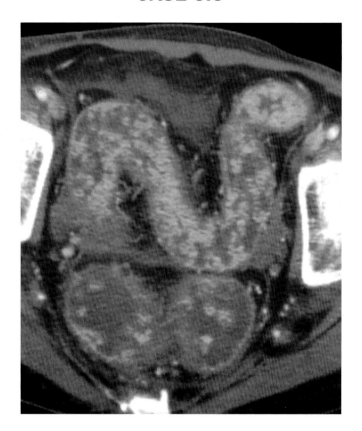

CASE 5.6

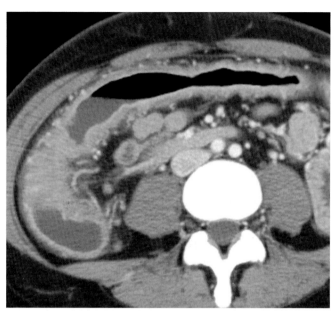

Findings

Case 5.5. Contrast-enhanced CT. Innumerable enhancing polypoid filling defects are present throughout the rectosigmoid colon. The wall of the colon is hyperenhancing and slightly irregular in contour.

Case 5.6. Contrast-enhanced CT. The wall of the colon is diffusely thickened. Multiple collaterals are present about the thick-walled colonic segments.

Differential Diagnosis
1. Ulcerative colitis
2. Polyposis syndrome

Diagnosis

Acute changes of ulcerative colitis (case 5.5 has innumerable inflammatory pseudopolyps)

Discussion

Detection of inflammatory diseases of the colon at CT depends on the severity of the disease and the quality of the examination. Usually, mild disease confined to the mucosa is not detectable at CT. Severe disease with inflammatory changes extending to the serosal surface causes bowel wall thickening and often soft tissue stranding in the pericolonic fat (as in these cases).

CASE 5.7

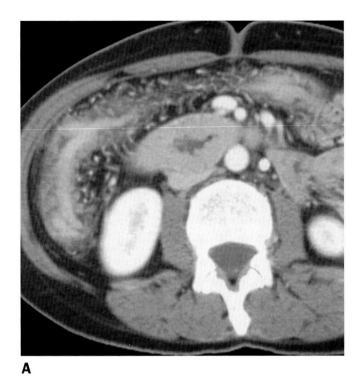

A

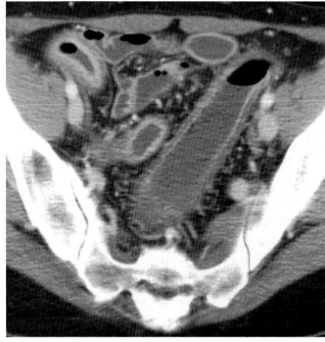

B

Findings

Contrast-enhanced CT. **A** and **B.** Diffuse thickening and hyperenhancement of the wall of the colon and terminal ileum. Engorgement of the vasa recti.

Differential Diagnosis

1. Acute colitis
2. Crohn disease
3. Ulcerative colitis
4. Infectious colitis
5. Pseudomembranous colitis

Diagnosis

Ulcerative colitis with backwash ileitis

Discussion

Ulcerative colitis can be suspected in patients with continuous, symmetric bowel wall thickening. Thickening of the terminal ileum in this patient raises the possibility of Crohn disease, but backwash ileitis was found at colonoscopy. Hyperenhancement of the bowel wall and vascular engorgement of the pericolonic tissues indicate active inflammatory changes.

CASE 5.8

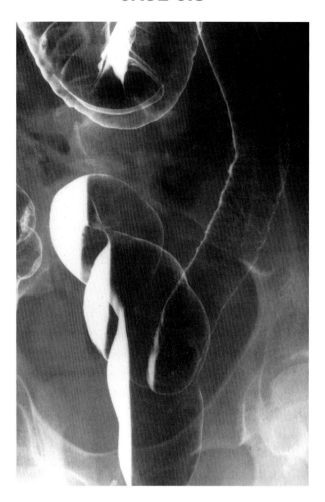

Findings
Double-contrast barium enema. Active ulcerations (stippled and linear) are present in the sigmoid colon. The rectum has a featureless mucosa with some mild loss of distensibility.

Differential Diagnosis
1. Ulcerative colitis
2. Infectious colitis
3. Crohn colitis

Diagnosis
Ulcerative colitis, healing pattern

Discussion
Rectal involvement is usually present in patients with ulcerative colitis, and in this patient it can be assumed to have occurred in the past because of the reduced distensibility of this bowel segment. Patients using corticosteroid enemas may have a normal-appearing rectal mucosa with active disease in the more proximal colon. This distribution of disease can also occur in patients with ulcerative colitis who have not used corticosteroid enemas because of segmental mucosal healing and repair. The distribution of mucosal healing is the same as that of active inflammation in patients with ulcerative colitis—beginning in the rectum and progressing proximally in a continuous manner. Therefore, when the healing process begins, the rectum nearly always appears normal first, with variable degrees of inflammation present in the more proximal colon. The most severe disease usually is found proximally in a colonic segment near the leading edge of ascending inflammation.

CASE 5.9

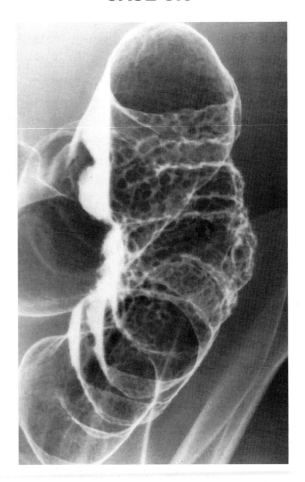

Findings
Double-contrast barium enema. Multiple nodules are present in the descending colon in this patient with a 22-year history of ulcerative colitis. The nodules abut each other and have flattened edges.

Differential Diagnosis
1. Inflammatory polyps in ulcerative colitis
2. Carcinoma
3. Lymphoma
4. Dysplasia

Diagnosis
Mucosal dysplasia

Discussion
Endoscopic biopsy showed that the nodules were formed of atypical colonic glands crowded within the lamina propria. This pattern is often found in dysplastic nodules. Patients with ulcerative colitis are at increased risk for development of colon cancer. Those patients at greatest risk have colonic epithelial dysplasia. Detection of dysplasia in a colitic colon should prompt endoscopic biopsy and possibly prophylactic colectomy. Unfortunately, most mucosal dysplasia is not visible radiographically and requires random endoscopic biopsy for detection.

Radiographically, dysplasia appears as a solitary nodule or multiple nodules. A close grouping of nodules with opposed flattened edges is most commonly (50% of time) associated with dysplasia. Inflammatory polyps may be indistinguishable from dysplastic nodules. Colitic carcinomas usually are associated with luminal narrowing. Lymphoma is not commonly associated with ulcerative colitis.

CASE 5.10

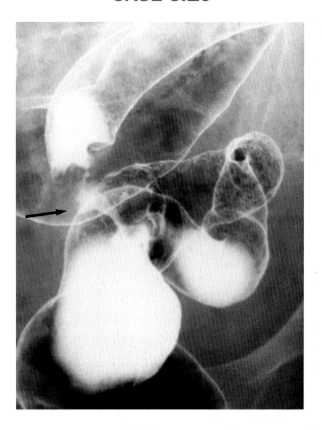

CASE 5.11

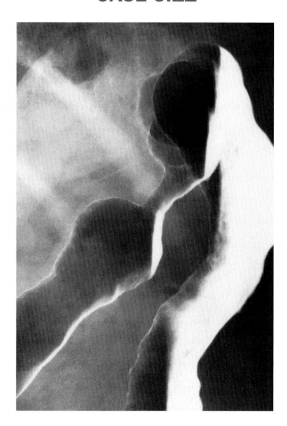

Findings

Case 5.10. Double-contrast barium enema. An annular segment of narrowing (arrow) is present in the sigmoid colon. Granular mucosal changes also are present.

Case 5.11. Double-contrast barium enema. A stricture is present in the region of the ahaustral splenic flexure of the colon.

Differential Diagnosis

Colitic cancer

Diagnosis

Colitic cancer

Discussion

Patients with ulcerative colitis have an increased risk for development of colorectal cancer (colitic cancer). The risk depends on the extent and duration of inflammation. Patients with pancolitis are at higher risk of colon cancer than patients with only limited disease. The risk of cancer developing begins after a patient has had the disease for 10 years, and it increases with time. The actual cancer risk varies from study to study—ranging from a 3% to 10% risk of malignancy after 10 years to a 13% to 25% risk after 25 years of ulcerative colitis. The clinical activity of the disease has little effect on the overall cancer risk.

Mucosal dysplasia is the precursor of carcinoma. Most cancers complicating ulcerative colitis are annular constricting lesions. Some carcinomas develop as flat, infiltrating tumors—extending into the submucosal tissues and causing either a smooth or an abruptly tapered stricture. About one-fourth of all cancers present as strictures. Multiple cancers are common. Polypoid masses are rare. Generally, these malignancies are high-grade, aggressive tumors.

Benign strictures also can develop in ulcerative colitis as a result of muscular hypertrophy or of severe inflammation. Because it is impossible to differentiate benign from malignant strictures radiographically, they should be regarded with suspicion.

CASE 5.12

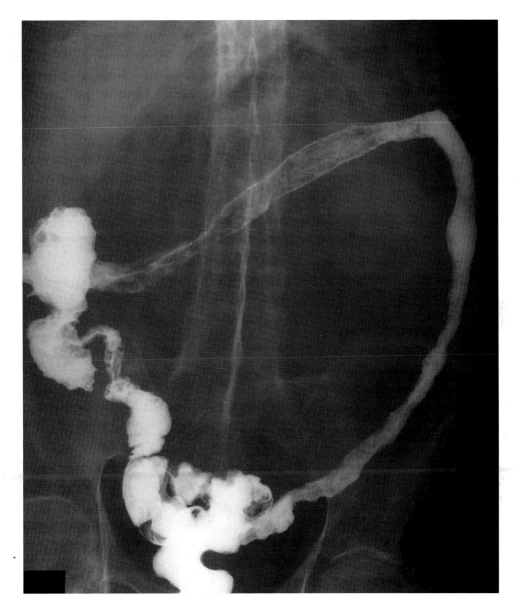

Findings

Single-contrast post-evacuation barium enema. The colon is ahaustral and shortened. Typical changes of ankylosing spondylitis also are present.

Differential Diagnosis

1. Chronic ulcerative colitis
2. Cathartic abuse

Diagnosis

Chronic ulcerative colitis

Discussion

Long-standing ulcerative colitis often results in a colon devoid of the normal haustral markings and a diffusely shortened and often narrowed colonic lumen. The colon usually appears featureless and rigid. Hypertrophy of the circular and longitudinal muscle fibers is now believed to be the most frequent cause of these changes.

Spondylitis often precedes the inflammatory bowel disease, whereas the symptoms of peripheral joint disease occur concurrently or after the onset of bowel symptoms.

CASE 5.13

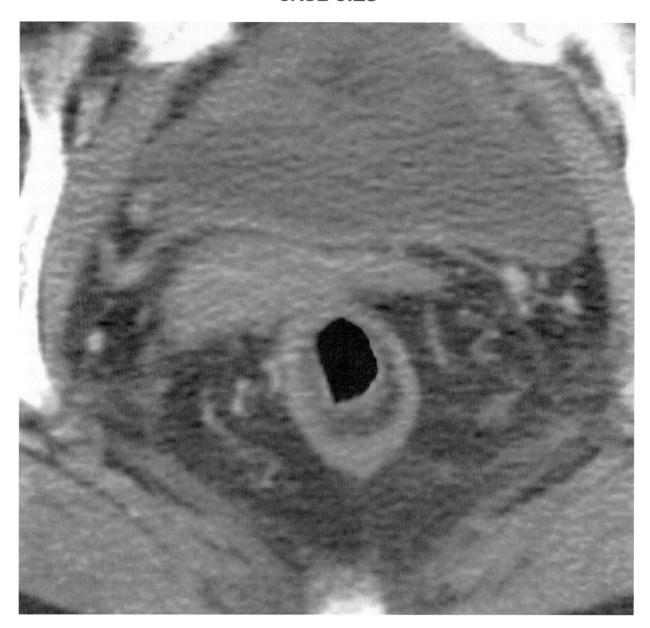

Findings
Contrast-enhanced CT. Diffuse thickening of the wall of the colon. The wall contains fat attenuation tissue.

Differential Diagnosis
1. Chronic ulcerative colitis
2. Crohn colitis

Diagnosis
Chronic ulcerative colitis

Discussion
Fat attenuation in the wall of the colon usually indicates long-standing disease that is inactive. The pancolitis in this case favors ulcerative colitis. There is mild soft tissue stranding in the pericolonic tissues in the ascending colon. At colonoscopy, mild changes of acute colitis were present in this patient with known chronic ulcerative colitis.

CASE 5.14

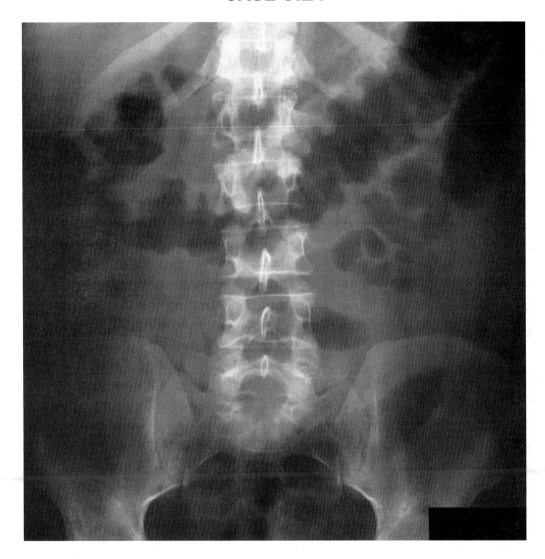

Findings
Abdominal radiograph. The haustral folds are diffusely thickened throughout the transverse colon.

Differential Diagnosis
1. Pseudomembranous colitis
2. Inflammatory bowel disease
3. Infectious colitis
4. Ischemic colitis

Diagnosis
Inflammatory bowel disease: acute Crohn colitis

Discussion
Most patients with acute colitis present with similar radiographic findings in the involved portions of the colon. Intramural edema and hemorrhage cause wall and haustral thickening (as in this case). Inflammatory polyps can be visible within the gas-filled colon in patients with inflammatory bowel disease (cases 5.4, 5.5, and 5.6). The splenic flexure is often an isolated segment of involved colon in elderly patients with ischemic colitis (case 5.42). A contrast enema usually is contraindicated in patients with acute colitis because of the risk of perforation. It can be performed safely after the acute episode has resolved. Proctoscopy is often useful for revealing the mucosal changes of ulcerative colitis or pseudomembranous colitis.

CASE 5.15

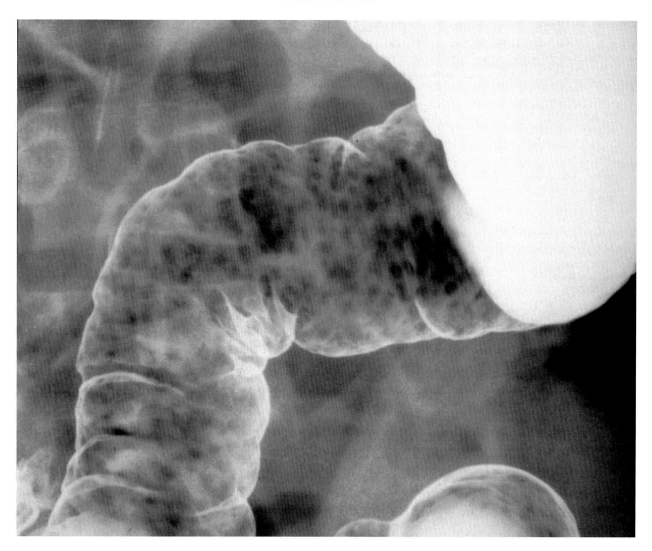

Findings
Double-contrast barium enema. A prominent lymphoid pattern is present in the sigmoid colon. Some of the nodules are mildly enlarged (>4 mm).

Differential Diagnosis
1. Prominent lymphoid pattern
2. Early Crohn disease
3. Polyposis syndrome

Diagnosis
Early Crohn disease

Discussion
The earliest change of Crohn colitis is submucosal granulomatous inflammation. Enlarged lymphoid follicles are often seen radiographically. These mucosal elevations usually have poorly defined borders and may contain a small central umbilication. The early changes of Crohn colitis are best depicted with the double-contrast technique. A lymphoid pattern can be seen in 10% to 15% of normal adults (cases 5.107 and 5.108). These nodules are uniformly small. In some patients it may be impossible to differentiate a normal lymphoid pattern from early Crohn disease. In these patients, either repeat double-contrast colon examination in several months or endoscopic biopsy is helpful.

CASE 5.16

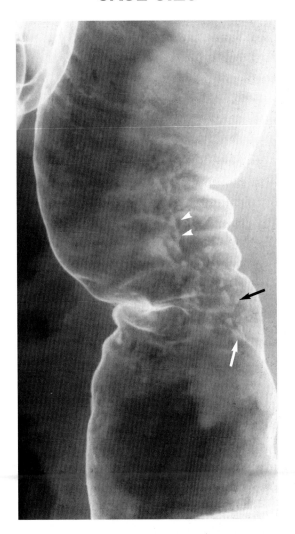

Findings

Double-contrast barium enema. Multiple discrete (aphthous) ulcers (arrows) are present within the descending colon. A halo of edema surrounds each ulceration. Many of the ulcers have become confluent, producing a linear ulceration (arrowheads). The intervening mucosa between ulcers appears normal. The distribution of ulcerations is circumferentially asymmetric.

Differential Diagnosis

1. Crohn colitis
2. Infectious colitis

Diagnosis

Crohn colitis: aphthous and confluent ulcerations

Discussion

Aphthous ulcers develop from enlarged lymphoid follicles that ulcerate centrally. These ulcers are very shallow lesions and usually are not seen in profile. Multiplicity of lesions is common. The central barium collection often varies in size and is always surrounded by a halo of edema. Although the aphthous ulcer is characteristic of Crohn disease, it is not diagnostic. These lesions also have been reported in infectious colitides, including *Yersinia* and amebic colitis.

CASE 5.17

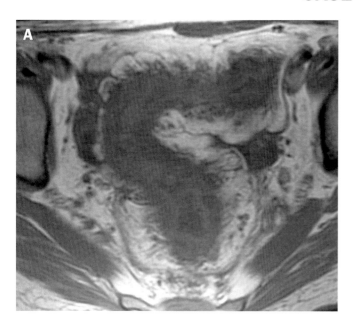

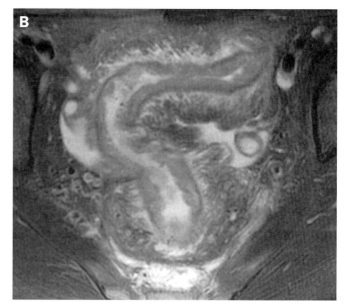

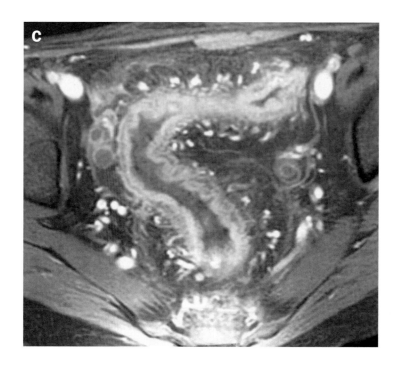

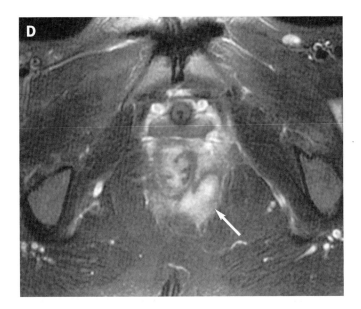 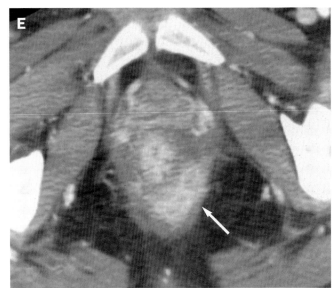

Findings

Unenhanced and enhanced MRI. **A.** T1-weighted image. Marked thickening of the wall of the rectosigmoid with pericolonic soft tissue stranding. **B.** T2-weighted image (with fat saturation). Thickening of the wall of the rectosigmoid with high-signal intensity changes in the pericolonic fat. **C.** Gadolinium-enhanced T1-weighted image (with fat saturation). Diffuse mural enhancement with submucosal edema. **D.** T2-weighted image (with fat saturation). Focal fluid collection (arrow) in the left perianal region. **E.** Contrast-enhanced CT. A fluid collection (arrow) is present in the left perianal region with surrounding inflammatory reaction.

Differential Diagnosis

1. Crohn colitis
2. Ulcerative colitis
3. Other types of acute colitis

Diagnosis

Crohn colitis with perianal abscess

Discussion

The extensive colonic inflammatory changes in this patient make it difficult to make a precise diagnosis. Any type of acute colitis could have this appearance. The perianal abscess is a characteristic feature of Crohn disease (in addition to perianal fistula, abscess, and creeping fat)—and a very helpful discriminator. MRI is a preferred method for evaluating patients with perianal abscess and fistulas.

CASE 5.18

A
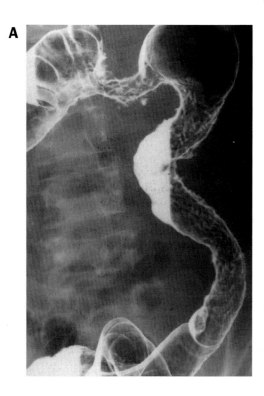

B
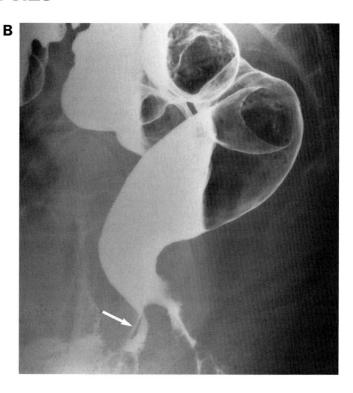

Findings

Double-contrast barium enema. **A.** Segmental regions of narrowing are present in the left transverse colon and in the descending colon. Polypoid mucosal (inflammatory polyps) changes and deep linear and thornlike ulcers are present in the affected segments. Circumferential asymmetry is present in the splenic flexure as a result of fibrosis and scarring in the medial wall of the colon. **B.** The mucosa in the rectum is normal, but there is a rectovaginal fistula (arrow) arising from the anterior wall of the distal rectum.

Differential Diagnosis

1. Crohn colitis
2. Ischemic colitis
3. Infectious colitis

Diagnosis

Crohn colitis

Discussion

Advanced Crohn colitis is characterized by discontinuous and asymmetric disease (as in this case). The rectum is often uninvolved. Deep ulcerations can appear as longitudinal and transverse collections of barium. These ulcers may crisscross, producing a cobblestone mucosal appearance. Solitary deep ulcers may appear thornlike or as a collar button. Inflammatory polyps often are present. Colonic strictures are due to transmural inflammation and fibrosis. These strictures do not have the same malignant potential as do those in patients with ulcerative colitis (cases 5.10 and 5.11).

Fistulas and perianal disease are common in Crohn disease. Fistulas can occur from the colon to another bowel loop(s), vagina, bladder, skin, or retroperitoneal organs.

The segmental disease, rectal sparing, fistula, and deep ulcerations makes ulcerative colitis unlikely. Ischemic colitis usually occurs in an older population, most commonly affecting the splenic flexure (cases 5.42, 5.43, and 5.44). Various infectious colitides (*Actinomyces, Yersinia, Campylobacter, Salmonella, Shigella, Chlamydia, Clostridium, Escherichia coli, Neisseria, gonorrhoeae,* and others) can affect the colon.

CASE 5.19

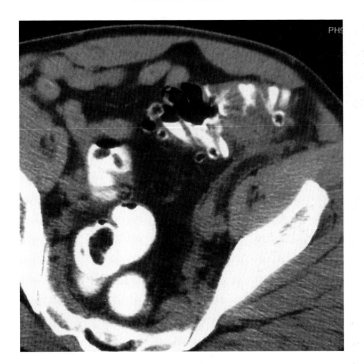

CASE 5.20

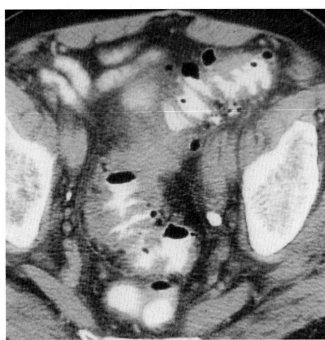

Findings
Cases 5.19 and 5.20. Contrast-enhanced CT. Focal thickening of the wall of the sigmoid colon. Soft tissue stranding and thickening are present within the adjacent soft tissues.

Differential Diagnosis
1. Diverticulitis
2. Colon cancer

Diagnosis
Diverticulitis

Discussion
These cases illustrate a mild form of diverticulitis. Soft tissue stranding alone about the colon represents the earliest radiographic findings at CT. Bowel wall thickening in combination with soft tissue stranding also can be seen. In patients with these findings, treatment with antibiotics usually is successful. Differentiation of diverticulitis from cancer is not always possible at CT. Follow-up CT, barium enema, or endoscopy can be used to exclude carcinoma.

CASE 5.21

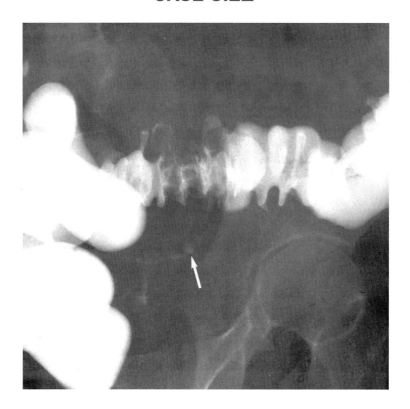

CASE 5.22

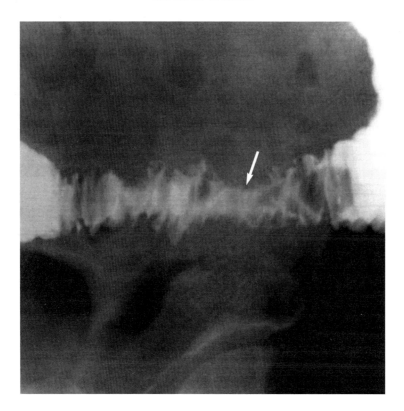

CASE 5.23

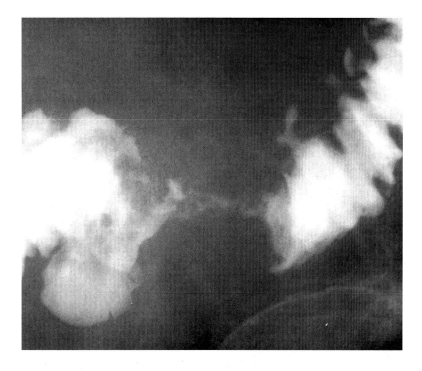

Findings

Case 5.21. Single-contrast barium enema. A segmental region of fold thickening is present in the mid-sigmoid colon. A tract (arrow) of barium extends inferiorly from the involved sigmoid. The mucosa is intact through the involved region.

Case 5.22. Single-contrast barium enema. The sigmoid colon is narrowed. Normal mucosal folds are present across this relatively long segment of involved colon. Mass effect (arrow) is present along the superior sigmoid.

Case 5.23. Single-contrast barium enema. A short focal segment of narrowing is present in the sigmoid colon. The margins of the focal abnormality are abrupt. Normal mucosal markings are difficult to identify.

Differential Diagnosis
1. Diverticulitis
2. Serosal metastases
3. Carcinoma

Diagnosis
Diverticulitis

Discussion

Diverticulitis is a result of inflammation of a solitary diverticulum and subsequent perforation and extravasation of colonic contents into pericolonic tissues. Usually the pericolonic inflammation is walled off. Rarely, peritonitis may develop. Diverticulitis may resolve spontaneously, often responding to antibiotic therapy and a soft diet. In some patients, the disease may be more severe; if an intramural or pericolonic abscess develops, it may require percutaneous or surgical drainage. Seeding of the mesenteric veins with microorganisms can result in sepsis, hepatic abscess, or mesenteric vein thrombosis. Fistulas can develop and communicate with the bladder, vagina, bowel loops, and other locations or organs.

Radiographic findings at contrast enema include narrowing of the colonic lumen (usually a longer segment is involved than in colon cancer), thickening of the mucosal folds (from the adjacent inflammation), mass effect with an intact overlying mucosa (due to the abscess), and extravasation of contrast material into the abscess cavity. Careful assessment of the mucosa is critical for excluding cancer.

CASE 5.24

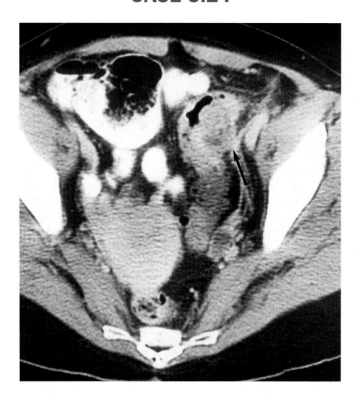

CASE 5.25

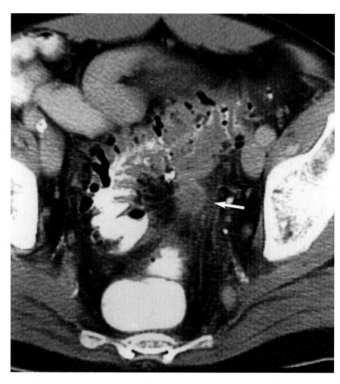

Findings

Case 5.24. Contrast-enhanced CT. Near the junction of the sigmoid and descending colon is a focal region of bowel wall thickening, luminal narrowing, and mesenteric soft tissue stranding. A small low-density mass (arrow) is present within the wall of the colon.

Case 5.25. Contrast-enhanced CT. The wall of the sigmoid colon is thickened, and a small low-density mass (arrow) and soft tissue stranding are present in the sigmoid mesentery. Extensive sigmoid diverticulosis is present.

Differential Diagnosis
1. Diverticulitis
2. Colon cancer

Diagnosis
Diverticulitis

Discussion

These cases exemplify diverticulitis with small abscesses. In case 5.25, the abscess is located in the mesentery; in case 5.24, it is intramural. In patients with pericolonic soft tissue stranding and a small (<3 cm) abscess, treatment with antibiotics usually is successful. If surgical intervention is deemed necessary, a single-stage sigmoid resection with primary reanastomosis often is possible. In both of these cases, the abscesses are too small for percutaneous drainage.

CASE 5.26

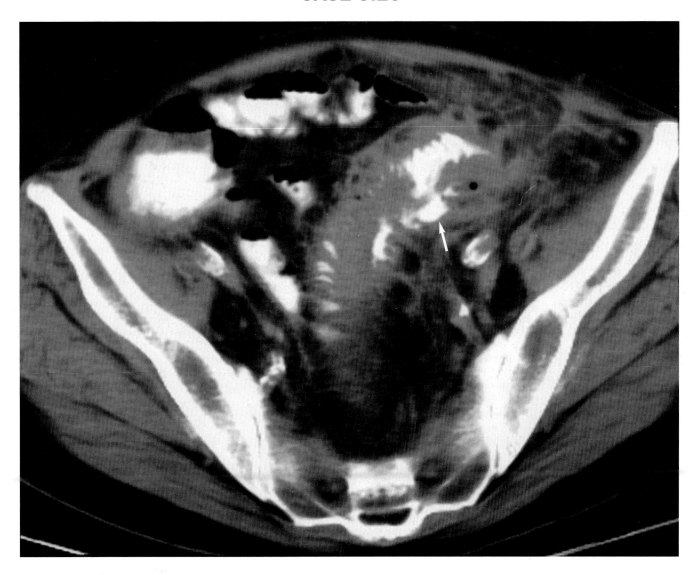

Findings

Contrast-enhanced CT. Intraluminal contrast material has extravasated into the bowel wall (arrow). Bowel wall thickening and mesenteric soft tissue stranding also are present.

Differential Diagnosis

1. Diverticulitis
2. Perforated colon cancer
3. Crohn disease

Diagnosis

Diverticulitis

Discussion

At CT, visualization of an intramural sinus tract or mesenteric abscess is considered diagnostic of diverticulitis. Perforated carcinoma, however, can present with a pericolonic fluid collection (abscess) (cases 5.90 and 5.91). Patients with perforated colon cancer also can have symptoms that mimic those of diverticulitis. If operation is not performed, it may be prudent to perform a barium enema or colonoscopy to assess the colonic mucosa and exclude carcinoma.

CASE 5.27

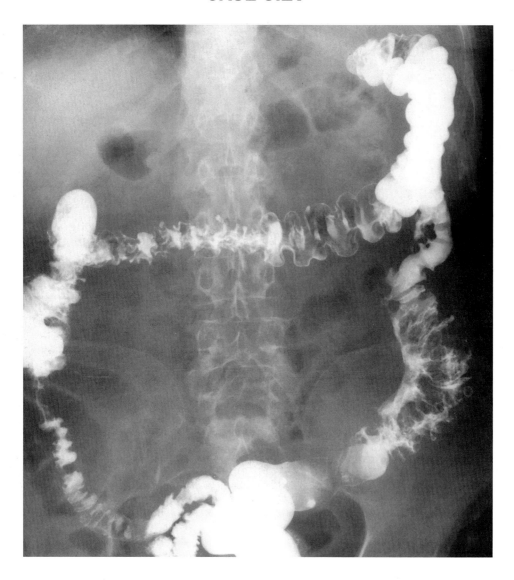

Findings
Single-contrast barium enema. Along the medial aspect of the sigmoid colon, there is an abnormal collection of barium within the wall of the colon. The collection communicates with the colonic lumen. Diverticulosis also is present.

Differential Diagnosis
1. Diverticulitis
2. Crohn disease

Diagnosis
Diverticulitis with intramural tracking

Discussion
In a patient with an intramural collection of fluid, distinguishing Crohn disease from diverticulitis requires assessment of the underlying colonic mucosa. In diverticulitis the mucosa is normal, whereas in Crohn disease the mucosa is often ulcerated and contains nodular features. In this patient, there is no indication of an abnormal underlying mucosa. Normal mucosal lines are seen throughout this colonic segment, as is diverticulosis.

CASE 5.28

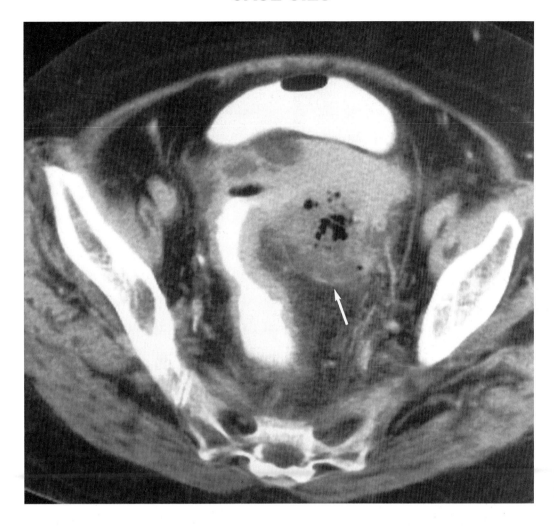

Findings

Contrast-enhanced CT. Bowel wall thickening, mesenteric soft tissue stranding, and a pericolonic abscess (arrow) involve the sigmoid colon.

Differential Diagnosis

1. Diverticulitis
2. Perforated colon cancer
3. Crohn disease

Diagnosis

Diverticulitis

Discussion

CT can be helpful for evaluating patients with suspected diverticulitis. The advantage of this technique is its ability to directly image the entire bowel wall and extraluminal tissues. CT findings of diverticulitis include bowel wall thickening, soft tissue stranding in the pericolonic fat, and a pericolonic abscess (fluid or gas collection). An actual abscess is found in fewer than half of the patients.

Percutaneous drainage of large abscesses can be helpful preoperatively. After much of the infection and inflammation have subsided with drainage and antibiotic therapy, a single-stage sigmoid resection often can safely be performed. More immediate operation is required if peritoneal signs are present, there is evidence of peritoneal spillage or abscess rupture, or the abscess is poorly defined and multiloculated.

CASE 5.29

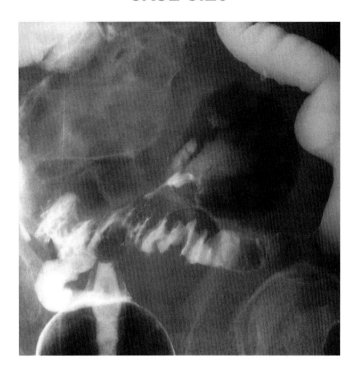

CASE 5.30

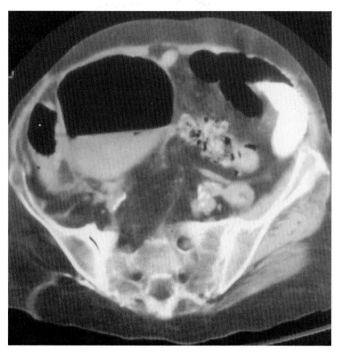

Findings

Case 5.29. Single-contrast barium enema. The folds of the sigmoid colon are thickened and tethered. A barium-filled tract arises from the superior aspect of the sigmoid and partially fills a well-defined gas-filled cavity. A fistulous tract also was present between the sigmoid and the destroyed right hip (not shown).

Case 5.30. Contrast-enhanced CT. A large, thin-walled cavity containing air and fluid is present in the pelvis. This cavity was found to arise from the sigmoid on adjacent images.

Differential Diagnosis
1. Diverticulitis with abscess
2. Giant sigmoid diverticulum

Diagnosis
Giant sigmoid diverticulum

Discussion

A giant sigmoid diverticulum develops as a result of diverticulitis. A persistent tract forms between the colonic lumen and the abscess cavity. The cavity develops a fibrous well-defined capsule over time. Usually, a ball-valve communication is present which allows air and contrast material into the cyst but incomplete emptying. Sometimes these cysts can reach gigantic proportions, occupying a large volume of the abdomen. Operative resection of the diverticulum and affected sigmoid usually is performed for cure and to prevent perforation, torsion, and infarction.

Findings and Treatment of Diverticulitis

CT Findings

- Bowel wall thickening
- Pericolonic soft tissue stranding
- Pericolonic or intramural fluid collection (abscess)

Contrast Enema Findings

- Luminal narrowing
- Intact mucosal folds
- Mass effect (from adjacent inflammatory mass with or without abscess)
- Extravasation of contrast material into pericolonic cavity

Treatment

- Soft tissue stranding, small ($"3$ cm) abscess: antibiotics
- Well-defined abscess (>3 cm): percutaneous drainage
- Poorly defined or multiloculated abscess: operation

CASE 5.31

CASE 5.32

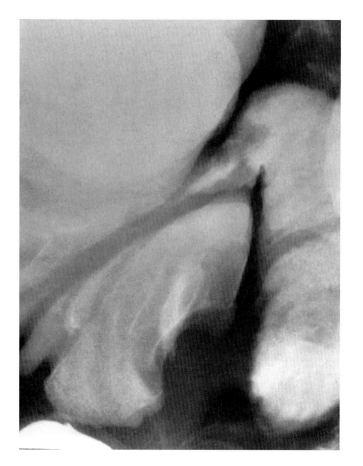

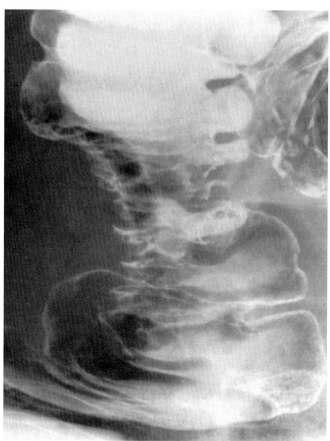

Findings

Case 5.31. Single-contrast barium enema. A smooth-surfaced filling defect is present at the base of the cecum. The appendix did not fill.

Case 5.32. Double-contrast barium enema. Mass effect is present along the lateral aspect of the mid ascending colon. There are thickened and tethered folds in this region.

Differential Diagnosis
1. Appendicitis
2. Serosal metastasis

Diagnosis

Appendicitis (retrocecal location in case 5.32)

Discussion

Appendicitis is caused by obstruction of the appendiceal lumen, with secondary dilatation, infection, inflammation, ischemia, and possible perforation. Clinically, patients usually complain of generalized abdominal discomfort that localizes to the right lower quadrant. Signs of peritoneal irritation or generalized peritonitis may be present. Early recognition of appendicitis is important because the mortality associated with the disease is low, 0.1%, if the appendix is only inflamed but increases to more than 13% with an appendiceal abscess not initially treated with appendectomy. The appendix can be located almost anywhere in the abdomen, and demonstration of the appendix in an unusual location may provide an explanation for confusing clinical signs and symptoms.

CASE 5.33

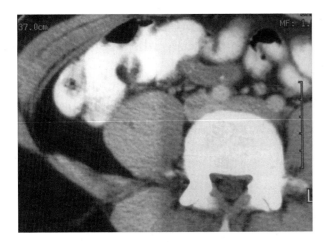

CASE 5.34

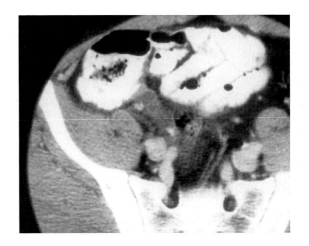

CASE 5.35

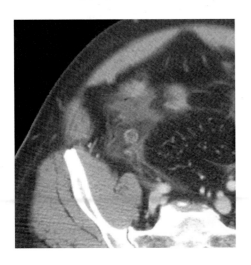

CASE 5.36

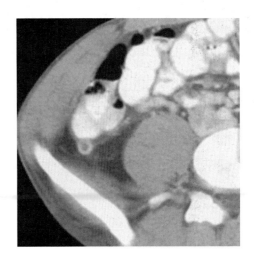

Findings

Case 5.33. Contrast-enhanced CT. The appendix is distended and thick-walled.

Case 5.34. Contrast-enhanced CT. Soft tissue stranding and fluid are present about the fluid-distended appendix.

Case 5.35. Contrast-enhanced CT. An enhancing tubular structure is present in the right lower quadrant. There is soft tissue stranding and fluid in the surrounding fat.

Case 5.36. Contrast-enhanced CT. A hyperenhancing tubular structure is present posterior to the colon with a small amount of surrounding soft tissue stranding.

Differential Diagnosis
1. Appendicitis
2. Mucocele

Diagnosis
Appendicitis

Discussion
The earliest changes of appendicitis include thickening of the walls of the appendix (which is often distended with water-attenuation material) and soft tissue stranding in the periappendiceal fat. Usually patients with appendicitis present with abdominal pain, fever, and leukocytosis. Patients with a mucocele usually do not have symptoms suggesting an acute inflammatory condition.

CASE 5.37

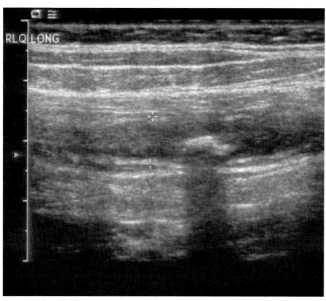

A

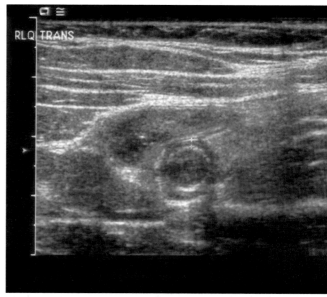

B

Findings

Transabdominal sonography. **A.** Dilated (8 mm), fluid-filled appendix containing an echogenic, posteriorly shadowing appendicolith is visible on this longitudinal sonogram of the right lower quadrant. **B.** Transverse view of the appendix also shows the dilated fluid-filled appendix. The wall of the appendix is thickened (2 mm). The appendix was not compressible.

Differential Diagnosis

Acute appendicitis

Diagnosis

Acute appendicitis

Discussion

Ultrasonography can be useful for directly visualizing the appendix in patients with equivocal clinical findings. Sonography is recommended as the first-line imaging test for children, ovulating women, and pregnant women. It is less useful in obese patients, patients whose abdomen is too tender for compression, and patients with overlying bowel gas.

Graded compression of the right lower abdomen is performed to empty the cecum and right colon of gas and fluid. The appendix usually is visualized at the base of the cecum. Normally, the appendiceal wall does not exceed 2 mm in thickness. Often the normal appendix is not visible, but an appendix that is abnormally distended (≥6 mm diameter) or has a thickened wall (>2 mm) is considered pathologic. A periappendiceal fluid collection can often be identified if the appendix is perforated.

Crohn disease can affect the appendix as part of the spectrum of granulomatous ileocolitis. Occasionally, the disease is localized solely to the appendix. It is usually not possible to distinguish acute appendicitis from Crohn appendicitis.

CASE 5.38

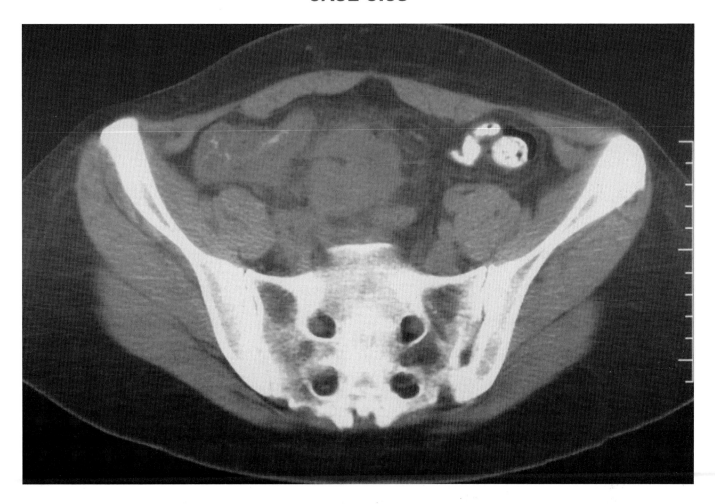

Findings

Unenhanced CT. A soft-tissue–density mass is present in the pelvic mesentery with surrounding inflammatory stranding. There is thickening of the wall of the cecum adjacent to this inflammatory mass.

Differential Diagnosis

Acute appendicitis

Diagnosis

Acute appendicitis (phlegmonous periappendiceal change)

Discussion

The appendix and periappendiceal region can be directly visualized at CT. CT findings of appendicitis include appendiceal mural thickening and enhancement, periappendiceal and mesenteric soft tissue stranding or a soft tissue mass, an appendicolith, thickening of the wall of the colon, fascial thickening, and a periappendiceal fluid collection (abscess). Direct visualization of the appendix is possible in a majority of patients.

CT also is useful for separating appendiceal abscess into three categories: 1) phlegmon, 2) well-defined abscess, and 3) poorly defined multicompartmentalized abscess. Phlegmons are best treated with antibiotics, well-defined abscess with percutaneous drainage, and multicompartmentalized abscess with operative drainage. Interval, elective appendectomy may be required in patients treated nonoperatively.

CASE 5.39

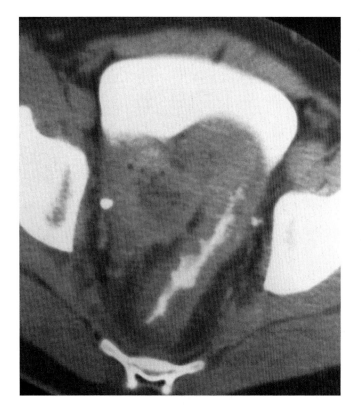

CASE 5.40

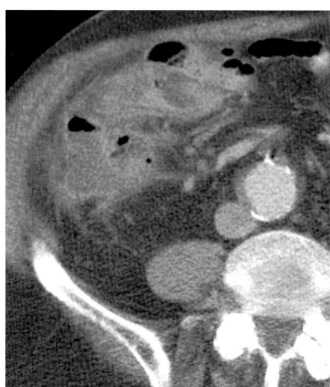

Findings

Case 5.39. Contrast-enhanced CT. A large mass is present in the right side of the pelvis; the center is the attenuation of water and has a thick soft tissue rind. The wall of the sigmoid colon is circumferentially thickened.

Case 5.40. Contrast-enhanced CT. A multicompartmentalized inflammatory mass is present adjacent to the cecum with multiple air-fluid levels.

Differential Diagnosis
1. Appendiceal abscess
2. Diverticular abscess
3. Pelvic inflammatory disease with abscess

Diagnosis
Appendiceal abscess

Discussion

Gangrenous appendicitis and a pelvic abscess were present at operation in both of these cases. Case 5.39 is an example of a well-defined periappendiceal abscess that could be drained percutaneously if safe access is possible. The multicompartmental periappendiceal abscess in case 5.40 usually requires operative drainage.

CASE 5.41

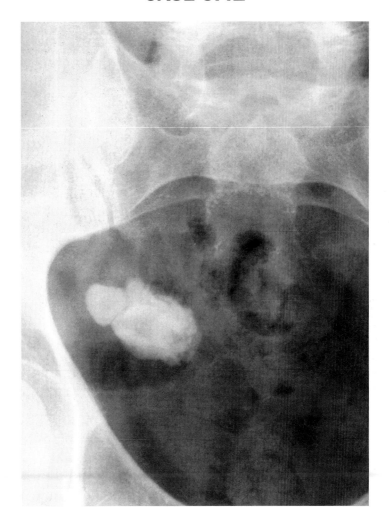

Findings
Abdominal radiograph. Two laminated calcific densities are present in the right lower quadrant.

Differential Diagnosis
1. Appendicolith
2. Calcified mesenteric lymph node
3. Ovarian dermoid tumor
4. Calcified uterine fibroid
5. Enterolith in Meckel diverticulum

Diagnosis
Appendicolith

Discussion
Appendicoliths develop as a result of calcification about an obstructing nidus of fecal debris within the appendiceal lumen. The calculus often has a lucent center and has an average diameter of 2 cm. Approximately 15% of all patients with appendicitis have a visible calculus. Approximately half of all symptomatic patients with a visible appendicolith already have a perforated appendix.

Other findings of appendicitis that may be present on abdominal plain radiography include an atonic gas-filled terminal ileum or cecum (sentinel loop) or a generalized adynamic ileus if peritonitis has developed. It may not be possible to exclude other differential considerations. Enteroliths often have a laminated appearance. Correlation with the clinical history is important. CT is invaluable for further evaluation of a suspicious finding.

Findings of Appendicitis

CT Findings

- Mural thickening >2 mm
- Appendiceal distention, ≥6 mm diameter
- Mural hyperenhancement
- Periappendiceal soft tissue stranding
- Periappendiceal fluid collection
- Appendicolith

Sonographic Findings

- Mural thickening >2 mm
- Appendiceal distention, ≥6 mm diameter
- Noncompressible appendix
- Pain with appendiceal compression
- Periappendiceal fluid collection
- Appendicolith

Contrast Enema Findings

- Nonfilling of the entire appendix (must see bulbous tip to be normal)
- Filling defect at the base of the cecum, without filling of the appendix
- Pain with compression over the appendix
- Appendicolith

CASE 5.42

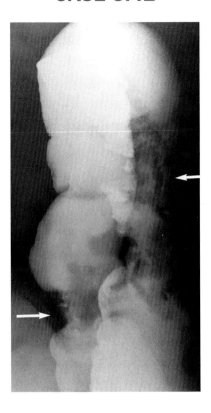

CASE 5.43

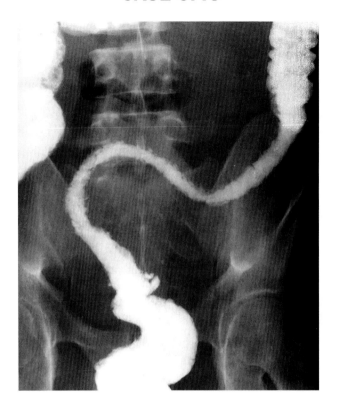

Findings

Case 5.42. Single-contrast barium enema. Two segments (arrows) of luminal narrowing, mucosal irregularity, and ulceration are present in the region of the splenic flexure of the colon.

Case 5.43. Single-contrast barium enema. The entire sigmoid colon is narrowed and irregular in contour.

Differential Diagnosis

1. Crohn disease
2. Ischemic colitis
3. Infectious colitis

Diagnosis

Ischemic colitis

Discussion

Ischemia of the colon can be caused by various events, including low perfusion states and arterial or venous occlusion. The elderly are at highest risk for this condition, but younger individuals also can be affected—especially those with a vasculitis or a coagulopathy. The splenic flexure is the commonest location for ischemic changes in patients with low perfusion states.

Normally, three events can ensue, depending on the degree of ischemia. 1. In mild ischemia, only mucosal sloughing occurs; after the blood supply is reconstituted or collateral blood supply is established, the colon can return to normal. 2. Moderate ischemia affects the deeper layers of the bowel wall with stricture formation after healing. 3. Severe ischemia affects the entire bowel-wall thickness, with transmural necrosis and possible perforation.

Conventional radiographic examination of the ischemic colon usually is limited to plain abdominal radiography in the severely ischemic patient. Adynamic ileus (case 5.125), pneumatosis coli (cases 5.117 and 5.118), pneumoperitoneum, and thickened haustral folds (often described as thumbprinting) (case 5.44) can be seen. Mild and moderate ischemia also may be identified by findings of thickened and edematous haustral folds on plain radiography or barium enema examination. After healing, a stricture may develop, with gradually tapering margins and a featureless mucosal pattern.

CASE 5.44

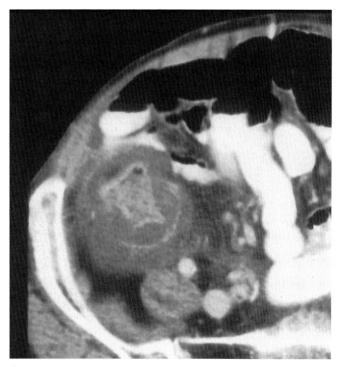

A

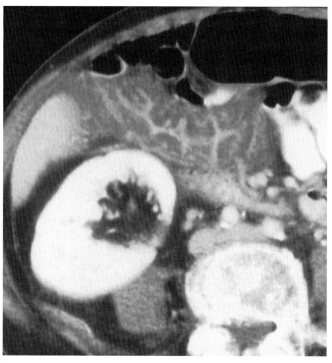

B

Findings
Contrast-enhanced CT. **A** and **B**. The right and transverse colon are thick-walled, with water attenuation changes within the wall. Pericolonic fluid also is present.

Differential Diagnosis
1. Inflammatory bowel disease
2. Pseudomembranous colitis
3. Neutropenic colitis
4. Ischemic colitis

Diagnosis
Ischemic colitis

Discussion
Colonic ischemia often presents with nonspecific findings at CT, including bowel wall thickening, mesenteric soft tissue stranding, ascites, and mesenteric hemorrhage. Secondary findings of arterial or venous occlusion should be sought, as should pneumatosis coli and mesenteric venous or portal venous gas. Clinical correlation often is needed.

CASE 5.45

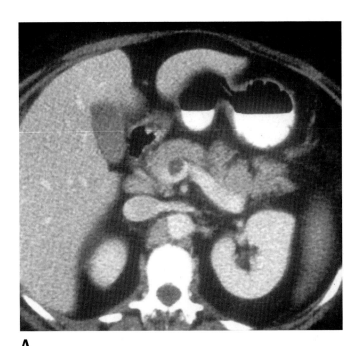

A

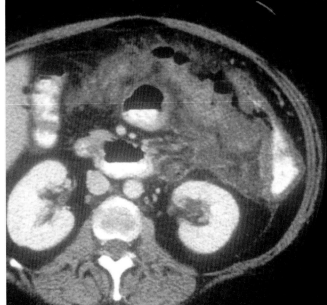

B

Findings

Contrast-enhanced CT. **A.** A filling defect is present in the superior mesenteric vein. **B.** A loop of bowel (transverse and hepatic flexure of the colon) in the upper abdomen has a thick wall, and there is considerable fluid and soft tissue stranding in the adjacent mesentery.

Differential Diagnosis

1. Ischemic colitis due to superior mesenteric vein thrombosis
2. Intra-abdominal abscess with ascending phlebitis and thrombosis of the superior mesenteric vein

Diagnosis

Ischemic colitis due to superior mesenteric vein thrombosis

Discussion

Ischemia can be due to low flow states, arterial emboli, or venous thrombosis. Contrast-enhanced CT has the capability of directly assessing the major blood supply of the splanchnic circulation. A filling defect in either the superior mesenteric artery or vein is a critical clue to the diagnosis of ischemia. Prolonged ischemia (as present in this case) can lead to bowel perforation and abscess. This complication leads to substantial increase in morbidity and mortality. Early diagnosis and treatment are critical for reducing these complications.

CASE 5.46

CASE 5.47

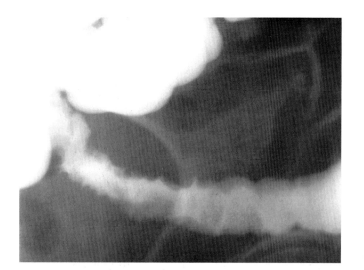

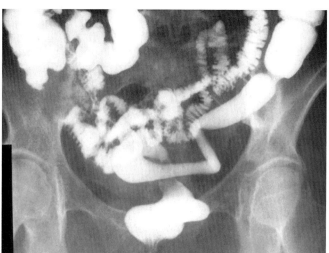

Findings

Case 5.46. Single-contrast barium enema. The sigmoid colon is diffusely narrowed. The luminal contour is irregular and the folds are markedly thickened (thumbprinting).

Case 5.47. Single-contrast barium enema. The proximal rectum and sigmoid colon are diffusely narrowed and featureless, devoid of haustral markings.

Differential Diagnosis
1. Radiation colitis
2. Ischemic colitis

Diagnosis
Radiation colitis

Discussion
Both patients had a history of radiation therapy. The patient in case 5.46 had recent therapy, and the patient in case 5.47 had treatment 26 years previously. Radiation

damage to the ileum and colon remains relatively common. Symptoms develop in patients after a total of 45 Gy has been administered. Most patients have a history of cervical, endometrial, ovarian, or bladder cancer. An occlusive endarteritis is the chief pathologic alteration. Acutely, edema and mucosal ulceration are present. The bowel often has a shaggy appearance, with fold thickening and luminal narrowing.

Radiation-induced strictures are common, developing more than 2 years after radiation treatment, and of variable lengths. Severe strictures (especially those in the small bowel) can cause luminal obstruction. The normal mucosal markings (haustral folds) are often absent, and there is a gradual tapering of the lumen from normal to abnormal. Patients may complain of diarrhea, cramping, or bleeding. Often the symptoms respond poorly to conservative therapy and operation is required. Surgical treatment can be difficult and associated with a high morbidity due to adherent loops, adhesions, poor tissues, and impaired healing.

CASE 5.48

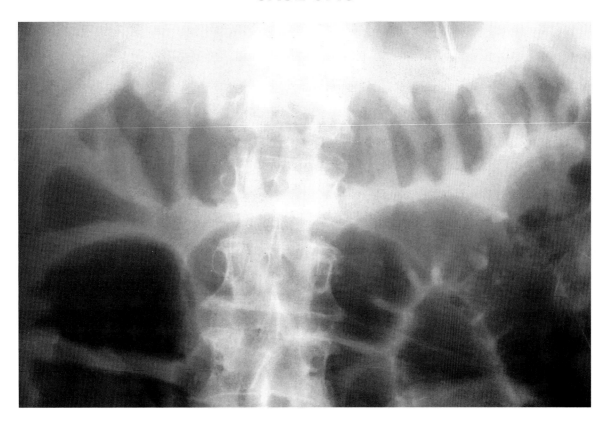

Findings
Abdominal radiograph. The transverse colon is gas-filled and the haustral markings are diffusely thickened.

Differential Diagnosis
1. Infectious colitis
2. Pseudomembranous colitis
3. Ischemic colitis
4. Acute inflammatory bowel disease
5. Neutropenic colitis

Diagnosis
Pseudomembranous colitis

Discussion
Pseudomembranous colitis is caused by the potent enterotoxins produced by *Clostridium difficile*, a gram-negative bacillus. Infection by this organism usually follows antibiotic therapy (originally described after lincomycin or clindamycin administration). Patients usually present with watery diarrhea. Sigmoidoscopy usually shows multiple yellowish white plaques covering the colonic mucosa. The diagnosis can be confirmed by performing a stool assay for *C. difficile* enterotoxin.

Radiographically, the disease often can be suggested on the basis of the plain abdominal radiograph. Haustral folds throughout the colon can appear thickened (as in this case). The disease occasionally can spare portions of the colon. Although usually involving the whole colon, it is possible for a patient with this disease to have a normal proctoscopic examination, with disease in the more proximal colon.

Inflammatory polyps may be visible within the colon in patients with inflammatory bowel disease (cases 5.4, 5.5, and 5.6). Ischemic colitis usually affects older persons and involves a segment of bowel (often the splenic flexure) rather than involving the bowel diffusely (case 5.43). A history of antibiotic use is helpful for diagnosing pseudomembranous colitis, and a history of profound neutropenia and administration of cytotoxic agents is helpful for diagnosing neutropenic colitis.

CASE 5.49

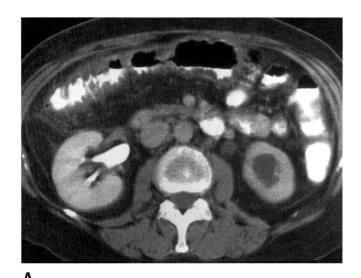

A

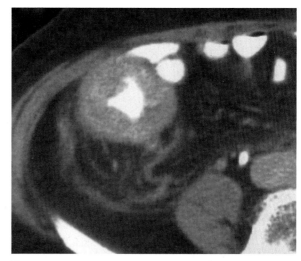

B

Findings

Contrast-enhanced CT. **A** and **B.** The wall of the right and transverse colon is circumferentially thickened. Pericolonic soft tissue stranding also is present.

Differential Diagnosis

1. Infectious colitis
2. Pseudomembranous colitis
3. Ischemic colitis
4. Acute inflammatory bowel disease
5. Neutropenic colitis

Diagnosis

Pseudomembranous colitis

Discussion

The findings are nonspecific and could be due to any type of acute colitis. Pseudomembranous colitis was proved by stool assay for *Clostridium difficile* enterotoxin. The CT findings in patients with pseudomembranous colitis usually are nonspecific, with colonic wall thickening. The wall thickening may be diffuse or segmental.

Because many patients with pseudomembranous colitis have fever, leukocytosis, and vague abdominal complaints, CT often is done to exclude an intra-abdominal abscess. The findings at CT can be helpful for directing further investigation of the colon, whereas endoscopy and stool assay can show the typical yellowish white plaques and the presence of the offending enterotoxin. Once the diagnosis is confirmed, the usual treatment is vancomycin.

CASE 5.50

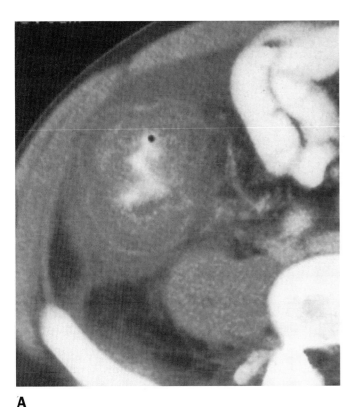

A

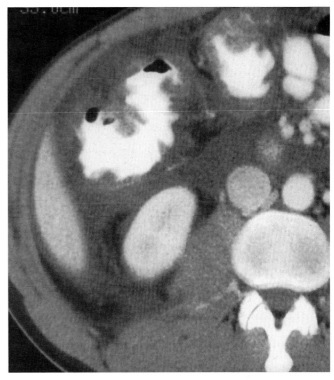

B

Findings

Contrast-enhanced CT. **A** and **B.** Marked thickening of the wall of the right colon and ascites are present.

Differential Diagnosis

1. Infectious colitis
2. Pseudomembranous colitis
3. Ischemic colitis
4. Acute inflammatory bowel disease
5. Neutropenic colitis

Diagnosis

Neutropenic colitis

Discussion

This patient was being treated for acute lymphocytic leukemia and was severely neutropenic at the time of this examination. Neutropenic typhlitis was suggested in view of the history. Neutropenic typhlitis develops in severely neutropenic patients (usually patients with leukemia or lymphoma who are undergoing chemotherapy) with an associated adynamic ileus. The ileus-induced stasis, distention, and possible ischemia; the direct cytotoxic effect on the mucosa from the medication; and the inability to mount an immunologic defense are important predisposing factors. Pathologically, mucosal and submucosal necrosis, edema, and hemorrhage are present. Perforation can occur. Radiographically, an adynamic ileus is present on abdominal plain radiographs (case 5.125). Thickening of the colon wall, fascial thickening, and pericolonic soft tissue stranding are typical findings at CT.

CASE 5.51

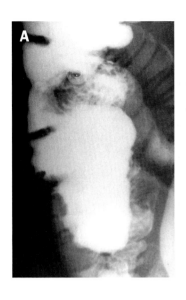
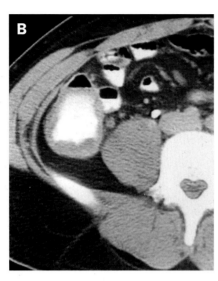
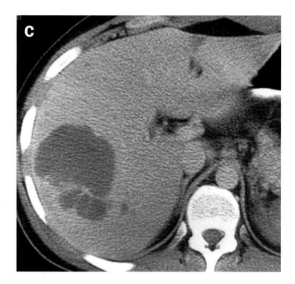

Findings

A. Single-contrast barium enema. The cecum is narrowed with an irregular contour.

B. Contrast-enhanced CT. The wall of the right colon is thickened.

C. Contrast-enhanced CT. A multiloculated, low (fluid)-density mass is present in the right lobe of the liver.

Differential Diagnosis

1. Amebiasis
2. Colon cancer
3. Inflammatory bowel disease

Diagnosis

Amebiasis

Discussion

Amebiasis is an infection by the protozoan *Entamoeba histolytica*, which is endemic throughout the world—particularly in tropical climates. Infection occurs by ingestion of the amebic cyst, which in the alkaline environment of the small bowel will shed its inner capsule and release trophozoites. Trophozoites burrow into the intestinal wall—most commonly the cecum and sigmoid colon. Multifocal or confluent ulcerations develop at the site of the bowel wall penetration. Secondary bacterial invasion of the bowel causes marked submucosal edema, bowel wall thickening, and even hemorrhage (as in this case). A focal mass (ameboma) can develop. The protozoan infection can spread from the bowel to any part of the body by direct extension and hematogenous and lymphatic dissemination. A hepatic abscess is the usual extraintestinal site for infection (as in this case). A liver abscess can erode through the diaphragm and result in pleural, pericardial, bronchial, or lung infection. Penetration of an ulcer through the bowel wall can result in a pericolonic abscess, fistula, peritonitis, or distant intraperitoneal abscess. Long-term changes of amebiasis usually include benign-appearing colonic strictures. Treatment of this disease is with antiamebic therapy. Surgical treatment of this disease is associated with high morbidity and mortality, often without cure.

Radiologically, the cecum and sigmoid colon are affected most often. Involvement of the terminal ileum occurs in a minority of patients. Initially, the patient may have mucosal changes resembling ulcerative colitis (granular-appearing mucosa with fine ulcerations and thickened and edematous haustra). Deeper and more extensive ulcerations may be seen as the disease progresses. The cecum often becomes nondistensible and conical in shape. Amebomas can be indistinguishable from colon cancer. Multiplicity of lesions, ulceration elsewhere in the colon, young age, and travel history may all be helpful for differentiating this disease from carcinoma.

CASE 5.52

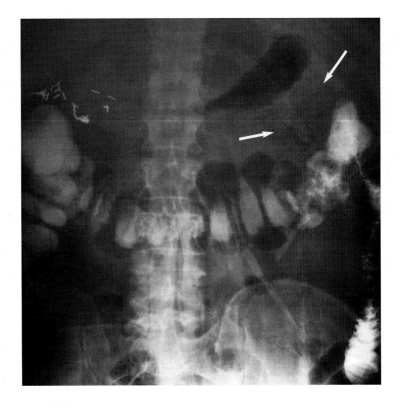

Findings

Abdominal radiograph. An extraluminal gas (arrows) collection (multiple small bubbles) is present in the region of the pancreatic bed. Luminal narrowing and thickened folds are present in the descending colon, which contains contrast material from a recent barium enema.

Differential Diagnosis

Pancreatic abscess

Diagnosis

Pancreatic abscess

Discussion

Imaging procedures are not necessary in all patients for making the diagnosis of acute pancreatitis. Imaging tests are invaluable for confirming a suggested diagnosis and for detecting a complication of acute pancreatitis (including a pancreatic abscess). CT and sonography have replaced abdominal plain radiography and intraluminal contrast studies when the diagnosis of acute pancreatitis is suggested. In some patients, however, symptoms may be nonspecific and abdominal plain radiography is used to assess for the presence of adynamic ileus, obstruction, or tube placements.

A pancreatic effusion is commonly associated with acute pancreatitis. Most often the effusion is located within the left anterior pararenal space and lesser sac. The mass effect from this fluid can displace the stomach anteriorly and the colon inferiorly. As the volume of the pancreatic effusion increases, it can extend inferiorly, adjacent to the descending colon and along the transverse mesocolon. Inflammatory changes (thickened folds, spasm, narrowing) of the transverse and descending colon can be seen. The splenic flexure of the colon usually is involved with inflammatory changes because of its proximity to the pancreatic tail. A pancreatic effusion also can dissect within the leaves of the small bowel mesentery and cause ascites in patients with severe disease. The colon cutoff sign has been regarded as a classic radiographic finding of acute pancreatitis. Patients with this sign have gaseous distention of the right and transverse colon, with little gas visible beyond the splenic flexure (as seen in this case). It can be impossible to exclude colonic obstruction on plain radiographs, and a contrast enema or CT may be required.

CASE 5.53

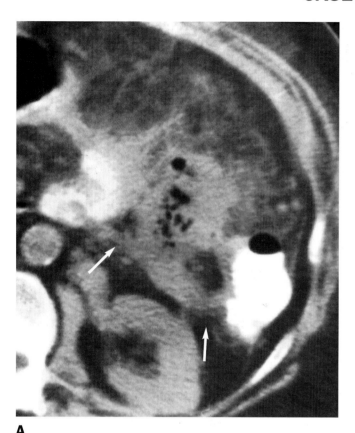

A

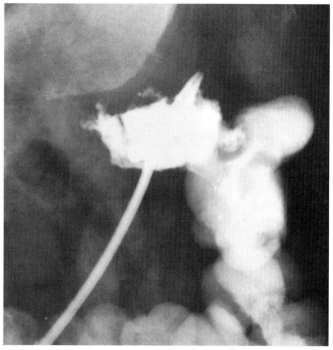

B

Findings

A. Contrast-enhanced CT. An abscess is present in the pancreatic bed. An inflammatory reaction and two tracts (arrows) to the splenic flexure of the colon can be identified.

B. Sinogram. A drainage catheter in the pancreatic abscess cavity is injected with contrast material. A fistula is present between the abscess and the splenic flexure of the colon.

Differential Diagnosis

Pancreatic abscess with pancreatico-colonic fistula

Diagnosis

Pancreatic abscess with pancreatico-colonic fistula

Discussion

A pancreatic abscess is a life-threatening complication of acute pancreatitis. CT and sonography are sensitive imaging methods for detecting peripancreatic fluid—which may or may not be infected. The finding of gas in the pancreatic bed is highly suggestive of infection but is not diagnostic. Correlation with clinical information and percutaneous aspiration of fluid are important steps for determining the proper diagnosis. Fistula formation between the pancreatic bed and splenic flexure of the colon is a relatively common complication of pancreatitis and can lead to a pancreatic abscess. Knowledge that a fistula is present is critical for planning proper therapeutic intervention. Colonic resection or percutaneous drainage may be necessary. If the fistula is not repaired operatively, long-term catheter drainage often is required.

CASE 5.54

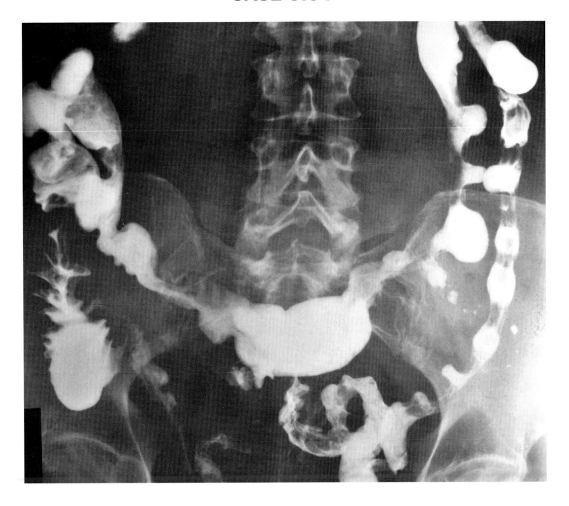

Findings
Single-contrast barium enema. Multiple wide-mouth sacculations are present along the antimesenteric border of the transverse colon.

Differential Diagnosis
1. Scleroderma
2. Crohn disease

Diagnosis
Scleroderma

Discussion
Scleroderma causes patchy replacement of the muscular layers of the colon with collagen and elastic fibers. Intimal proliferation of the feeding arteries with possible ischemia also can occur.

Radiographically, the antimesenteric border of the colon may develop sacculations or pseudodiverticula as a result of the limp supporting tissues in the wall of the colon. The mesenteric side is not affected because the tissues and vessels in this region continue to support the bowel wall. Haustral markings may be lost, and redundancy (due to dilatation and elongation) may be present. Localized areas of narrowing also may be seen as a result of ischemia.

The main differential consideration is Crohn colitis, with multiple areas of asymmetric bowel wall involvement and pseudodiverticula (case 5.18). The asymmetric changes in Crohn disease usually are segmental, with normal intervening colon. The pseudodiverticula in patients with Crohn disease may affect either the mesenteric or the antimesenteric border of the colon. The clinical history is often revealing.

CASE 5.55

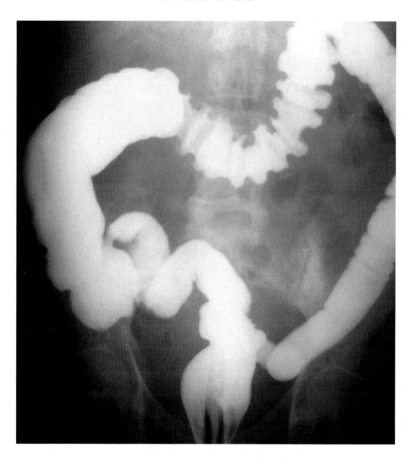

Findings
Single-contrast barium enema. Segmental, haustral fold thickening is present in the transverse colon.

Differential Diagnosis
1. Ischemic colitis
2. Acute radiation colitis
3. Pancreatitis
4. Crohn disease
5. Mastocytosis

Diagnosis
Mastocytosis

Discussion
This finding is nonspecific and could be the result of several diseases causing bowel wall edema or inflammation or infiltration. This patient was found to have mastocytosis.

Mastocytosis is a rare condition of abnormal deposition of mast cells, often within the skin (urticaria pigmentosa) and less commonly within other organs (liver, spleen, bones, alimentary tract). Gastrointestinal symptoms usually include nausea, vomiting, and diarrhea. The incidence of peptic ulcer disease is increased in mastocytosis, presumably due to histamine-mediated acid secretion. Malabsorption also can occur with diffuse small bowel involvement. Many patients experience an intolerance to alcohol, which can exacerbate symptoms.

Pathologically, cellular infiltration (mast cells) and edema usually are present within the bowel wall. The small bowel is most commonly affected, but potentially any portion of the gut can be involved.

Radiographically, fold thickening and distortion are usually present (as in this case). Occasionally, a diffuse, fine nodular pattern of sandlike lucencies is seen. Urticarial lesions also have been described. Skeletal sclerosis also may be a helpful clue.

CASE 5.56

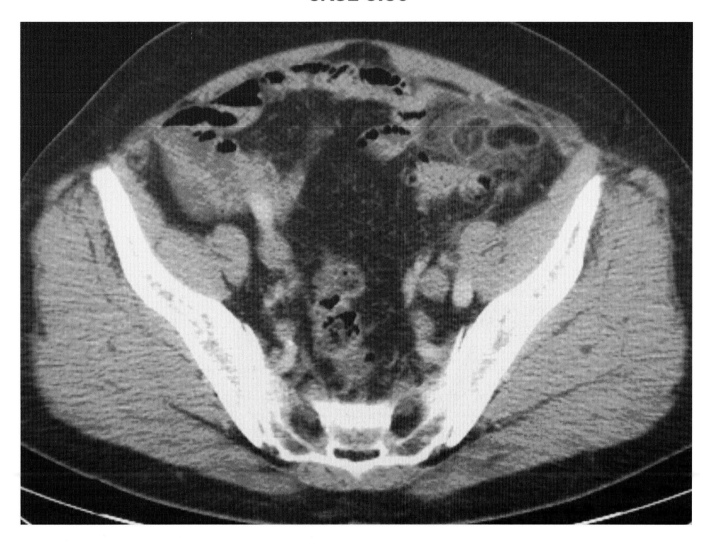

Findings

Contrast-enhanced CT. A fat-attenuation mass with a peripheral rim of higher attenuation and surrounding inflammatory changes is present in the mesentery anterior to the sigmoid colon. There is sigmoid diverticulosis, but the wall of the adjacent colon is not thickened.

Differential Diagnosis

1. Epiploic appendagitis
2. Diverticulitis
3. Omental torsion
4. Mesenteric panniculitis

Diagnosis

Epiploic appendagitis

Discussion

Epiploic appendages are peritoneal outpouchings that arise from the serosal surface of the colon and usually measure 2 to 5 cm in length. Epiploic appendagitis is caused by torsion of the epiploic appendages with secondary ischemia. The most common part of the colon involved by acute appendagitis is the sigmoid colon. The disorder usually is self-limited and treated symptomatically with pain relief. This disorder usually is differentiated from diverticulitis by absence of bowel wall thickening and the epicenter of the inflammatory process centered away from the colon. Mesenteric panniculitis usually is centered in the root of the mesentery. Omental torsion usually involves a larger fatty region and often is located on the right side of the abdomen.

Inflammatory Diseases of the Colon

		Case
Ulcerative colitis	Circumferential, symmetric involvement starting in the rectum and progressing proximally. Granular mucosa acutely; rigid, shortened colon chronically	5.1–5.13
Crohn disease	Asymmetric involvement with skip areas, aphthous ulcers, or cobblestone appearance. Usually rectal sparing. Perianal disease is common	5.14–5.18
Diverticulitis	Long-segment colonic thickening and inflammatory changes in region with diverticula. Abscess should be sought	5.19–5.30
Appendicitis	Acute abdomen, lumen ≥6 mm in diameter, wall >2 mm in diameter with mural enhancement, periappendiceal stranding or fluid collection, appendicolith	5.31–5.41
Ischemic colitis	Low-perfusion states and arterial or venous occlusion. Often seen at splenic flexure. Pneumatosis and portal venous gas should be sought	5.42–5.45
Radiation colitis	Acute changes include fold thickening and shaggy appearance. Rigidity and strictures are seen chronically. Restricted to radiation port	5.46 and 5.47
Pseudomembranous colitis	*Clostridium difficile* infection after antibiotic therapy. Usually pancolitis with marked mural thickening	5.48 and 5.49
Neutropenic colitis	Usually patients with leukemia or lymphoma undergoing chemotherapy. Usually right-sided colonic involvement	5.50
Infectious colitis	Variable colonic involvement, travel history, stool cultures	5.51
Pancreatitis	Inflammatory thickening and narrowing of transverse and proximal descending colon adjacent to pancreatic tail	5.52 and 5.53
Scleroderma	Sacculations or pseudodiverticula on antimesenteric border of colon	5.54
Mastocytosis	Small bowel most commonly affected. Usually fine nodular pattern	5.55
Epiploic appendagitis	Caused by torsion of epiploic appendices with secondary ischemia. Pericolonic fat stranding with no colonic wall thickening	5.56

CASE 5.57

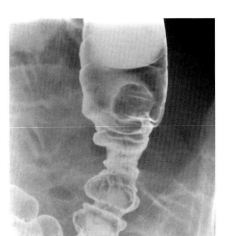

CASE 5.58

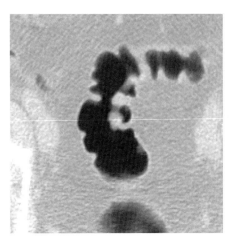

CASE 5.59

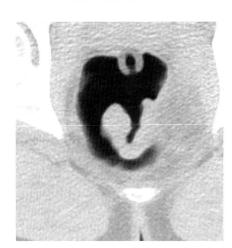

Findings

Case 5.57. Double-contrast barium enema. A pedunculated filling defect is present in the mid transverse colon.

Case 5.58. CT colonography. Pedunculated filling defect in mid sigmoid colon.

Case 5.59. CT colonography. Pedunculated filling defect in rectum.

Differential Diagnosis

Polyp, pedunculated

Diagnosis

Polyp, pedunculated

Discussion

Polyps of the colon can be classified by histologic type: hyperplastic (retention), adenomatous, and hamartomatous. There are no reliable radiographic findings to distinguish adenomatous polyps from the other types. Hyperplastic polyps generally are small (<1 cm diameter), and these small lesions are believed not to have malignant potential.

Adenomatous polyps can be further classified into three histologic subtypes: tubular, tubulovillous, and villous adenomas. Most authorities now believe that the majority of adenocarcinomas of the colon arise from preexisting adenomas. Polyps with a higher percentage of villous features are at a higher risk for malignant transformation than are tubular adenomas. Polyp diameter is also a key factor in assessing the risk of malignancy in an adenomatous polyp because the larger the polyp, the higher the risk. Muto et al. tabulated these data as follows:

Malignant Potential of Colorectal Adenomas

Histologic type	% Malignant potential, by size		
	<1 cm	1-2 cm	>2 cm
Tubular	1.0	10.2	34.7
Tubulovillous	3.9	7.4	45.8
Villous	9.5	10.3	52.5

Modified from Muto T, Bussey HJR, Morson BC: The evolution of cancer of the colon and rectum. Cancer. 1975;36:2251-70. By permission of the American Cancer Society.

Hamartomatous polyps are associated with Peutz-Jeghers syndrome (case 5.68) and with juvenile polyposis (case 5.73).

CASE 5.60

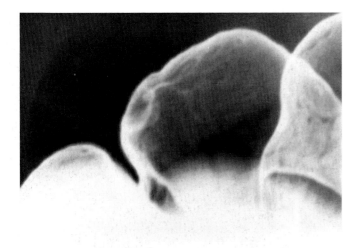

CASE 5.61

A

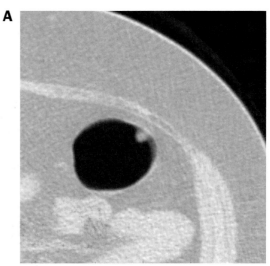

B

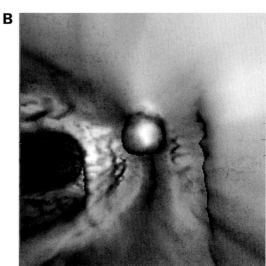

Findings

Case 5.60. Double-contrast barium enema. A sessile filling defect is present in the colon.

Case 5.61. CT colonography. **A** and **B**. A small half-sphere filling defect is present in the colon on both the two- and three-dimensional endoluminal views.

Differential Diagnosis
1. Polyp
2. Stool

Diagnosis
Polyp

Discussion

Polyps are commonly multiple, and synchronous lesions are seen in 25% to 50% of patients. Nearly half of all polyps are located in the rectosigmoid, 20% in the right colon, and 29% to 35% in the transverse and descending colon. Polyps at CT should be homogeneous soft tissue attenuation, whereas stool often is inhomogeneous internally, containing air or fat attenuation.

CASE 5.62

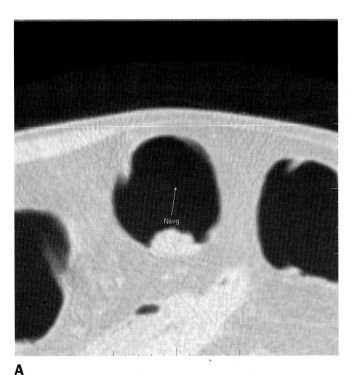

A

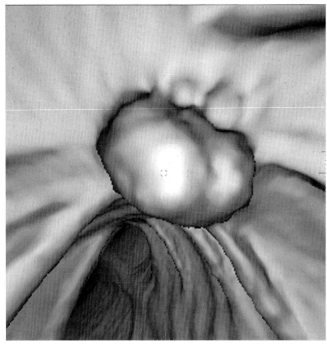

B

Findings

CT colonography. **A.** A 2-cm filling defect is present in the colon. **B.** Three-dimensional endoluminal view shows the filling defect as a lobulated mass, distinct from the nearby haustral fold.

Differential Diagnosis

1. Polyp
2. Cancer
3. Stool

Diagnosis

Large adenomatous colon polyp

Discussion

The incidence of malignancy increases with increasing polyp size and is less than 1% in polyps less than 1 cm in diameter, 10% in polyps 1 to 2 cm in diameter, and 40% in polyps more than 2 cm in diameter.

CASE 5.63

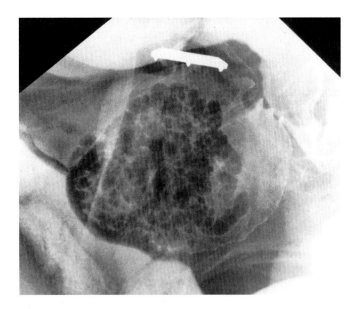

CASE 5.64

A

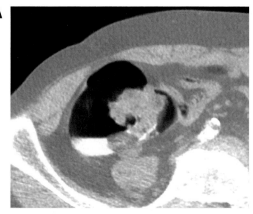

B

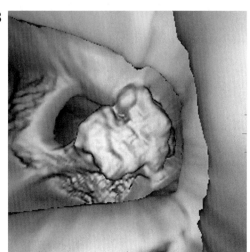

Findings

Case 5.63. Single-contrast barium enema. A large polypoid mass is present in the base of the cecum. Barium fills the interstices of the mass. Its surface appearance resembles a cauliflower or raspberry.

Case 5.64. CT colonography. **A.** Axial two-dimensional image. An irregular-shaped filling defect is present in the ascending colon. **B.** Three-dimensional endoluminal image. The surface of the lesion is markedly irregular.

Differential Diagnosis

1. Villous adenoma
2. Retained stool

Diagnosis

Villous adenoma

Discussion

Villous adenomas can be recognized if the typical surface features are visible. Characteristically, barium fills the interstices of the tumor between the individual fronds. Unfortunately, it is usually not possible to detect villous features within small polyps. Usually, polyps must be nearly 2 cm in diameter before the typical features are recognizable. Villous tumors usually are soft and compressible, and rectal lesions can easily be missed on digital examinations. Because villous tumors have a high risk of malignancy, they should be removed.

CASE 5.65

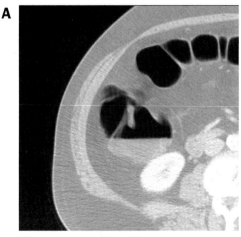

A

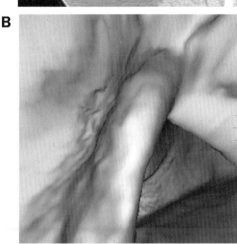

B

CASE 5.66

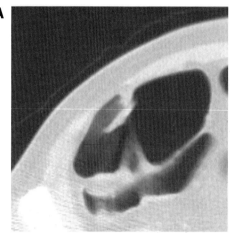

A

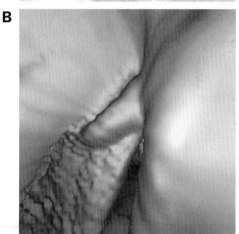

B

Findings

Case 5.65. CT colonography. **A** and **B.** A cigar-shaped filling defect is present within the ascending colon lumen. The abnormality is more difficult to see on three-dimensional endoluminal view.

Case 5.66. CT colonography. **A** and **B.** A flat, somewhat lobulated filling defect is present within the ascending colon. The filling defect is less conspicuous on the three-dimensional endoluminal view.

Differential Diagnosis

1. Flat polyp
2. Stool

Diagnosis

Flat polyp (adenoma)

Discussion

Flat polyps can be difficult to detect and can be either adenomatous or hyperplastic. Flat adenomas may have a higher prevalence of malignancy than sessile and pedunculated polyps. They are most commonly found in the right colon. Focal regions of soft tissue thickening identified on two-dimensional axial images can be an important clue for the presence of a flat polyp.

CASE 5.67

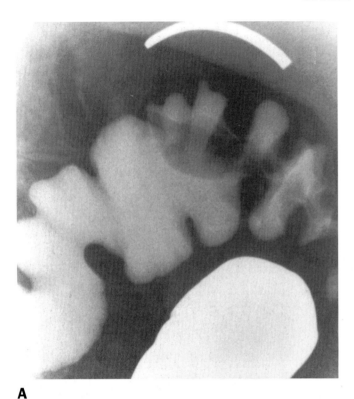

A

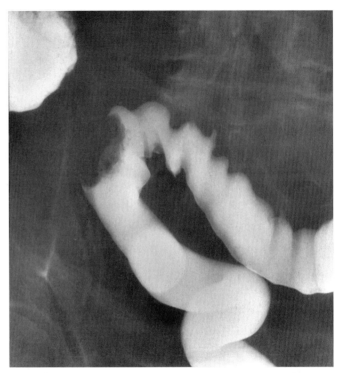

B

Findings
Single-contrast barium enema. **A.** A large pedunculated polyp is present in the sigmoid colon. **B.** Almost 8 years later, a large sessile carcinoma has developed at the site of the previous polyp.

Differential Diagnosis
Adenoma to carcinoma transformation

Diagnosis
Adenoma to carcinoma transformation

Discussion
Today, most researchers believe that the majority of colon cancers arise from preexisting polyps. This case supports that hypothesis. The role of radiologists is to detect all polypoid colonic lesions with the hope that they can be removed successfully before malignant degeneration. Risk factors for the development of colorectal polyps include increasing age, history of previous polyps, and family history of colon polyps or carcinoma. Patients with ulcerative colitis also have a higher incidence of colon cancer developing.

American Cancer Society Guidelines for the Early Detection of Colon Cancer

Beginning at age 50 years,* the American Cancer Society recommends men and women follow one of the following five testing options:

1. Yearly fecal occult blood test (FOBT)
2. Flexible sigmoidoscopy every 5 years
3. Yearly FOBT and flexible sigmoidoscopy every 5 years†
4. Double-contrast barium enema every 5 years
5. Colonoscopy every 10 years

*Persons known to be at increased risk for colorectal cancer (because of inflammatory bowel disease, personal or family history of polyps or cancer, familial syndromes such as familial adenomatous polyposis or hereditary nonpolyposis colorectal cancer) need to begin screening at an early age and may need more frequent screening.
†The combination of FOBT and flexible sigmoidoscopy is preferred over either test alone. Note: A digital rectal examination is not an acceptable substitute for the above-recommended tests.

CASE 5.68

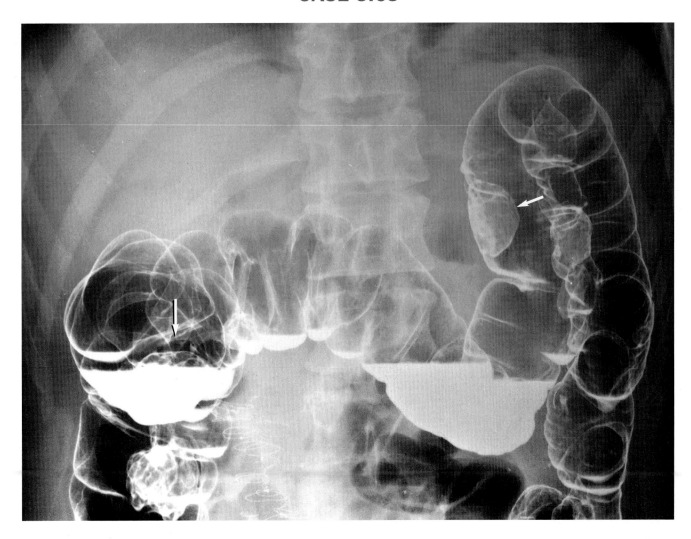

Findings

Double-contrast barium enema. Multiple large polyps (arrows) are present in the colon. The patient had multiple mucocutaneous pigmentations at physical examination.

Differential Diagnosis

Peutz-Jeghers syndrome

Diagnosis

Peutz-Jeghers syndrome

Discussion

Peutz-Jeghers syndrome is a disease of mucocutaneous pigmentation and gastrointestinal polyposis. Patients usually present with symptoms of abdominal cramping, rectal bleeding, melena, or anemia. Cramping often is due to transient intussusceptions within the small bowel.

Gastrointestinal polyps in Peutz-Jeghers syndrome most frequently are found in the small bowel (95%) (cases 4.7 and 4.8), but they also can be identified in the colon and rectum (30%) and stomach (25%). The polyps can vary in size and usually are less numerous in the stomach and colon. Polyps in the stomach and small bowel are hamartomatous, but colonic polyps usually are adenomatous (and potentially malignant). Alimentary tract malignancies develop in 2% to 3% of patients with Peutz-Jeghers syndrome.

CASE 5.69

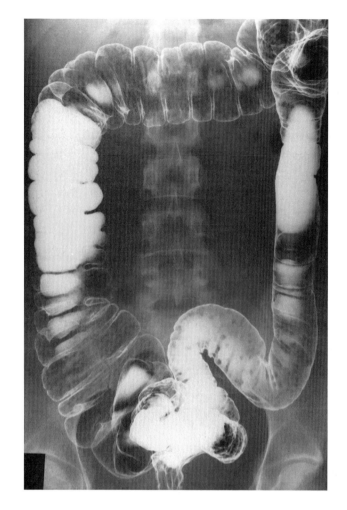

CASE 5.71

A

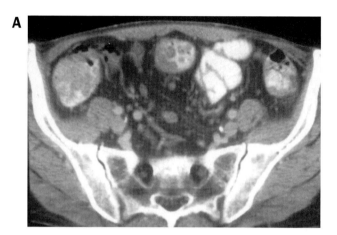

B

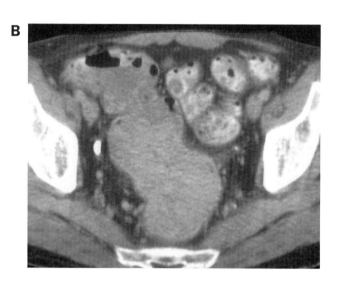

CASE 5.70

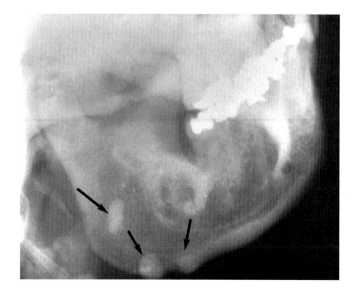

CASE 5.72

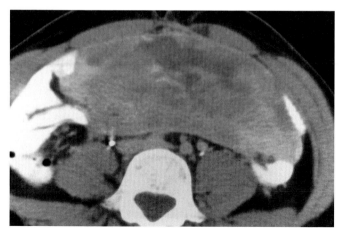

Findings

Case 5.69. Double-contrast barium enema. Multiple polypoid filling defects are present throughout the colon. These findings are characteristic of a polyposis syndrome.

Case 5.70. Radiograph of the mandible. Multiple osteomas (arrows) are visible arising from the mandible.

Case 5.71. Contrast-enhanced CT. **A** and **B.** Multiple filling defects are present throughout the colon, including a very large filling defect that occupies most of the lumen of the rectosigmoid colon.

Case 5.72. Contrast-enhanced CT. A huge soft tissue tumor occupies a large portion of the abdomen.

Differential Diagnosis

Polyposis syndrome—familial adenomatous polyposis syndrome

Diagnosis

Polyposis syndrome—familial adenomatous polyposis syndrome

Discussion

Familial adenomatous polyposis is the commonest of the polyposis syndromes, characterized by large numbers of adenomatous polyps that often carpet the entire colon. Patients often present with rectal bleeding in their early 30s; if colectomy is not performed, they will die of adenocarcinoma of the colon in their early 40s. Family screening should be performed in sporadic cases. Radiographically, innumerable polyps are identified throughout the entire colon and may be found in the small bowel and stomach. Occasionally, the polyps may conglomerate and appear as bizarre filling defects in the colon.

Gardner syndrome is a variant of familial polyposis, with various mesenchymal-derived extraintestinal manifestations. Soft tissue tumors in patients with Gardner syndrome include 1) sebaceous cysts; 2) benign mesenchymal tumors, such as fibromas, lipofibromas, lipomas, leiomyomas, and neurofibromas; 3) malignant mesenchymal tumors; and 4) fibrous tissue proliferation producing desmoid tumors, keloids, peritoneal adhesions, and mesenteric and retroperitoneal fibrosis. Large abdominal desmoid tumors (as in case 5.72) usually occur after total colectomy. Localized areas of dense bone (osteomas) commonly are present, often involving the skull, mandible, and maxilla. Long bone cortical thickening and dental abnormalities also are common.

CASE 5.73

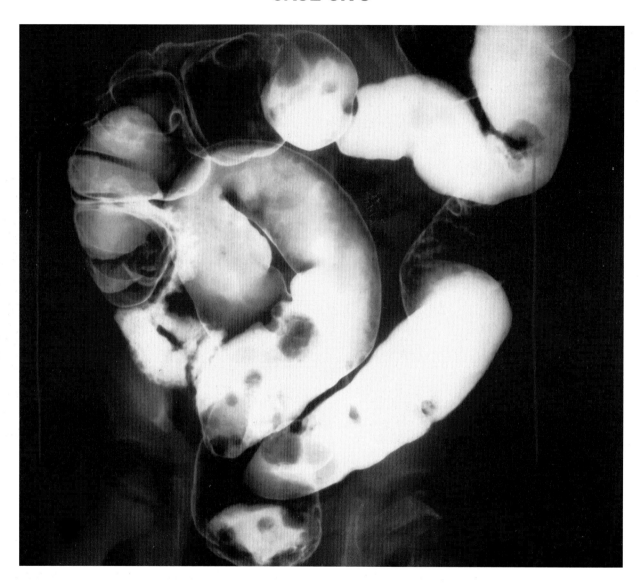

Findings
Double-contrast barium enema. Multiple variable-sized polyps are present in the colon.

Differential Diagnosis
Polyposis syndrome—unknown type

Diagnosis
Juvenile polyposis syndrome

Discussion
Juvenile polyposis is usually a disorder of children which includes solitary or multiple hamartomatous polyps. Histologically, these polyps have abundant connective tissue stroma containing mucin-filled cystic spaces lined with epithelium. Sporadic cases usually are associated with only a few polyps, whereas the hereditary form is associated with multiple polyps (juvenile polyposis coli). In the hereditary disease, polyps can be found throughout the alimentary tract. Juvenile polyps may coexist with adenomatous polyps in patients with familial adenomatous polyposis syndrome. The commonest symptoms and signs are rectal bleeding, anemia, and anal prolapse of a polyp.

CASE 5.74

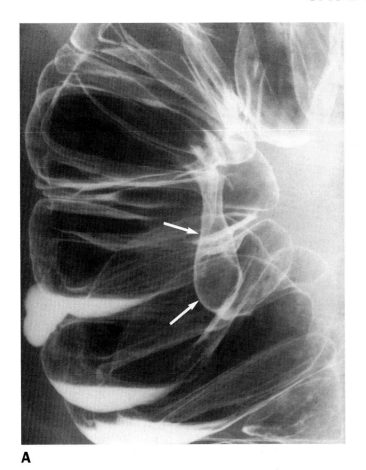

A

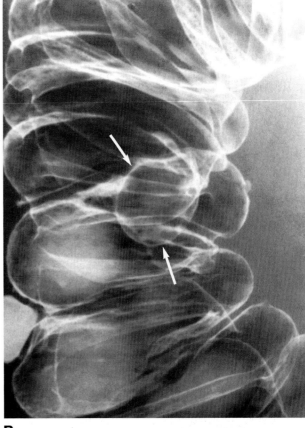

B

Findings

Double-contrast barium enema. **A.** A pedunculated, smooth-surfaced polyp (arrows) is present along the medial aspect of the ascending colon. **B.** The polyp (arrows) has changed shape with a change in position and distention. It now appears as a broad-based submucosal mass.

Differential Diagnosis

1. Pedunculated polyp
2. Lipoma

Diagnosis

Lipoma

Discussion

The smooth surface of this lesion indicates its submucosal origin. Its changeable shape favors a lipoma, which was verified histologically. Colonic lipomas are the most frequent submucosal tumors of the colon. They are slow-growing, benign neoplasms that are most commonly found in the right side of the colon. Most lipomas are asymptomatic and found incidentally. Occasionally, lipomas can be the lead point for an intussusception, and patients may present with abdominal pain and rectal bleeding (case 5.76).

A filling defect (usually >3 cm) with a very smooth surface is most often seen at contrast enema. The tumor is pliable and readily changes shape with compression or with collapse of the colonic lumen. Within the distended colon, the mass often is round, elliptical, or ovoid. It is common for the tumor to elongate and become sausage-shaped within the evacuated colon. The ileocecal valve also may become lipomatous. Often the valve appears enlarged, with a very smooth surface. Pliability and distensibility are key features of a lipomatous tumor which distinguish it from other submucosal lesions.

CASE 5.75

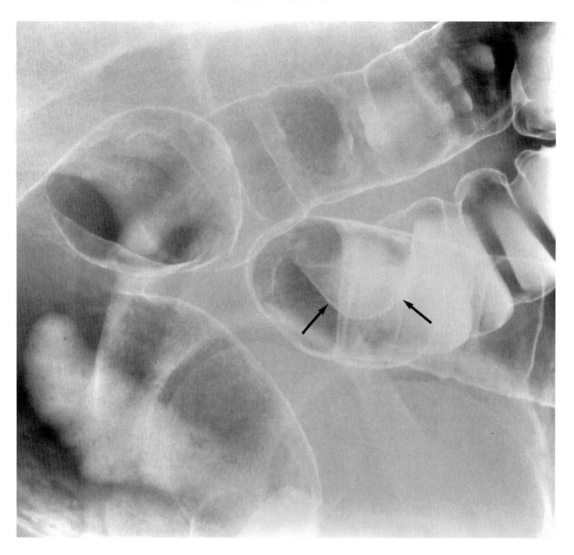

Findings

Double-contrast barium enema. A 3-cm smooth-surfaced filling defect (arrows) in the sigmoid colon. The mass appears to make obtuse angles with the normal colon wall, but it does not displace the lumen of the colon and appears intraluminal in location.

Differential Diagnosis

1. Lipoma
2. Gastrointestinal stromal tumor
3. Serosal metastasis

Diagnosis

Lipoma

Discussion

Lipomas are the commonest submucosal tumor of the colon. Although they most often occur in the right colon, they can be found anywhere. The smooth surface and changeable shape are characteristic findings. Stromal tumors rarely arise in the colon, but when they do the rectum is the commonest location. Serosal metastasis indicates a tumor that has spread to the peritoneum. A history of a primary tumor, multiple lesions, and the presence of tethering of the colon are helpful additional features that strongly suggest this diagnosis.

CASE 5.76

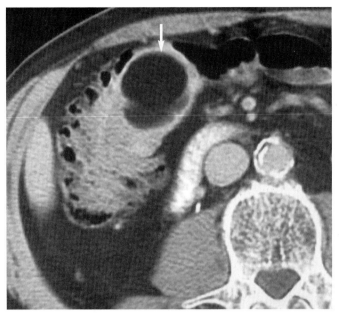

A

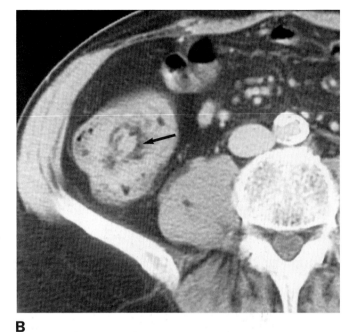

B

Findings

Contrast-enhanced CT. **A.** An intraluminal mass (arrow) is present within the right colon. The mass is of fatty density. **B.** At a slightly more caudal level, a ring of mesenteric fat (arrow) is seen within the colon.

Differential Diagnosis

Intussuscepting colonic lipoma

Diagnosis

Intussuscepting colonic lipoma

Discussion

Most patients with a colonic lipoma are asymptomatic; however, occasionally large intraluminal lipomas cause intussusception, ulceration, or hemorrhage. Lipomas have no risk of malignant degeneration. If the lesion is asymptomatic, no treatment is required.

CASE 5.77

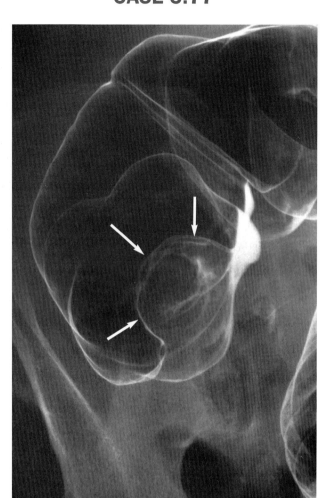

CASE 5.78

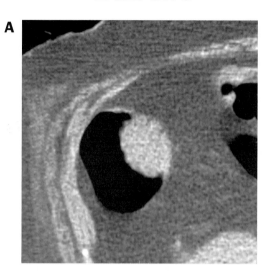

A

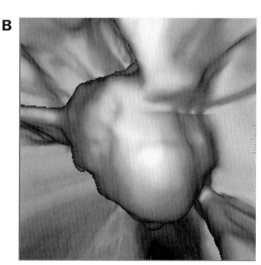

B

Findings

Case 5.77. Double-contrast barium enema. A polypoid mass (arrows) is present in the mid ascending colon. No contrast material passed proximal to the obstructing mass.

Case 5.78. CT colonography. **A** and **B.** A large polypoid mass is present within the hepatic flexure of the colon.

Differential Diagnosis
1. Colon carcinoma
2. Large colon polyp

Diagnosis
Polypoid colon cancer

Discussion

Colon cancer is the most frequent cause of large bowel obstruction. An enema with contrast material or CT colonography is a rapid and accurate method to determine the cause of the obstruction. Colitis has been reported to occur proximal to an obstructing lesion in some patients. High-grade obstruction and a competent ileocecal valve also can lead to increased intraluminal pressure, decreased venous flow, and possible colonic ischemia.

CASE 5.79

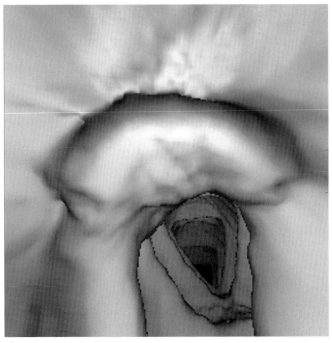

A

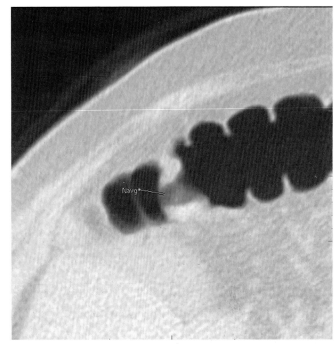

B

Findings
CT colonography. **A** and **B**. Focal, lobulated thickening of a haustral fold.

Differential Diagnosis
1. Colon cancer
2. Asymmetric haustral fold thickening

Diagnosis
Colon cancer

Discussion
Colon cancer at CT colonography can present as a focal area of haustral fold thickening. Often the surface of the tumor is irregular in contour and distinctly thicker than neighboring folds. The focal thickening is fixed and usually can be identified on both supine and prone views.

CASE 5.80

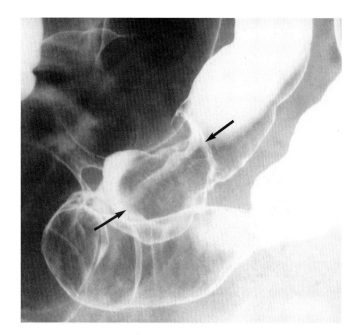

CASE 5.81

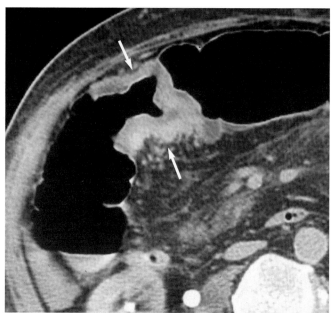

Findings

Case 5.80. Double-contrast barium enema. A nearly annular, ulcerative mass (arrows) is present in the mid sigmoid colon. The lesion has margins that are abrupt and shouldered, resembling a napkin ring.

Case 5.81. Contrast-enhanced CT. A short segment of circumferential bowel wall thickening (arrows) is present in the hepatic flexure of the colon. The wall thickening abruptly meets the normal colonic wall.

Differential Diagnosis

Annular carcinoma

Diagnosis

Annular carcinoma

Discussion

Advanced colon cancers often appear as annular, constricting lesions. Most tumors are less than 6 cm long. These tumors are thought to arise from a flat, plaquelike growth that extends circumferentially around the bowel lumen. Most small cancers are indistinguishable from benign polyps. Thus, most polyps 1 cm or more in diameter are removed.

CASE 5.82

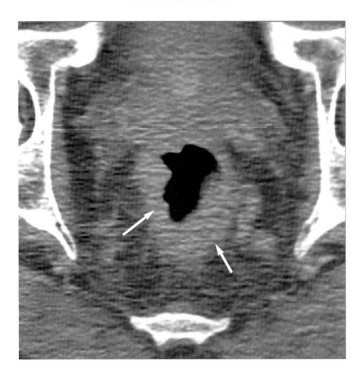

CASE 5.83

A

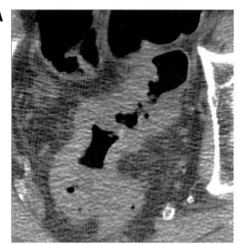

B

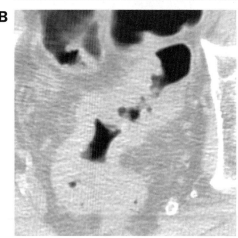

Findings

Case 5.82. CT colonography. Circumferential thickening (arrows) is present about the rectum. The margins between the wall thickening and perirectal fat are poorly defined.

Case 5.83. CT colonography. **A** and **B.** Axial images. A long segmental region of bowel wall thickening is present in the sigmoid colon. The soft tissue windows are optimal for visualizing the abnormality.

Differential Diagnosis

1. Annular cancer
2. Segmental luminal collapse

Diagnosis

Annular cancer

Discussion

Rectal cancers can be difficult to diagnose at CT colonography, especially those in the distal rectum, which can mimic the collapsed anus. Rectal tumors also can be obscured by an inflated balloon-tipped enema tube. Generally, the rectum is best seen with the patient in the prone position. Larger, more extensive neoplasms (as in case 5.83) can mimic a segmental region of collapse. Viewing the segment in two views, with use of glucagon (a spasmolytic) or by reinflating and rescanning, may be helpful to demonstrate the fixed nature of the tumor. Cancers often are best depicted with soft tissue windows, whereas polyps are most conspicuous with lung windows.

CASE 5.84

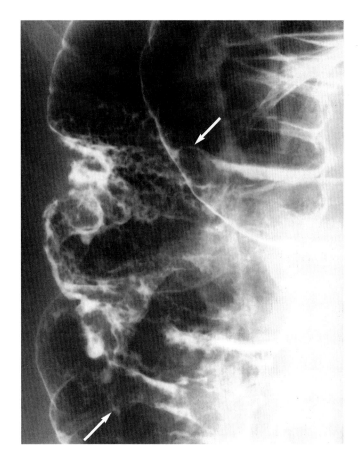

CASE 5.85

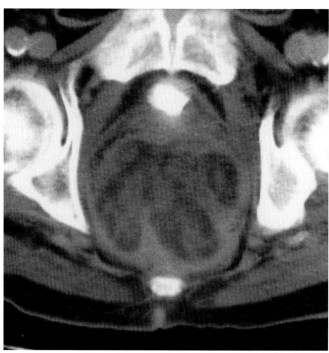

Findings

Case 5.84. Double-contrast barium enema. A mass (arrows) is present along the lateral wall of the mid ascending colon. The mass contains a frondlike surface.

Case 5.85. Contrast-enhanced CT. The rectal lumen is markedly distended, and the rectal wall is unevenly thickened. Multiple intraluminal soft tissue masses are present within the rectum.

Differential Diagnosis

Villous adenoma, probably containing carcinoma

Diagnosis

Villous adenoma containing invasive carcinoma

Discussion

Villous adenomas have the highest incidence of malignant transformation of all adenomatous polyps. The villous nature of these lesions can be suspected by identifying a lacelike or raspberrylike surface contour. It is unusual to visualize the villous features of a colonic tumor at CT. Usually, only localized bowel wall thickening or a focal mass is seen. In these patients, the large size and the morphologic features of the mass were helpful for predicting the histologic type.

CASE 5.86

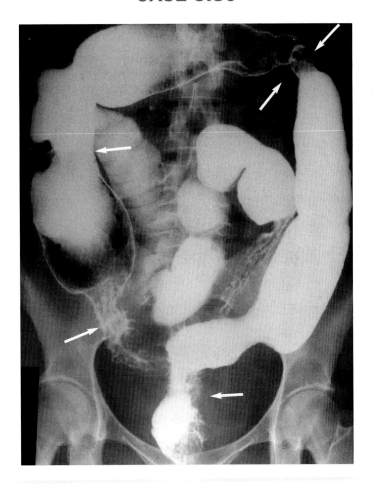

Findings
Barium enema. There are at least four regions (arrows) of colonic narrowing: cecum, ascending colon, splenic flexure, and rectosigmoid. The colon is diffusely ahaustral and appears shortened.

Differential Diagnosis
1. Chronic ulcerative colitis
2. Chronic ulcerative colitis with multiple cancers

Diagnosis
Chronic ulcerative colitis with multiple cancers

Discussion
This patient had a long history of ulcerative colitis. At operation, multiple colon cancers were present, as was peritoneal carcinomatosis. Patients with long-standing (>10 years) ulcerative colitis have an increased risk for development of colon cancer. These cancers can be multicentric (as in this patient) and appear as either typical annular cancers (case 5.10) or regions of tapered narrowing (case 5.11).

Approximately 5% of patients with an ordinary colon carcinoma have another synchronous cancer. Therefore, it is important to examine the entire colon—even after the discovery of an unsuspected lesion. In one series, less than one-third of synchronous lesions were palpable at operation. The proximal colon should not be examined at barium enema only if a patient has a high-grade obstruction from the cancer. In that case, CT colonography can be helpful to examine the colon proximal to the obstruction. Polyps more commonly are found in patients with either a synchronous polyp or cancer or a history of a previous polyp or cancer. Metachronous cancers, those developing at a later date in patients with a previous history of colorectal cancer, occur in about 5% of patients.

CASE 5.87

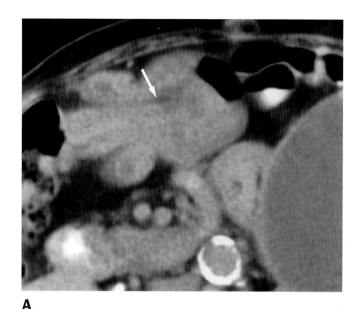

A

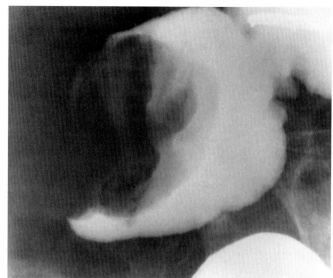

B

Findings

A. Contrast-enhanced CT. An intussusception is present within the right transverse colon. A linear band of low-density mesenteric fat is visible within the mass (arrow). A lead point for the intussusception is not seen. There is also a thick-walled cystic mass arising from the left kidney.

B. Single-contrast barium enema. A follow-up barium enema showed a polypoid colon cancer acting as the lead point for the reducible intussusception.

Differential Diagnosis
1. Colocolic intussusception
2. Ileocolic intussusception

Diagnosis
Colon carcinoma with colocolic intussusception

Discussion
At operation in this patient, both a colon cancer and cystic renal adenocarcinoma were removed. Colon cancer is the most frequent cause of a colocolic intussusception in adults. The radiographic appearance at barium enema and CT usually is diagnostic. As in the small bowel, a sausage-shaped filling defect is seen within a shortened colon. A coiled-spring appearance often is visible at the proximal end of the mass. Sometimes it is possible to fully reduce the intussusception and to identify the offending mass at contrast enema. In many patients, the cancer is located in the cecum. Visualization of mesenteric fat and occasionally vessels within the mass is pathognomonic (as in this case) of an intussusception at CT.

CASE 5.88

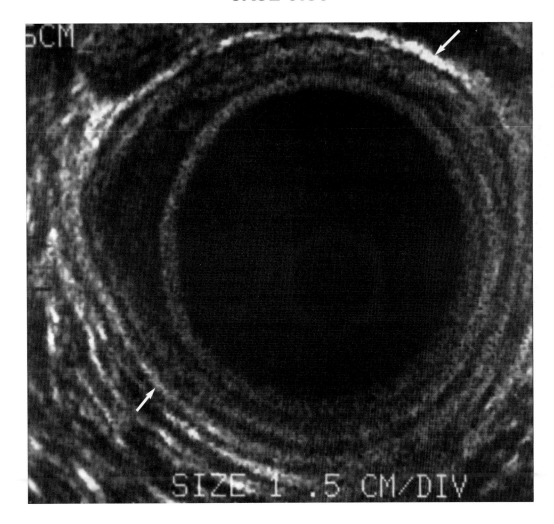

Findings

Endorectal ultrasonography. The normal bowel wall layers are visible except for a localized area of hypoechoic bowel wall thickening at the 9- to 10-o'clock position. The outermost echogenic layer (muscularis propria and perirectal fat interface) is intact (arrows) overlying this mass. (From Jochem RJ, Reading CC, Dozois RR, Carpenter HA, Wolff BG, Charboneau JW: Endorectal ultrasonographic staging of rectal carcinoma. Mayo Clin Proc. 1990;65:1571-7. By permission of Mayo Foundation for Medical Education and Research.)

Differential Diagnosis

Localized rectal cancer (confined to bowel wall)

Diagnosis

Localized rectal cancer (confined to bowel wall)

Discussion

The intact outermost echogenic layer indicates that the tumor is confined to the bowel wall (Dukes stage B1 lesion). Endorectal sonography routinely can display the five normal layers of the bowel. The innermost echogenic layer represents the balloon-mucosal interface; the next hypoechoic layer, the muscularis mucosa; the middle echogenic layer, the submucosa; the fourth hypoechoic ring, the muscularis propria; and the outer echogenic ring, the muscularis propria-perirectal fat interface. The outer echogenic layer is the key ring for distinguishing tumors confined to the bowel wall from those extending into the perirectal fat. Endorectal sonography also is sensitive for detecting perirectal lymph nodes, but it is nonspecific for distinguishing metastatic from inflammatory nodes.

CASE 5.89

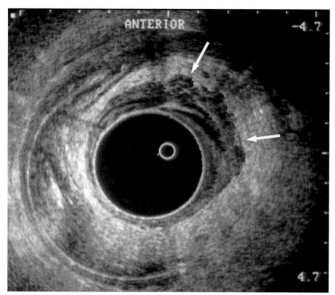

A

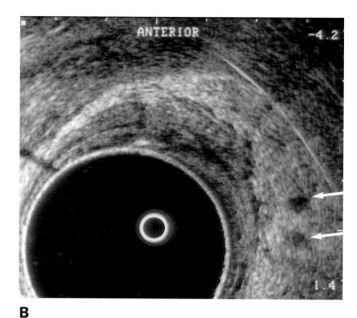

B

Findings

Endorectal ultrasonography. **A.** The anterolateral aspect of the rectal wall (from 11-o'clock to 3-o'clock position) is abnormally thickened, with loss of the normal echogenic bowel layers. In addition, the mass (arrows) can be seen to extend deeply into the perirectal fat through the muscularis propria-perirectal fat interface. **B.** Coned-in view shows two small hypoechoic lymph nodes (arrows) in the perirectal fat at the level of the invasive rectal mass.

Differential Diagnosis

Invasive colon cancer with extension into perirectal fat

Diagnosis

Invasive colon cancer with extension into perirectal fat

Discussion

Colorectal cancers appear as hypoechoic or isoechoic masses that disrupt the bowel wall layers. The staging accuracy of endorectal ultrasonography is 85% to 90%. Evaluation of lymph nodes remains a challenge, because reactive lymph nodes can be enlarged and discrimination of benign from malignant nodes is impossible. Endoscopic ultrasonography can be helpful for detecting recurrent tumor adjacent to the anastomosis, a finding not visible at endoscopy.

CASE 5.90

A

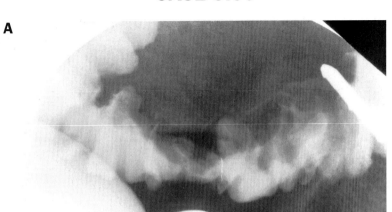

B

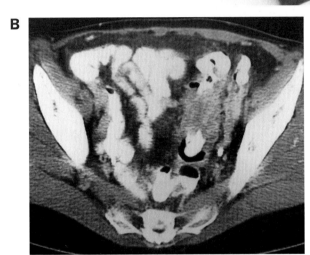

C

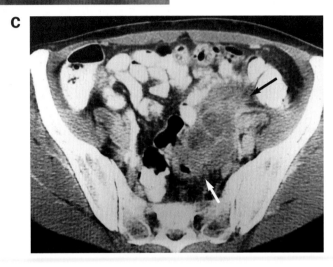

Findings

A. Single-contrast barium enema. The sigmoid lumen is narrowed, and there is a lobulated mass deforming the superior sigmoid contour. The lobulated contours are worrisome for neoplasm, but mucosal destruction or ulceration is not identified.

B and **C.** Contrast-enhanced CT. A mixed-density (fluid and soft tissue) mass (arrows) is present within the perisigmoidal tissues.

Differential Diagnosis
1. Diverticulitis
2. Perforated colon cancer

Diagnosis
Perforated colon cancer

Discussion

Perforated colon cancers are unusual, constituting 2.5% to 8% of all colorectal cancers. The importance of this entity lies in the fact that patients may present with signs suggesting diverticulitis and receive suboptimal therapy. In addition, curative resection is less likely and operative mortality is higher. In cases of gross perforation with peritoneal contamination (found in a minority of patients), the 5-year survival rate is only 7%.

A contrast enema usually does not show the site of colonic perforation. Common findings on contrast enema include a long area of segmental narrowing and extrinsic mass effect or obstruction. Mucosal ulceration can be difficult to evaluate because of the associated inflammatory changes. Findings at CT include a colorectal mass associated with an abscess the density of fluid or phlegmon. Metastatic disease often is identified. Endoscopy often is necessary to obtain a tissue diagnosis.

CASE 5.91

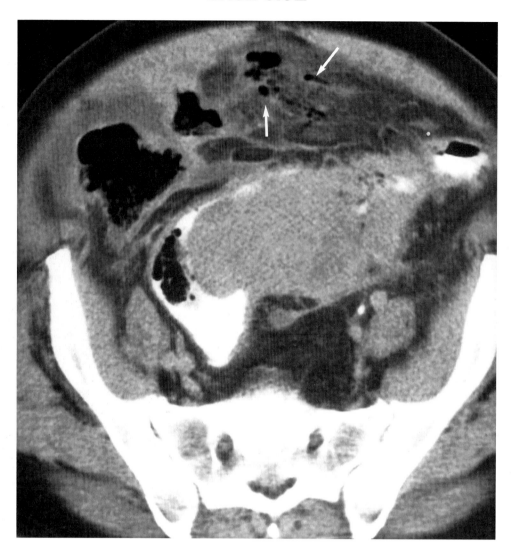

Findings
Contrast-enhanced CT. A large soft tissue mass narrows and deforms the sigmoid colon. Contrast material is visible within the sigmoid lumen. Soft tissue stranding is present throughout the perisigmoidal fat. Extraluminal gas (arrows) is present in the soft tissues anterior to the sigmoid colon.

Differential Diagnosis
1. Diverticulitis
2. Perforated colon cancer

Diagnosis
Perforated colon cancer

Discussion
Differentiating a perforated colon cancer from a complicated case of diverticulitis with pericolonic phlegmon or abscess is often difficult. The marked wall thickening and short segment of involved colon in this case favor perforated cancer over complicated diverticulitis. Often, however, it is necessary to recommend endoscopy after antibiotic therapy for presumed cases of diverticulitis to exclude an underlying cancer.

CASE 5.92

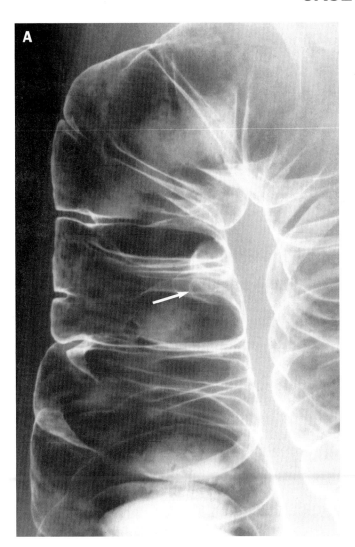

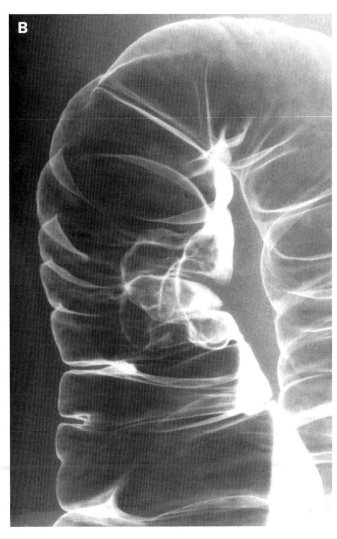

Findings
Double-contrast barium enema. **A.** A sessile polyp (arrow) is present along the medial wall of the ascending colon. The polyp was removed endoscopically.
B. Follow-up barium enema 3 years later shows a polypoid mass at the site of the previous polyp.

Differential Diagnosis
1. Colon polyp with growth
2. Colon polyp with recurrence at index site

Diagnosis
Villous adenoma with recurrence as adenocarcinoma

Discussion
Among patients who have undergone curative resection for colon cancer, 30% to 50% have a recurrence within 2 years. Locally recurrent colorectal cancers can occur at sites of surgical anastomosis, within pericolic or pelvic fat near the surgical site, or at previous sites of endoscopic removal. Local recurrence developing at the anastomosis is best evaluated with an intraluminal study (i.e., barium enema, CT colonography, or endoscopy). Extraluminal and distant disease are best detected at CT. The usual radiographic appearance of an anastomotic recurrence is either a polypoid mass or irregular and eccentric narrowing of the lumen.

CASE 5.93

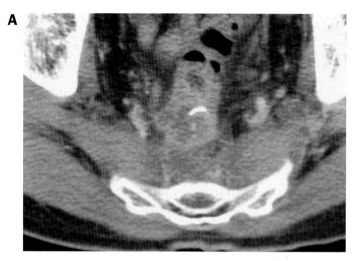

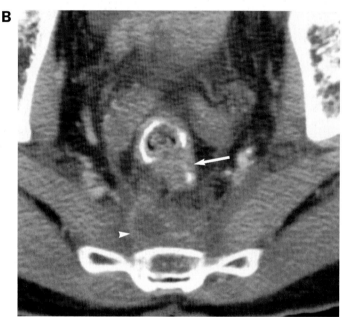

Findings

Contrast-enhanced CT. **A** and **B.** An opaque staple line is seen at the colorectal anastomosis. Soft tissue (arrow) is present adjacent to the anastomosis, and there is abnormal soft tissue in the presacral space (arrowhead).

Differential Diagnosis

Recurrent colorectal cancer

Diagnosis

Recurrent colorectal cancer

Discussion

Incomplete resection of rectal cancer can lead to recurrent tumor at or near the anastomosis and in the presacral space. In this case, recurrent tumor is present in both locations. Histologic confirmation can be obtained with a CT-directed biopsy.

CASE 5.94

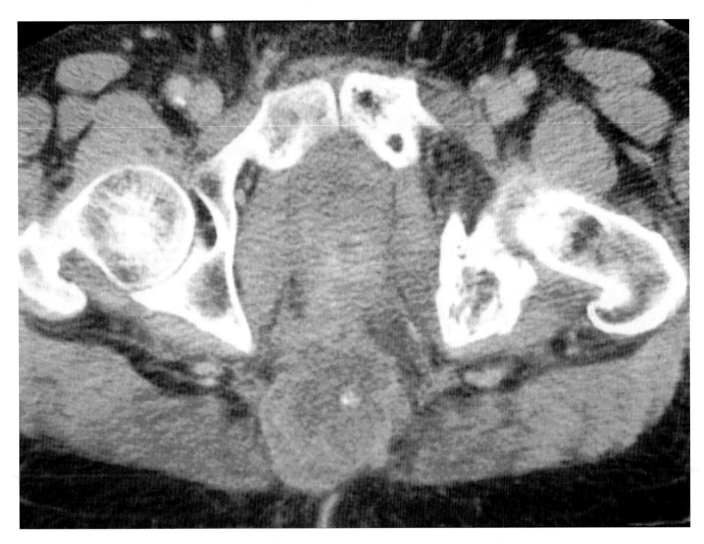

Findings

Contrast-enhanced CT. The rectum has been removed. A large soft tissue mass is present in the old rectal bed and presacral region. The heterogeneous mass contains calcification.

Differential Diagnosis

1. Recurrent rectal cancer
2. Metastases

Diagnosis

Recurrent colorectal cancer

Discussion

CT findings of recurrent tumor in the pelvis usually include an expanding presacral soft tissue mass with indistinct margins. Local invasion, lymphadenopathy, and distant metastases (liver, lung, retroperitoneum) can be seen. Recurrent neoplasm is most likely in a patient with a history of rectal cancer. Percutaneous biopsy with CT is helpful for confirming the diagnosis.

CASE 5.95

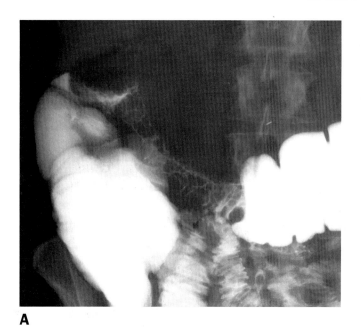

A

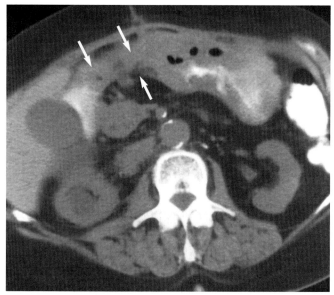

B

Findings

A. Single-contrast barium enema. A long segment of circumferential narrowing is present in the right transverse colon. The mucosa through much of the involved region appears distorted but intact.

B. Unenhanced CT. The wall of the gastric antrum is thickened. A contiguous soft tissue mass (arrows) extends from the stomach and engulfs (on lower slices) the colon. The right kidney is obstructed.

Differential Diagnosis

1. Gastric cancer with extension to the colon
2. Colon cancer with extension to the stomach
3. Peritoneal carcinoma involving colon and stomach

Diagnosis

Gastric cancer with extension to the colon

Discussion

Metastatic disease to the colon can occur by several routes: intraperitoneal spread, direct extension, and hematogenous dissemination. Meyers described the patterns of malignant spread by each route. Understanding these patterns allows the radiologist to diagnose metastases and to predict the possible origin of the primary tumor.

Direct extension of malignancies is most common in patients with ovarian or uterine carcinoma, prostate cancer, and renal carcinoma. Pelvic malignancies often cause mass effect on the anterior wall of the rectum and on the inferior aspect of the sigmoid. The affected bowel can be narrowed and nodular and contain tethered folds. Prostatic tumors often involve only the anterior aspect of the rectum, but they also can extend circumferentially around the rectum, causing annular narrowing resembling a primary rectal cancer. Renal adenocarcinoma usually does not incite a desmoplastic response, as occurs in most other metastases. These tumors (either primary or locally recurrent tumors) can invade the colon and appear as a large intraluminal, nonobstructing polypoid mass. Gastric (as in this case) and pancreatic malignancies often invade the transverse colon by extending into the gastrocolic ligament and transverse mesocolon. Classically, gastric malignancies cause narrowing, mass effect, and tethering of the superior aspect of the transverse colon. Pancreatic malignancies usually involve the inferior aspect of the transverse colon.

CASE 5.96

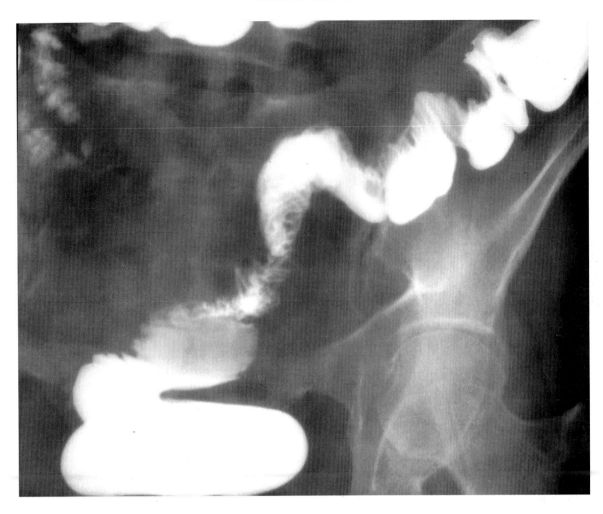

Findings

Single-contrast barium enema. The sigmoid colon is narrowed from mass effect, and mucosal tethering is present along its superior surface. This patient had ovarian cancer.

Differential Diagnosis

Serosal metastases to the colon

Diagnosis

Serosal metastases to the colon

Discussion

Intraperitoneal metastases implant on peritoneal surfaces in regions where the ascitic flow is arrested. The four common sites of intraperitoneal seeding are 1) the pouch of Douglas, the most dependent and common location in the abdomen; 2) the ileocecal region, a region where fluid and cells collect after cascading down the small bowel mesentery into the right lower quadrant; 3) the superior aspect of the sigmoid colon; and 4) the right paracolic gutter, the main channel for fluid traveling from the pelvis into the upper abdomen.

Hematogenous spread to the colon is relatively infrequent. Breast cancer can invade the submucosal tissues and resemble linitis plastica in the affected segment. Narrowing and lack of distensibility are the commonest findings.

CASE 5.97

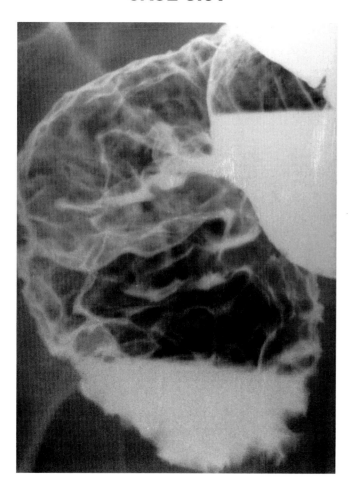

CASE 5.98

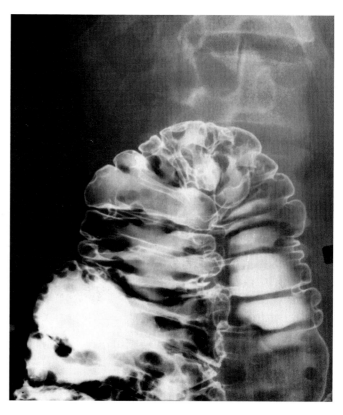

Findings

Case 5.97. Double-contrast barium enema. Multiple smooth-surfaced filling defects are present in the rectum.

Case 5.98. Double-contrast barium enema. Multiple smooth-surfaced filling defects are present throughout the colon.

Differential Diagnosis
1. Lymphoma
2. Colitis cystica profunda
3. Polyposis syndrome

Diagnosis
Non-Hodgkin lymphoma

Discussion

Primary lymphoma of the colon usually occurs in patients older than 50 years and most often among men. Symptoms usually include abdominal pain, weight loss, weakness, anorexia, and fever.

Radiologically, early diffuse lymphoma presents with submucosal nodules that involve only a limited portion of the colon. The cecum and rectum are the sites most often involved. Later, innumerable diffuse filling defects with concomitant haustral thickening are seen.

Colitis cystica profunda is limited to the rectum. Polyposis syndromes have well-defined filling defects arising from the mucosa. Usually these conditions affect younger patients.

CASE 5.99

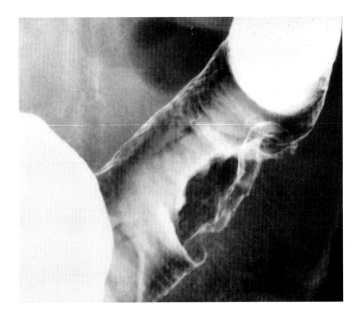

CASE 5.100

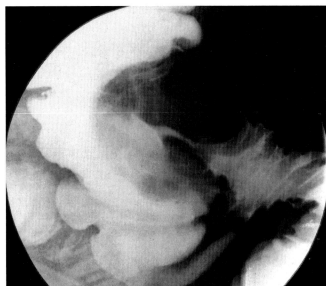

Findings

Case 5.99. Double-contrast barium enema. A broad-based sessile mass is present at the junction of the sigmoid and descending colon.

Case 5.100. Single-contrast barium enema. The ileocecal valve is markedly enlarged, and the folds of the terminal ileum are thickened.

Differential Diagnosis

1. Colon carcinoma
2. Lymphoma

Diagnosis

Lymphoma

Discussion

Localized lymphomas can have three radiographic presentations: a localized polypoid mass indistinguishable from a polypoid carcinoma (as in these cases), a region of narrowing resembling carcinoma (usually without evidence of obstruction), and an aneurysmal segment of colon with luminal dilatation and mucosal ulceration. Intussusception can occur with bulky intraluminal masses.

CASE 5.101

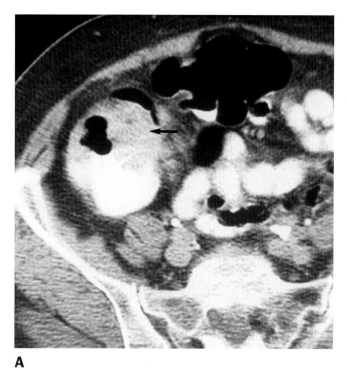

A

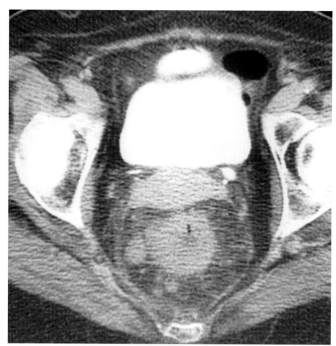

B

Findings
Contrast-enhanced CT. **A.** A localized soft tissue mass (arrow) is present in the medial wall of the cecum with several small lymph nodes in the cecal mesentery.
B. The rectal wall is diffusely thickened and several enlarged lymph nodes are visible in the perirectal fat.

Differential Diagnosis
1. Lymphoma
2. Metastases

Diagnosis
Multifocal lymphoma

Discussion
The CT finding of lymphoma is usually focal or diffuse bowel wall thickening. Perforation is an important complication of this disease and develops because of the lack of the usual desmoplastic reaction that occurs with most other tumors. This complication has been reported in 9% to 47% of patients and is often clinically silent. Identification of gas or fluid within a lymphomatous mass may indicate the presence of perforation. CT is excellent for determining the amount of bowel wall thickening, extent of disease, and presence of associated adenopathy.

CASE 5.102

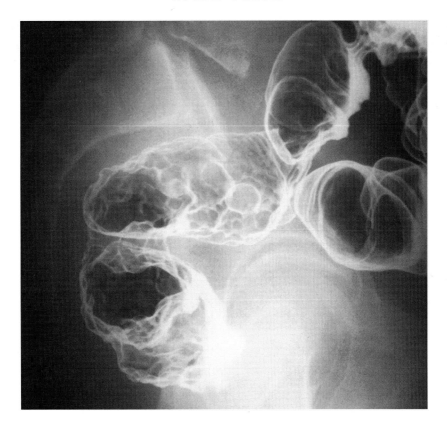

Findings
Double-contrast barium enema. Multiple round submucosal filling defects are present within the rectum.

Differential Diagnosis
1. Lymphoma
2. Colitis cystica profunda
3. Ulcerative colitis with multiple inflammatory polyps
4. Polyposis syndrome

Diagnosis
Colitis cystica profunda

Discussion
Colitis cystica profunda is a disease of unknown cause characterized by multiple mucin-filled cysts within the mucosa and submucosa of the rectum and, rarely, the sigmoid colon. Patients may complain of rectal bleeding, diarrhea, abdominal pain, and prolapse of the rectum. Large cysts can cause obstruction.

Radiographically, multiple round submucosal cystlike filling defects are seen in the rectum. Occasionally the cysts can simulate a large mass and resemble a villous tumor (case 5.84).

Colitis cystica superficialis is a condition in which the mucosa is diffusely involved with mucus-filled bullae. It is believed to be of no clinical significance, except that it may be associated with pellagra and celiac disease.

Lymphoma could have a similar appearance but rarely is confined to the rectum. Similarly, evidence of more proximal disease would be likely in a patient with ulcerative colitis. A polyposis syndrome is never confined to the rectum, and the filling defects are sharply defined because of their mucosal origin.

CASE 5.103

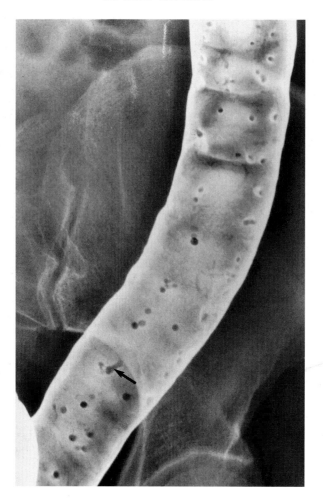

Findings
Double-contrast barium enema. Multiple polypoid filling defects are present in the colon. Some of the polyps are elongated (arrow). The background mucosal pattern is otherwise normal.

Differential Diagnosis
Postinflammatory polyps

Diagnosis
Postinflammatory polyps

Discussion
This is the typical appearance of postinflammatory polyps in this patient with known ulcerative colitis. Postinflammatory polyps develop during the healing phase in patients with either Crohn colitis or ulcerative colitis. In the process of epithelial regeneration, true polyps develop (containing submucosa and mucosa). These polyps are often long and thin (wormlike) and may branch. They often are referred to as filiform polyps (from the Latin word *filum*, meaning "thread"). The background mucosa is nearly always normal in appearance without evidence of acute inflammation.

Polypoid changes are usually multiple and may involve the colon either locally or diffusely. Rarely, a masslike collection of postinflammatory polyps can simulate a villous adenoma or carcinoma. These giant postinflammatory polyps are usually found in the right colon and are associated with other areas of typical filiform polyps.

CASE 5.104

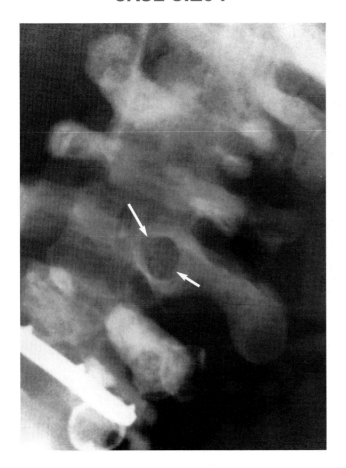

CASE 5.105

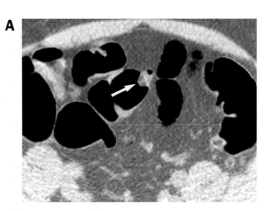

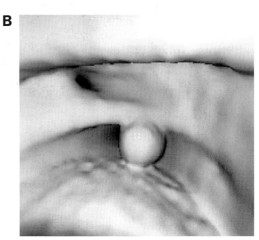

Findings

Case 5.104. Single-contrast barium enema. A round filling defect (arrows) is present in the sigmoid colon. Sigmoid diverticulosis is present. The filling defect has a bright white ring of barium around it.

Case 5.105. CT colonography. **A.** Two-dimensional axial soft tissue window. Heterogeneous density material (arrow) fills a diverticulum and protrudes into the lumen. **B.** Three-dimensional endoluminal image. A polypoid filling defect is present.

Differential Diagnosis

1. Pseudopolyp
2. Polyp

Diagnosis

Pseudopolyp

Discussion

Diverticulosis is a common finding, especially among older persons. Stool may fill a diverticulum and remain lodged within it despite proper cathartics and cleansing enemas. When viewed en face, the stool-filled diverticulum can simulate a polyp. Identifying the rim of barium around the pseudopolyp is key to excluding a real polyp. If tangential views are possible, stool often can be seen within the diverticulum.

At CT, with two-dimensional images, the filling defect can be seen to reside within a diverticulum and protrude into the lumen. The filling defect may be homogeneous or inhomogeneous in internal attenuation. Three-dimensional endoluminal images are usually not helpful for differentiating stool from polyps.

CASE 5.106

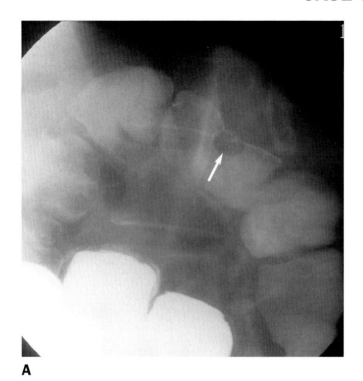

A

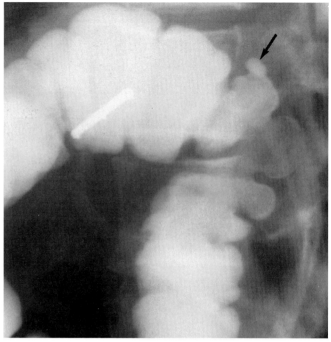

B

Findings
Single-contrast barium enema. **A.** An approximately 2-cm filling defect (arrow) is present in the splenic flexure of the colon. **B.** A single diverticulum (arrow) is present at the site of the prior filling defect.

Differential Diagnosis
Inverted colonic diverticulum

Diagnosis
Inverted colonic diverticulum

Discussion
An inverted diverticulum can simulate a polyp and may be indistinguishable from a polyp on a barium enema or CT colonography examination. Complete distention of the colon minimizes its occurrence.

CASE 5.107

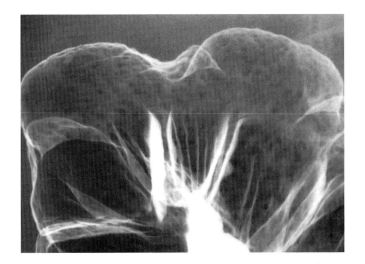

CASE 5.108

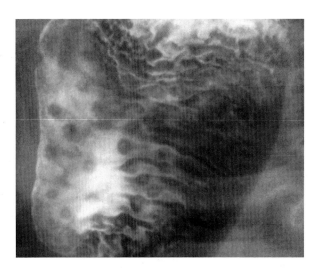

Findings

Case 5.107. Double-contrast barium enema. Multiple tiny submucosal nodular filling defects are uniformly distributed in the colon.

Case 5.108. Double-contrast barium enema. A central collection of barium (umbilication) is visible within several of the nodules.

Differential Diagnosis

1. Normal lymphoid pattern
2. Polyposis syndrome
3. Crohn disease
4. Diffuse lymphoma
5. Retained stool

Diagnosis

Normal lymphoid follicular pattern

Discussion

The lymphoid follicular pattern is a common finding in normal children and in 10% to 15% of normal adults. The double-contrast technique usually is needed to identify the subtle textural changes of this entity. The key finding is the small size (<4 mm diameter) of the filling defects that are uniformly distributed in the colon. Usually the right side of the colon is affected more than the left. A polyposis syndrome (cases 5.68 through 5.73) usually has filling defects of larger and more variable size, and some are pedunculated. The lymphoid nodules and aphthous ulcers in Crohn disease are usually somewhat larger and often in a patchy segmental distribution (cases 5.15 and 5.16). Diffuse lymphoma has submucosal nodules of larger (>4 mm) and variable size (cases 5.97 and 5.98). Retained stool has angular margins, whereas lymphoid nodules are smooth and rounded.

Umbilication of lymphoid nodules (as in case 5.108) can be a normal finding. The main differential consideration is Crohn colitis with multiple aphthous ulcers (case 5.16). It may be impossible to exclude inflammatory bowel disease on the basis of the radiographic findings alone. Clinical correlation is always suggested, and follow-up studies to assess for disease progression or endoscopic biopsy also can be helpful.

CASE 5.109

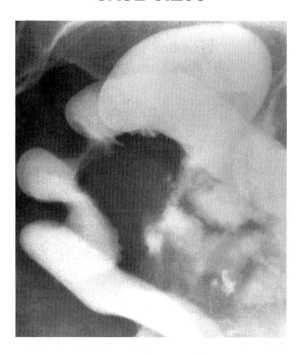

CASE 5.110

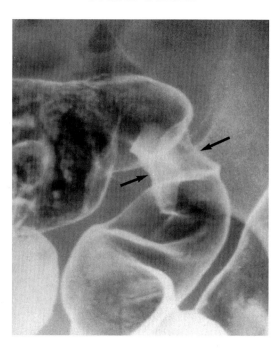

Findings

Case 5.109. Single-contrast barium enema. There is an extrinsic mass on the anterior wall of the rectosigmoid. Tethered colonic folds are associated with the mass.

Case 5.110. Double-contrast barium enema. A focal region of annular constriction (arrows) is present in the mid sigmoid colon.

Differential Diagnosis

1. Serosal metastases
2. Colon carcinoma
3. Endometriosis

Diagnosis

Endometriosis

Discussion

In a woman in her reproductive years without a prior malignancy, endometriosis is an important diagnostic consideration with the radiographic findings shown here. Endometriosis was found at operation.

Endometriosis is the third most common cause of benign filling defects in the colon (after adenomas and lipomas). Intestinal implants are estimated to occur in 4% of all women between the ages of 20 and 40 years. Endometrial tissue extruded from the fallopian tubes can implant on the peritoneal surface, usually in the pouch of Douglas or on the sigmoid colon (most commonly on its inferior surface). The implants invade muscular and submucosal bowel layers and often stimulate local smooth muscle proliferation of the colon, secondary inflammatory changes, and a variable degree of fibrosis. Symptoms include constipation, pelvic pain, diarrhea, and, rarely, rectal bleeding. Typically, the symptoms are cyclical, but not always.

Radiographically, an intramural or extrinsic filling defect is present with an intact overlying mucosa. Sometimes the mucosa may appear pleated or tethered because of the associated desmoplastic reaction (as in case 5.109). Rarely, a constricting lesion is seen with smooth margins and an intact mucosa (case 5.110).

CASE 5.111

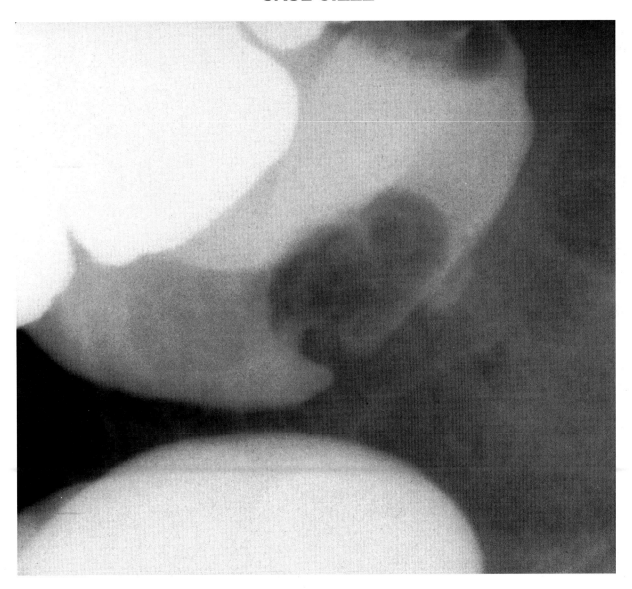

Findings

Single-contrast barium enema. A small filling defect is present in the base of the cecum.

Differential Diagnosis

1. Colon polyp
2. Lipoma
3. Mucocele
4. Endometrioma

Diagnosis

Endometriosis

Discussion

The radiographic appearance of an endometrioma depends on its anatomical location—serosal or submucosal. The mucosa is rarely involved, but in some cases (as in this example) the filling defect can resemble a mucosal mass. Filling defects usually range from 2 to 7 cm in diameter.

CASE 5.112

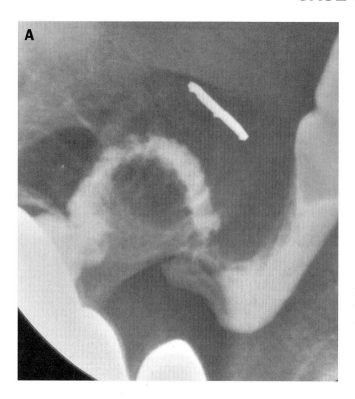

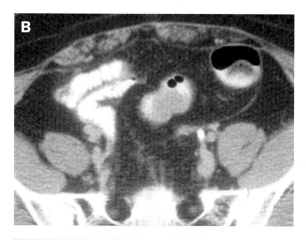

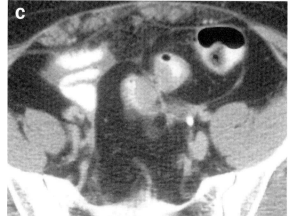

Findings

A. Single-contrast barium enema. The sigmoid is narrowed, and there is mass effect on its inferior border. Tethered folds are visible about the mass.

B and **C.** Contrast-enhanced CT. A soft tissue mass is present on the inferior aspect of the sigmoid colon. Minimal soft tissue stranding is present in the pericolonic tissues. No other pelvic mass is present.

Differential Diagnosis

1. Endometriosis
2. Ovarian tumor
3. Pelvic inflammatory disease
4. Diverticulitis

Diagnosis

Endometriosis

Discussion

The soft tissue mass due to an endometrioma can be directly visualized at CT in some cases. Occasionally, it is difficult to detect. Lesions developing on the inferior aspect of the sigmoid are most likely to arise from organs in the pelvis. In females during their reproductive years, endometriosis should be a primary consideration. CT in this case was very helpful for excluding a primary pelvic tumor or changes of diverticulitis.

CASE 5.113

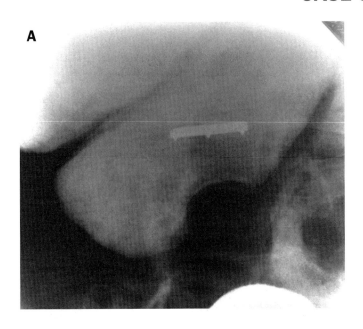

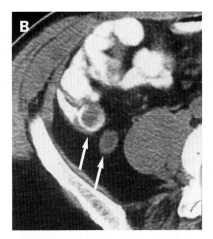

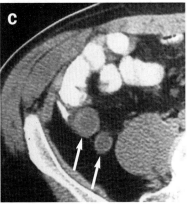

Findings

A. Single-contrast barium enema. A smooth-surfaced filling defect is present on the base of the cecum. The appendix is not seen. A compression device containing a 2-cm marker is visible.

B and **C.** Unenhanced CT. The appendix (arrows) is distended and fluid-filled. Linear calcification is present within part of the wall of the appendix. Findings are typical of a mucocele.

Differential Diagnosis
Mucocele

Diagnosis
Mucocele

Discussion

A mucocele of the appendix is regarded by some authors as a mucus-distended appendix due to luminal obstruction by a fecalith, foreign body, adhesions, or volvulus. Other authors include tumorous conditions of the appendix. These conditions include focal or diffuse mucosal hyperplasia, mucinous cystadenoma, and mucinous cystadenocarcinoma. Carcinoid tumors of the appendix are not classified with the epithelial-derived adenoma and adenocarcinoma tumors. They rarely are associated with appendiceal mucoceles.

At contrast enema, a mucocele usually presents with findings of a smooth filling defect on the base of the cecum. CT has improved the ability to diagnose a mucocele. Findings at CT include a thin-walled, cystic, and tubular structure with internal contents of low density. Wall calcification is common. CT also is helpful in assessing for metastases in patients with an appendiceal cystadenocarcinoma.

CASE 5.114

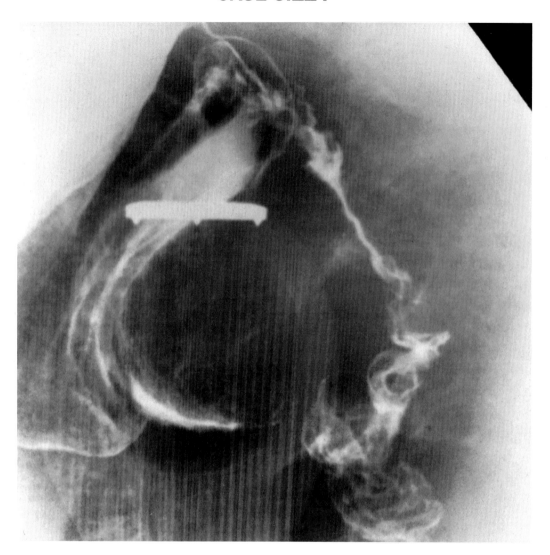

Findings

Single-contrast barium enema. A large smooth-surfaced filling defect is present on the base of the cecum. A compression device containing a 2-cm marker is visible.

Differential Diagnosis

1. Mucocele
2. Lipoma
3. Appendiceal abscess
4. Lymphoma
5. Endometrioma

Diagnosis

Mucocele: appendiceal adenocarcinoma

Discussion

Patients with appendiceal tumors often (50%) present clinically with symptoms of acute appendicitis. Approximately 15% of these tumors are discovered incidentally on histologic examination of the appendix. Metastatic mucinous cystadenocarcinoma often results in diffuse peritoneal carcinomatosis that produces large quantities of mucinous material that can calcify. This condition is often referred to as pseudomyxoma peritonei.

Lipomas are soft and deformable at fluoroscopy. Younger patients are most likely to have appendicitis or endometriosis—and the clinical presentation also is different. Lymphoma is most often found in older patients.

CASE 5.115

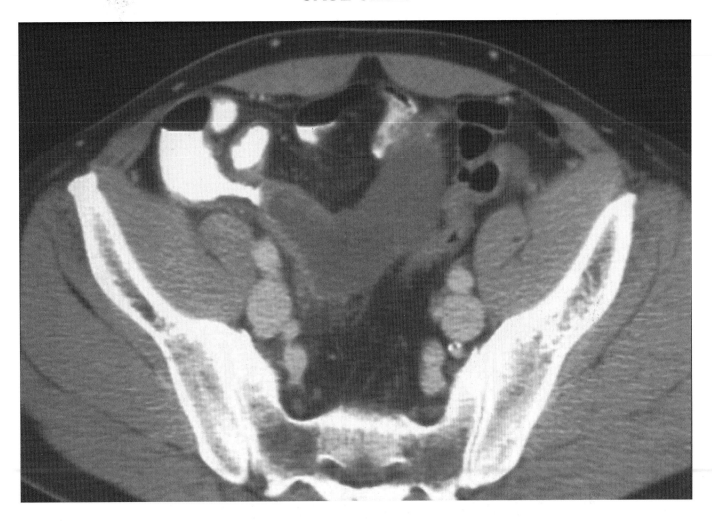

Findings
Contrast-enhanced CT. A large tubular, water-attenuation–filled stricture is present in the pelvis. The stricture arises from the base of the cecum.

Differential Diagnosis
1. Appendicitis
2. Mucocele
3. Meckel diverticulum
4. Duplication cyst

Diagnosis
Mucocele

Discussion
Mucoceles can occasionally be large. The appendiceal shape and attachment to the cecum are key findings to suggest a mucocele. Appendicitis is unlikely without inflammatory changes in the periappendiceal fat and without appendiceal wall thickening. Meckel diverticulum arises from the small bowel, not the cecum. A duplication cyst usually has no communication or attachment to the bowel.

CASE 5.116

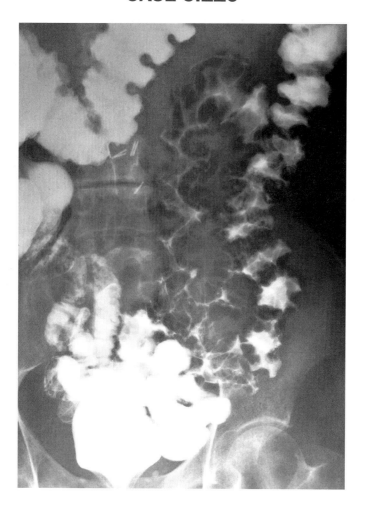

Findings

Single-contrast barium enema. Multiple intramural cystic gas collections are present throughout most of the left colon.

Differential Diagnosis

Pneumatosis cystoides coli

Diagnosis

Pneumatosis cystoides coli

Discussion

Pneumatosis coli refers to intramural air within the colon. Intramural air within the small bowel is referred to as pneumatosis intestinalis or pneumatosis cystoides intestinalis (if the air collections are cystlike). Patients with pneumatosis cystoides coli have endothelial-lined gas-filled cysts within the bowel wall which do not communicate with the lumen. The cysts may vary in size, reaching up to several centimeters in diameter. The cause is unknown, but some patients have associated collagen vascular disorders, ischemia, diabetes, or a history of trauma. This condition often is discovered incidentally in patients without symptoms.

The radiologic diagnosis is dependent on recognizing the radiolucent collections of gas within the bowel wall. Often the collections are rounded and grapelike. The left side of the colon is affected more often than the right (excluding the rectum).

Once the gas density of the collections is recognized, no further diagnostic considerations are necessary. The intraluminal protrusions may simulate polyps, lymphoma, segmental colitis (Crohn colitis), and ischemic colitis. Colitis cystica profunda usually affects the rectum, and the filling defects are not the lucency of gas (case 5.102).

CASE 5.117

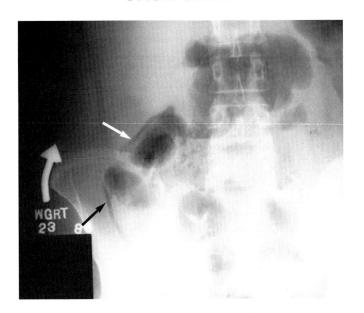

CASE 5.118

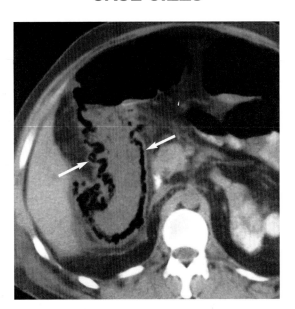

Findings

Case 5.117. Abdominal radiograph. A linear band of intramural gas (arrows) is present within the right colon. This patient had recently undergone colonoscopy with biopsy.

Case 5.118. Contrast-enhanced CT. Linear and cystic intramural pneumatosis is present in the right colon (arrows).

Differential Diagnosis

Pneumatosis coli

Diagnosis

Pneumatosis coli

Discussion

Pneumatosis coli can be due to the same underlying conditions as are found in pneumatosis intestinalis (cases 4.77 through 4.80). The intramural gas may appear cystic (case 4.78), but often it is linear (as in these cases). Patients receiving corticosteroid therapy, those with an underlying collagen vascular disease, those who have had a recent mucosal biopsy, or those with a history of chronic obstructive pulmonary disease are most likely to have this condition. These benign causes usually do not require any particular treatment. Ischemic colitis is the most important condition to exclude clinically, because emergency operation would be required to prevent perforation.

Intraluminal gas is always in a nondependent location, whereas pneumatosis can be present in any intramural location, including the dependent portions of the bowel.

Colonic Masses and Filling Defects

Benign tumors		Case
Polyp	Pedunculated, sessile, or flat, multiple polyps in hereditary nonpolyposis colorectal cancer or familial adenomatous polyposis	5.57–5.73
Lipoma	Commonest submucosal tumor, pliable (changes shape with compression or luminal changes)	5.74–5.76
Malignant tumors		
Adenocarcinoma	Annular, polypoid, or villous, 5% synchronous tumors	5.77–5.94
Metastases	Usually multiple masses, history of malignancy, direct tumor extension, serosal implants, or hematogenous or lymphatic spread	5.95 and 5.96
Lymphoma	Solitary, multiple or diffuse, look for adenopathy	5.97–5.101
Other benign conditions		
Colitis cystica profunda	Multiple smooth, round filling defects in rectum only	5.102
Postinflammatory polyps	Wormlike filiform polyps, in either ulcerative colitis or Crohn disease. Background mucosa normal	5.103
Pseudopolyps	Usually caused by stool or inverted diverticulum, angular margins and inhomogeneous internal attenuation	5.104–5.106
Normal lymphoid follicular pattern	Small (<4 mm) filling defects uniformly distributed in colon, common in children and occurs in 10%-15% of adults	5.107 and 5.108
Endometriosis	Intramural or extrinsic filling defect(s) in young women, common on inferior surface of sigmoid colon	5.109–5.112
Mucocele	Smooth filling defect at base of cecum, appendix obstructed by appendicolith or tumor	5.113–5.115
Pneumatosis coli	Linear or cystlike intramural gas collections, often benign cause, but ischemia should be ruled out	5.116–5.118

CASE 5.119

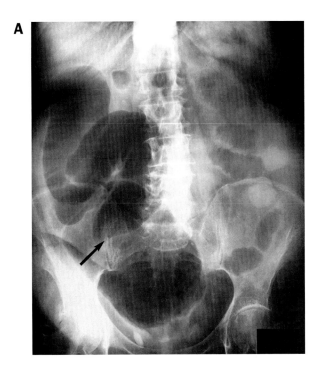

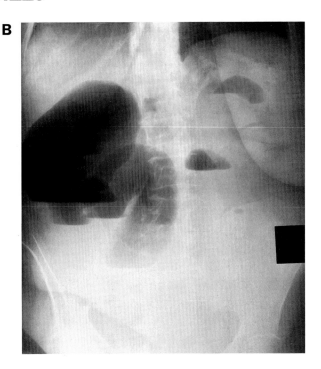

Findings

A. Supine abdominal radiograph. The cecum, ascending and proximal transverse colon are distended with gas. No gas is seen distal to the mid transverse colon (arrow). Mildly dilated small bowel loops are present.

B. Upright radiograph. Multiple air-fluid levels are seen in the right side of the colon and in two small bowel loops.

Differential Diagnosis
Mechanical colonic obstruction

Diagnosis
Mechanical colonic obstruction

Discussion
These findings are typical of a mechanical colonic obstruction involving the transverse colon. At operation, an incarcerated loop of transverse colon was found to be obstructed within a midline incisional hernia.

Mechanical colonic obstruction is most often due to carcinoma. Diverticulitis, volvulus, mass effect from an extracolonic pelvic neoplasm, fecal impaction, and, rarely, a hernia or adhesion also can cause large bowel obstruction. The radiographic findings include dilatation of the colon to the level of obstruction. The colon may be filled with gas (as in this case), fluid, or stool. The small bowel is also often dilated if the ileocecal valve is incompetent. If the valve remains competent, the colon will continue to distend. Perforation can occur with prolonged and marked cecal dilatation. A contrast enema or CT is often necessary to determine the cause of the obstruction. Only a small amount of barium should be passed beyond a high-grade obstruction so that inspissated barium does not cause a problem later (including obstipation and possible obstruction). Chronic obstruction can be recognized on abdominal radiographs by the presence of haustral thickening and the presence of gray and granular-appearing fluid within the colon proximal to the obstruction.

CASE 5.120

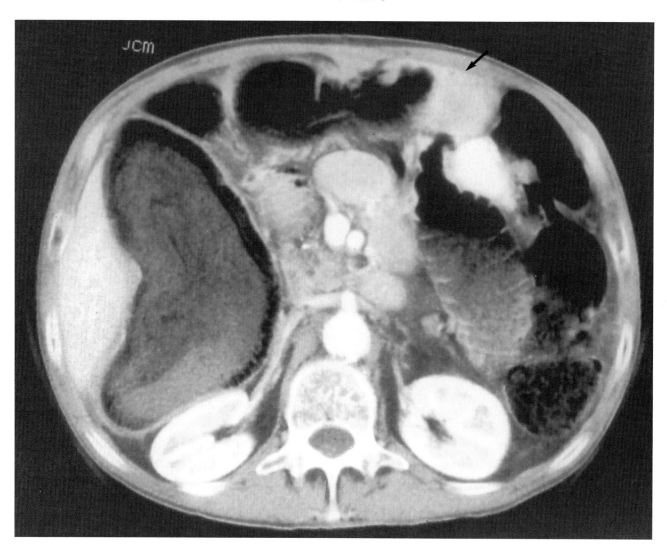

Findings
Contrast-enhanced CT. The colon is dilated to the level of the mid transverse colon. A soft tissue mass (arrow) encases the colon and causes partial colonic obstruction (normal-caliber descending colon).

Differential Diagnosis
1. Mechanical colonic obstruction
2. Primary colon cancer
3. Metastases

Diagnosis
Mechanical colonic obstruction due to metastatic gastric cancer

Discussion
CT is helpful for identifying dilated bowel, the level of obstruction, and in many cases the cause of obstruction. This patient with gastric cancer had tumor spread along the greater omentum to the transverse colon—a common route for gastric cancer to spread locally.

CASE 5.121

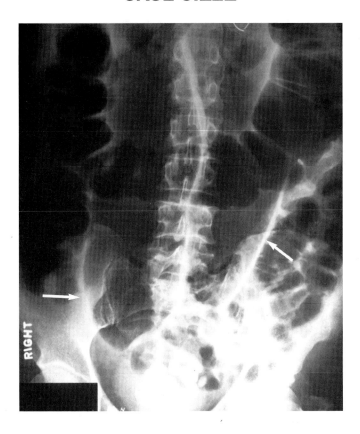

CASE 5.122

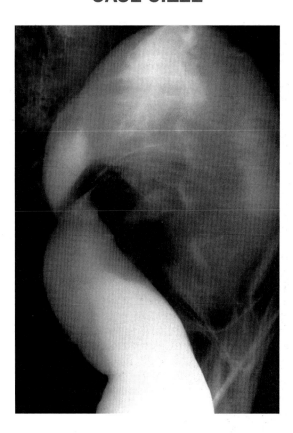

Findings

Case 5.121. Abdominal radiograph. The entire colon is moderately distended with gas, and there is a dilated, inverted U-shaped loop (arrows) arising from the pelvis.

Case 5.122. Water-soluble enema. The sigmoid colon gradually tapers and narrows to a region of high-grade obstruction. The colon proximal to the obstruction is dilated. Beaking (twisting) of the colon is visible at the level of the obstruction.

Differential Diagnosis

Sigmoid volvulus

Diagnosis

Sigmoid volvulus

Discussion

Sigmoid volvulus occurs as a result of a redundant sigmoid colon on a loose mesentery that twists on itself and obstructs. Patients are often older and have a history of chronic constipation. Acute abdominal pain, distention, and vomiting often occur.

Radiographically, the diagnosis usually is made by identifying a prominent bean-shaped, dilated loop of colon arising from the pelvis on abdominal plain radiographs. Gas often is present in the colon proximal to the sigmoid twist. If the diagnosis is equivocal, the obstruction can be confirmed with a contrast enema.

It is often helpful and possible to pass a rectal tube across the obstruction into the dilated sigmoid loop. This will decompress the volvulus and provide the opportunity for elective operative repair of the sigmoid (reduction sigmoid colocolostomy). If tube decompression is not possible, then urgent operation is required to prevent sigmoid infarction and perforation. Recurrence of the volvulus is common without operative repair.

CASE 5.123

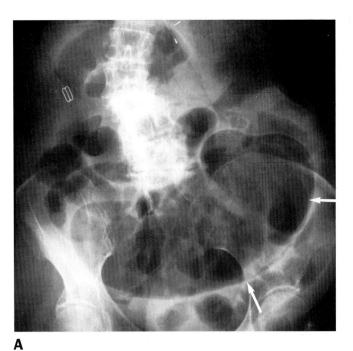

A

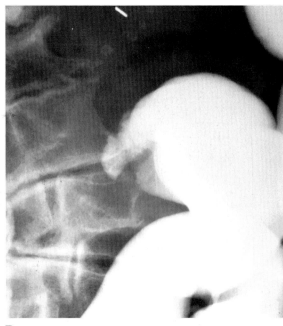

B

Findings

A. Supine abdominal radiograph. A dilated, gas-filled viscus (arrows) fills a large portion of the pelvis and extends slightly into the left upper abdomen. This organ has the shape of an abnormally positioned right colon. Dilated small bowel loops also are present throughout the abdomen. The transverse and left colon are not identified.

B. Single-contrast barium enema (spot radiograph). There is gradual narrowing of the colon to the point of obstruction in the right colon.

Differential Diagnosis

Cecal volvulus

Diagnosis

Cecal volvulus

Discussion

Cecal volvulus occurs as a result of a redundant right colonic mesentery, allowing all or part of the right colon to twist on itself. As the colon twists, it moves into an abnormal location within the abdomen, often in the midline or within the left upper quadrant. The twist causes mechanical obstruction of the colon and often vascular insufficiency of the affected loop. Patients may have a history of intermittent abdominal pain, perhaps due to periodic twisting and untwisting of the colon. Treatment invariably is operative because the risk of cecal perforation is high, and if perforation does occur it is associated with a high morbidity and high mortality.

The initial radiologic examination is usually abdominal radiography. Typically, a dilated (>9 cm) cecum is identified in an abnormal location, often the left upper quadrant. Depending on the duration of symptoms, the colon distal to the obstructing twist has little or no remaining gas within it. Dilated, gas-filled small bowel often is identified. The abdominal radiograph should be scrutinized for evidence of perforation (free air and a rapidly decompressing cecum) and of ischemia (portal venous gas and cecal intramural pneumatosis) (cases 5.117, 5.118, and 4.75 through 4.82). The diagnosis can be rapidly and easily confirmed with a contrast enema. The finding of obstruction in the right colon with a beaklike appearance at the site of the twist is typical.

CASE 5.124

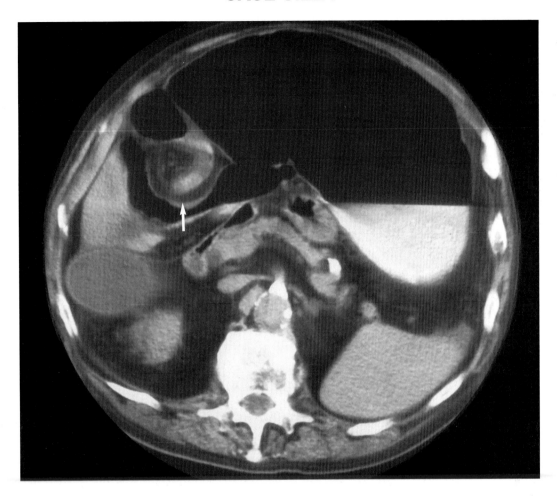

Findings

Contrast-enhanced CT. A dilated gas- and contrast-filled viscus (cecum) fills the upper abdomen. A twisted or whorled appearance of the mesentery is present in the right upper abdomen (arrow). Intestines encircle the mesenteric vessels.

Differential Diagnosis

1. Midgut volvulus
2. Cecal volvulus

Diagnosis

Cecal volvulus

Discussion

Usually the diagnosis of volvulus is suggested on the basis of abdominal radiographic findings (case 5.123) and confirmed with an intraluminal examination with contrast material. A volvulus may be found in the course of a CT examination in patients with indeterminate, intermittent abdominal pain. Midgut volvulus can be suspected when a rotational anomaly of the gut is identified (jejunum in the right upper quadrant) and the superior mesenteric artery is located to the right of the superior mesenteric vein (reversal of the normal anatomical relationships). Cecal volvulus can be more difficult to identify. The cecum is located in an abnormal position in the mid or left abdomen. In the region of the right colon, both bowel and mesentery are twisted and encircle each other (as in this case). Equivocal cases may require a contrast enema to confirm the diagnosis.

CASE 5.125

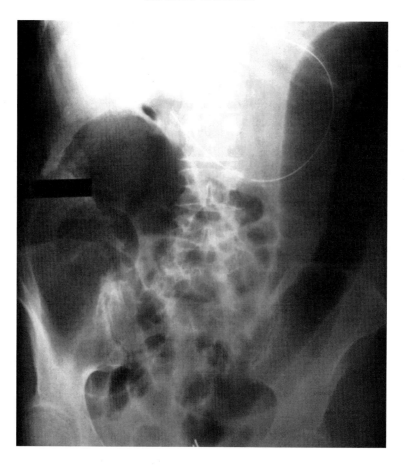

Findings

Abdominal radiograph. Gas is present in mildly dilated loops of small and large bowel. A continuous column of gas fills the colon. The cecum is located normally in the right lower quadrant.

Differential Diagnosis

1. Adynamic ileus
2. Distal mechanical colonic obstruction

Diagnosis

Adynamic ileus

Discussion

Adynamic ileus of the colon is a condition in which the colon becomes atonic and often dilated. There are numerous causes of this condition, including postoperative and postanesthesia states, trauma, adjacent inflammation or infection, various medications, various systemic illnesses, and other conditions. Clinically, patients may have poorly localized abdominal distress and pain, a distended abdomen, and diminished bowel sounds.

Radiographically, the colon usually is distended with air and fluid. Gas fills the colon as a continuous column; however, often the low descending and sigmoid colon are not air-filled as a result of their dependent location in the peritoneal cavity. Radiographs with the patient decubitus or prone can be helpful for demonstrating the gas-filled portions of the colon in equivocal cases. If a contrast-enema study is performed, no obstruction will be identified.

The main differential consideration is mechanical colonic obstruction (cases 5.119 through 5.124). If a continuous column of gas throughout the colon is not present, then a limited contrast enema (contrast material is administered up to the level where a continuous air column is present) can be performed to assess for a distal colonic obstruction.

CASE 5.126

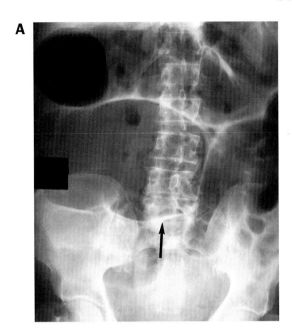

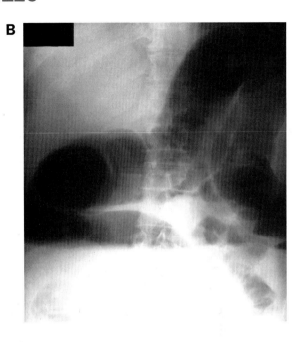

Findings

Supine (**A**) and upright (**B**) abdominal radiographs.
The cecum (arrow) is mobile, dilated, and positioned in
the right and middle abdomen. Air-fluid levels are present
in the cecum and descending colon. Two gas-filled small
bowel loops are visible inferior and lateral to the cecum.
There is a continuous column of gas throughout the colon.

Differential Diagnosis

1. Cecal ileus
2. Cecal volvulus

Diagnosis

Cecal ileus

Discussion

Cecal ileus can develop in patients with a mobile cecum
(10% of the general population) and an underlying colonic
adynamic ileus. The mobile cecum rotates anteromedially
in the abdomen and gradually distends (to a diameter in
excess of 9 cm). Because of the nondependent cecal
location when patients are supine for prolonged periods,
gas does not empty into the less dilated distal colon.
Recognition of this entity is important because excessive
cecal distention for longer than 2 or 3 days has a significant
risk of cecal perforation and possible death. Cecal

perforation occurs more frequently in patients with cecal
ileus than in those with cecal volvulus, mechanical colonic
obstruction, or typical colonic ileus, probably because
patients with obstruction of the colon (cecal volvulus,
mechanical colonic obstruction) usually present with
symptoms that demand an urgent diagnosis and treatment.
Patients with cecal ileus often have nonspecific abdominal
complaints, and cecal distention may go unnoticed for
days. The duration of cecal distention (longer than 2-3 days)
is an important factor in determining the risk of perforation.
Actual cecal size (≥9 cm) does not correlate well with risk
of perforation. If conservative therapy (rectal tubes and
cathartics) is not successful, more aggressive therapy with
either a surgically placed cecostomy tube or colonoscopic
decompression should be instituted. Colonoscopic
decompression may have to be repeated several times
until the ileus resolves.

Radiographically, there is a continuous column
of gas throughout most of the colon (colonic ileus) with
disproportionate dilatation of the cecum, which is abnormally
positioned, often in the mid abdomen. There is no
obstruction at the time of a contrast enema.

Cecal volvulus usually presents radiographically with
absence of gas in the colon distal to the twist and
obstruction in the right colon at contrast enema.

Colonic Obstruction and Ileus

		Case
Mechanical colonic obstruction	Most commonly caused by carcinoma, can be caused by diverticulitis, volvulus, extrinsic mass, fecal impaction, hernia, or adhesions	5.119 and 5.120
Sigmoid volvulus	Inverted U-shaped loop extends into upper abdomen, beaking at level of obstruction	5.121 and 5.122
Cecal volvulus	Dilated cecum extending into left upper quadrant, colon distal to obstruction decompressed	5.123 and 5.124
Adynamic ileus	Distended air and fluid-filled colon with a continuous column to the rectum, often occurs postoperatively or with narcotic medications	5.125 and 5.126

CASE 5.127

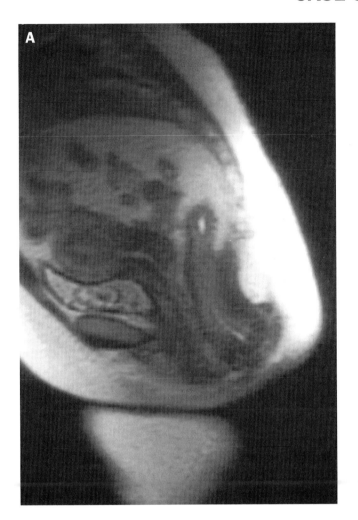

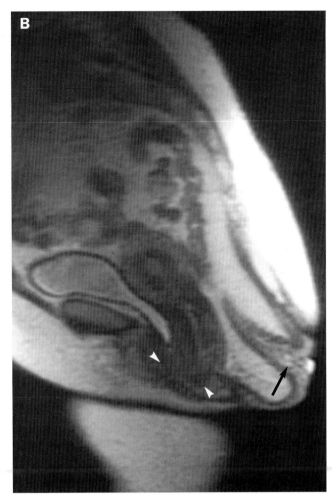

Findings

Dynamic MRI proctogram. **A.** Single-shot fast-spin echo sagittal image of the pelvis shows abnormal pelvic floor descent at rest.

B. Image during straining shows prolapse of the rectal mucosa out of the anal canal (arrow) and abnormal descent of the uterus and bladder into the vagina (arrowheads).

Differential Diagnosis

Rectal prolapse (uterine prolapse and cystocele)

Diagnosis

Rectal prolapse (uterine prolapse and cystocele)

Discussion

Rectal prolapse is protrusion of the rectal mucosa through the anus. Patients present with constipation, incontinence, and rectal ulcerations. Rectal prolapse is six times more common in females. The exact cause is unknown, but it often is associated with long-standing constipation. If the protruding rectal mass is visible with straining on physical examination, proctography is not necessary for diagnosis. As the disease progresses, the rectum may no longer spontaneously retract after defecation, and patients may have to replace it manually. Among patients with rectal prolapse, 10% to 20% have uterine or bladder prolapse, and 35% have an associated cystocele. Rectopexy often is required for treatment. An incarcerated rectal prolapse is rare, but it may require emergency resection if the viability of the bowel is in question.

CASE 5.128

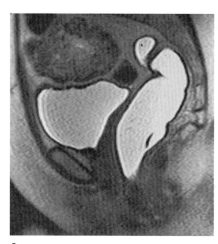

A

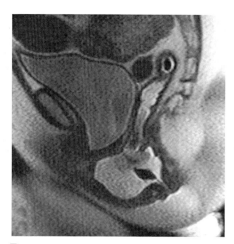

B

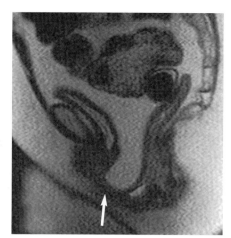

C

Findings

Dynamic MRI proctogram. **A.** Single-shot fast-spin echo sagittal image of the pelvis at rest shows the uterus is surgically absent. The bladder and rectum appear in normal position. **B.** Image obtained during attempted defecation shows abnormal pelvic floor descent with a large anterior bulge of the rectum into the vagina. The bladder also bulges posteriorly into the vagina. None of the rectal contrast material could be expelled despite multiple attempts. **C.** After defecation, with Valsalva maneuver. The rectum and bladder are empty. Abnormal pelvic floor descent. A peritoneocele (arrow) exists with pelvic fat filling the rectovesical space.

Differential Diagnosis

Rectocele (and cystocele)

Diagnosis

Rectocele, cystocele, peritoneocele

Discussion

A rectocele is a bulge of the anterior wall of the rectum into the vagina. Rectoceles may present without any other abnormalities or as part of a generalized weakness of the pelvic floor coexisting with cystoceles, enteroceles, uterine prolapse, or rectal prolapse. Women with multiple deliveries, difficult deliveries, perineal tears, episiotomies, or hysterectomies are at increased risk for development of a rectocele. Patients often present with constipation, difficulty evacuating stool with straining, and the sensation of a mass in the vagina during a bowel movement. Some women find that pressing against the back wall of the vagina helps to empty the rectum. Rectoceles are diagnosed with barium defecating proctography or, more recently, with MRI proctography. Conservative treatment for rectoceles includes stool softeners or a pessary. In more extreme cases, surgical repair may be necessary.

CASE 5.129

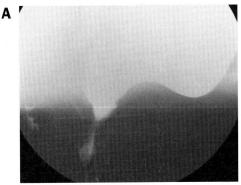

A

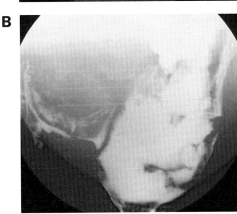

B

CASE 5.130

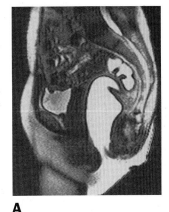 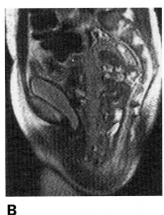

A   B

Findings

Case 5.129. Defecating proctogram, lateral view.
A. Squeeze image. Normal anorectal angle and puborectalis muscle impression. The vagina contains contrast material anteriorly. **B.** During evacuation and straining. A large enterocele containing multiple contrast-filled small bowel loops has entered the space between the rectum (posteriorly) and the vagina (anteriorly). The pelvic floor has descended to an abnormally low position.

Case 5.130. MRI proctogram. **A.** During defecation. Abnormal descent of the pelvic floor. **B.** After defecation with Valsalva maneuver. The pelvic floor has descended further, and an enterocele has developed within the rectovesical space.

Differential Diagnosis

Enterocele

Diagnosis

Enterocele

Discussion

An enterocele refers to herniation of a peritoneal sac along the ventral rectal wall into the cul-de-sac. If the small bowel loops have not been opacified, separation of the opacified vagina and upper rectum during straining suggests this abnormality. An enterocele can contain sigmoid colon, omentum and mesenteric fat, and small intestine. This can be associated with vaginal and rectal prolapse and other pelvic floor abnormalities.

CASE 5.131

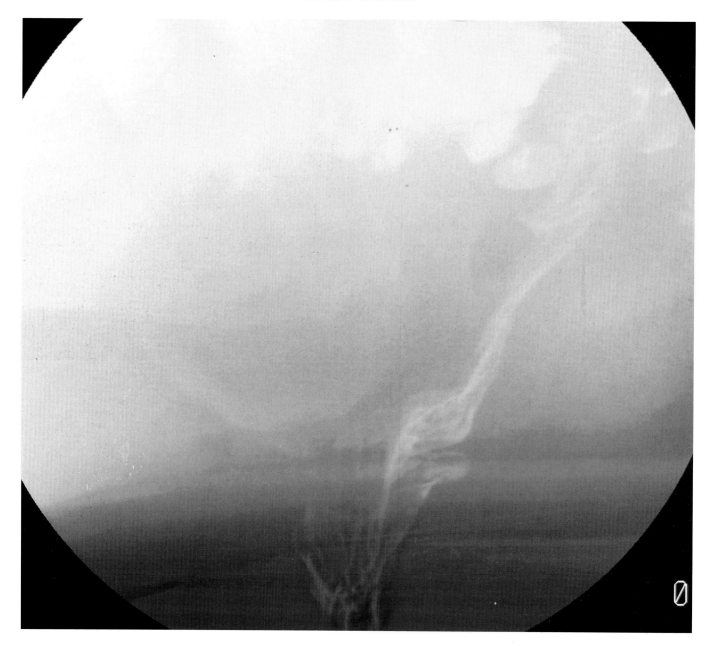

Findings
Defecating proctogram. A small amount of rectal intussusception is present during defecation.

Differential Diagnosis
Rectal intussusception

Diagnosis
Rectal intussusception

Discussion
Rectal intussusception is concentric invagination of the rectal wall that starts in the upper or mid rectum and progresses toward the anal canal. If the intussusception reaches through the anal sphincter, it results in rectal prolapse (case 5.127). Patients often present with constipation and incomplete defecation. Surgical treatment with perineal rectopexy may be necessary in some cases.

CASE 5.132

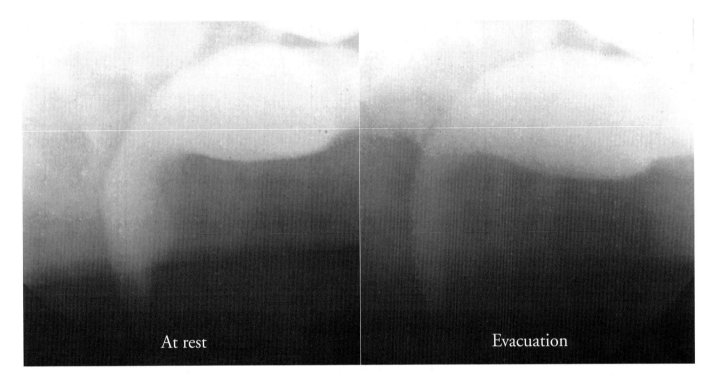

At rest

Evacuation

Findings
Defecating proctogram. No change in the anorectal angle or perineal descent between the images taken at rest and at evacuation. The puborectalis muscle impression is prominent in both images.

Differential Diagnosis
1. Spastic pelvic floor syndrome (anismus)
2. "Stage fright"

Diagnosis
Spastic pelvic floor syndrome (anismus)

Discussion
Spastic pelvic floor syndrome involves the inability to relax the puborectalis muscle, which explains the lack of change in the two images shown here. Retraining of pelvic floor muscles is required to overcome this problem. Coaching and giving the patient enough time (and privacy) may be required to ensure that embarrassment has not led to "stage fright," in which the patient is unable to relax these muscles at the time of examination.

CASE 5.133

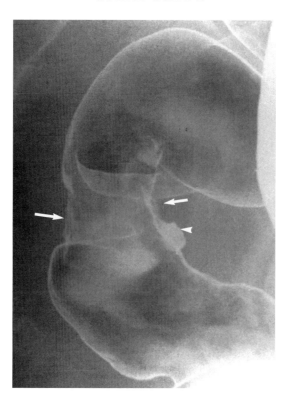

Findings

Double-contrast barium enema. A circumferential ulceration (arrows) is present in the mid rectum, with a focal ulcer crater (arrowhead) anteriorly.

Differential Diagnosis

1. Rectal carcinoma
2. Metastases
3. Solitary rectal ulcer syndrome

Diagnosis

Solitary rectal ulcer syndrome

Discussion

The solitary rectal ulcer syndrome is found in patients with chronic defecation difficulties and abnormalities of the rectal wall. Patients also may complain of rectal bleeding. Defecation abnormalities include either repeated episodes of rectal intussusception or failure of the puborectalis muscle to relax normally (spastic pelvic floor syndrome). Pathologically, one or more rectal ulcers may be present, but they are not necessary for the diagnosis. In addition, thickening of the muscularis mucosa and fibroblastic proliferation within the lamina propria are specific features.

Findings at barium enema include thickened rectal folds, mucosal granularity, rectal stricture, and ulceration. Intussusception, rectal prolapse, failure of the puborectalis muscle to relax, and abnormal perineal descent may be visible at defecating proctography.

Differential considerations include annular neoplasms (case 5.80) and metastases to the colon. The diagnosis of solitary rectal ulcer syndrome should be considered in patients with a long history of straining at stool. Defecating proctography is the method of choice for making the diagnosis.

Disorders of Defecation

		Case
Rectal prolapse	Mucosa extends beyond anal opening at evacuation	5.127
Rectocele	Anterior bulge of rectal wall	5.128
Enterocele	Abnormal descent of small bowel loops into rectal fossa	5.129 and 5.130
Rectal intussusception	Can be normal in 30% of patients	5.131
Spastic pelvic floor syndrome (anismus)	Lack of change of puborectalis muscle and pelvic floor between rest and evacuation	5.132
Solitary rectal ulcer syndrome	Traumatic ulceration from recurrent prolapse or intussusception	5.133

CASE 5.134

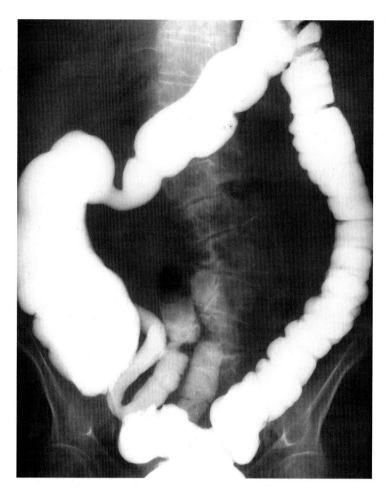

Findings

Single-contrast barium enema. The right and transverse colon are relatively ahaustral; the left colon appears normal.

Differential Diagnosis

1. Cathartic colon
2. Ulcerative colitis
3. Ischemic colitis

Diagnosis

Cathartic colon

Discussion

Cathartic colon is a term used to describe the radiographic changes that occur after prolonged use of irritant cathartics such as cascara, senna, phenolphthalein, and castor oil. The proximal colon usually is affected initially, but left-sided involvement also can occur.

Findings include lack of haustrations (most common in the right colon), shortening, and inconsistent luminal constrictions. It is believed that the strictures are due to muscular hypertrophy. Observation of these areas at fluoroscopy or on sequential radiographs shows the slow, changeable nature of these narrowed segments. The terminal ileum may appear gaping and resemble "backwash" ileitis. This entity usually can be differentiated from ulcerative colitis by obtaining a history. In addition, the distal colon appears to be of normal size and contour in cathartic colon. Shortening of the colon in ulcerative colitis usually is associated with lack of distensibility and narrowing (case 5.12). In cathartic colon, the wall remains distensible. Chronic changes from ischemia can result in a featureless colon segment, but usually there is luminal narrowing and a history consistent with ischemia.

CASE 5.135

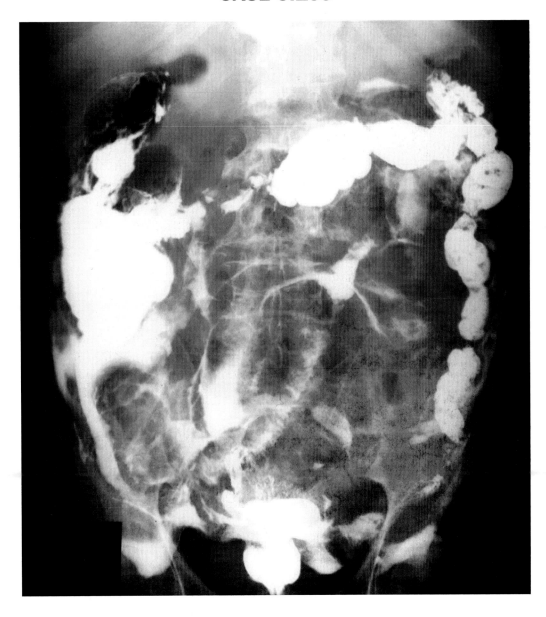

Findings
Water-soluble contrast enema. A large amount of contrast material is present within the peritoneal space. Contrast material is present in the colon and also outlines the serosal surface of many small bowel loops.

Differential Diagnosis
Peritoneal extravasation of contrast material

Diagnosis
Peritoneal extravasation of contrast material

Discussion
This patient had a polyp fulgurated on the day before this examination. The colonic defect was repaired at operation.

If a colonic perforation is suspected, a water-soluble agent should be used instead of barium. Barium is difficult to remove surgically and can elicit a granulomatous reaction in the peritoneal cavity.

CASE 5.136

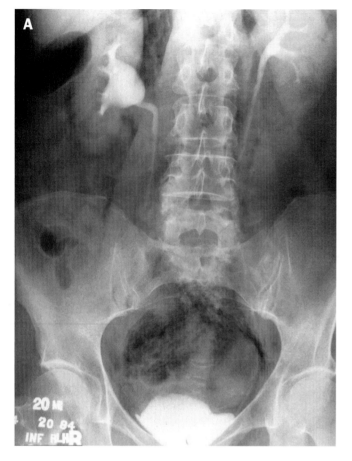

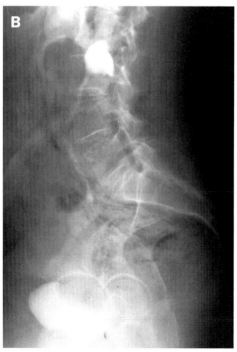

CASE 5.137

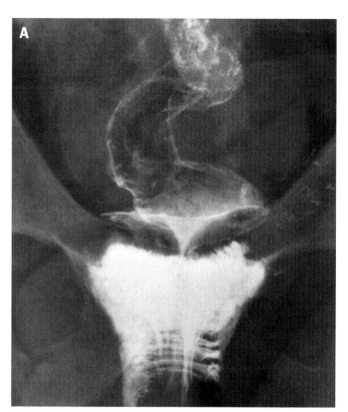

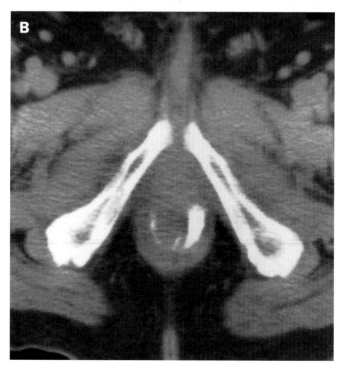

Findings

Case 5.136. Abdominal radiograph. **A** and **B.** Retroperitoneal gas is present in a perirectal and paraspinal location. The majority of the gas resides in the pelvis.

Case 5.137. A. Single-contrast barium enema. A collection of contrast material is present around the rectum. Transverse striations are present within this collection.

B. Unenhanced CT. A linear collection of barium is present within the rectal wall.

Differential Diagnosis

Rectal perforation

Diagnosis

Rectal perforation

Discussion

The patient in case 5.136 recently had had a colonoscopic examination with perforation of the sigmoid. Surgical repair was required. The patient in case 5.137 had an enema tip improperly placed. Colonoscopic perforations are reported to occur in approximately 1 in 1,000 examinations, and the mortality rate is approximately 1 in 10,000. These colonic leaks may not be appreciated at the time of the procedure. Pain often develops, and patients seek medical care within a few hours after the examination. Usually, a plain abdominal radiograph shows peritoneal, retroperitoneal, or intramural gas (cases 5.117 and 5.118) if a significant leak has developed. CT is more sensitive than plain radiography for detecting small amounts of extraluminal gas or pneumatosis. A water-soluble enema sometimes is required to clarify an equivocal finding or to show the site of the leak.

Perforations after a barium enema are unusual, occurring in fewer than 1 in 25,000 examinations. An improperly placed enema tip or an overinflated rectal balloon (particularly in patients with an abnormal, nondistensible rectum, i.e., ulcerative colitis or a rectal cancer) are the most common causes. If an enema tip is difficult to insert, it is prudent to perform a rectal examination to determine the anorectal angle, to determine whether a rectal tumor is present, and to lubricate the anal canal. Balloon inflation should be performed so as not to distend the rectum. If patients complain of pain, the balloon should be deflated until it can be retained comfortably.

CASE 5.138

CASE 5.139

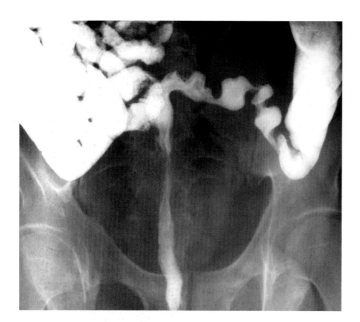

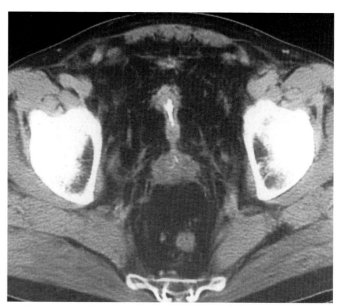

Findings

Case 5.138. Single-contrast barium enema. The rectum is narrowed and straightened. The soft tissues in the pelvis are hyperlucent.

Case 5.139. Enhanced CT. Excessive fatty tissue is present in the pelvis with associated soft-tissue stranding. The fatty tissue has elevated the prostate anteriorly and narrowed the rectum and bladder from side to side.

Differential Diagnosis
Pelvic lipomatosis

Diagnosis
Pelvic lipomatosis

Discussion

Pelvic lipomatosis is a condition of unknown origin with fat and fibrous tissue proliferation in the pelvis. The fibrofatty tissue envelops the rectum and bladder. Patients may complain of backache, constipation, or dysuria. Males are affected more often than females.

Abdominal plain radiography shows a hyperlucent pelvis. Contrast studies show a narrowed and less distensible rectum that resembles a straight tube rising out of the pelvis. The luminal contours and mucosal pattern are otherwise normal. The presacral space often is widened by fat. Similar fatty compression of the bladder often occurs, resulting in a teardrop shape. The ureters may be displaced and mildly to moderately dilated. Clinically significant ureteral or rectal obstruction is uncommon.

CT is the most helpful examination for evaluating patients with suspected pelvic lipomatosis and for excluding other soft tissue abnormalities. The density of the deforming tissues (fat) is diagnostic of this condition.

CASE 5.140

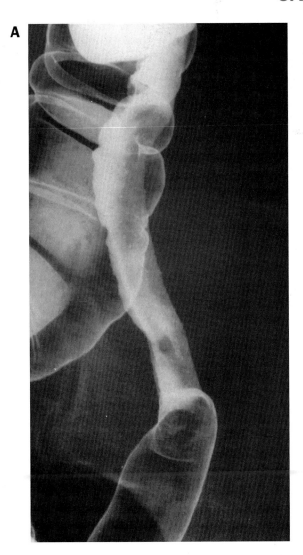

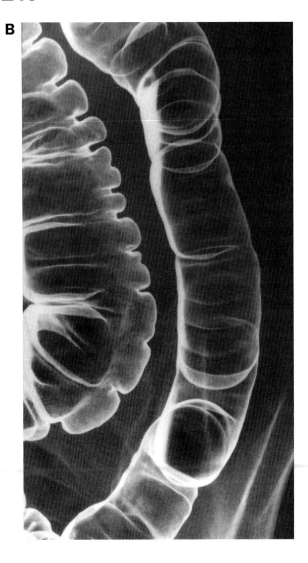

Findings

Double-contrast barium enema. **A.** Multiple spiculations and collections of barium are present in the partially collapsed descending colon. **B.** Air-distended view of the same colonic segment is normal and without evidence of ulceration.

Differential Diagnosis

1. Innominate grooves
2. Ulcerative colitis
3. Infectious colitis

Diagnosis

Innominate grooves

Discussion

Innominate lines (grooves) represent collections of barium within the crevices of the normally collapsed colon. The lines are seen only within the partially filled colon and disappear with complete distention (as seen in this case). Their importance lies in differentiating these normal lines from mucosal ulcerations found in patients with inflammatory bowel disease or infectious colitis. Real mucosal ulcers persist and are well shown on views of the colon with air distention.

Miscellaneous Colon Conditions

		Case
Cathartic colon	Lack of haustrations in right colon. History of laxative abuse	5.134
Rectal perforation	Intramuscular, transverse striations. Peritoneal, outlines bowel loops and space	5.135–5.137
Lipomatosis	Hyperlucent pelvis. Straightening and narrowing of colon and bladder	5.138 and 5.139
Innominate grooves	Granular mucosa in partially distended colon. Disappears with full distention	5.140

DIFFERENTIAL DIAGNOSES

Solitary Filling Defects

Ileocecal valve
Polyp
Adenocarcinoma
Lipoma
Endometrioma
Lymphoma
Appendicitis
Mucocele
Metastases

Multiple Filling Defects

Stool or bubbles or pseudopolyps
Polyps
Carcinomas
Lymphoid follicular pattern
Inflammatory polyps
Polyposis syndrome
Lymphoma
Metastases
Pneumatosis coli
Amebiasis
Colitis cystica profunda

Narrowing

Colonic spasm
Diverticulitis
Carcinoma
Metastases
Crohn colitis
Ulcerative colitis
Ischemia
Pancreatitis
Radiation enteritis
Endometriosis
Cathartic colon
Pelvic lipomatosis

Thickened Folds

Diverticulitis
Pseudomembranous colitis
Neutropenic colitis
Ulcerative colitis
Crohn colitis
Ischemic colitis
Pancreatitis
Appendicitis
Mastocytosis
Radiation enteritis
Crohn colitis

COLONIC FILLING DEFECTS

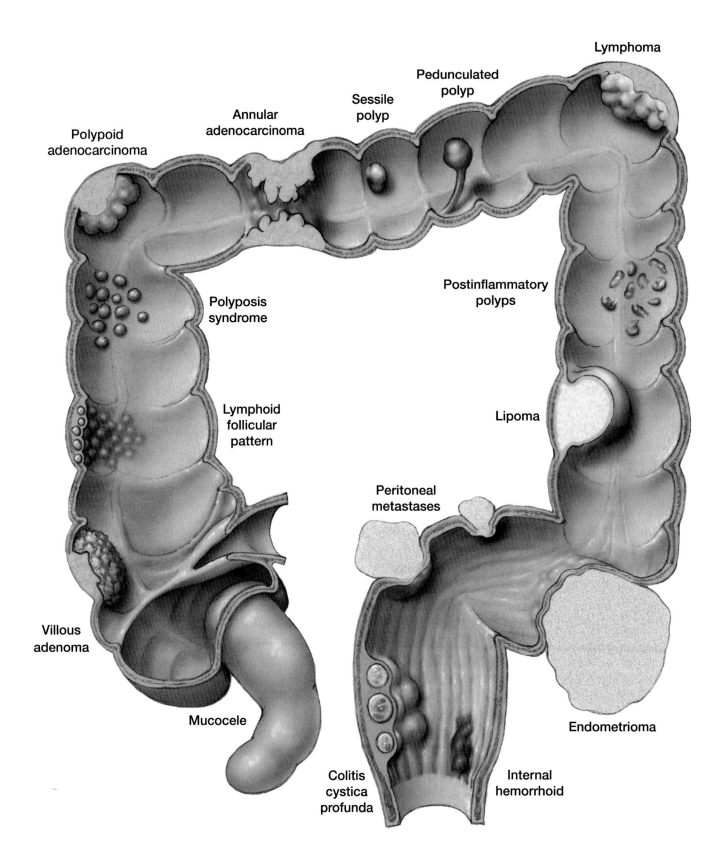

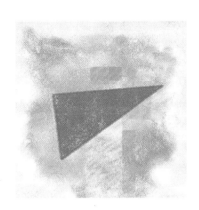

CHAPTER 6
LIVER

CASE 6.1

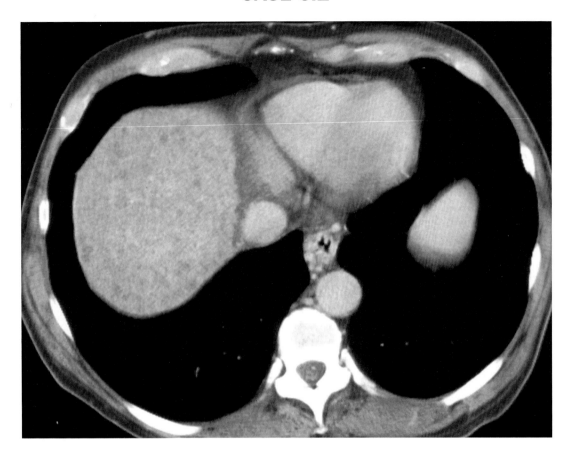

Findings

Contrast-enhanced CT of the liver. The liver is heterogeneously perfused. Multiple tiny low-density nodules are seen throughout the liver parenchyma. Esophageal varices also are present.

Differential Diagnosis

1. Cirrhosis
2. Infection—candidiasis

Diagnosis

Cirrhosis

Discussion

Cirrhosis of the liver refers to diffuse hepatic parenchymal injury with resulting fibrosis, nodular regeneration of the liver, and disorganization of the lobular and vascular anatomy. Cirrhosis can be classified as micronodular or macronodular. Micronodular cirrhosis (Laënnec cirrhosis) has tiny regenerative nodules 3 mm or less in diameter (as in this case). Alcoholic cirrhosis is the commonest cause. Macronodular cirrhosis (postnecrotic cirrhosis) has variably sized regenerative nodules from 3 mm to several centimeters in diameter. Viral hepatitis is the commonest cause of this type. Mixed patterns also exist.

Complications of cirrhosis include hepatic failure, portal venous hypertension (with esophageal varices and bleeding), ascites, renal failure, bacterial peritonitis, and hepatocellular carcinoma.

Microabscesses from candidiasis (case 6.26) are usually fewer in number and of water density. Many times, the spleen has similar-appearing lesions. Patients with candidiasis are immunosuppressed and often febrile.

CASE 6.2

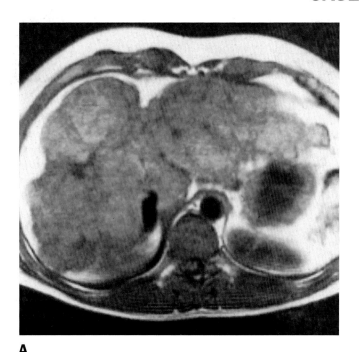

A

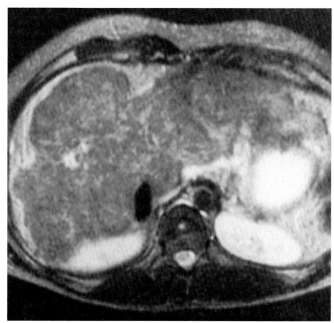

B

Findings

A. T1-weighted unenhanced MRI. The liver has a nodular contour, and large masses bulge the surface. The right lobe of the liver is smaller than expected, and the left lobe is prominent in size. Multiple large nodules are seen throughout the liver, some with higher signal intensity than others.

B. T2-weighted unenhanced MRI. The hepatic parenchyma is slightly heterogeneous in signal. All of the nodules throughout the liver are isointense with the liver.

Differential Diagnosis

Macronodular cirrhosis

Diagnosis

Macronodular cirrhosis

Discussion

The lobar changes in this case are typical of advanced cirrhosis with atrophy of the right lobe and hypertrophy of the left lobe. Often the caudate lobe is spared and appears enlarged because of its dual arterial blood supply and because of its short intrahepatic portal veins. Viral hepatitis was the likely underlying cause of this patient's cirrhosis, because of the macronodular appearance of the liver. MRI is effective for examining the liver for complicating hepatocellular carcinoma. Although several different pulse sequences need to be performed for a complete liver examination, the absence of a high-signal intensity mass on a T2-weighted image is good evidence that the masses are benign nodules rather than hepatocellular carcinoma. The high-signal intensity of some nodules on the T1-weighted images indicates the nodule contains either fat or copper. In-phase and out-of-phase T1-weighted imaging could help make this distinction. Some dysplastic nodules contain fat.

CASE 6.3

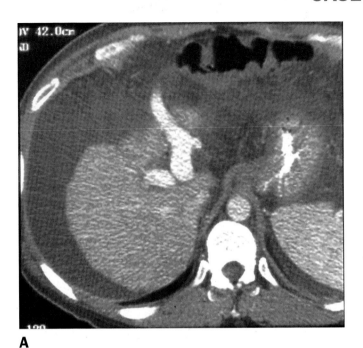

A

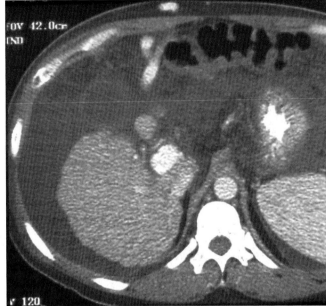

B

Findings
Contrast-enhanced CT. **A** and **B.** The liver is small and has a finely nodular contour. A recanalized umbilical vein leads from the left branch of the portal vein through the falciform ligament to a location posterior to the anterior abdominal wall.

Differential Diagnosis
Cirrhosis with recanalized umbilical vein

Diagnosis
Cirrhosis with recanalized umbilical vein

Discussion
The umbilical vein closes soon after birth, and it never reopens. A recanalized umbilical vein actually is an enlarged collateral vein that runs adjacent to the obliterated umbilical vein carrying hepatofugal-flowing blood. Some authors refer to this vein as the paraumbilical vein. This vein normally is insignificant, but it can be enlarged in patients with portal hypertension. It runs caudad from the liver along the falciform ligament to the umbilicus. In some patients, large collaterals develop in the region of the umbilicus. When these enlarged collaterals are visible on physical examination, they are referred to as caput medusae. Additional collaterals usually form to provide a connection with the systemic venous system (usually with pelvic veins).

CASE 6.4

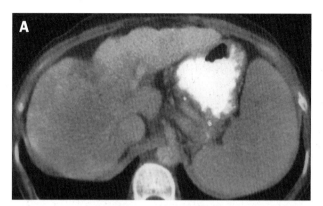

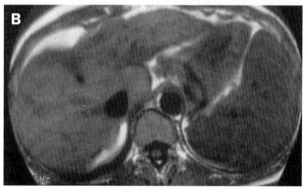

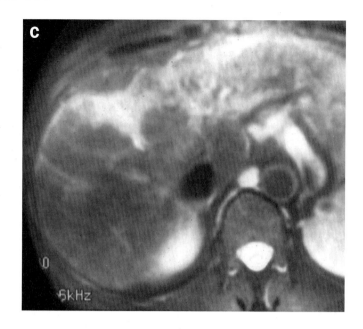

Findings

A. Contrast-enhanced CT. The contour of the liver is nodular. There is retraction of the capsule near the junction of the right and left lobes. There is a low-attenuation region within the liver subjacent to the area of retraction. Splenomegaly.

B. T1-weighted MRI. The area of low attenuation at CT corresponds to a poorly defined region of low-signal intensity.

C. T2-weighted MRI. The area of low-signal intensity on the T1-weighted image is of high-signal intensity. Ill-defined high-signal intensity changes also are present in the left lobe of the liver.

Differential Diagnosis

1. Cirrhosis with diffuse hepatocellular carcinoma
2. Cholangiocarcinoma
3. Cirrhosis with confluent fibrosis

Diagnosis

Cirrhosis with confluent fibrosis

Discussion

Confluent hepatic fibrosis usually manifests as a wedge-shaped region extending from the porta hepatis to the capsule. It most commonly involves the anterior segment of the right lobe and the medial segment of the left lobe. Capsular retraction is seen in 90% of cases. An ill-defined band of abnormal signal (low intensity on T1-weighted images and high signal on T2-weighted images) is characteristic of confluent hepatic fibrosis.

Differentiating confluent hepatic fibrosis from diffuse or infiltrating hepatocellular carcinoma or cholangiocarcinoma can be difficult. Usually a tumor is expansive and bulges the hepatic contour. In patients with confluent hepatic fibrosis, there is no venous invasion and the size of the area does not change over time.

CASE 6.5

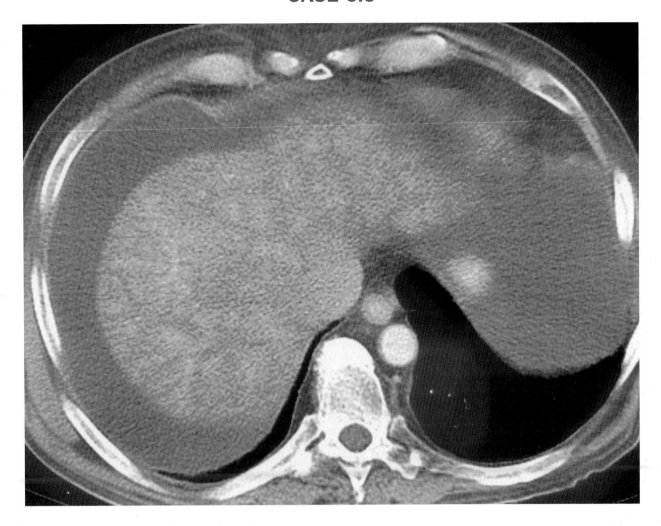

Findings

Contrast-enhanced CT. The liver enhances heterogeneously. The inferior vena cava is dilated. Ascites.

Differential Diagnosis

1. Hepatic cirrhosis
2. Cardiac cirrhosis

Diagnosis

Cardiac cirrhosis

Discussion

Cardiac failure and constrictive pericarditis lead to increased central venous pressure, increased hepatic venous pressure, sinusoidal engorgement, diminished hepatic arterial flow, and hepatocellular hypoxia. If the increased central venous pressure persists for long periods, changes of cirrhosis develop. Liver enzyme values can be increased, but frank liver failure develops rarely. Because the cardiac findings usually overshadow the liver failure, the diagnosis usually is apparent.

CT findings of hepatic congestion include reflux of contrast material into dilated hepatic veins and the inferior vena cava. Enhancement of the liver is often mottled and resembles early changes of Budd-Chiari syndrome (case 6.13). Other findings include cardiomegaly, hepatomegaly, intrahepatic periportal lucency, ascites, and pleural and pericardial effusions. At sonography, the Doppler waveform of the portal vein also may be abnormal. There is loss of the normal continuous flow pattern and increased pulsatility that represents direct transmission of the fluid wave from the heart through the hepatic sinusoids.

CASE 6.6

A
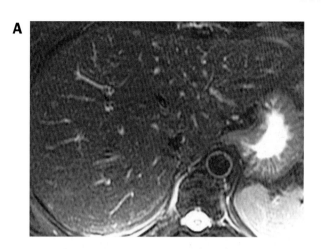

B
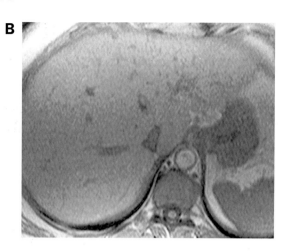

C
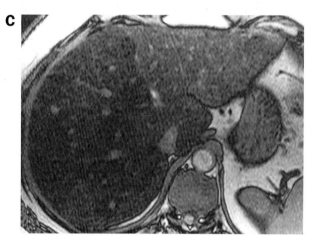

Findings

A. T2-weighted MRI. The liver is normal in appearance.

B. T1-weighted (in-phase) MRI. The liver is diffusely higher in signal intensity than normal.

C. T1-weighted (out-of-phase) MRI. The liver is diffusely lower in signal intensity than normal.

Differential Diagnosis
Diffuse fatty infiltration

Diagnosis
Diffuse fatty infiltration

Discussion

Fatty infiltration of the liver is associated with various conditions, including excessive alcohol consumption, obesity, parenteral nutrition, diabetes, corticosteroid use, and nonalcoholic steatohepatitis. Fatty changes also can be present in 25% of healthy persons. Fatty infiltration of the liver may be diffuse or focal. MRI accurately differentiates fatty infiltration from tumors. On T1-weighted images, fatty infiltration appears as regions of increased signal intensity. Chemical shift imaging (using in- and out-of-phase T1-weighted images) exploits the difference in resonance frequency between the protons present in fat and water. Loss of signal intensity of hepatic parenchyma between the in-phase and out-of-phase images indicates the presence of microscopic lipid. The absence of abnormal signal on the T2-weighted image is reassuring that an underlying mass is absent.

CASE 6.7

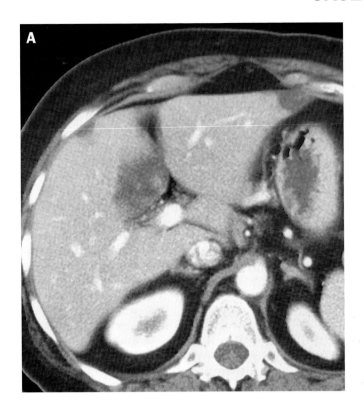

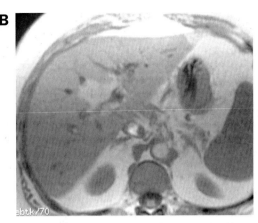

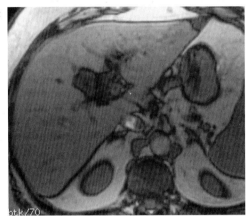

Findings

A. Contrast-enhanced CT. There is a focal low-attenuation mass within the medial segment of the left lobe of the liver and a similar-appearing smaller region within the lateral segment of the left lobe.

B and **C.** In- and out-of-phase T1-weighted MRI. The two regions are of high-signal intensity on the in-phase image and of low-signal intensity on the out-of-phase image.

Differential Diagnosis

Focal fatty infiltration of the liver

Diagnosis

Focal fatty infiltration of the liver

Discussion

Focal steatosis most often is found in the liver tissue adjacent to the fissure of the ligamentum teres, but it can occur anywhere, be any size, and be solitary or multiple. Focal steatosis is assumed to be related to regional differences or disturbances in hepatic blood flow. This mechanism explains why focal fatty changes are common in patients with trauma or ischemic insults to the liver. They can appear as a focal hepatic low-attenuation mass and can mimic a primary or metastatic liver tumor(s).

Noncontrast-enhanced scans are most helpful for CT diagnosis. Normally, the attenuation of the liver is similar or slightly higher than paraspinal muscle. Fatty infiltration of the liver results in attenuation values of the liver to decrease below the normal 50 to 75 Hounsfield units.

The findings of focal fat at MRI are the same as those of diffuse fatty infiltration. At sonography, a fatty liver is diffusely echogenic. The degree of echogenicity is roughly equivalent to the level of steatosis. Fat causes increased attenuation of the ultrasound beam and poorer visualization of deeper structures.

CASE 6.8

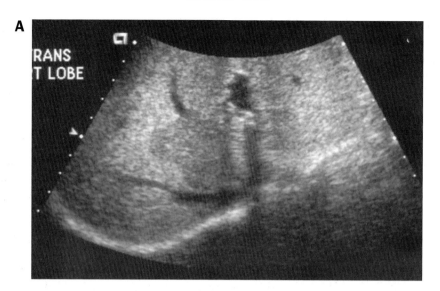

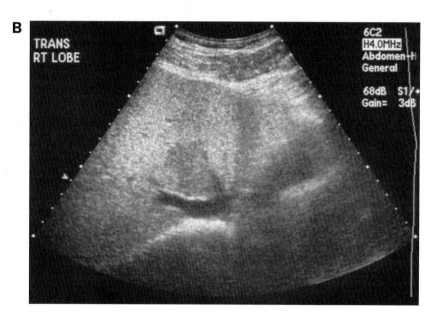

Findings
Hepatic sonogram. **A** and **B.** The liver is diffusely echogenic. A geographic hypoechoic region is present within the right lobe of the liver.

Differential Diagnosis
1. Hepatic neoplasm
2. Fatty infiltration of the liver with focal normal liver

Diagnosis
Fatty infiltration of the liver with focal normal liver

Discussion
Fatty infiltration of the liver is a relatively common finding. It can present as diffuse or focal fatty infiltration. Occasionally an island(s) of normal liver is present in a liver that is otherwise fat-infiltrated. The region of focal normal liver can simulate a neoplasm. The key in recognizing this entity is to identify the diffusely increased echogenicity of the underlying liver. In addition, the normal liver does not cause mass effect, and vessels often can be seen to course normally through this region.

CASE 6.9

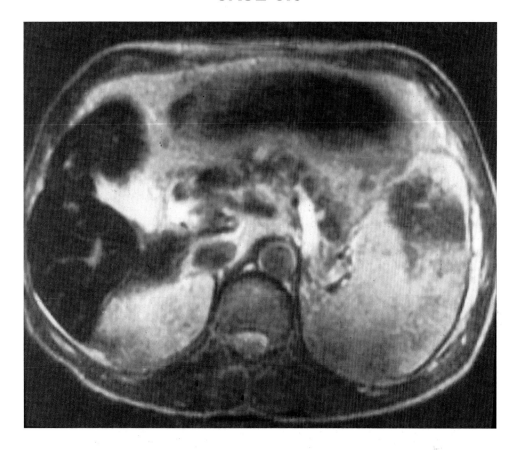

Findings

T2-weighted MRI of the liver. The liver and pancreas are of diffusely low-signal intensity. The spleen is enlarged and is predominantly of high-signal intensity.

Differential Diagnosis

1. Hemochromatosis
2. Hemosiderosis

Diagnosis

Hemochromatosis

Discussion

Primary hemochromatosis (hereditary hemochromatosis or idiopathic hemochromatosis) is an autosomal recessive disorder. Abnormal absorption and deposition of iron occur. In primary hemochromatosis, the liver is the main organ for abnormal iron deposition, consisting of ferritin and hemosiderin. Early deposition is located in periportal hepatocytes. This progresses to perilobular fibrosis with iron deposition in the biliary epithelium, Kupffer cells, and fibrous septa. In patients with advanced disease, the liver is cirrhotic with broad fibrous septa surrounding large areas of relatively normal liver parenchyma. Other sites of abnormal iron deposition include the pancreas and heart.

One-third of deaths from hemochromatosis are the result of hepatocellular carcinoma. Cardiomyopathy, diabetes, and arthropathy also can occur. Screening for hemochromatosis usually involves measurement of serum ferritin and transferrin saturation. Definitive diagnosis of primary hemochromatosis can be made with genetic testing or liver biopsy with quantitative determination of liver iron concentration. MRI can be used to assess for complicating hepatocellular carcinoma and, in specialized centers, to quantitate the amount of hepatic iron. Low-signal intensity of the liver and pancreas with normal signal in the spleen is characteristic. Because the liver also is involved in secondary hemochromatosis (hemosiderosis), involvement of the pancreas is a key finding.

CASE 6.10

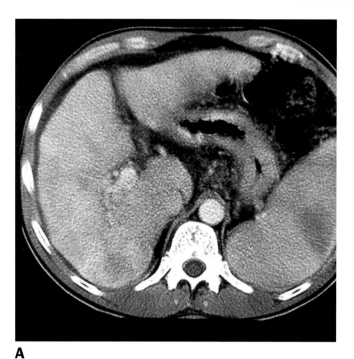

A

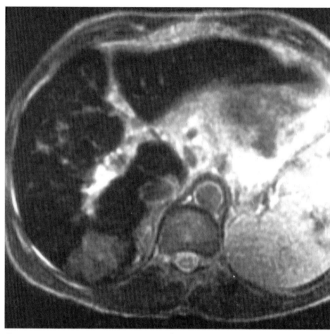

B

Findings

A. Contrast-enhanced CT. There is a focal, approximately 5-cm mass in the posterior aspect of the right lobe of the liver. The caudate lobe is prominent in size, and the right lobe appears small. The spleen is also prominent in size and contains a focal hypoattenuating region.

B. T2-weighted MRI. The mass in the posterior aspect of the right lobe of the liver is well defined and of uniformly high-signal intensity compared with the very low-signal intensity of the liver parenchyma. The spleen is of normal signal intensity.

Differential Diagnosis

1. Cirrhosis with complicating hepatocellular carcinoma
2. Hemochromatosis with complicating hepatocellular carcinoma
3. Hepatic metastasis

Diagnosis

Hemochromatosis with complicating hepatocellular carcinoma

Discussion

The liver is of lower than expected signal intensity on the T2-weighted sequence. On T2-weighted images, the paraspinal muscles are a good internal control to consider whether the liver is of abnormal signal intensity. Generally, the signal of normal liver is not lower than that of muscle. In primary hemochromatosis, iron deposition occurs within the hepatocytes rather than the Kupffer cells (reticuloendothelial system). Because the spleen in this patient is of normal signal intensity, primary hemochromatosis is most likely. The mass in the liver should represent a complicating hepatocellular carcinoma. If primary hemochromatosis is untreated, a hepatocellular carcinoma will develop in approximately one-third of patients.

Patients with increased hepatic iron have diffuse increased attenuation of the liver, usually more than 75 Hounsfield units on unenhanced CT examinations. Hepatomegaly also may be seen on CT. The focal abnormality in the spleen in this case was due to an infarct.

CASE 6.11

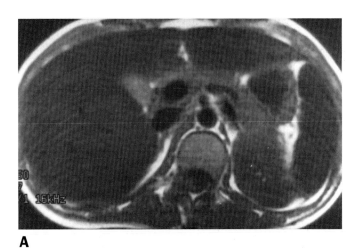

A

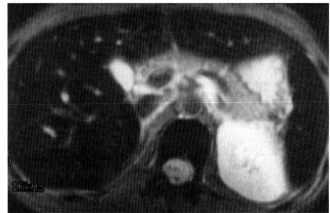

B

Findings
A. T1-weighted MRI. The liver is of diffusely abnormal lower-signal intensity.

B. T2-weighted MRI. The liver, spleen, and bone marrow are of abnormally decreased signal intensity. The pancreas has a normal appearance. No focal masses are present.

Differential Diagnosis
1. Hemosiderosis (secondary hemochromatosis)
2. Primary hemochromatosis

Diagnosis
Hemosiderosis

Discussion
Secondary hemochromatosis (hemosiderosis) can be caused by multiple factors, such as parenteral administration of iron (from transfusions), increased absorption of normal dietary iron, and increased dietary iron load. Normally, iron is stored in the body as hemosiderin or ferritin in the reticuloendothelial cells of the liver, spleen, and bone marrow. Usually, no organ damage occurs. Involvement of the pancreas and heart is unusual, unless the iron load exceeds the capacity of the reticuloendothelial system.

Differentiating hemosiderosis from primary hemochromatosis is important because the treatments and natural history of the disease are very different (case 6.9). Both diseases cause a loss of signal in the liver at MRI, but, commonly, primary hemochromatosis also results in iron deposition in the pancreas and heart (and loss of parenchymal signal). Hemosiderosis spares the pancreas and heart, but iron deposition in the spleen and bone marrow usually is obvious at MRI. T2-weighted gradient echo sequences are most sensitive for visualizing iron deposition.

CASE 6.12

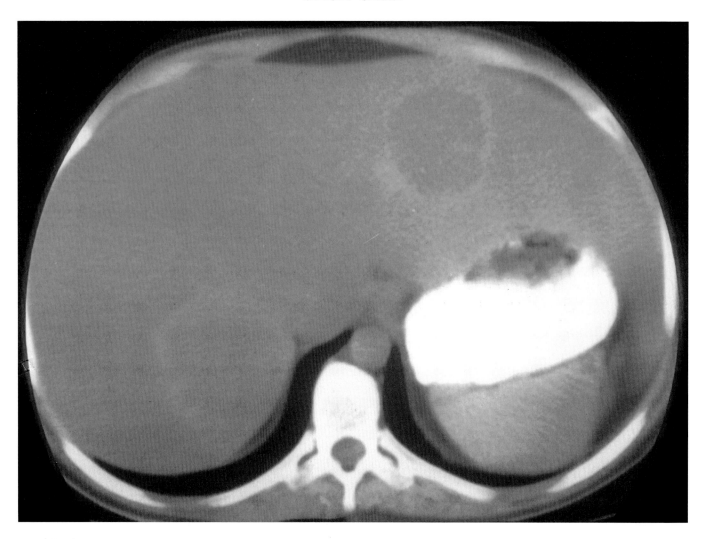

Findings
Contrast-enhanced CT. The liver is of diffusely low
attenuation. Two low-attenuation masses are seen.

Differential Diagnosis
1. Diffuse fatty infiltration with metastases
2. Glycogen storage disease with multiple hepatic adenomas

Diagnosis
Glycogen storage disease with multiple hepatic adenomas
(von Gierke disease)

Discussion
The glycogen storage diseases are inherited disorders of
metabolism. Most of the disorders involve an abnormality
breaking down glycogen into glucose. In glycogen storage
disease type I (von Gierke disease), there is an accumulation
of glycogen within the hepatocytes and proximal tubules
of the kidney. Although glycogen accumulation usually
results in a hyperattenuating liver, the effects of fatty
infiltration predominate in this disease as a result of
chronic hormonal stimulation of the liver. One of the
complications of this disease is an increased incidence of
hepatic cell adenomas. Unlike solitary adenomas, there is
an increased incidence of hepatocellular carcinoma arising
from these adenomas.

CASE 6.13

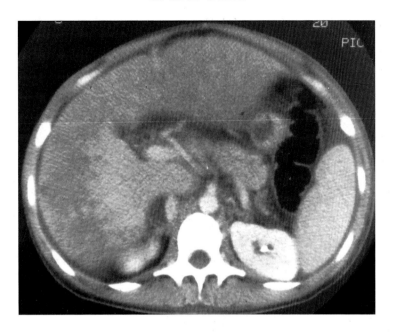

Findings

Contrast-enhanced CT. Heterogeneous enhancement of the liver parenchyma. There appears to be normal, uniform enhancement of the caudate lobe.

Differential Diagnosis

1. Budd-Chiari syndrome
2. Hepatic congestion from cardiac failure
3. Portal vein thrombosis

Diagnosis

Budd-Chiari syndrome

Discussion

Budd-Chiari syndrome refers to a group of conditions with hepatic venous outflow obstruction. Obstruction can occur at the hepatic vein level or within the supradiaphragmatic portion of the inferior vena cava. The clinical symptoms of acute Budd-Chiari syndrome are usually ascites, abdominal pain, vomiting, and hypotension. Other biochemical evidence of hepatic failure also often is present. Primary Budd-Chiari syndrome refers to a membranous (wafer-thin to several-centimeter–thick membrane) obstruction of the hepatic veins. This cause is common in the Far East, Israel, and South Africa. Membranous obstruction is associated with hepatocellular carcinoma in 20% to 40% of patients.

Secondary Budd-Chiari syndrome is most common in North America and Europe and can be classified further as occurring at the central and sublobular venous level or involving the major hepatic veins. Various drugs or treatments are implicated for sublobular venous occlusion, whereas a coagulopathy is often the cause of large vein occlusion.

Angiography is the standard for diagnosis. Pressure measurements within the inferior vena cava and hepatic veins are helpful to exclude a membranous obstruction. A wedged hepatic venogram that shows the spider-web pattern of intrahepatic collaterals is pathognomonic of sublobular venous occlusion. The CT and MRI findings can vary depending on the duration and extent of the condition. Findings in acute and subacute Budd-Chiari syndrome include hepatomegaly, ascites, acute hyperdense thrombus, patchy enhancement (often with normal enhancement of the central portion of the liver and caudate lobe), portal vein thrombosis (in approximately 20% of cases), and compression of the inferior vena cava. Chronically, the hepatic veins may become invisible, and the peripheral portions of the liver (with hypertrophy of the caudate lobe) often atrophy. If a single hepatic vein remains patent, intrahepatic collateral veins may be visible carrying blood from the segments with occluded veins to the sole patent outflow vein.

CASE 6.14

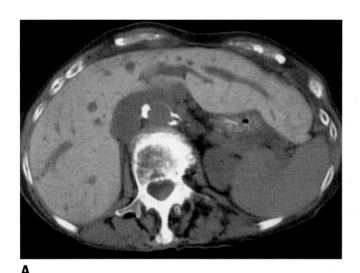

A

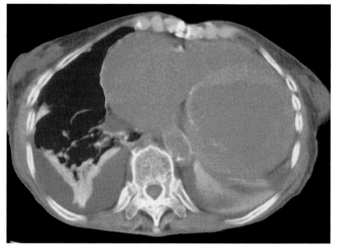

B

Findings

Unenhanced CT. **A.** The liver is diffusely hyperattenuating. It is significantly higher in attenuation than either the spleen or paraspinal muscle. **B.** Cardiomegaly with high-attenuation changes involving atelectatic lung in the lung bases.

Differential Diagnosis

1. Hemochromatosis
2. Amiodarone therapy
3. Previous thorium dioxide therapy
4. Glycogen storage disease
5. Gold therapy

Diagnosis

Amiodarone therapy

Discussion

There are few imaging findings in patients with drug-induced liver disease. Several drugs have been implicated in liver disease or failure. These drugs cause at least 40% of hospital admissions for acute hepatitis and 2% to 5% of all hospital admissions. The most commonly implicated drugs in liver disease include halothane, acetaminophen, α-methyldopa, and phenytoin.

Amiodarone is an antiarrhythmic cardiac medication in which the drug or its iodine-containing metabolites are concentrated in the liver—leading to an abnormally high attenuation of liver parenchyma. There also can be hyperattenuation within the lung parenchyma and secondary interstitial lung disease.

Large amounts of iron stores also can lead to a hyperattenuation of the liver parenchyma in patients with primary and secondary hemochromatosis. Thorium dioxide, a discontinued vascular contrast agent, is concentrated in Kupffer cells and can lead to abnormal liver attenuation. Glycogen storage disease leads to an accumulation of glycogen within hepatocytes. The high glycogen content leads to high liver attenuation. Some patients with glycogen storage disease have concomitant fatty infiltration that actually leads to a lower than normal liver attenuation (case 6.12). Gold used for therapy in rheumatoid arthritis is accumulated by the reticuloendothelial system and causes an increase in liver attenuation.

CASE 6.15

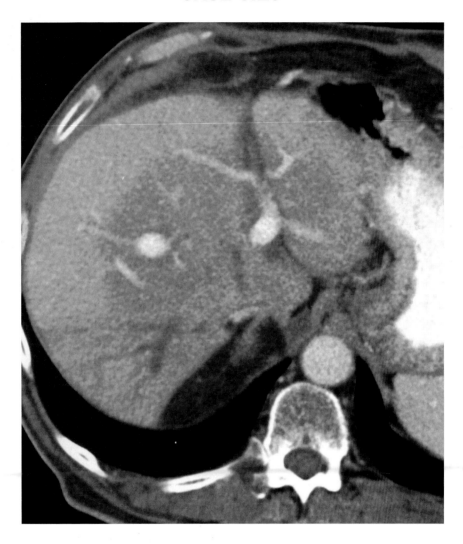

Findings
Contrast-enhanced CT. There is a large central low-attenuation region in the liver. The patient had a history of radiation therapy for cholangiocarcinoma in this region.

Differential Diagnosis
Radiation-induced liver disease

Diagnosis
Radiation-induced liver disease

Discussion
Radiation can cause liver changes in patients treated for esophageal, gastric, pancreatic, or breast malignancies. Radiation hepatitis can develop in patients receiving more than 12 Gy as a single dose or more than 40 Gy in fractionated doses.

Findings at CT are usually a straight, sharply defined zone of different attenuation that corresponds to the treatment port. The irradiated area is usually of lower attenuation than normal liver because of the edema and fatty infiltration that occur. With time, the sharply defined zone may become more indistinct, and hepatic atrophy can develop. At sonography, the acutely irradiated zone appears hypoechoic. At MRI, acute radiation injury is of low-signal intensity on the T1-weighted images and of increased signal intensity on the T2-weighted images. Chronically, fatty change often develops in these regions of injury.

Diffuse Diseases of the Liver

		Case
Cirrhosis	Nodular contour, atrophic right lobe, hypertrophic left and caudate lobes	6.1–6.5
Fatty infiltration	Diffuse or focal. Low attenuation at CT. Usually geographic with vessels coursing through area. Chemical shift changes at MRI	6.6–6.8
Hemochromatosis	Iron deposition in liver, pancreas, heart. Cirrhosis and hepatocellular carcinoma can occur	6.9 and 6.10
Hemosiderosis	Iron deposition in liver, spleen, marrow. No organ damage	6.11
Glycogen storage disease	High attenuation or fatty changes at CT. Predisposes to multiple adenomas	6.12
Budd-Chiari syndrome	Hepatic venous or inferior vena cava occlusion. Heterogeneous liver with normal-appearing central portion and caudate lobe	6.13
Amiodarone therapy	Iodine-containing antiarrhythmic. High-attenuation liver and lung parenchyma	6.14
Radiation-induced disease	Edema or fatty changes correspond to radiation port	6.15

CASE 6.16

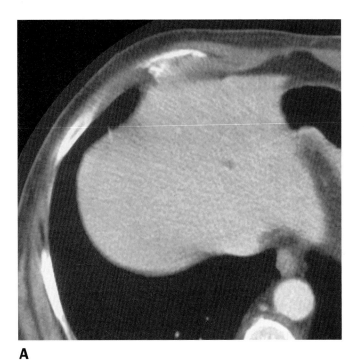

A

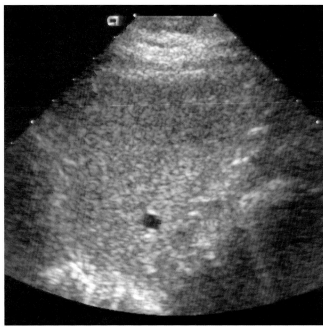

B

Findings

A. Contrast-enhanced CT. A tiny low-attenuation lesion is present in the superior aspect of the liver.

B. Sonogram. A tiny anechoic liver lesion with posterior acoustic enhancement is seen, corresponding to the lesion on CT.

Differential Diagnosis

1. Tiny hepatic cyst
2. Metastases
3. Von Meyenburg complex

Diagnosis

Hepatic cyst

Discussion

Low-attenuation liver lesions are commonly found on CT of the abdomen. When the lesions are large, it is often possible to diagnose them as cysts (fluid density on CT).

However, tiny lesions (such as the one in this case) are often too small to characterize confidently and are considered indeterminate. Most of these tiny low-attenuation lesions are inconsequential liver cysts or even hemangiomas, but tiny metastases can have an identical CT appearance. In cases of high clinical concern, such as a history of malignancy, ultrasonography is often invaluable for differentiating hepatic cysts from solid liver tumors.

A liver cyst is defined as an epithelial-lined fluid-filled space. Hepatic cysts are extremely common, occurring in up to 5% of the population. The precise cause of hepatic cysts is unclear, as is the explanation of why these lesions usually do not develop until middle age. On sonographic examination, simple hepatic cysts are anechoic with a thin wall and posterior acoustic enhancement. Very rarely, a cyst may become symptomatic as a result of infection or hemorrhage into the cyst. Von Meyenburg complex (case 6.19) is a biliary hamartoma, often containing fat. Like cysts, it has no known clinical sequelae.

CASE 6.17

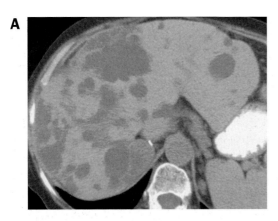

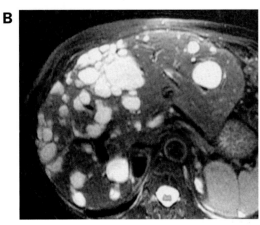

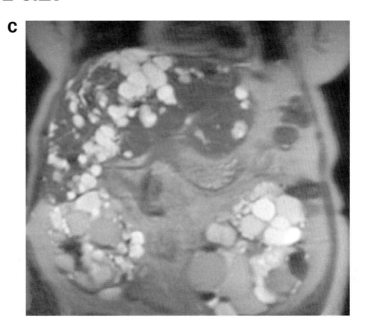

Findings

A. Unenhanced CT. Multiple cysts are present in the liver with confluent cystic change in the right lobe of the liver.

B and C. Unenhanced MRI. T2-weighted axial (B) and coronal (C) images. Multiple cysts are present in the liver. Near complete replacement of both kidneys with cysts is seen on the coronal image.

Differential Diagnosis

1. Autosomal dominant polycystic disease
2. Multiple hepatic cysts

Diagnosis

Autosomal dominant polycystic disease

Discussion

Autosomal dominant polycystic disease (adult polycystic disease) is inherited in an autosomal dominant pattern, presenting clinically in adulthood. The renal parenchyma is progressively replaced by cysts of varying sizes, and most patients present between ages 30 and 50 years with hypertension and renal failure. Cysts often occur in the liver (50%-75% of cases), pancreas (10% of cases), spleen (5% of cases), and other organs. No correlation exists between the severity of renal disease and the extent of liver involvement. The liver cysts in autosomal dominant polycystic disease rarely cause hepatic dysfunction. Unlike autosomal recessive polycystic disease (infantile polycystic disease), there is no association with hepatic fibrosis.

When liver function values are increased, biliary obstruction, cyst infection, or tumor should be excluded. Multiple large cysts can rarely cause compression of the portal vein, resulting in portal hypertension. Cardiovascular abnormalities associated with autosomal dominant polycystic disease include intracranial berry aneurysms (10% of cases), mitral valve prolapse (25% of cases), bicuspid aortic valve, aortic aneurysms, and aortic dissections.

CASE 6.18

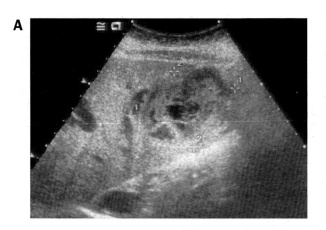

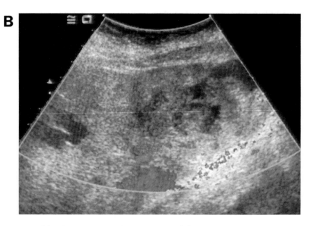

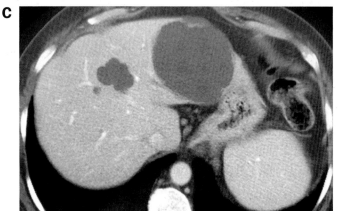

Findings

Sonogram. **A** and **B.** A complex cystic liver mass is present within the left lobe of the liver. The lesion contains significant internal echoes, consistent with a mixed solid and cystic mass. No blood flow is seen within the mass on color Doppler interrogation.

C. Contrast-enhanced CT. Two fluid-density liver masses are present, the larger of which is in the lateral segment of the left lobe of the liver.

Differential Diagnosis

1. Infected cyst or abscess
2. Hemorrhagic cyst
3. Cystic hepatocellular carcinoma
4. Cystic metastasis

Diagnosis

Hemorrhagic liver cyst

Discussion

This patient underwent CT of the abdomen for acute abdominal pain. The superiority of ultrasonography over CT for the evaluation of cystic lesions is clearly shown in this case. Aspiration of this complex cyst revealed hemorrhagic products and resulted in relief of the pain. Because hepatic cysts have an epithelial lining and invariably recur, aspiration is not indicated for asymptomatic cysts.

An infected hepatic cyst could have a similar sonographic appearance, but the patient would likely present clinically with a fever and an increased leukocyte count. A cystic liver tumor can be excluded, given the lack of an enhancing rim at CT and lack of internal blood flow at sonography.

CASE 6.19

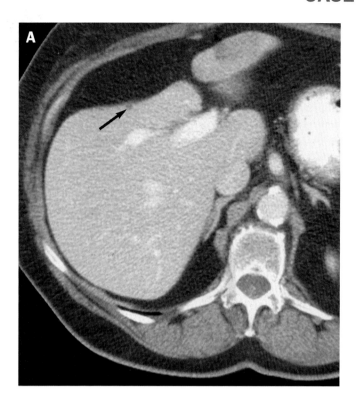

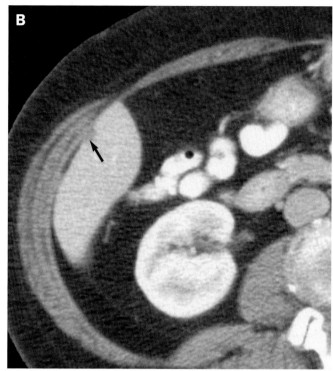

Findings

Contrast-enhanced CT. **A** and **B.** Two tiny low-attenuation lesions (arrows) are present in the periphery of the liver.

Differential Diagnosis

1. Simple hepatic cysts
2. Tiny hepatic metastases
3. Von Meyenburg complexes

Diagnosis

Von Meyenburg complexes

Discussion

This patient with a history of colon cancer had several tiny hypodense liver lesions that were thought likely to be metastases. They were surgically resected and found to be von Meyenburg complexes. Von Meyenburg complexes

(also known as biliary hamartomas) are composed of a cluster of proliferated bile ducts embedded in a fibrous stroma. These small (usually <1 cm) benign lesions are detected incidentally in 1% to 5% of reported autopsies and are often multiple. They are of no clinical significance except that they can be easily mistaken for metastases on CT and ultrasonography. Von Meyenburg complexes are usually uniformly hypoechoic on ultrasonography but may contain echogenic foci with ringdown artifact related to the presence of cholesterol crystals in the dilated tubules. Von Meyenburg complexes usually can be differentiated from metastases at MRI with very high signal on T2-weighted images. No enhancement or only a rim of enhancement is visible on post-gadolinium images. This rim enhancement is thought to be caused by compressed liver parenchyma surrounding the biliary hamartoma.

CASE 6.20

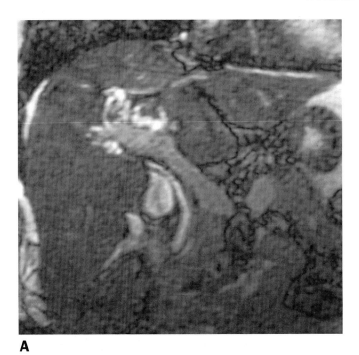

A

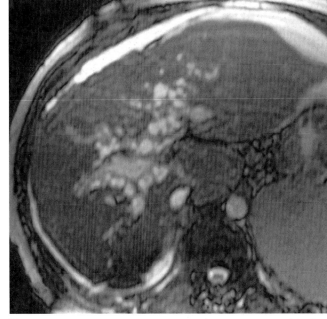

B

Findings

Coronal (**A**) and axial (**B**) MRCP. Numerous small cystic lesions encase the bile ducts throughout the liver. The common bile duct and intrahepatic ducts are normal. The liver has a cirrhotic configuration, and the left and caudate lobes are enlarged. A small amount of ascites is seen around the liver.

Differential Diagnosis

1. Peribiliary cysts
2. Caroli disease
3. Multiple simple hepatic cysts
4. Von Meyenburg complexes

Diagnosis

Peribiliary cysts

Discussion

Peribiliary cysts develop in patients with severe liver disease and dilated intrahepatic peribiliary glands. They can occur as discrete cysts, clustered cysts, or strings of cysts (as in this case) along the portal tracts. The development of peribiliary cysts seems to be related to disturbances in hepatic circulation. These cysts most commonly occur in the setting of cirrhosis, portal venous hypertension or thrombosis, hepatic transplantation, cholangitis, or autosomal dominant polycystic disease. Peribiliary cysts usually are asymptomatic and rarely result in biliary duct dilatation. The intrahepatic and extrahepatic bile ducts remain normal in uncomplicated cases. Peribiliary cysts can be identified by CT, MRI, or ultrasonography. Cholangiographic-enhanced CT can be very helpful in some cases to differentiate peribiliary cysts from intrahepatic bile duct dilatation or Caroli disease (cases 7.31 and 7.32). Other hepatic cystic lesions such as von Meyenburg complexes (case 6.19) or simple hepatic cysts (case 6.16) arise independently from the bile ducts.

Liver Cysts

		Case
Simple cyst	Well-circumscribed, water attenuation, no enhancement	6.16
Polycystic disease	Multiple benign cysts, some hemorrhagic—kidneys, liver, pancreas	6.17
Hemorrhagic cyst	Complex cyst. High attenuation at CT, high-signal intensity T1-weighted MRI, mixed solid and cystic at sonography	6.18
Von Meyenburg complexes	Tiny water attenuation masses resemble tiny simple cysts. May be fat attenuation	6.19
Peribiliary cysts	Multiple tiny cysts clustered, or discrete cysts adjacent to biliary tree; usually associated with cirrhosis	6.20

CASE 6.21

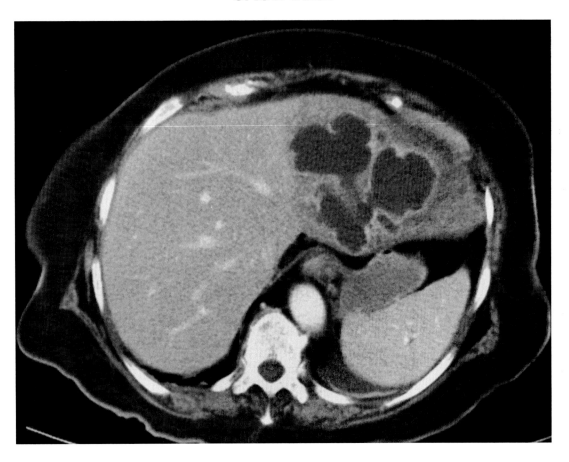

Findings

Contrast-enhanced CT. Several low-attenuation masses with hyperattenuating rings are present within the lateral segment of the left lobe of the liver.

Differential Diagnosis

1. Hepatic abscess
2. Cystic hepatocellular carcinoma
3. Cystic metastases
4. Biliary cystadenoma

Diagnosis

Hepatic abscess

Discussion

Pyogenic hepatic abscesses most commonly are due to diverticulitis, appendicitis, or cholecystitis. Other causes include ascending cholangitis with biliary obstruction, hepatic arterial septicemia from bacterial endocarditis or pneumonitis, direct extension from an adjacent infection, trauma or penetrating injuries with infection, or infected tumor. *Escherichia coli* is the most common organism cultured in adults, whereas *Staphylococcus* organisms are most common in children.

Many hepatic abscesses communicate and can be drained by a single drainage catheter. These types of abscesses may have the appearance of a cluster of water density masses (as in this case). The presence of air within a hepatic abscess is unusual. Definitive diagnosis usually requires percutaneous aspiration and assessment of the fluid for organisms.

Not all hepatic abscesses are pyogenic in origin. Amebic abscess caused by the organism *Entamoeba histolytica* is a common infection worldwide. The presentation is usually nonspecific, but patients may present with a unilocular water-density mass with a low-density ring (case 6.22). Echinococcal disease is discussed in cases 6.23 through 6.25.

CASE 6.22

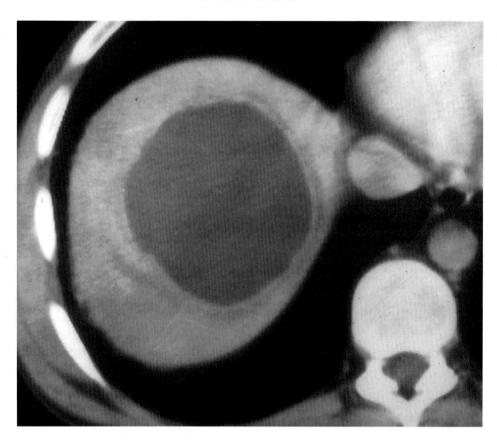

Findings

Contrast-enhanced CT. There is a large water-attenuation mass within the liver. The mass is well demarcated. A low-attenuation ring partially surrounds the mass.

Differential Diagnosis

1. Amebic abscess
2. Cystic hepatocellular carcinoma
3. Cystic metastases
4. Biliary cystadenoma
5. Pyogenic abscess

Diagnosis

Amebic abscess

Discussion

Entamoeba histolytica affects nearly 10% of the world's population. Most people are asymptomatic carriers. It is commonly found in the stool of homosexual men. The life cycle of this parasite begins by oral ingestion of the cystic form. Invasive trophozoites develop from the cyst as they pass through the digestive tract. Most invade the bowel in the cecum. Invasion can result in a local infection with formation of an ameboma, amebic appendicitis, thickening of the wall of the cecum, and fistulization. Distal spread of the parasite to liver or lungs occurs when it gains access to either the splanchnic veins or the lymphatics. The hepatic abscess usually is solitary and most often affects the right lobe. Symptoms often are nonspecific and include right upper quadrant pain. Serologic testing is helpful because stool specimens usually are negative.

This case shows the typical appearance of an amebic abscess—solitary water-density mass with a low-attenuation rim. The fluid obtained on percutaneous aspiration of an amebic abscess is thick, dark reddish brown, and the consistency of anchovy paste. Major complications include pleuropulmonary involvement (consolidation, abscess, effusion, empyema, fistula), abscess rupture into the peritoneal space or pericardial sac, and renal involvement.

CASE 6.23

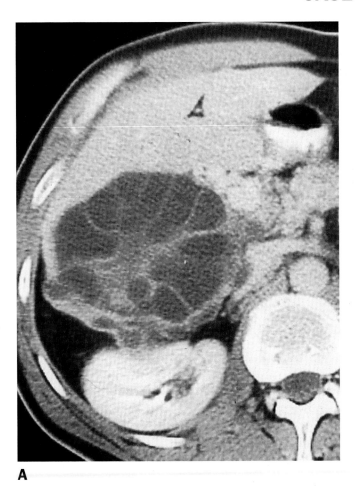

A

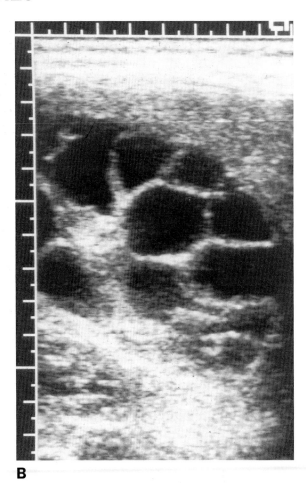

B

Findings
Contrast-enhanced CT (**A**) and hepatic sonogram (**B**). A multiloculated mass is present within the right lobe of the liver. Multiple smaller cysts are seen within a large mass.

Differential Diagnosis
1. Echinococcal hepatic abscess
2. Pyogenic abscess
3. Biliary cystadenoma

Diagnosis
Echinococcal hepatic abscess

Discussion
Echinococcal disease is most prevalent in Greece, Uruguay, Argentina, New Zealand, and Australia—areas where dogs are used to herd livestock. The disease is caused by two different types of tapeworms: *Echinococcus granulosus* and *E. multilocularis*. For *E. granulosus* (as in this case), dogs are the primary host. The tapeworm lives in the dog and sheds eggs that, when ingested by humans, activate an embryo that invades the intestinal wall and enters the splanchnic venous system. Usually the embryo is carried to the liver, where it develops into a growing cyst containing larvae. For *E. multilocularis* (*alveolaris*), cats and rodents are the primary host. Human infection follows the same course, except the larvae proliferate outside the hepatic cyst and penetrate liver tissue. They induce a granulomatous reaction about the cyst.

CASE 6.24

CASE 6.25

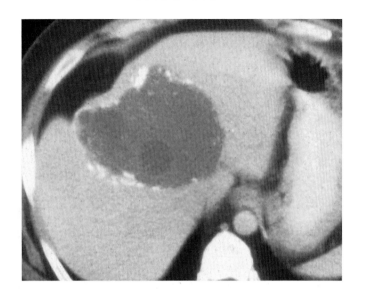

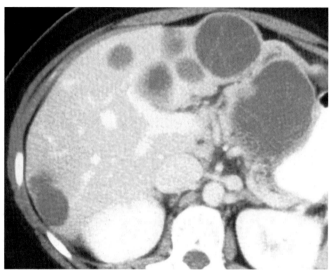

Findings

Case 6.24. Contrast-enhanced CT. There is a peripherally calcified water-attenuation mass in the liver. Within the mass are several cysts that are lower attenuation than the remaining internal fluid.

Case 6.25. Contrast-enhanced CT. Multiple low-density masses are present throughout the liver. The largest mass in the left lobe appears to be septated.

Differential Diagnosis

1. Echinococcal cyst
2. Autosomal polycystic disease
3. Multiple simple hepatic cysts

Diagnosis

Echinococcal cyst

Discussion

The lesion in case 6.24 is typical for an echinococcal cyst with the visible daughter lesions and peripheral calcification. The lesions in case 6.25 are less typical and show that echinococcal disease also can present as a unilocular mass or as multiple masses. The larger masses in case 6.25

contain daughter cysts but only appear to be septated; in this case, a high level of clinical suspicion would be required to make the correct diagnosis.

Most patients are infected during childhood and remain asymptomatic until adulthood. The cyst(s) enlarges slowly at about 1 cm per year. Serologic tests are the most helpful to establish the diagnosis. Complications include rupture of the cyst into the biliary system or peritoneal cavity.

At CT, *Echinococcus granulosus* presents as either a unilocular or a multilocular cyst. The walls can be of variable thickness. Daughter cysts usually are located in the periphery of the mother cyst, and they usually are of lower attenuation. Calcification of the wall is common. *E. multilocularis* presents with geographic, infiltrating regions of hypoattenuation. Invasive, poorly defined solid masses are present.

Therapy of *E. granulosus* cysts is usually with a combination of surgery and antibiotics. Recently, percutaneous therapy has been described with the addition of either hypertonic saline or alcohol. There is a risk of anaphylaxis if the cyst fluid escapes into the peritoneal cavity; however, new devices have been developed to prevent this problem.

CASE 6.26

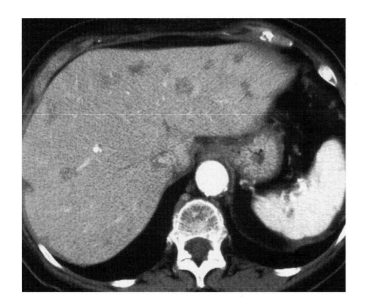

CASE 6.27

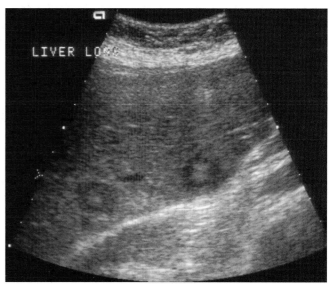

Findings

Case 6.26. Contrast-enhanced CT. Multiple small, low-attenuation masses are present in the liver and spleen.

Case 6.27. Sonogram. Multiple bull's-eye lesions are present in the liver.

Differential Diagnosis

1. Hepatosplenic candidiasis
2. Lymphoma
3. Leukemic infiltration

Diagnosis

Candidiasis

Discussion

Candidiasis is the commonest systemic fungal infection, usually affecting immunocompromised patients. Patients receiving chemotherapy and those with acquired immunodeficiency syndrome are particularly at risk. Diagnosis can be difficult because only about 50% of affected patients have a positive blood culture.

Findings at sonography include the following:

1. Bull's-eye pattern that includes a hyperechoic center with a hypoechoic rim
2. Wheel within a wheel, which describes a three-layer lesion consisting of a central hypoechoic nidus surrounded by a hyperechoic rim surrounded by another hypoechoic rim
3. Uniformly hypoechoic liver due to progressive fibrosis
4. Echogenic liver caused by scar formation

Findings at CT are usually multiple small, hypoattenuating masses. Occasionally, scattered calcification can be identified. Increased periportal fibrosis can be identified as hyperattenuating periportal regions seen on delayed enhancement scanning.

Hepatic Abscesses

		Case
Pyogenic abscess	Solitary or multiple (clustered) water-attenuation masses with rim enhancement	6.21
Amebic abscess	Solitary, low-attenuation ring, right lobe	6.22
Echinococcal abscess	*Echinococcus granulosus.* Solitary low-attenuation mass with internal daughter cysts	6.23–6.25
Candidiasis	Multiple small, low-attenuation masses in liver and spleen. Immunocompromised host. Bull's-eye lesions at sonography	6.26 and 6.27

CASE 6.28

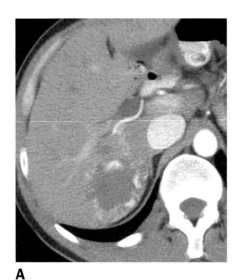

A

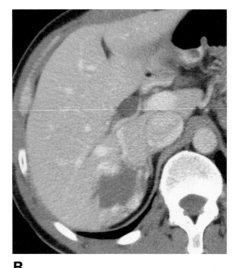

B

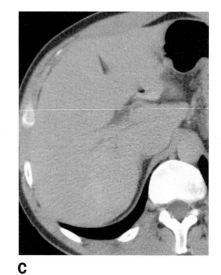

C

Findings

Contrast-enhanced CT. Arterial phase (**A**), portal-venous phase (**B**), and delayed (**C**) images of the liver show a low-attenuation lesion in the posterior right lobe of the liver with peripheral globular enhancement with progressive fill-in on later images. The enhancing tissue is isoattenuating or hyperattenuating compared with the aorta.

Differential Diagnosis

Hepatic hemangioma

Diagnosis

Hepatic hemangioma

Discussion

Except for benign cysts, hepatic hemangiomas are the most common benign tumor of the liver, found in approximately 5% of the population. Hemangiomas can occur at any age, but frequently they are found in middle-aged women (female:male ratio, 5:1). Hemangiomas are usually solitary but can be multiple in up to one-third of patients. Approximately 90% of hemangiomas are less than 4 cm

in size. These small hemangiomas are rarely symptomatic and often are found incidentally on radiographic examinations of the abdomen. Giant cavernous hemangiomas (typically defined as larger than 4 cm, case 6.33) can rarely cause symptoms due to mass effect on adjacent structures, consumptive coagulopathy (Kasabach-Merritt syndrome), thrombosis of the vascular spaces, or even spontaneous or traumatic rupture.

Hemangiomas arise from vascular endothelial cells and consist of vascular channels of varying size supported by fibrous septae. Blood, supplied by the hepatic artery, constitutes the bulk of the internal contents.

The typical CT findings of a hemangioma are present in this case. The peripheral globular enhancement that is isoattenuating or hyperattenuating compared with the aorta (because blood supply is arterial) with progressive centripetal fill-in is considered pathognomonic. Hemangiomas also can be diagnosed confidently at MRI (case 6.30), nuclear medicine-tagged red blood cell scanning (case 6.32), and sonography (case 6.31). Atypical hemangiomas (cases 6.34 and 6.35) can be mistaken for other primary liver tumors or metastases.

CASE 6.29

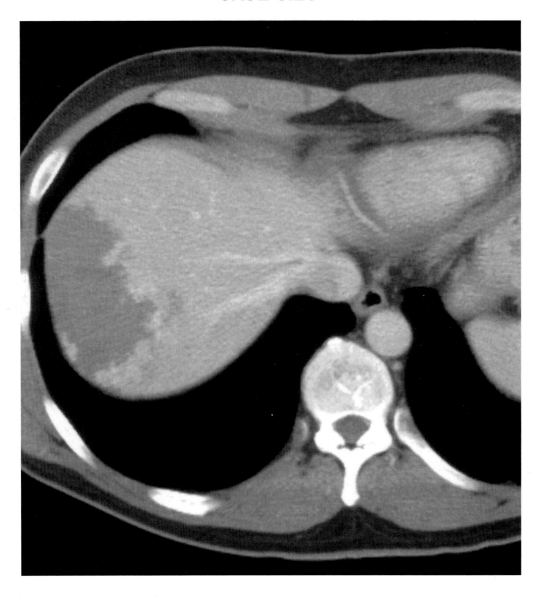

Findings
Contrast-enhanced CT. A large hypodense mass is present in the right lobe of the liver with peripheral high-attenuation globular enhancement.

Differential Diagnosis
Hemangioma

Diagnosis
Hemangioma

Discussion
This case illustrates the typical enhancement pattern of a hemangioma at CT. Hemangiomas are composed of large vascular channels filled with slow-moving blood. These vascular channels are fed by the hepatic arteries and result in peripheral nodular enhancement on early phases of imaging with progressive centripetal fill-in that usually occurs after 5 to 30 minutes. The enhancement of a hemangioma should always parallel the aorta. Hemangiomas often have central areas of fibrosis (especially in larger tumors), and complete fill-in of the tumor on delayed images is not necessary for confident diagnosis.

CASE 6.30

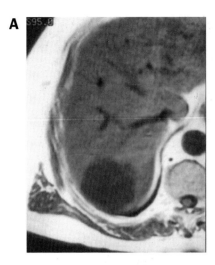

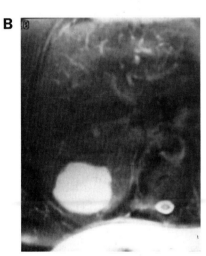

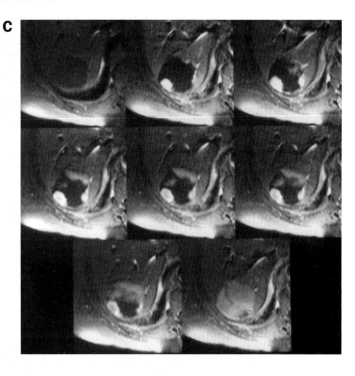

Findings

Unenhanced and post-gadolinium MRI. **A.** T1-weighted sequence. A mass with low-signal intensity is present in the posterior right lobe of the liver. **B.** T2-weighted (fat-suppressed) sequence. The mass is of markedly increased signal. The signal intensity of the mass mimics the signal intensity of the cerebrospinal fluid. **C.** Precontrast and multiple delayed post-gadolinium images show peripheral globular enhancement with progressive centripetal fill-in.

Differential Diagnosis

Hemangioma

Diagnosis

Hemangioma

Discussion

MRI is a sensitive and specific imaging method for the diagnosis of hemangiomas. The markedly high signal seen on T2-weighted images (approaching that of a cyst) is due to the extremely long relaxation time of free fluid—in this case, slowly moving blood. If the signal intensity on T2-weighted images is not as high as that of the cerebrospinal fluid, gadolinium-enhanced images can be very helpful. These images provide information similar to that of contrast-enhanced CT.

CASE 6.31

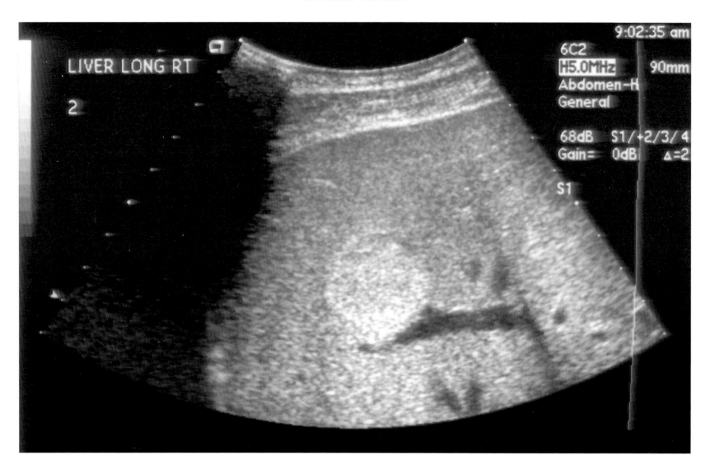

Findings

Sonogram. A well-defined, homogeneously hyperechoic mass with increased through transmission is present in the right lobe of the liver.

Differential Diagnosis

1. Hemangioma
2. Hyperechoic metastasis
3. Focal fatty infiltration

Diagnosis

Hemangioma

Discussion

This mass has the typical homogeneous hyperechoic sonographic appearance of a hemangioma. Two-thirds of hemangiomas have this appearance. The increased echogenicity within these lesions is related to the numerous acoustical interfaces (multiple vascular channels) within them. The increased through transmission in this case is a nonspecific finding, but it is seen in approximately 75% of hemangiomas. Because of the extremely slow blood flow within these vascular tumors, flow will not routinely be identified within a hemangioma on color or duplex Doppler imaging. Atypical sonographic appearances of hemangiomas (case 6.35) are relatively common and often require additional imaging (CT or MRI) for confident diagnosis. Echogenic metastases can mimic a hemangioma but often have a hypoechoic halo, raising the suspicion of malignancy. Focal fatty infiltration of the liver usually presents as a geographic hyperechoic region rather than a rounded mass.

CASE 6.32

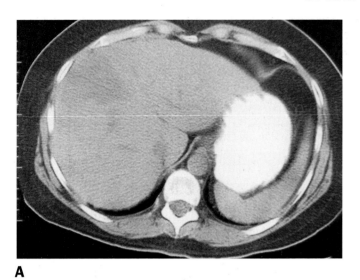

A

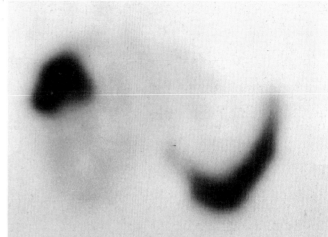

B

Findings

A. Unenhanced CT. A large indeterminate low-attenuation mass is present in the periphery of the liver.

B. Technetium-99m–labeled red blood cell scintigraphy (1 hour delayed axial single-photon emission CT image). The mass has markedly increased tracer uptake compared with the rest of the liver.

Differential Diagnosis

Hepatic hemangioma

Diagnosis

Hepatic hemangioma

Discussion

Hemangiomas such as this one are common incidental findings on CT and ultrasonography. In this patient, the mass was evaluated with red blood cell scintigraphy because of an increased creatinine value and pacemaker (contraindications to contrast-enhanced CT and MRI). Single-photon emission CT tagged red blood cell scintigraphy has an extremely high specificity (approximately 95%) for the diagnosis of hemangiomas. The sensitivity of single-photon emission CT red blood cell scintigraphy is also high for hemangiomas more than 2 cm in diameter.

Hemangiomas typically have decreased or no red blood cell-labeled tracer uptake immediately after tracer injection. Delayed imaging at 1 to 2 hours typically shows markedly increased tracer uptake within a hemangioma compared with the normal liver. Liver metastases, alternatively, typically have early tracer uptake with quick washout.

CASE 6.33

A
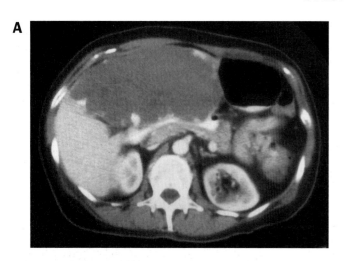

B
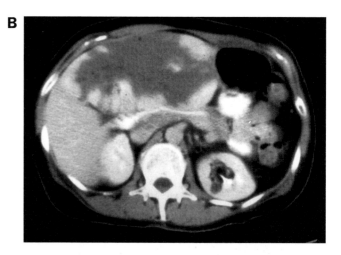

C
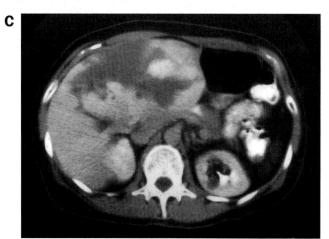

D
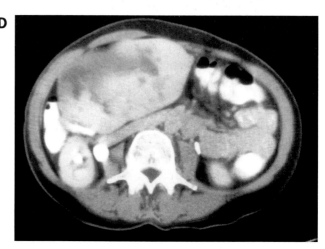

Findings

Contrast-enhanced CT. **A** through **D.** Progressively delayed post-contrast images show a very large low-density mass replacing the majority of the left lobe of the liver and extending into the right lobe. This mass has peripheral globular enhancement equal to that of the aorta with progressive centripetal fill-in on delayed images.

Differential Diagnosis

Giant hemangioma

Diagnosis

Giant hemangioma

Discussion

Giant hemangiomas usually are defined as those more than 4 cm in diameter; they constitute only 10% of all hemangiomas. Most hemangiomas are asymptomatic, but giant hemangiomas may cause pain from mass effect on adjacent structures or, rarely, intratumoral thrombosis. Giant hemangiomas are at increased risk of bleeding with trauma and have been reported to rupture spontaneously. Giant hemangiomas can result in thrombocytopenia or an intrahepatic consumptive coagulopathy (Kasabach-Merritt syndrome). Biliary obstruction and Budd-Chiari syndrome can even occur as a result of mass effect from these large lesions.

Symptomatic or complicated giant hemangiomas often are treated with surgical enucleation. Hepatic arterial embolization of these tumors is an alternative therapy in symptomatic patients who are poor surgical candidates. Observation is reserved for asymptomatic patients.

CASE 6.34

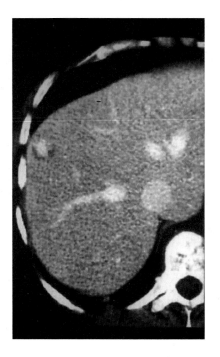

CASE 6.35

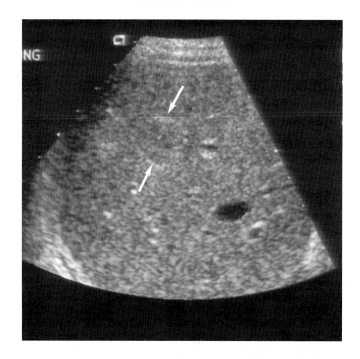

Findings

Case 6.34. Contrast-enhanced CT. A single slice from a portal-venous phase CT shows a small low-density lesion in the right lobe of the liver with central enhancement.

Case 6.35. Sonogram. An isoechoic liver lesion with a thin echogenic rim (arrows) is present.

Differential Diagnosis

1. Atypical hemangioma
2. Metastasis
3. Primary liver tumor

Diagnosis

Atypical hemangioma

Discussion

Approximately 15% of hemangiomas have atypical enhancement at CT, which presents a significant diagnostic challenge. These atypical hemangiomas may present with diffuse early arterial enhancement and rapid washout ("flash" hemangioma). This enhancement pattern usually is seen in small lesions. Occasionally, as in case 6.34, hemangiomas have central enhancement with centrifugal fill-in on delayed images.

Atypical features of hemangiomas on ultrasonography are common (approximately one-third of cases) and include inhomogeneous hyperechoic masses, isoechoic or hypoechoic masses with a thin hyperechoic rim (as in case 6.35), or hypoechoic masses in the setting of a diffusely hyperechoic (fatty) liver.

MRI (especially for small lesions) or red blood cell scintigraphy (for lesions >2 cm) are often used as primary diagnostic or problem-solving tools for atypical lesions. Radiographically indeterminate lesions can be observed with close (6-month) follow-up imaging or with biopsy. Percutaneous biopsy with a 20-gauge needle is a safe and effective method for diagnosing hemangioma.

CASE 6.36

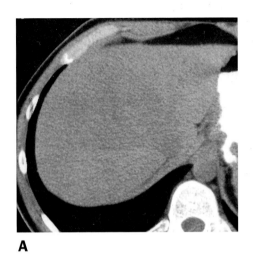

A

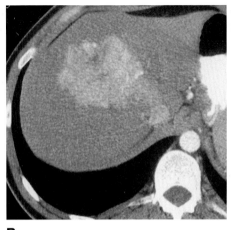

B

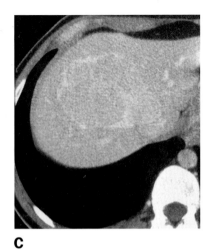

C

Findings

A. Unenhanced CT. An isodense mass is present in the right lobe of the liver.

B and **C.** Biphasic contrast-enhanced CT. A large homogeneously enhancing mass is present within the right lobe of the liver. A central scar is visible. The mass is nearly isodense with the liver on the portal venous phase of imaging with prominent peripheral enhancement.

Differential Diagnosis

1. Focal nodular hyperplasia
2. Hepatic adenoma
3. Hepatocellular carcinoma

Diagnosis

Focal nodular hyperplasia

Discussion

Focal nodular hyperplasia (FNH) is a solid mass consisting of abnormally arranged hepatocytes, bile ducts, and Kupffer cells (hepatic hamartoma). It is the second most common liver tumor, surpassed only by hemangiomas. FNH is believed to arise as a result of locally increased hepatic blood flow from a hepatic arteriovenous malformation. FNH is most common in women in their 30s and 40s. It is nearly always clinically silent and is discovered incidentally with cross-sectional imaging.

The key finding of FNH is *homogeneous* enhancement during the arterial phase of imaging. Visualization of a central scar (cases 6.37 and 6.39) is helpful.

Although FNH has no capsule, increased enhancement around the lesion can be seen (as in this case) as a result of large peripheral draining veins.

Hepatic adenoma (cases 6.42 through 6.45) can be seen in the same patient population, but it enhances heterogeneously without a central scar. In most instances, FNH can be diagnosed with confidence. Hepatocellular carcinomas (cases 6.51 through 6.58) usually are found in patients with underlying cirrhosis and can have features similar to those of hepatic adenomas. The extremely rare fibrolamellar hepatocellular carcinoma (case 6.65) can have CT and MRI findings similar to those of FNH, including a central scar, but often other evidence of malignancy is present, including adenopathy and angioinvasion.

CASE 6.37

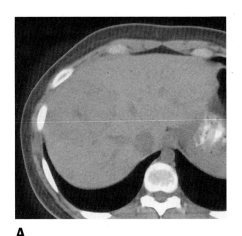

A

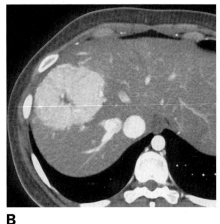

B

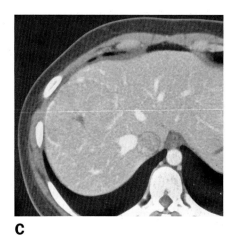

C

Findings

A. Unenhanced CT. An almost isodense mass is present in the periphery of the right lobe of the liver with a hypodense structure centrally.

B and C. Biphasic contrast-enhanced CT. A homogeneously enhancing mass is present on the arterial phase of enhancement with a stellate central scar. The mass is isodense with the surrounding liver during the portal venous phase of enhancement. The hypodense central scar is still visible with a thin rim of hyperenhancing veins around the mass.

Differential Diagnosis

1. Focal nodular hyperplasia
2. Fibrolamellar hepatocellular carcinoma

Diagnosis

Focal nodular hyperplasia

Discussion

This case has the classic CT appearance of focal nodular hyperplasia (FNH). The intense, uniform, early enhancement in this case is typical of FNH, as is its barely perceptible appearance on unenhanced and delayed post-contrast CT imaging. The hallmark feature of FNH is homogeneous arterial-phase enhancement, a central stellate scar, and radiating fibrous septa dividing the tumor into lobules. The central scar contains the supplying arteries and bile ductules. The central stellate scar sometimes is more easily visualized on MRI (case 6.39). When imaging studies are inconclusive, biopsy sometimes is necessary. Histologically, the presence of abnormal vessels in a scar or septa, as well as the abnormally organized hepatocytes, bile ductules, and Kupffer cells, is typical.

The presence of a central scar is not pathognomonic for FNH because it can be identified in various benign and malignant neoplasms. Only when it is found in combination with homogeneous arterial enhancement should FNH be diagnosed. Some fibrolamellar hepatocellular carcinomas also contain a scar, but their enhancement is usually inhomogeneous and other signs of a malignancy may be present.

CASE 6.38

A

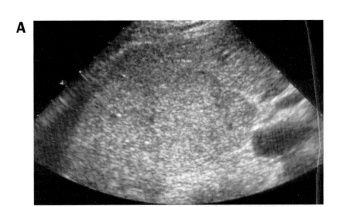

B

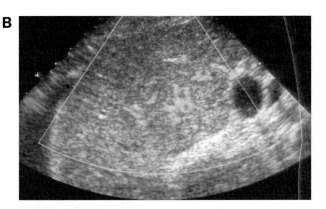

C

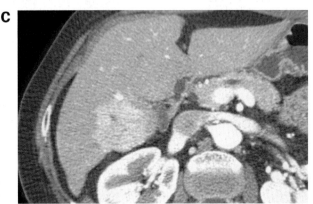

Findings

A and **B.** Sonogram with color-Doppler evaluation. A large isoechoic mass is present in the right lobe of the liver. The mass is extremely vascular (especially centrally) compared with the normal surrounding liver on the color-Doppler image.

C. Contrast-enhanced CT. Corresponding arterial-phase image shows the gently lobulated homogeneously enhancing mass. The central scar is better shown on CT than ultrasonography.

Differential Diagnosis

1. Focal nodular hyperplasia
2. Other solid liver mass

Diagnosis

Focal nodular hyperplasia

Discussion

Focal nodular hyperplasia (FNH) is often a subtle liver mass on ultrasonography, consistent with its description as a "stealth" lesion. FNH usually is isoechoic to normal liver parenchyma and may be seen only because of subtle contour abnormalities and displacement of normal vascular structures. The central scar, when visualized, usually is hypoechoic. Doppler features of FNH are highly specific for the diagnosis because of the prominent central vessels arranged in a stellate pattern.

FNH is most commonly found incidentally in women in their 30s and 40s. It is important to differentiate this benign lesion that does not require any treatment from other, more serious masses. Hepatic adenomas usually enhance heterogeneously and may have a capsule.

Oral contraception is not thought to cause development of FNH, but it may exert an effect on its growth. This is in contrast to the clearly proven risk for development of a hepatic adenoma with the use of oral contraceptive agents. Hepatic adenomas are also at a high risk for bleeding, in contradistinction to FNH.

CASE 6.39

A
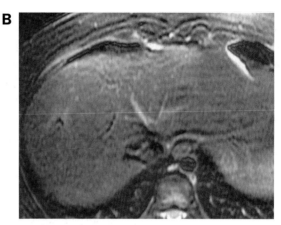

B
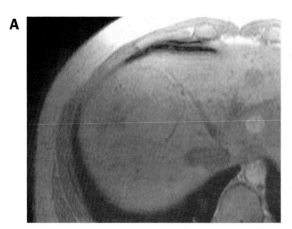

C
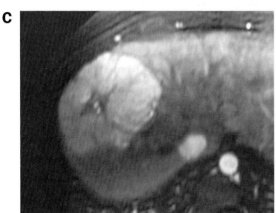

D
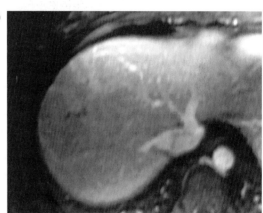

Findings

Unenhanced and dynamic gadolinium-enhanced images of the liver. **A.** T1-weighted MRI. An isointense mass with a hypointense central scar is present in the periphery of the right lobe of the liver. **B.** T2-weighted MRI. The mass is nearly isointense to the liver parenchyma with a hyperintense central scar. **C.** Arterial-phase post-gadolinium MRI. Marked homogeneous enhancement of the mass with a central hypointense stellate scar. Enhancing peripheral veins also are present. **D.** Post-gadolinium portal venous phase MRI. The mass is nearly isointense compared with the surrounding liver.

Differential Diagnosis

Focal nodular hyperplasia

Diagnosis

Focal nodular hyperplasia

Discussion

This case has almost all of the classic MRI findings of focal nodular hyperplasia (FNH). FNH typically is isointense on T1- and T2-weighted images. The central scar is typically hypointense on T1-weighted images and hyperintense on T2-weighted images. Post-gadolinium homogeneous enhancement pattern mirrors that at contrast-enhanced CT (case 6.40).

Typical features of FNH at CT and MRI are diagnostic. Follow-up imaging can be avoided. Unfortunately, often FNH has atypical findings at unenhanced MRI (hypointense or hyperintense on either T1- or T2-weighted images or both). Gadolinium enhancement then is recommended to show the homogeneous arterial perfusion of the mass. Sulfur colloid scintigraphy can be helpful in the minority of cases that remain equivocal. Lesions must be 2 cm or more. Tracer uptake within the Kupffer cells (reticuloendothelial system) can be identified in approximately two-thirds of the masses.

CASE 6.40

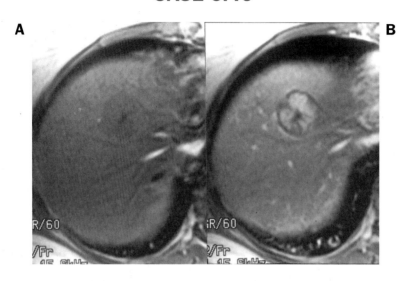

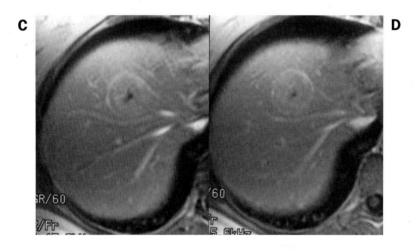

Findings

A through **D.** Unenhanced and sequential post-gadolinium, fat-saturated T1-weighted MRI. A slightly hypointense 3-cm mass with hypointense central scar is seen on the pre-contrast image (**A**). The mass is homogeneously hyperenhancing with central to peripheral septations on arterial-phase post-gadolinium images. Gradual enhancement of the stellate central scar is visible on delayed images.

Differential Diagnosis

Focal nodular hyperplasia

Diagnosis

Focal nodular hyperplasia

Discussion

This case has the typical appearance and enhancement pattern of focal nodular hyperplasia (FNH) at MRI. A central scar may be easier to detect at MRI than at CT. The scar is typically hypointense on T1-weighted images and hyperintense on T2-weighted images.

In addition, the typical lobulation (segmentation) of FNH is shown. Often, these tumors are segmented by fibrous septa—analogous to the segmentation found in an orange. These usually are identified most easily during the early phases of contrast enhancement. Their presence can be very helpful for suggesting the diagnosis.

CASE 6.41

A

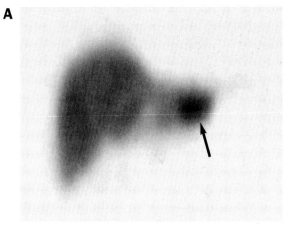

B

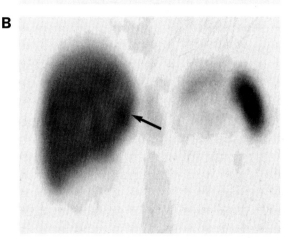

C

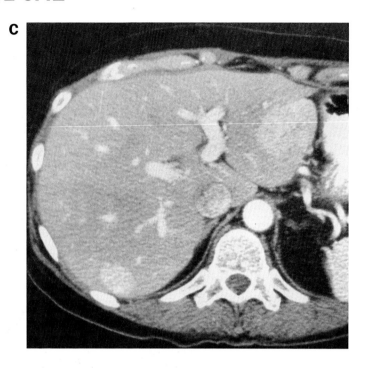

Findings

A and B. Coronal single-photon emission CT images from sulfur colloid scintigraphy. A rounded area of focally increased tracer uptake is seen in the lateral segment of the left lobe of the liver (arrow in **A**) with a smaller focus of increased uptake in the posterior right lobe of the liver (arrow in **B**).

C. Contrast-enhanced CT. Two hyperenhancing masses are seen on this late arterial-phase image, which correspond to the two areas of increased tracer uptake on the sulfur colloid scan.

Differential Diagnosis

Multiple focal nodular hyperplasia

Diagnosis

Multiple focal nodular hyperplasia

Discussion

Sulfur colloid scintigraphy is often helpful for the diagnosis of focal nodular hyperplasia (FNH). FNH contains functioning reticuloendothelial cells (Kupffer cells). These cells normally take up radiolabeled sulfur colloid. When a liver mass has uptake of sulfur colloid equal to (60% of cases of FNH) or greater than (10% of cases of FNH) that of normal liver, the findings are pathognomonic of FNH. In 30% of cases of FNH, there will not be uptake of sulfur colloid, and these lesions remain indeterminate. Hepatic adenomas often contain dysfunctional Kupffer cells but sulfur colloid uptake is in very low quantities when it occurs and rarely is isointense with liver.

FNH is multiple in 20% of cases. Multiple FNH is associated with vascular malformations in the liver (hepatic hemangiomas in 25% of cases) and in other organs.

CASE 6.42

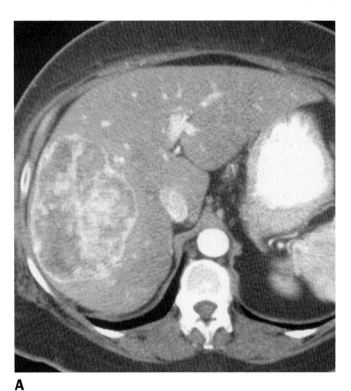

A

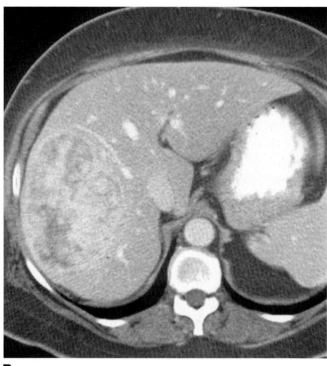

B

Findings
Contrast-enhanced CT. **A** and **B**. Arterial and portal venous-phase images show a large, well-defined, heterogeneously enhancing mass in the right lobe of the liver with an enhancing capsule.

Differential Diagnosis
1. Hepatic adenoma
2. Hepatocellular carcinoma

Diagnosis
Hepatic adenoma

Discussion
Hepatic adenomas are rare, benign primary tumors composed of cords of hepatocytes with an abnormal architecture. These tumors are most commonly found in young women and have an increased incidence in patients using oral birth control. Hepatic adenomas often present as large solitary masses (such as in this case), reaching up to 30 cm in diameter. They usually have heterogeneous enhancement and a well-defined capsule. No imaging methods can reliably differentiate hepatic adenoma from hepatocellular carcinoma. Because of their propensity to hemorrhage and their potential for malignant transformation into hepatocellular carcinoma, hepatic adenomas usually are removed surgically. Alternatively, if the patient is taking oral contraceptives, use of the medication may be stopped to determine whether the tumor regresses on its own.

CASE 6.43

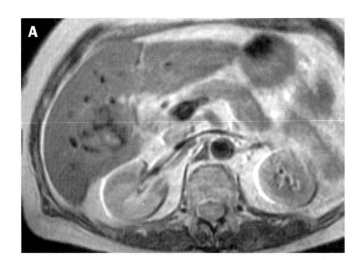

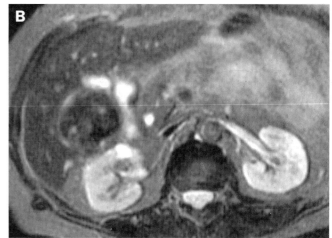

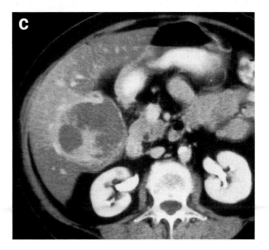

Findings
A. T1-weighted MRI. A mixed low- and high-signal intensity mass is present in the right lobe of the liver.

B. T2-weighted MRI. The mass is of heterogeneous intensity with a high-intensity capsule.

C. Contrast-enhanced CT. The mass and capsule are heterogeneously enhancing.

Differential Diagnosis
1. Hepatic adenoma
2. Hepatocellular carcinoma

Diagnosis
Hepatic adenoma

Discussion
Hepatic adenomas usually have a heterogeneous, mosaic (multicompartment) appearance on CT and MRI. An enhancing capsule also is frequently observed. Areas of increased T1 signal intensity are often present within hepatic adenomas (as in this case) and may be caused by fat content or intratumoral hemorrhage. Although hepatocellular carcinoma can have an identical radiographic appearance, hepatic adenoma is the favored diagnosis in young patients with no radiographic evidence or clinical history of cirrhosis.

CASE 6.44

A

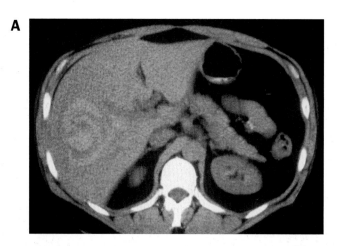

B

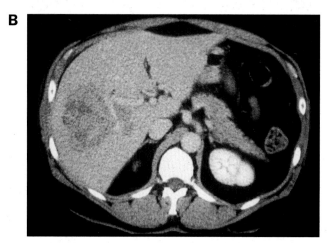

Findings

A. Unenhanced CT. A high-attenuation mass with a whorled appearance is present in the right lobe of the liver.

B. Contrast-enhanced CT. An underlying mixed-attenuation mass is present on portal venous-phase imaging. The high-attenuation whorled regions on the pre-contrast image are difficult to identify on the enhanced image.

Differential Diagnosis

1. Hemorrhagic hepatic adenoma
2. Hemorrhagic hepatocellular carcinoma
3. Hemorrhagic metastasis

Diagnosis

Hepatic adenoma, hemorrhagic

Discussion

This 33-year-old woman who was taking oral contraceptives presented to the emergency department with acute pain in the right upper quadrant. At operation, a hemorrhagic hepatic adenoma was found. Unenhanced images are important for identifying hyperattenuating areas of acute hemorrhage associated with hepatic adenoma. Rupture of a peripheral hepatic adenoma with hemoperitoneum may be life-threatening.

CASE 6.45

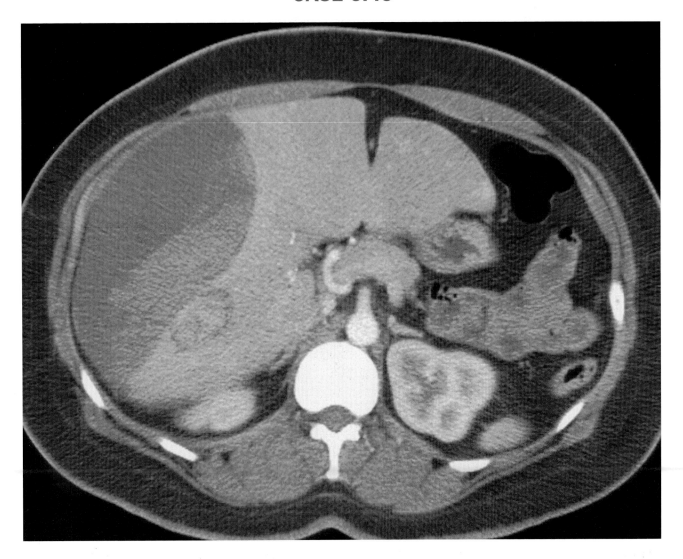

Findings

Contrast-enhanced CT. A large subcapsular hematoma is present along the lateral right lobe of the liver with layering blood products. A 4-cm, heterogeneously enhancing mass is present in the periphery of the right lobe of the liver, adjacent to the hematoma.

Differential Diagnosis

1. Hepatic adenoma (with subcapsular hemorrhage)
2. Hemorrhagic hepatocellular carcinoma
3. Hemorrhagic metastasis

Diagnosis

Ruptured hepatic adenoma with subcapsular hematoma

Discussion

Even asymptomatic hepatic adenomas usually are resected, primarily to avoid potential life-threatening hemorrhages, such as in this case. Although hepatic adenomas cannot be differentiated radiographically from hepatocellular carcinoma or hepatic metastases, hepatic adenoma was correctly favored as a cause of the large subcapsular hemorrhage because the patient was a young woman taking oral contraceptives.

CASE 6.46

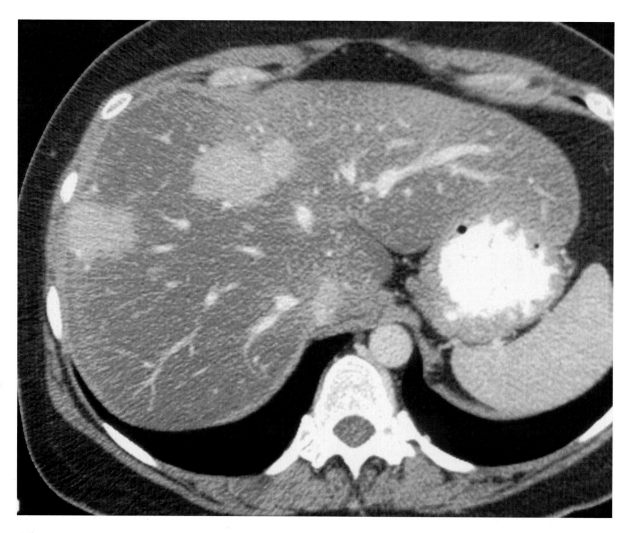

Findings

Contrast-enhanced CT. Two hypervascular liver masses are present during the portal venous phase of contrast enhancement. The liver is of low attenuation compared with the spleen and paraspinal muscles.

Differential Diagnosis

1. Multiple hepatic adenomas (in setting of glycogen storage disease)
2. Metastases

Diagnosis

Glycogen storage disease with multiple hepatic adenomas (von Gierke disease)

Discussion

Hepatic adenomas are multiple in approximately one-third of cases. Cases of solitary or multiple hepatic adenomas are more common in women taking oral birth control pills. Hepatic adenomas also are more common in patients with glycogen storage disease, anabolic steroid use, or familial diabetes mellitus. This patient had a history of von Gierke disease (type Ia glycogen storage disease). The steatohepatitis commonly associated with von Gierke disease accounts for the hepatomegaly and diffuse low attenuation of the liver parenchyma on CT. One or more hepatic adenomas are reported to be present in up to 40% of patients with von Gierke disease. Malignant degeneration of hepatic adenomas into hepatocellular carcinoma can occur and should be considered if there is rapid growth of a liver lesion.

CASE 6.47

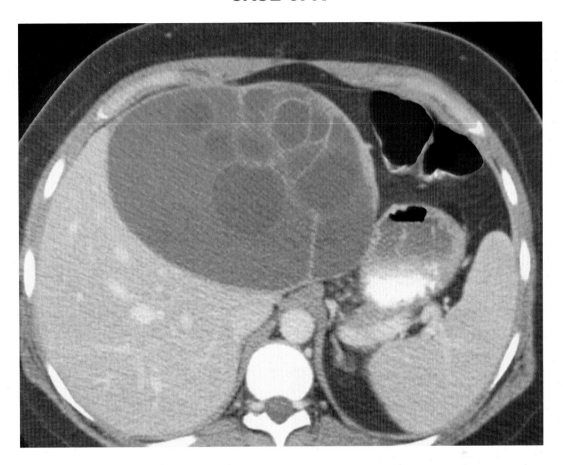

Findings

Contrast-enhanced CT. There is a large multilocular cystic mass in the left lobe of the liver.

Differential Diagnosis

1. Echinococcal cyst
2. Biliary cystadenoma or carcinoma
3. Metastatic mucinous cystadenocarcinoma
4. Hepatic abscess

Diagnosis

Biliary cystadenoma

Discussion

Biliary cystadenomas are rare, premalignant hepatic cystic tumors that originate from biliary duct precursors, lined by mucin-secreting columnar epithelium. These tumors usually are multilocular with a well-defined thick capsule (as in this case). Biliary cystadenomas are most commonly found in middle-aged white women (female:male ratio, 4:1). Because these tumors can be large, patients can present with chronic abdominal pain and a palpable abdominal mass. Many are discovered incidentally.

Several other pathologic entities can have a similar radiographic appearance. Patients with echinococcal disease of the liver (case 6.23) usually have peripheral intracystic cysts and wall calcification with a history of travel to an endemic area. Patients with hepatic abscesses (case 6.21) often have multiple well-defined cystic masses with rim hyperenhancement and present with fevers and leukocytosis. Metastatic cystadenocarcinoma should be considered; however, the cyst-within-a-cyst appearance is atypical.

No reliable clinical or radiographic criteria differentiate biliary cystadenoma from cystadenocarcinoma, and because of the malignant potential of biliary cystadenomas, these lesions should be removed surgically. The finding of mural nodules or thick, irregular, enhancing septations should raise concern for cystadenocarcinoma.

CASE 6.48

A

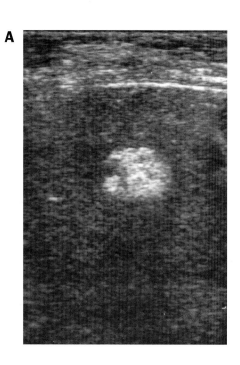

B

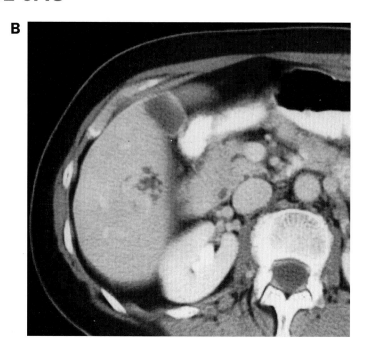

Findings
A. Sonogram. A 2.5-cm, well-defined, predominantly hyperechoic mass is present in the right lobe of the liver.

B. Contrast-enhanced CT. The mass contains discrete areas of fat with enhancement along the posterolateral aspect of the mass.

Differential Diagnosis
1. Angiomyolipoma
2. Lipoma
3. Hepatic adenoma
4. Hepatocellular carcinoma

Diagnosis
Angiomyolipoma

Discussion
Because of concern over a primary hepatic malignancy in this patient, a right hepatic wedge resection was performed. Angiomyolipoma was proven histologically. Angiomyolipomas are rare, benign mesenchymal tumors composed of varying proportions of fat, smooth muscle, and vascular elements. Typically, these tumors are asymptomatic and discovered incidentally.

Angiomyolipomas of the liver may occur as either a solitary mass (as in this case) or as multiple masses in association with tuberous sclerosis. Hepatic angiomyolipomas are much rarer than their renal counterparts and occur in only 5% of patients with tuberous sclerosis with renal angiomyolipomas.

Grossly, hepatic angiomyolipomas are well-circumscribed masses ranging in size from 1 to 20 cm. They typically present as a hyperechoic mass on ultrasonography and can easily be mistaken for a hemangioma. Demonstration of fat within the mass is imperative for making the diagnosis. Unfortunately, angiomyolipomas arising in the liver do not consistently have the high fat content of renal angiomyolipomas. Lipomatous tissue may make up less than 5% of hepatic angiomyolipomas. As a rule, fatty tumors of the liver are benign (angiomyolipoma, lipoma, hepatic adenoma); however, hepatocellular carcinomas (case 6.53) or metastatic liposarcoma also can contain fat. These conditions usually have evidence of cirrhosis or a history of a liposarcoma. Percutaneous needle biopsy or surgical biopsy may be required for equivocal cases. Spontaneous hemorrhage of hepatic angiomyolipomas is less common than with their renal counterparts.

Benign Liver Tumors

		Case
Hemangioma	Globular peripheral enhancement isodense to aorta. Always follows blood characteristics	6.28–6.35
Focal nodular hyperplasia	Homogeneous arterial-phase enhancement. Central scar	6.36–6.41
Hepatic adenoma	Heterogeneous enhancement. Hemorrhage in symptomatic lesions. Oral contraceptives causative	6.42–6.46
Biliary cystadenoma	Large cystic mass with septations. Resembles complicated benign cyst	6.47
Angiomyolipoma	Internal fat. Increased in tuberous sclerosis	6.48
Cyst	Homogeneous fluid contents without enhancement. Posterior acoustic enhancement	6.16

CASE 6.49

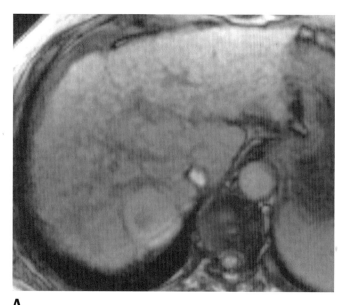

A

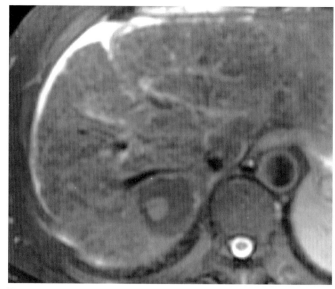

B

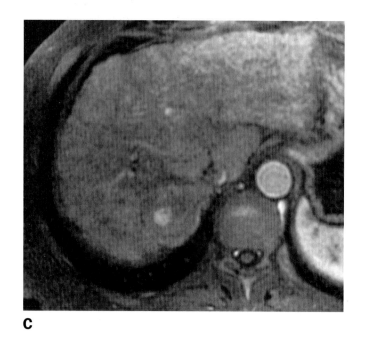

C

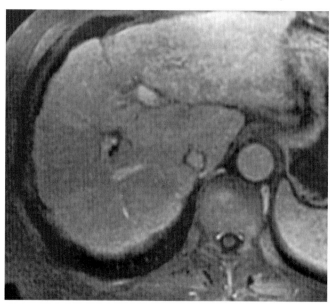

D

Findings

A. T1-weighted out-of-phase MRI of the liver. Cirrhotic changes in the liver with a nodular surface contour and a hyperintense mass within the posterior segment of the right hepatic lobe. The mass contains a capsule and a low-intensity nodule.

B. T2-weighted MRI. The mass is isointense to the liver except for a small hyperintense internal focus.

C. Dynamic contrast-enhanced MRI. The mass enhances homogeneously with the remainder of the liver except a small focus of hyperenhancing tissue that corresponds to the hyperintense focus on the T2-weighted image.

D. Delayed contrast-enhanced MRI. The mass is entirely isointense with the remainder of the hepatic parenchyma.

Differential Diagnosis

1. Dysplastic nodule
2. Dysplastic nodule with a focus of hepatocellular carcinoma
3. Regenerative nodule
4. Indeterminate hepatic mass

Diagnosis

Dysplastic nodule with a focus of hepatocellular carcinoma (early HCC)

Discussion

The primary reason for screening patients with cirrhosis is to assess for a complicating hepatocellular carcinoma (HCC). A dominant "nodule" or mass should be an important clue that a problem exists. The two main possibilities if a mass is found are a dysplastic nodule or HCC. In the case shown here, the dominant mass is of high intensity on the T1-weighted images—a common finding for dysplastic nodules (usually due to internal fat or copper). The presence of a capsule is unusual for a benign mass and is worrisome for a malignancy. In addition, a focus of high signal intensity on the T2-weighted images is an important finding to differentiate benign (isointense) nodules from malignant (hyperintense) nodules. Enhancement of the abnormal T2-focus is further evidence that malignant transformation has occurred.

This case represents a nodule-within-a-nodule appearance for early HCC. Because the dysplastic nodule is larger than the enhancing tumor, this tumor likely arose as a regenerative nodule, transformed into a dysplastic nodule, and later developed a small focus of HCC. A dysplastic nodule should remain isointense on the T2-weighted and contrast-enhanced sequences. A regenerative nodule is usually isointense on both the T1- and T2-weighted images. Although tumors other than HCC can develop in a cirrhotic liver, it is much less common than in a noncirrhotic liver.

CASE 6.50

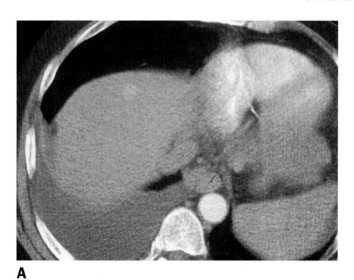

A

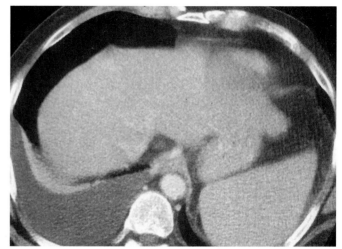

B

Findings

A. Contrast-enhanced CT, arterial phase. There is a small, hyperenhancing mass within the liver near the diaphragmatic dome.

B. Contrast-enhanced CT, portal venous phase. The hyperattenuating mass is no longer visible.

Differential Diagnosis

1. Hepatocellular carcinoma
2. Dysplastic nodule
3. Flash hemangioma
4. Focal nodular hyperplasia
5. Hypervascular metastasis

Diagnosis

Early hepatocellular carcinoma

Discussion

Hepatocellular carcinoma (HCC) is the most common primary hepatic tumor worldwide. Most of these tumors develop as a complication of hepatic cirrhosis. In sub-Saharan Africa and Asia, the tumor is common because of the high incidence of hepatitis and exposure to aflatoxins. In the Western Hemisphere, the incidence is relatively low and the tumor usually is due to alcoholic liver disease. The traditional classification of HCC is useful only for large tumors. Before helical CT scanning, small HCC was rarely detected. With the advent of CT scanners that can acquire images at different phases of contrast enhancement, detection of smaller and earlier HCC has been possible. HCC derives its blood supply from the hepatic artery and in most cases is a hypervascular lesion. Screening of cirrhotic patients at risk for the development of HCC requires scanning during the arterial phase of contrast enhancement as well as during the portal venous phase. Approximately 15% to 20% of tumors are seen only as hyperenhancing masses on the arterial phase of enhancement (as in this case). Hemangiomas and focal nodular hyperplasia are uncommon in cirrhotic livers. Dysplastic nodules occasionally enhance during the arterial phase, and MRI may be helpful to differentiate dysplastic nodules from HCC. Patients with a history of a malignancy (islet cell carcinoma, carcinoid tumor, renal adenocarcinoma, melanoma) also can present with a similar-appearing lesion.

CASE 6.51

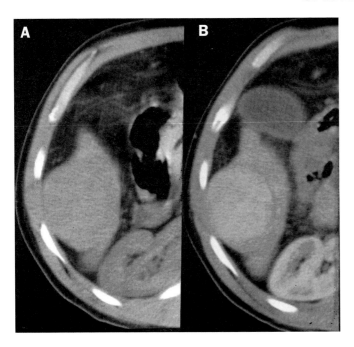

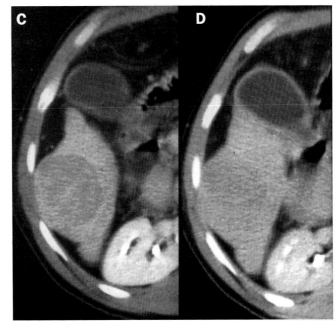

Findings

A. Unenhanced CT. A large mass arises from the inferior tip of the right lobe of the liver. The mass is slightly hypoattenuating compared with normal liver.

B. Contrast-enhanced CT, late arterial phase. The mass is enhancing, and there is a hypoattenuating circumferential capsule.

C. Contrast-enhanced CT, portal venous phase. The capsule is hyperattenuating compared with the hypoattenuating mass.

D. Contrast-enhanced CT, delayed. The capsule and mass are isoattenuating.

Differential Diagnosis

1. Hepatocellular carcinoma
2. Amebic abscess
3. Metastasis

Diagnosis

Focal hepatocellular carcinoma

Discussion

Advanced hepatocellular carcinoma (HCC) usually is classified as focal, multifocal, or diffuse. Focal tumors have the most favorable biologic behavior-favoring expansion rather than invasion. Typical features of a focal HCC include the presence of a capsule, fat, or a mosaic architecture.

The presence of a capsule about a mass is highly suggestive of focal HCC. The appearance of the capsule depends on the phase of contrast enhancement. HCC is a hypervascular lesion that usually enhances briskly during the arterial phase of contrast enhancement and washes out quickly during the portal venous phase (arterial-venous shunting). The capsule is predominantly fibrous and enhances slowly—usually maximal enhancement occurs in the late portal venous or delayed phases of contrast enhancement. The difference in vascularity explains the changing appearance of both tumor and capsule. Capsules usually are found in well-differentiated HCC and often indicate a more favorable prognosis than poorly marginated tumors.

CASE 6.52

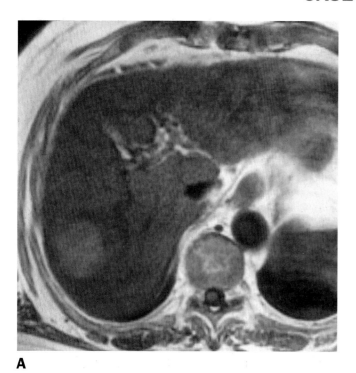

A

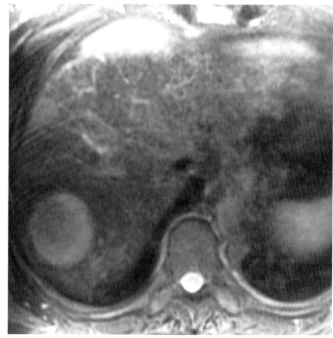

B

Findings
A. T1-weighted MRI. A hyperintense mass is present in the posterior segment of the right lobe. A low signal intensity capsule is visible about the mass.

B. T2-weighted MRI. The mass is homogeneously hyperintense. The liver has a micronodular pattern.

Differential Diagnosis
1. Hepatocellular carcinoma
2. Hepatic adenoma
3. Hematoma

Diagnosis
Focal hepatocellular carcinoma—intralesional fat

Discussion
Approximately 40% of hepatocellular carcinomas (HCCs) contain internal fat that can be detected at MRI. Because this is an unusual finding except in rare hepatic lesions (lipomas and angiomyolipomas), it is a very helpful finding to suggest HCC. This lesion can be distinguished from a lipoma because of its high intensity on the T2-weighted image. Hematomas would not be expected to have a capsule, and there would likely be a history of trauma. Hepatic adenomas, benign primary hepatocellular tumors, can be indistinguishable from well-differentiated, solitary HCC. Correlation with a patient's age (HCC in the Western Hemisphere is more common in older patients), history of cirrhosis (nearly always present in patients with HCC), or oral contraceptive use (common among patients with hepatic adenoma) can be helpful. Dysplastic nodules can contain fat, but usually they are isointense to liver on T2-weighted images.

CASE 6.53

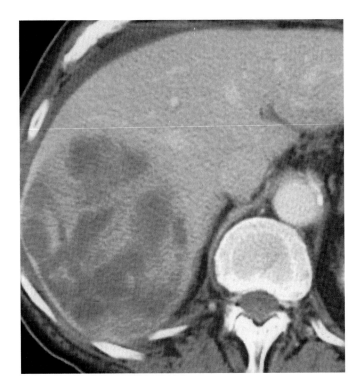

CASE 6.54

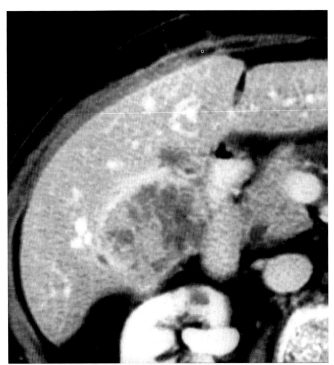

Findings

Case 6.53. Contrast-enhanced CT. There is a large mass in the right lobe of the liver. The internal architecture of the mass is heterogeneous with a multicompartmentalized appearance.

Case 6.54. Contrast-enhanced CT. A solitary mass with a mosaic internal appearance and hyperattenuating capsule is present in the region of the caudate lobe of the liver.

Differential Diagnosis

1. Hepatocellular carcinoma
2. Echinococcal cyst
3. Cystic metastasis

Diagnosis

Focal hepatocellular carcinoma—mosaic appearance

Discussion

These hepatocellular carcinomas (HCCs) have the classic mosaic internal architecture. The term "mosaic" refers to a multicompartmentalized tumor with multiple discrete solid and cystic regions. In most cases, cystic regions are present in the periphery of the tumor as commonly as in the central regions. The hypoattenuating regions are often small, rounded regions but can assume various shapes. These regions correspond to areas of necrosis and hemorrhage pathologically. The mosaic appearance is highly suggestive of HCC.

CASE 6.55

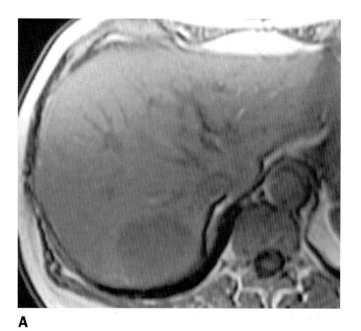

A

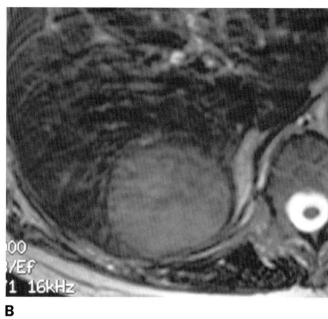

B

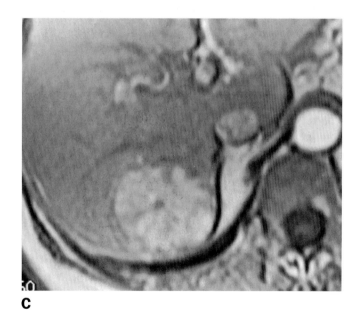

C

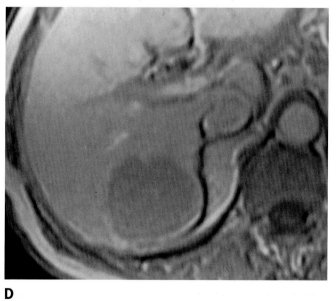

D

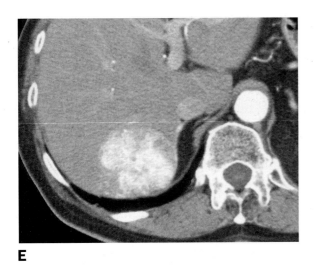

E

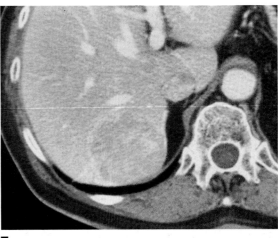

F

Findings

A. T1-weighted MRI. The well-circumscribed mass is of low signal intensity compared with the liver parenchyma.

B. T2-weighted MRI. The mass is fairly homogeneous and hyperintense.

C. Contrast-enhanced MRI (early phase). The mass enhances briskly and inhomogeneously during the early phases of contrast enhancement.

D. Delayed-enhancement MRI (3 minutes). The mass is hypointense compared with normal liver.

E. Contrast-enhanced CT, arterial phase. Heterogeneously enhancing mass is in the right hepatic lobe. An enhancing capsule is visible.

F. Contrast-enhanced CT, portal venous phase. The mass is now heterogeneously hypoattenuating. The capsule remains hyperattenuating.

Differential Diagnosis

1. Hepatic cell adenoma
2. Hepatocellular carcinoma
3. Focal nodular hyperplasia

Diagnosis

Focal hepatocellular carcinoma

Discussion

This case has classic imaging findings of a focal hepatocellular carcinoma (HCC). At unenhanced MRI, the lesion has nonspecific imaging characteristics (hypointense on T1- and hyperintense on T2-weighted images). The lesion is hypervascular and has intratumoral shunting (rapid washout of contrast material) after contrast enhancement. Typical capsular enhancement is seen during portal venous-phase CT.

It may be impossible to distinguish a well-differentiated, solitary HCC from an adenoma. Usually, the clinical history of a young woman taking oral contraceptives strongly suggests an adenoma. HCC should be strongly considered if the patient has a history of cirrhosis and is older than 50 years. Focal nodular hyperplasia should enhance homogeneously during the arterial phase of contrast enhancement and should not have a late-enhancing capsule.

CASE 6.56

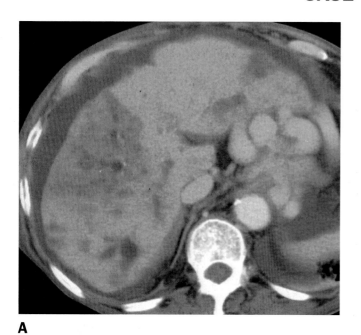

A

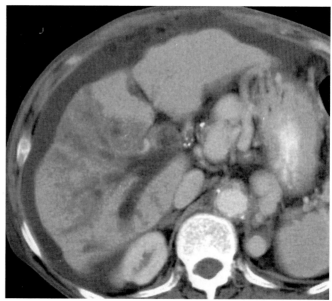

B

Findings
Contrast-enhanced CT. **A.** A poorly defined mass is present within the right lobe of the liver. A smaller, indeterminate mass is present within the left lobe. **B.** Thrombus fills the main and right branches of the portal vein. The liver is cirrhotic in configuration, and multiple large varices and ascites are present.

Differential Diagnosis
Hepatocellular carcinoma

Diagnosis
Focal hepatocellular carcinoma

Discussion
In many cases hepatocellular carcinoma (HCC) may not have a typical appearance and presents as an indeterminate hepatic mass. In these cases, the presence of secondary signs of HCC are key to suggesting the correct diagnosis. Secondary signs include angioinvasion with portal venous or hepatic venous thrombus, morphologic changes of hepatic cirrhosis, hemochromatosis, or prior thorium dioxide exposure. In the case shown here, a hypoattenuating nondescript mass and the presence of cirrhosis and portal vein thrombosis are key findings to suggest the correct diagnosis of HCC.

CASE 6.57

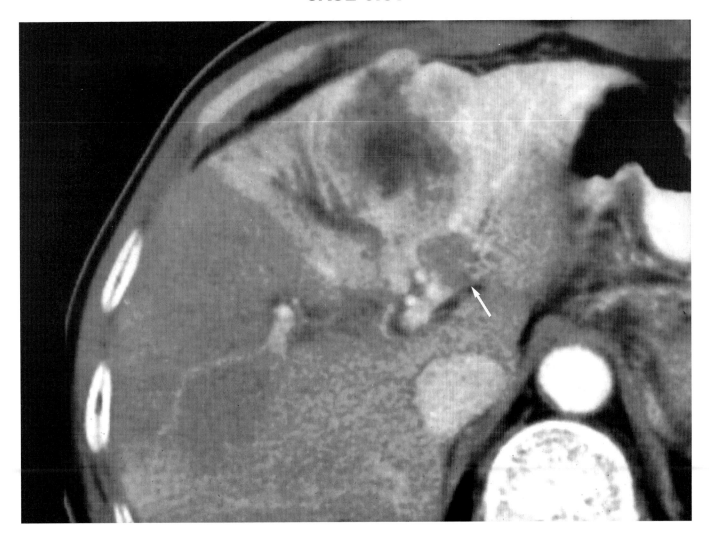

Findings

Contrast-enhanced CT. There is a mass within the lateral segment of the left lobe of the liver. The mass has components that are both hyperattenuating and hypoattenuating. About the mass is a wedge-shaped region of hyperattenuation. There is a nodular filling defect within the left lateral segmental portal vein (arrow).

Differential Diagnosis

1. Hepatocellular carcinoma
2. Metastasis

Diagnosis

Focal hepatocellular carcinoma—transient hepatic attenuation defect

Discussion

Local hepatic perfusion differences allow transient hepatic attenuation defects (THAD) to be seen in the liver. The presence of a THAD should prompt the search for an underlying neoplasm causing compression or obstruction of the supplying portal vein. Because the liver receives the majority of its blood supply from the portal vein, portal venous obstruction results in the recruitment of arterial blood to supply the ischemic region. The additional arterial supply explains the hyperenhancement seen during the early phases of contrast enhancement. In the case shown here, a tumor thrombus is seen to occlude the supplying portal vein. Occlusive tumor thrombus accounts for the THAD, and the presence of angioinvasion suggests that the underlying tumor is hepatocellular carcinoma.

CASE 6.58

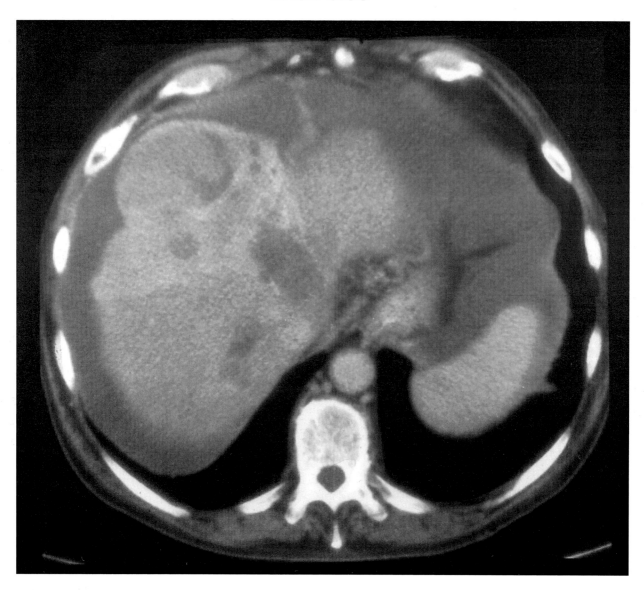

Findings

Contrast-enhanced CT. A heterogeneously enhancing mass bulges the hepatic contour. A wedge-shaped region of hyperattenuation surrounds the mass. Filling defects expand the hepatic veins. Ascites.

Differential Diagnosis

Hepatocellular carcinoma

Diagnosis

Focal hepatocellular carcinoma

Discussion

This case exemplifies the importance of secondary findings for diagnosing hepatocellular carcinoma (HCC). Although the primary tumor does not have any specific features of HCC (capsule, fat, mosaic appearance), the presence of a transient hepatic attenuation defect, ascites (due to cirrhosis), and angioinvasion of the hepatic veins (with thrombus) are typical secondary findings. These findings in combination make HCC the only real consideration. Angioinvasion can occur within the portal veins or hepatic veins or both. The same aggressive growth characteristics also can lead to biliary invasion in rare instances.

CASE 6.59

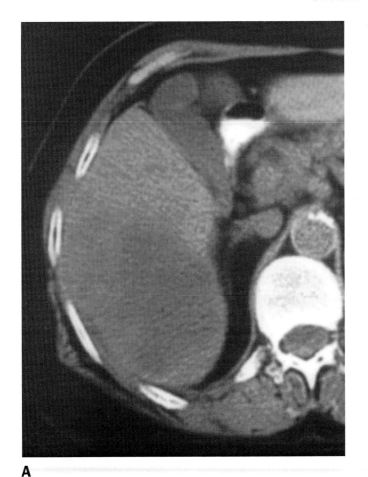

A

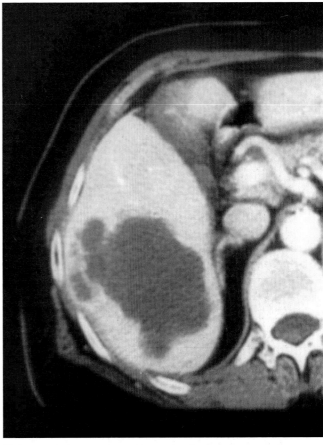

B

Findings
A. Unenhanced CT. A large hypoattenuating mass is present within the right lobe of the liver.

B. Contrast-enhanced CT. The mass does not enhance and appears cystic.

Differential Diagnosis
1. Abscess
2. Biliary cystadenoma
3. Cystic metastasis
4. Cystic hepatocellular carcinoma

Diagnosis
Cystic hepatocellular carcinoma

Discussion
Although the typical hepatocellular carcinoma (HCC) is a hypervascular tumor, occasional tumors are cystic in appearance and mimic an abscess. The diagnosis can be suggested by the presence of secondary signs of HCC (none are seen in this case). Patients with a pyogenic abscess (case 6.21) of this size usually are symptomatic (fevers and leukocytosis). Although possible, a solitary metastasis is rarely this large. A biliary cystadenoma (case 6.47) generally has enhancing septations.

CASE 6.60

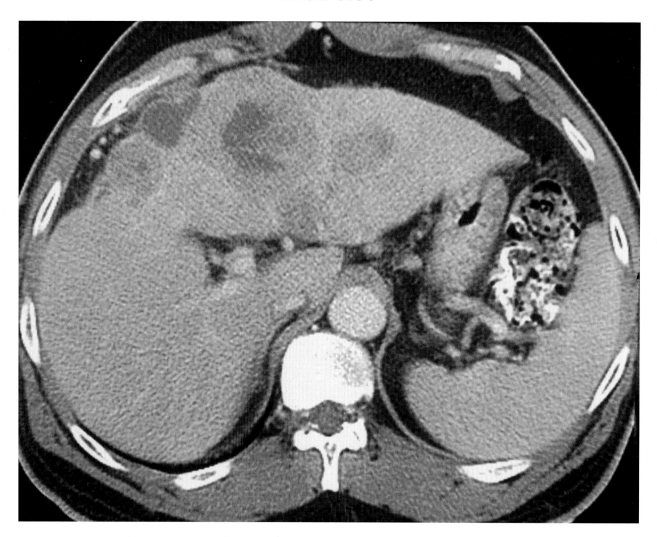

Findings

Contrast-enhanced CT. The left lobe of the liver is enlarged and contains several masses of varying size. One larger mass is dominant compared with the smaller peripheral masses.

Differential Diagnosis

1. Metastases
2. Multifocal hepatocellular carcinoma

Diagnosis

Multifocal hepatocellular carcinoma

Discussion

This is a common presentation for advanced hepatocellular carcinoma (HCC). Although multifocal disease can be indistinguishable from metastases, two findings should raise suspicion that the masses could be HCC: 1) a dominant (larger) mass with surrounding smaller satellite masses, and 2) masses that are hyperattenuating during the early phases of contrast enhancement compared with normal liver. In the case shown here, the CT image was obtained during the late phase of portal venous enhancement, and the tumor is hypoattenuating compared with normal liver because of arterial-venous shunting that often is found in patients with HCC. Satellite masses are believed to occur from portal venous metastases that seed adjacent hepatic parenchyma.

CASE 6.61

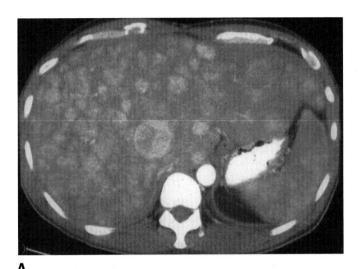

A

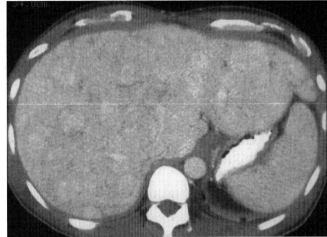

B

Findings

A. Contrast-enhanced CT, arterial phase. The liver enhances inhomogeneously. There are multiple ill-defined, nodular, enhancing masses throughout the liver.

B. Contrast-enhanced CT, portal venous phase. The liver remains slightly inhomogeneous in attenuation. The nodular masses are not well seen, although the contour of the liver is nodular and the left lobe is enlarged.

Differential Diagnosis

1. Diffuse hepatocellular carcinoma
2. Diffuse hypervascular metastases
3. Budd-Chiari syndrome

Diagnosis

Diffuse hepatocellular carcinoma

Discussion

Diffuse hepatocellular carcinoma (HCC) is the least common presentation of HCC. The tumor usually infiltrates throughout the liver, and the borders of the individual nodules are poorly defined. Arterial-phase scanning can be key to detection, because these tumors may be difficult to identify on portal venous and delayed enhancement images. Diffuse hypervascular metastases (neuroendocrine tumor, renal adenocarcinoma) could have a similar appearance, but usually portions of the tumor appear masslike and have heterogeneous internal changes. Budd-Chiari syndrome (case 6.13) can present with an inhomogeneous liver—but usually the central portions of the liver (including the caudate lobe) are spared. Biopsy may be required to confirm the presence of the tumor.

CASE 6.62

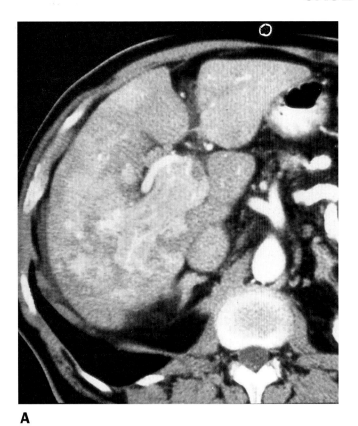

A

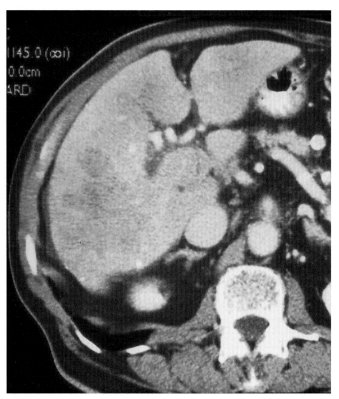

B

Findings

A. Contrast-enhanced CT, arterial phase. The liver enhances inhomogeneously. Hyperattenuating, enhancing soft tissue is present within the portal vein.

B. Contrast-enhanced CT, portal venous phase at a level caudad to A. Poorly defined, low-attenuation region within the posterior segment of the right lobe.

Differential Diagnosis

Hepatocellular carcinoma with portal venous tumor thrombus

Diagnosis

Advanced hepatocellular carcinoma with portal venous tumor thrombus

Discussion

A liver mass in combination with portal venous thrombus is highly suggestive of the diagnosis of hepatocellular carcinoma (HCC). Portal venous thrombosis is common because of the propensity for angioinvasion by HCC. It is not always possible to determine whether the filling defect is bland or tumor thrombus. Contrast enhancement at CT (as in this case) or the presence of an arterial Doppler waveform at sonography is diagnostic for tumor thrombus. Tumor thrombus adds to the likelihood that the hepatic mass is HCC, and it has grave prognostic significance.

CASE 6.63

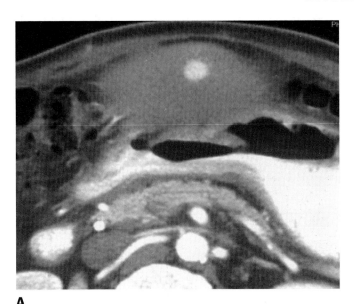

A

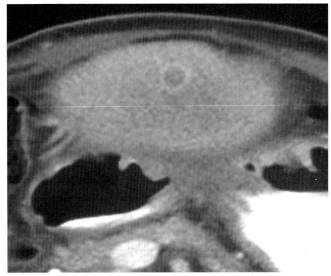

B

Findings

A. Contrast-enhanced CT, arterial phase. There is a small enhancing nodule within the left lobe of the liver. This patient had a prior right hepatectomy for hepatocellular carcinoma.

B. Contrast-enhanced CT, portal venous phase. The nodule is no longer hyperattenuating, but a small capsule about the mass is hyperattenuating.

Differential Diagnosis

1. Recurrent hepatocellular carcinoma
2. Focal nodular hyperplasia
3. Flash hemangioma

Diagnosis

Recurrent hepatocellular carcinoma

Discussion

Benign tumors are unusual in a cirrhotic liver. As a general rule, any mass in a cirrhotic liver is HCC until proved otherwise. In this patient with a history of HCC, the likelihood that this hypervascular mass represents HCC is even greater. The characteristic late-enhancing capsule also is supportive of this diagnosis. CT scanning during both the arterial and the portal venous phases of contrast enhancement is important for optimal detection and characterization of these lesions.

CASE 6.64

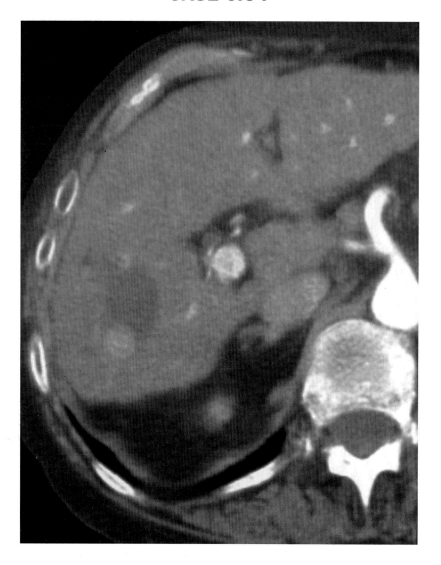

Findings

Contrast-enhanced CT. There is a hypoattenuating mass within the right lobe of the liver with an enhancing nodule in its inferior pole. The left lobe of the liver is enlarged, and the right lobe appears atrophic.

This patient had a prior percutaneous radiofrequency ablation of a small hepatocellular carcinoma in the right lobe of the liver.

Differential Diagnosis

Recurrent hepatocellular carcinoma

Diagnosis

Recurrent hepatocellular carcinoma

Discussion

CT is used routinely to assess for recurrent tumor immediately after an ablation for hepatocellular carcinoma (HCC) and at interim follow-up. A successful ablation results in a water-attenuation mass without evidence of enhancement. Hyperattenuating nodules within or adjacent to the ablation zone are consistent with recurrent or residual HCC (as seen in this case).

CASE 6.65

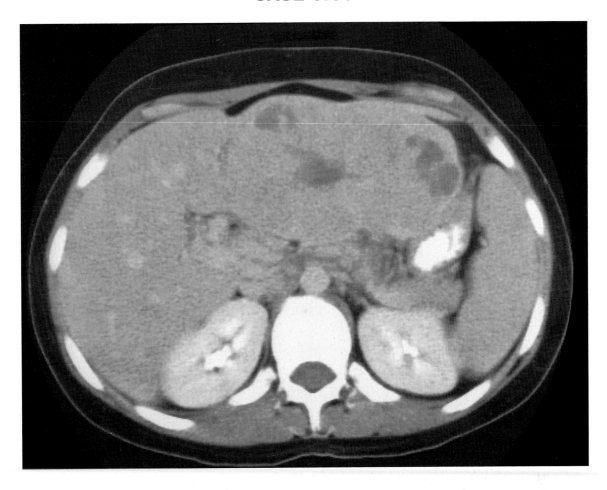

Findings

Contrast-enhanced CT. A large, well-circumscribed mass replaces the medial and lateral segments of the left lobe of the liver. The mass has a central scar, and there are several peripheral regions of low attenuation.

Differential Diagnosis

1. Hepatocellular carcinoma
2. Fibrolamellar hepatocellular carcinoma
3. Metastasis

Diagnosis

Fibrolamellar hepatocellular carcinoma

Discussion

Fibrolamellar hepatocellular carcinoma (HCC) is a type of primary hepatocellular malignancy that usually develops in young adults without underlying cirrhosis. Because these tumors often are discovered late in the course of the disease, they are large and of advanced stage at diagnosis. At one time, the prognosis for these tumors was believed to be better than that with usual HCC—but despite heroic attempts at surgical cure, most patients die as a result of the tumor. The classic radiographic features include a large mass containing a central scar and calcification. Although these features may be present in these tumors, they also can be present in many other benign and malignant tumors. For example, approximately 10% of usual HCCs contain calcification, and most large hemangiomas have a central scar. In most patients, a large, radiographically indeterminate mass is discovered in the liver. The nature of the mass is determined after surgical removal or biopsy.

Variable Appearance of Hepatocellular Carcinoma

The radiographic appearance of hepatocellular carcinoma (HCC) depends on the stage of the tumor at the time of detection and on the biologic aggressiveness of the neoplasm. The following classification and radiographic findings are helpful for understanding the varied appearance of this tumor.

		Case
Early HCC	Hyperenhancing mass, nodule within a nodule	6.49 and 6.50
Advanced HCC		
Focal	Internal fat, mosaic internal architecture, capsule	6.51–6.59
Multifocal	May simulate metastases, dominant mass with satellites	6.60
Diffuse	Innumerable masses	6.61

Secondary findings:

Portal vein or hepatic vein thrombosis	6.56–6.58, 6.62
Intratumoral shunting	6.57 and 6.58
Hemochromatosis	6.10
Prior thorium dioxide exposure	6.70

CASE 6.66

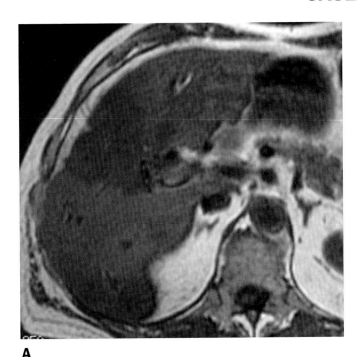

A

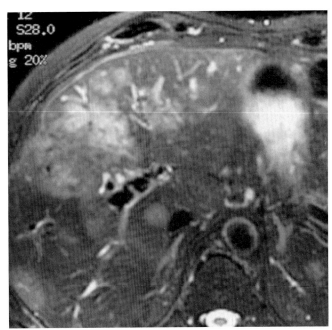

B

Findings

A. T1-weighted MRI. A large intrahepatic mass is located between the right and left lobes of the liver.

B. T2-weighted MRI. The mass is of high signal intensity compared with the liver, and there are multiple additional similar-appearing masses.

Differential Diagnosis

1. Metastases
2. Hepatocellular carcinoma
3. Cholangiocarcinoma

Diagnosis

Intrahepatic cholangiocarcinoma

Discussion

Cholangiocarcinoma arising from an intrahepatic bile duct can become large before becoming clinically apparent because of the large reserve capacity of the liver. In some cases, the mass remains small and chronically obstructs the bile duct and lobar atrophy occurs. In the case shown here, the mass is a large polypoid-type tumor that has replaced most of the surrounding liver tissue. Its appearance is nonspecific—and without the clinical history of a known risk factor it would be impossible to be certain of its nature. Because there are many masses in all hepatic segments, resection is not possible. Percutaneous biopsy could be performed to obtain tissue for histologic assessment.

Risk factors for cholangiocarcinoma include primary sclerosing cholangitis, choledochal cyst, familial polyposis syndrome, congenital hepatic fibrosis, infection with *Opisthorchis* (formerly *Clonorchis*) *sinensis* (liver fluke), and prior exposure to thorium dioxide.

Additional examples of cholangiocarcinoma are found in cases 7.20 through 7.26.

CASE 6.67

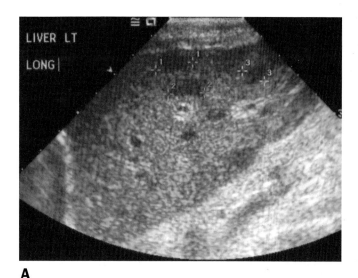

A

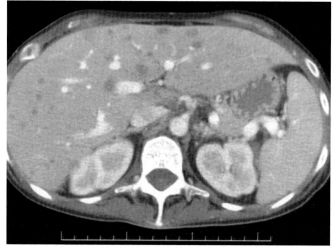

B

Findings

A. Longitudinal sonogram. Multiple hypoechoic masses are present in both lobes of the liver.

B. Contrast-enhanced CT. Multiple low-density lesions are seen in both lobes of the liver, corresponding to the hypoechoic masses on ultrasonography.

Differential Diagnosis

1. Hepatic metastasis
2. Hepatic lymphoma
3. Fungal abscesses (candidiasis)

Diagnosis

Hepatic lymphoma

Discussion

Liver biopsy led to the diagnosis of non-Hodgkin lymphoma in this case. The liver is a common secondary site for lymphomatous involvement, which is detected at autopsy in 60% of patients with Hodgkin lymphoma and 50% of patients with non-Hodgkin lymphoma. Secondary hepatic lymphoma typically presents radiologically as multiple small, hypoechoic lesions at sonography and multiple small, low-attenuation lesions at CT (as in this case). Secondary lymphomatous involvement of the liver is often difficult to detect radiographically because lymphomatous implants are often tiny and diffuse. Bulky abdominal adenopathy may favor the diagnosis of secondary hepatic lymphoma, but biopsy often is required to exclude metastatic disease or hepatic candidiasis (cases 6.26 and 6.27).

Primary lymphoma of the liver is extremely rare, constituting only 0.4% of all extranodal non-Hodgkin lymphomas and 0.016% of all non-Hodgkin lymphomas. The most common presentation of primary hepatic lymphoma is a solitary mass. Hepatic resection with additional chemotherapy or radiation therapy is advocated for these rare tumors. There appears to be a relationship between chronic liver disease and the development of primary hepatic lymphoma. This relationship is strongest in patients with human immunodeficiency virus and hepatitis C.

CASE 6.68

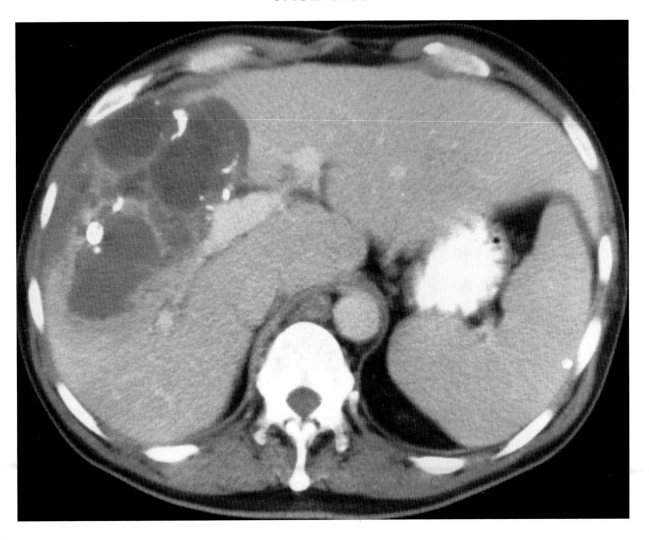

Findings

Contrast-enhanced CT. A complex, multilocular cystic mass is present in the right lobe of the liver with thick, nodular, enhancing septations and coarse calcifications.

Differential Diagnosis

1. Liver abscess
2. Biliary cystadenoma or cystadenocarcinoma
3. Echinococcal cyst

Diagnosis

Biliary cystadenocarcinoma

Discussion

Biliary cystadenocarcinomas are very rare primary liver neoplasms arising from the biliary epithelium. The thick septae, enhancing nodular components of this mass, and calcifications favor biliary cystadenocarcinoma over cystadenoma (case 6.47). Pathologists have begun to separate biliary cystadenomas and cystadenocarcinomas into those that contain ovarian stroma (found only in women) and those that do not (men and women). Those containing ovarian stroma tend to have a better prognosis. A liver abscess (case 6.21) would present in a patient with fever and increased leukocyte count, and the associated calcifications would be extremely unusual. Echinococcal cysts (cases 6.24 and 6.25) usually have thin septations, daughter cysts, and delicate peripheral calcifications.

CASE 6.69

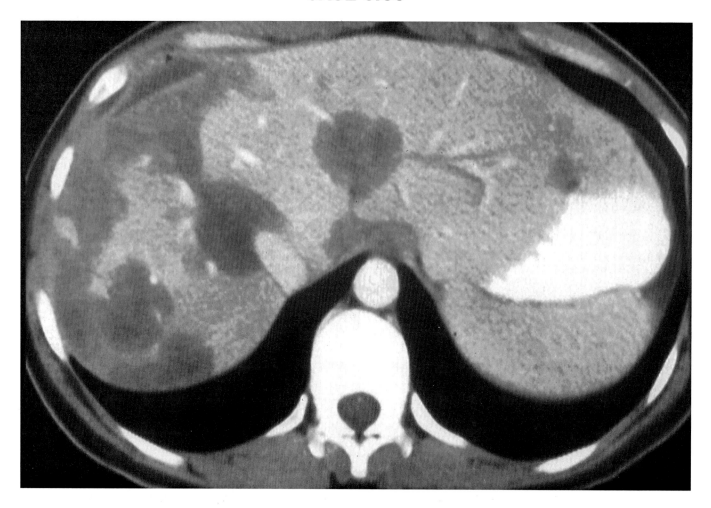

Findings

Contrast-enhanced CT. There are multiple masses throughout the liver, greater within the right lobe and periphery of the liver. The masses appear to be growing together into confluent regions of hypoattenuation.

Differential Diagnosis

1. Epithelioid hemangioendothelioma
2. Metastases
3. Multicentric hepatocellular carcinoma

Diagnosis

Epithelioid hemangioendothelioma

Discussion

This tumor is a rare malignant tumor of vascular origin. The tumor is believed to begin as multiple solitary masses that grow together to form a large confluent mass(es). Typically, the lesions are located in the periphery of the liver, and there may be capsular retraction at the level of the mass. Distinguishing this lesion from more common metastases or hepatocellular carcinoma may not be possible.

CASE 6.70

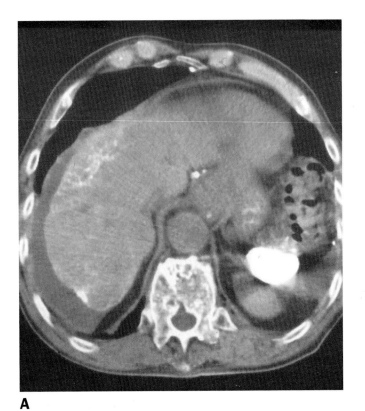

A

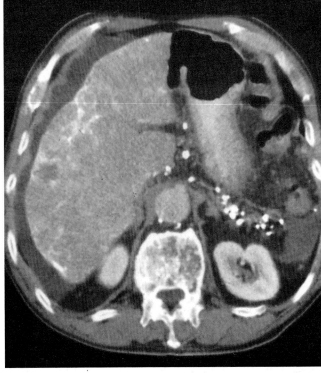

B

Findings

Unenhanced CT (**A**) and contrast-enhanced CT (**B**). The liver is of heterogeneous attenuation. High-attenuation material is seen throughout the liver in a lacelike pattern, especially about the capsular and subcapsular regions. The spleen is small and hyperdense. Multiple hyperdense lymph nodes are seen in the peripancreatic and gastrohepatic regions.

Differential Diagnosis

1. Thorium dioxide–induced angiosarcoma
2. Thorium dioxide–induced cholangiocarcinoma
3. Thorium dioxide–induced hepatocellular carcinoma
4. Thorium dioxide–induced cirrhosis

Diagnosis

Thorium dioxide–induced angiosarcoma

Discussion

Thorium dioxide was an intravascular contrast agent that emitted alpha radiation. The long half-life of the radioactive agent exposes patients to chronic radiation during their lifetimes. It was used in various radiologic procedures between 1920 and the 1950s, usually neuroangiography. After leaving the vascular space, the agent is taken up by the reticuloendothelial system (liver, spleen, bone marrow). The spleen usually becomes atrophic and hyperattenuating. Uptake of the agent in upper abdominal lymph nodes is also common. There is an increased incidence of liver cancers (angiosarcoma, hepatocellular carcinoma, and cholangiocarcinoma), cirrhosis, blood diseases, lung cancer, peritoneal tumors, and other neoplasms.

The patient in this case had an angiosarcoma, but other infiltrating neoplasms could have a similar appearance. Heterogeneity of the liver parenchyma is the key finding to suggest a complicating tumor. Percutaneous biopsy is necessary to confirm the diagnosis.

CASE 6.71

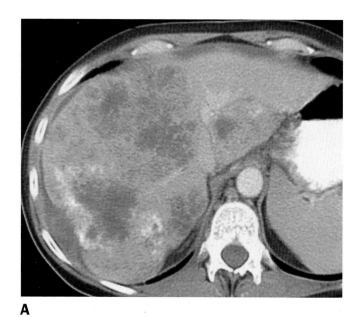

A

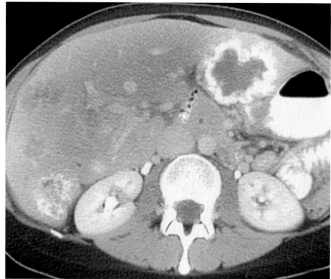

B

Findings
Contrast-enhanced CT. **A** and **B.** Multiple hypoattenuating and partially calcified masses are present throughout the liver.

Differential Diagnosis
Metastases

Diagnosis
Calcified metastases—colon primary

Discussion
Metastases are the commonest malignant tumor to involve the liver. One-fourth to one-half of all patients who die of cancer have liver metastases. Colon metastases are the commonest, and they usually present as expansile, hypoattenuating masses. Well-differentiated colon metastases that produce mucin may calcify (as in this case). Stomach and small bowel adenocarcinoma can present similarly—but calcify less often. Breast and lung cancers usually are smaller and often diffuse or infiltrative. Pancreatic cancer metastases usually are smaller and variable in number. Patients with pancreatic cancer do not usually live long enough for these metastases to reach a large size. Hypovascular metastases (as discussed above) usually are detected most accurately during the portal venous phase of contrast enhancement. Hypervascular metastases include tumors arising from the neuroendocrine system (carcinoid, islet cell, pheochromocytoma), melanoma, choriocarcinoma, breast cancer, thyroid cancer, and renal adenocarcinoma. If hypervascular metastasis is suspected, acquiring a scan during the arterial phase of contrast enhancement can be helpful.

CASE 6.72

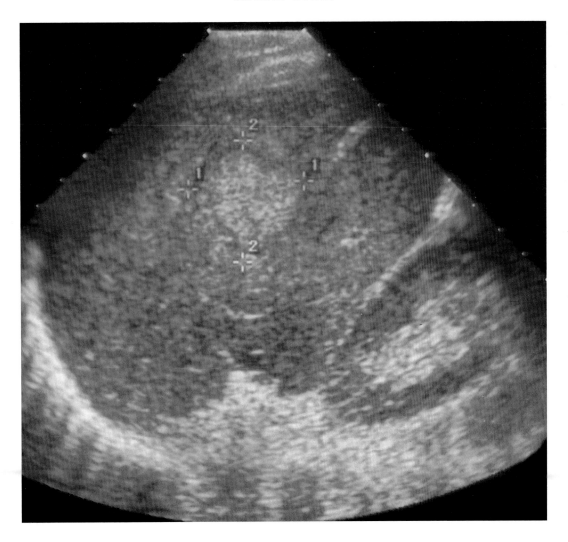

Findings

Sonogram. A 3.5-cm hyperechoic mass is present in the right lobe of the liver with a hypoechoic halo.

Differential Diagnosis

1. Hepatic metastasis
2. Hepatocellular carcinoma
3. Hepatic adenoma

Diagnosis

Hepatic metastasis

Discussion

This patient had a history of sigmoid adenocarcinoma, and needle biopsy of the liver mass was positive for metastasis.

Two common patterns for hepatic metastases on ultrasonography are multiple hypoechoic masses or multiple isoechoic or hyperechoic masses with hypoechoic halos. Although not absolutely indicative of malignancy, a hypoechoic halo around a liver mass is an ominous sign. This halo usually is seen with metastases or hepatocellular carcinoma; however, hepatic adenomas and atypical focal nodular hyperplasia also can present with hypoechoic halos. As a general rule, hepatic masses with hypoechoic halos should be treated as malignant until proved otherwise.

The hypoechoic halo has been shown histologically to usually represent compressed normal liver parenchyma caused by a rapidly expanding tumor. Less often, it can be due to peripheral tumor fibrosis or vascularization.

CASE 6.73

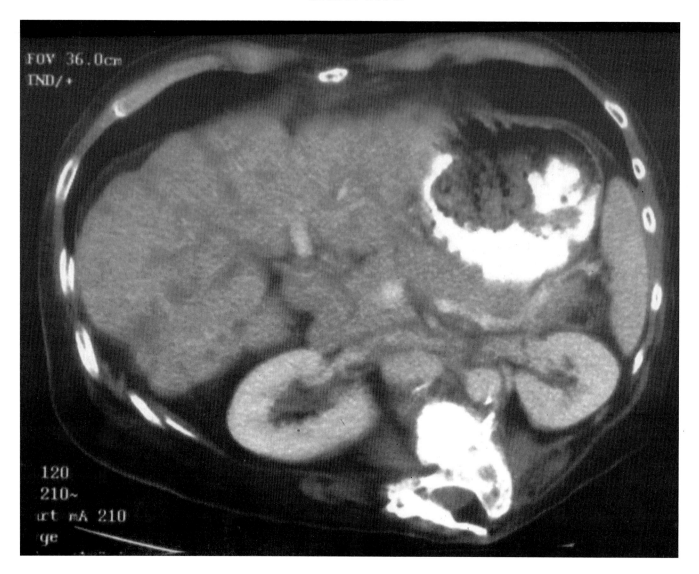

Findings

Contrast-enhanced CT. The liver appears shrunken, and the contour is nodular. There are several focal masses in the liver. Food is visible in the stomach.

Differential Diagnosis

1. Cirrhosis with multicentric hepatocellular carcinoma
2. Breast metastases to the liver with chemotherapy-induced pseudocirrhosis

Diagnosis

Breast metastases to the liver with chemotherapy-induced pseudocirrhosis

Discussion

In patients with breast cancer who are taking chemotherapeutic drugs, morphologic changes of the liver can develop which resemble cirrhosis. Pseudocirrhosis includes a lobular hepatic contour, segmental volume loss, and enlargement of the caudate lobe. Retraction of the capsular surface of the liver can be seen at the site of subjacent metastases. These changes can develop over several months. Pathologically, nodular regenerative hyperplasia without cirrhosis has been found.

CASE 6.74

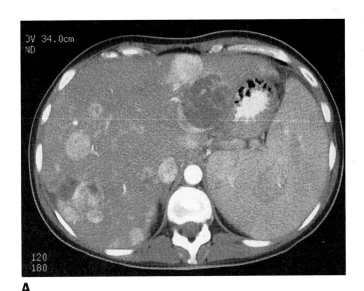

A

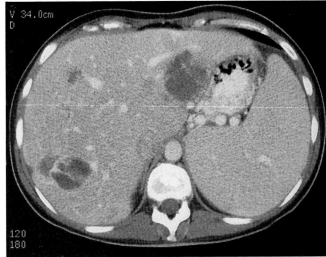

B

Findings

Contrast-enhanced CT. **A.** Arterial phase. Multiple hyperenhancing and cystic masses are present in the liver. **B.** Portal venous phase. The hypervascular masses have become isoattenuating with the liver. Splenomegaly.

Differential Diagnosis

1. Hypervascular metastases
2. Multifocal hepatocellular carcinoma
3. Multiple benign liver tumors (flash hemangiomas, adenomas, focal nodular hyperplasia)

Diagnosis

Hypervascular metastases (metastatic carcinoid tumor)

Discussion

Hypervascular metastases, such as a carcinoid tumor, can be isoattenuating to liver on unenhanced and portal venous-phase imaging. This case shows the importance of arterial-phase imaging when evaluating for hypervascular metastases (islet cell, carcinoid, melanoma, renal cell, thyroid, breast, sarcoma). Clinical history is important in this case because other benign and malignant tumors can have a similar CT appearance. The multiplicity of lesions favors metastatic disease in this case.

CASE 6.75

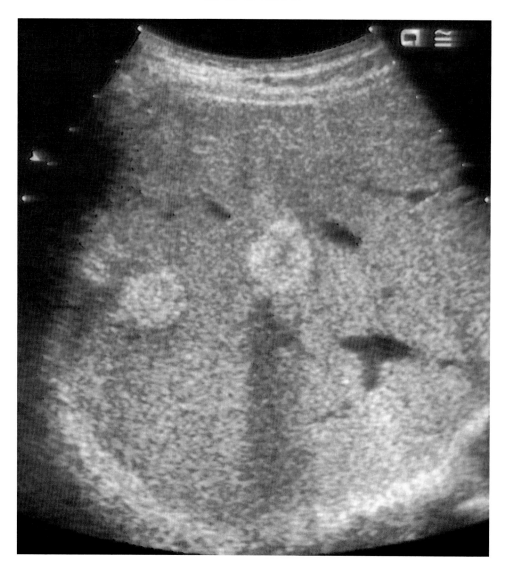

Findings

Sonogram. Rounded hyperechoic masses are seen in the right lobe of the liver. The masses have associated posterior acoustic shadowing.

Differential Diagnosis

1. Hyperechoic metastases
2. Hemangiomas
3. Fat-containing liver tumors (lipoma, angiomyolipoma)
4. Multifocal hepatocellular carcinoma

Diagnosis

Hyperechoic metastases (renal adenocarcinoma)

Discussion

The more vascular a tumor, the more likely it is to be echogenic. For this reason, metastases from renal cell carcinoma, carcinoid, sarcomas, and islet cell carcinomas tend to be hyperechoic. This patient had metastatic renal adenocarcinoma. The posterior acoustic shadowing behind these masses should be a tip-off that they are unlikely to be hemangiomas (case 6.31). Hemangiomas often have slight increased through transmission.

Malignant Liver Masses

		Case
Hepatocellular carcinoma	Capsule, mosaic and fatty internal contents. Cirrhosis, usually hypervascular	6.49–6.65
Cholangiocarcinoma	Scirrhous or polypoid. Klatskin tumor at bifurcation most common	6.66, 7.20–7.26
Lymphoma	Multiple, diffuse tiny lesions. Usually not specific appearance	6.67
Biliary cystadenocarcinoma	Large cystic mass containing thick septations	6.68
Epithelioid hemangioendothelioma	Peripheral mass, conglomerate. Capsular retraction	6.69
Angiosarcoma	Associated with thorium dioxide	6.70
Metastases	Multiple or solitary. Calcification, central necrosis, hemorrhage can occur	6.71–6.75

CASE 6.76

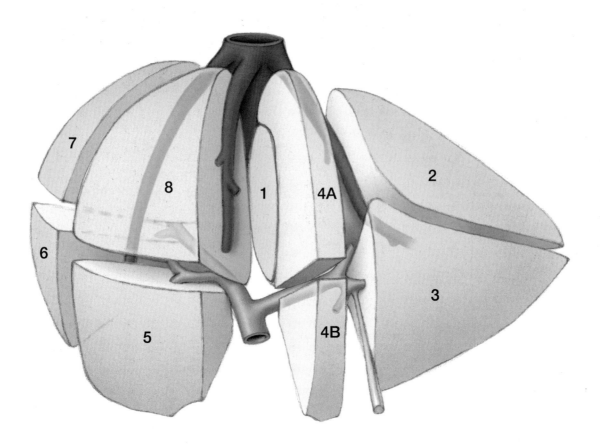

Findings

The liver is divided into eight sectors according to the Couinaud classification. This classification is useful to hepatic surgeons because it divides the liver according to the portal venous and hepatic venous supply. Sector 1 corresponds to the caudate lobe. Sectors 2 (superior) and 3 (inferior) represent the lateral segment of the left hepatic lobe. Sector 4 corresponds to the medial segment of the left hepatic lobe and often is divided into a superior (A) and inferior (B) subsector. The right lobe of the liver is divided into four sectors. The inferior (inferior to the main portal vein) segments are divided into anterior (sector 5) and posterior (sector 6) sectors. The superior segments are divided into anterior (sector 8) and posterior (sector 7) sectors. The anterior segment of the right lobe consists of sectors 5 and 8, and the posterior segment consists of sectors 6 and 7.

CASE 6.77

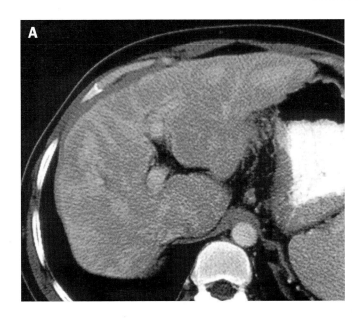

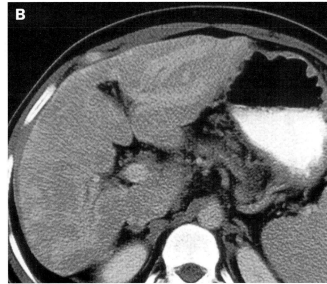

Findings

A and **B.** Contrast-enhanced CT. Diffuse hyperenhancement within the distribution of the portal tracts that result in abnormal linear branching structures throughout the liver.

Differential Diagnosis

1. Infectious disorders: tuberculosis, histoplasmosis, schistosomiasis, toxoplasmosis
2. Sarcoidosis
3. Drug reaction
4. Primary biliary cirrhosis

Diagnosis

Schistosomiasis

Discussion

Schistosomiasis (bilharziasis) is the second most prevalent tropical disease in the world, second only to malaria. More than 200 million people are infected. The main forms of human schistosomiasis are caused by five species of flatworm (blood flukes) in the genus *Schistosoma: S. haematobium, S. mansoni, S. japonicum, S. intercalatum,* and *S. mekongi.*

Adult worms mate and lay eggs. When the ova reach fresh water, miracidia are released and penetrate the snail. They asexually multiply cercariae. The cercariae leave the snail and swim to a human or nonhuman animal, where they penetrate the skin. Once inside, cercariae travel to the portal veins, where they develop into adult worms. Humans excrete approximately 50% of the eggs. The rest are trapped in various parts of the body.

Disease occurs as a result of the immunologic reaction to *Schistosoma* eggs trapped in tissues. Antigens released from the egg stimulate a granulomatous reaction. In the later stages of the disease, collagen deposition and fibrosis result in organ damage that may not be reversible. The most common gastrointestinal complication is periportal fibrosis that can lead to portal hypertension and gastrointestinal hemorrhage. Imaging findings, due to the abundant periportal fibrosis, include thickening of the portal tracts and hyperenhancement during the portal venous and delayed phases of contrast enhancement (as in this case).

Many other causes of liver granulomas could present similarly. Infectious conditions are most common, including bacterial (mycobacterial infections, brucellosis, tularemia, actinomycosis), fungal (histoplasmosis, cryptococcosis, blastomycosis), parasitic (toxoplasmosis), and others. Sarcoidosis is the most important noninfectious cause. Various drugs (quinidine, sulfonamides, allopurinol, phenylbutazone) also can be responsible. Primary biliary cirrhosis is the only important primary cause of hepatic granulomas.

Miscellaneous Liver Conditions

		Case
Liver segments (sectors)	1: caudate	6.76
	2: superior subsegment, left lateral segment	
	3: inferior subsegment, left lateral segment	
	4A: superior subsegment, left medial segment	
	4B: inferior subsegment, left medial segment	
	5: anterior-inferior subsegment, right lobe	
	6: posterior-inferior subsegment, right lobe	
	7: posterior-superior subsegment, right lobe	
	8: anterior-superior subsegment, right lobe	
Schistosomiasis	Thickening of portal tracts, delayed enhancement due to abundant fibrosis	6.77

DIFFERENTIAL DIAGNOSES

Cystic Masses

Benign
Simple cyst
Polycystic disease
Von Meyenburg complexes
Peribiliary cysts
Biliary cystadenoma
Biloma
Pyogenic abscess
Amebic abscess
Echinococcal cyst

Malignant
Biliary cystadenocarcinoma
Cystic cholangiocarcinoma
Cystic metastases (mucinous)
Necrotic tumors

Solid Masses

Benign
Hemangioma
Focal nodular hyperplasia
Hepatic adenoma
Lipoma
Angiomyolipoma
Regenerative nodules
Dysplastic nodules
Focal fatty infiltration

Malignant
Hepatocellular carcinoma
Cholangiocarcinoma
Metastases
Lymphoma

Increased Density on CT

Hemochromatosis
Drugs: amiodarone, cisplatin
Glycogen storage disease
Wilson disease
Gold therapy

Hypervascular Masses

Benign
Hemangioma
Focal nodular hyperplasia
Hepatic adenoma

Malignant
Hepatocellular carcinoma
Metastases (islet cell, carcinoid, renal adenocarcinoma, breast, thyroid, sarcoma)

Hyperechoic Masses

Benign
Hemangioma
Focal fatty infiltration
Lipoma
Angiomyolipoma

Malignant
Hepatocellular carcinoma
Hypervascular metastases (islet cell, carcinoid, renal adenocarcinoma, breast, thyroid, sarcoma)
Calcified metastases

LIVER MASSES

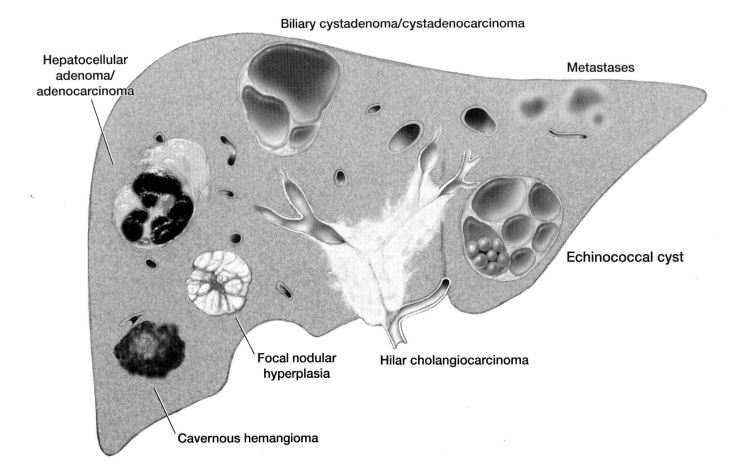

Biliary cystadenoma/cystadenocarcinoma

Metastases

Hepatocellular adenoma/adenocarcinoma

Echinococcal cyst

Focal nodular hyperplasia

Hilar cholangiocarcinoma

Cavernous hemangioma

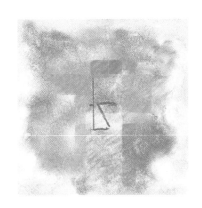

CHAPTER 7

BILE DUCTS AND GALLBLADDER

BILE DUCTS

GALLBLADDER

CASE 7.1

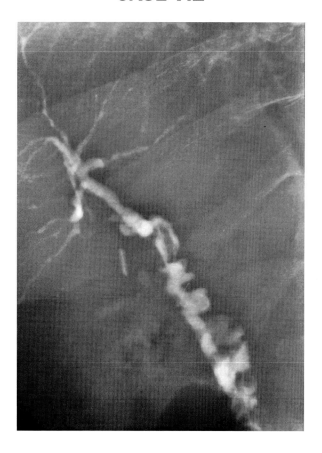

Findings
ERCP. The intrahepatic and extrahepatic bile ducts are irregularly narrowed. Bandlike strictures affect the extrahepatic duct. Alternating areas of normal and narrowed duct affect the intrahepatic bile ducts.

Differential Diagnosis
Primary sclerosing cholangitis

Diagnosis
Primary sclerosing cholangitis

Discussion
Primary sclerosing cholangitis (PSC) is a cholestatic disease of unknown origin most often affecting young (<45 years) males who have ulcerative colitis. The natural history of PSC is one of chronic progression; the median duration of survival is approximately 12 years from diagnosis. Pathologically, fibrosing inflammation is the key finding. The disease usually follows a progression from initial cholangitis to periportal hepatitis, to septal fibrosis, to bridging necrosis, and finally to cirrhosis. The disease most commonly affects both the intrahepatic and the extrahepatic ducts; however, intrahepatic involvement alone is visible at cholangiography in about 20% of patients. Direct gallbladder involvement is present in about 15% of patients.

Cholangiographic features of PSC include the following:

1. Band strictures (as in this case) leading to a beaded appearance
2. Nonuniform, segmental strictures 1 to 2 cm long
3. Pruned-tree appearance of intrahepatic ducts (due to obliteration of ducts)
4. Diverticular outpouchings
5. Mural irregularity—this can vary from fine to shaggy contour changes
6. Combinations of the above

CASE 7.2

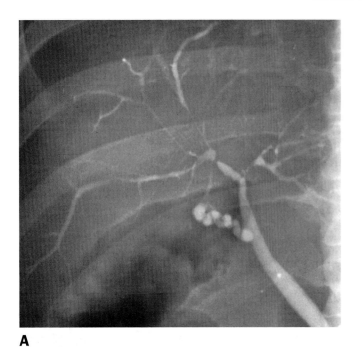

A

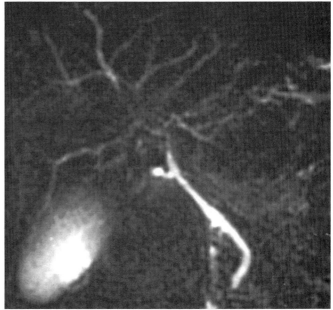

B

Findings
A. ERCP. **B.** MRCP. Diffuse long strictures are present throughout the intrahepatic ducts. The extrahepatic ductal system is normal in appearance.

Differential Diagnosis
Primary sclerosing cholangitis

Diagnosis
Primary sclerosing cholangitis

Discussion
This case illustrates long strictures that occasionally occur in primary sclerosing cholangitis (PSC). The case also shows the normal appearance of the extrahepatic ducts, a finding in up to 20% of patients with PSC. Even with a normal radiographic appearance of the extrahepatic ducts, the vast majority of patients with PSC have histologic changes of the disease in the extrahepatic ducts.

CASE 7.3

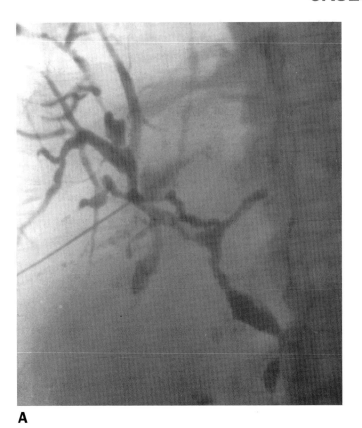

A

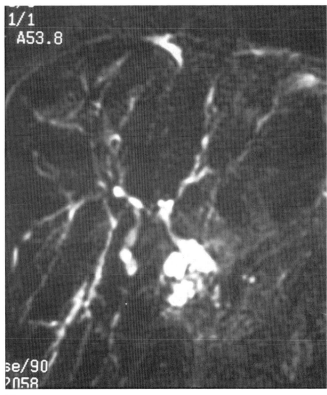

B

Findings

A. Percutaneous cholangiogram. Multiple strictures of varying length involve both the intrahepatic and the extrahepatic biliary system. The left intrahepatic ductal system is not opacified.

B. MRCP. Multiple biliary strictures correlate with those seen on the cholangiogram. The left intrahepatic ducts are visible and have an appearance similar to that of the right ducts. There is a high-grade stricture of the proximal left ductal system near the bifurcation of the common hepatic duct.

Differential Diagnosis

Primary sclerosing cholangitis

Diagnosis

Primary sclerosing cholangitis

Discussion

This case is a good example of random segmental strictures (1-2 cm in length) commonly seen in primary sclerosing cholangitis (PSC). In this case, nonfilling of the left ductal system is present on the percutaneous cholangiogram. Because MRCP does not depend on opacification of the bile ducts, the ductal system beyond an obstruction can be visualized. The dominant stricture, in this case in the main left bile duct, should raise concern that a complicating cholangiocarcinoma may be present.

CASE 7.4

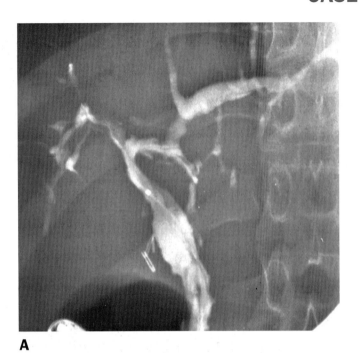

A

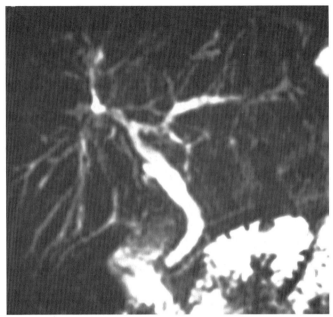

B

Findings
A. ERCP. The intrahepatic and extrahepatic bile ducts are diffusely abnormal and have regions of narrowing and mural irregularity.

B. MRCP. Changes are similar to those on the ERCP; however, multiple intrahepatic ducts are better visualized.

Differential Diagnosis
1. Primary sclerosing cholangitis
2. Ascending cholangitis

Diagnosis
Primary sclerosing cholangitis

Discussion
This case illustrates the mural irregularity that often occurs in primary sclerosing cholangitis. Although the same changes can be seen on both ERCP and MRCP, the spatial resolution at MRI is inferior to that at ERCP. Fine changes of mural irregularity could be overlooked at MRCP. Therefore, if clinical suspicion of the disease is high, ERCP is indicated despite a normal MRCP. MRCP is superior to ERCP for identifying bile ducts that are isolated from the main ductal system. These dilated, obstructed ducts may be a source of infection. MRCP can be a helpful study before a biliary drainage procedure to evaluate for an isolated duct(s). ERCP allows biopsy and brushings of dominant strictures to assess for a complicating cholangiocarcinoma.

CASE 7.5

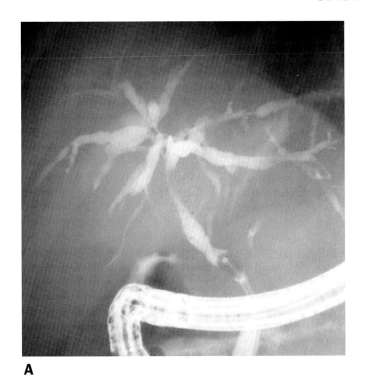

A

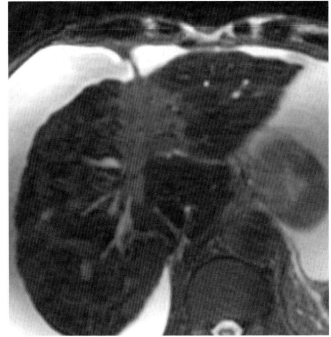

B

Findings

A. ERCP. The bile ducts are diffusely irregular and have areas of stricture and dilatation. A dominant stricture involves the proximal common hepatic duct.

B. T2-weighted MRI. A large, hyperintense mass arises at the junction of the medial and lateral hepatic segments and extends into the porta hepatis.

Differential Diagnosis

Cholangiocarcinoma complicating primary sclerosing cholangitis

Diagnosis

Cholangiocarcinoma complicating primary sclerosing cholangitis

Discussion

Cholangiocarcinoma is a dreaded complication of primary sclerosing cholangitis (PSC). Because of the diffuse and unpredictable ductal changes in patients with PSC, distinguishing benign strictures from cholangiocarcinoma often is difficult. Dominant strictures, those strictures that are most severe and critical in their location, should be considered suspicious for cholangiocarcinoma. Comparison of the cholangiogram with prior studies, ERCP-guided brushings for histologic analysis, and MRI can be helpful to assess the nature of a new stricture.

CASE 7.6

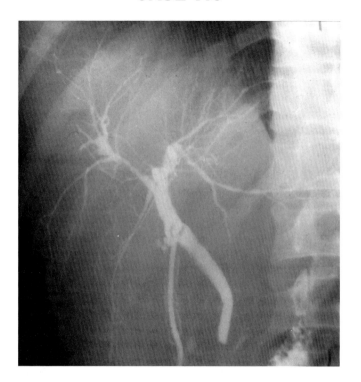

CASE 7.7

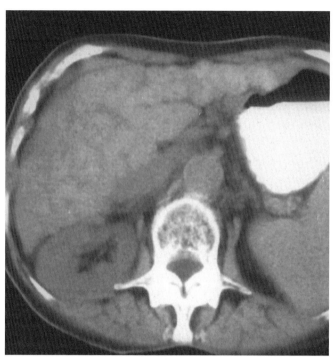

Findings

Case 7.6. T-tube cholangiogram. The intrahepatic bile ducts appear crowded and pruned, and there is some tortuosity and deformity of the peripheral ducts.

Case 7.7. Unenhanced CT. The liver has a diffusely nodular appearance without bile duct dilatation.

Differential Diagnosis
1. Hepatic cirrhosis
2. Small-duct primary sclerosing cholangitis
3. Primary biliary cirrhosis

Diagnosis
Primary biliary cirrhosis

Discussion

Primary biliary cirrhosis (PBC) is a cholestatic disease of unknown origin. T-cell–mediated immune response plays an important role in bile duct injury. Other autoimmune diseases often are associated (rheumatoid arthritis, Sjögren syndrome, Hashimoto thyroiditis, and others). Serologic markers, including antimitochondrial antibody, often are present. The disease predominantly affects females. Small duct destruction with an inflammatory cellular infiltrate is characteristic of PBC histologically.

Early in the disease, cholangiograms are normal. Later, the cholangiographic features are those of cirrhosis with crowding, tortuosity, and deformity of the bile ducts (as in this case). Enlarged benign reactive lymph nodes in the hepatic portal are common and can cause mass effect on the extrahepatic ducts. Although primary sclerosing cholangitis (PSC) affecting the large ducts (cases 7.1 through 7.4) has many features that are different from those of PBC, small-duct PSC may be indistinguishable. Further, other causes of hepatic cirrhosis also may result in a similar appearance. Correlation of the imaging studies with the clinical and laboratory findings is critical to a correct diagnosis. In many cases, a liver biopsy is necessary.

CASE 7.8

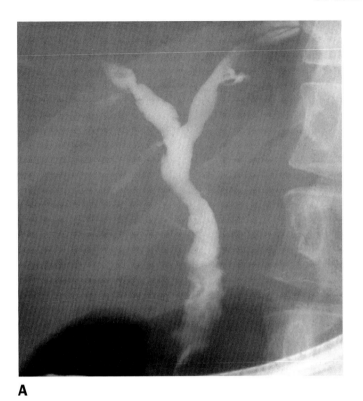

A

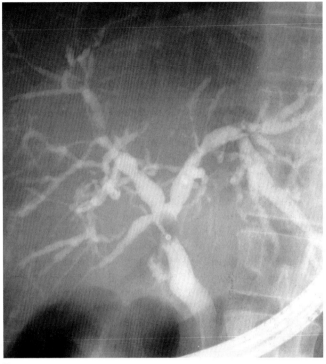

B

Findings
ERCP. **A** and **B**. The extrahepatic bile duct is mildly dilated, and the duct is diffusely irregular. The intrahepatic ducts are mildly dilated and have multiple segmental strictures. Endoscopic balloon in the common bile duct (**B**).

Differential Diagnosis
1. Primary sclerosing cholangitis
2. Ascending cholangitis
3. Acquired immunodeficiency syndrome cholangiopathy

Diagnosis
Acquired immunodeficiency syndrome cholangiopathy

Discussion
Acquired immunodeficiency syndrome (AIDS) is due to the human immunodeficiency virus, which destroys CD4 (T helper-inducer) lymphocytes. Affected persons have progressive loss of cellular immunity and become susceptible to opportunistic infection and tumors. Infectious organisms found in the gastrointestinal tract which can be clinically important in these patients include *Candida albicans,* cytomegalovirus, herpes simplex virus, *Cryptosporidium, Mycobacterium tuberculosis,* and *Mycobacterium avium-intracellulare.* Common tumors in these patients include Kaposi sarcoma and non-Hodgkin lymphoma.

Biliary tract abnormalities in patients with AIDS are related to infection with either *Cryptosporidium* or cytomegalovirus. Patients present with right upper quadrant abdominal pain, fever, leukocytosis, and abnormal liver function tests. The characteristic cholangiographic features of AIDS cholangiopathy include segmental strictures of the biliary system which are identical to those in patients with primary sclerosing cholangitis. In addition, some patients have papillary stenosis alone or in combination with the bile duct strictures. The combination of intrahepatic ductal strictures and papillary stenosis is unique to AIDS-related cholangitis. Acalculous cholecystitis also has been reported. Treatment of this condition is based on eradication of infectious agents. Endoscopic papillotomy can provide relief of symptoms and improve results of liver function tests.

CASE 7.9

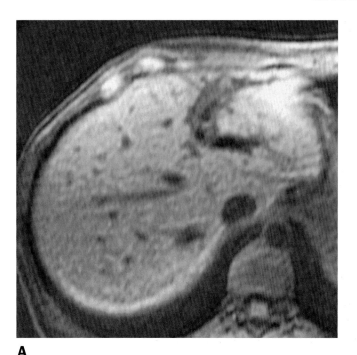

A

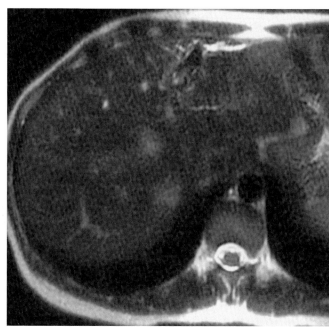

B

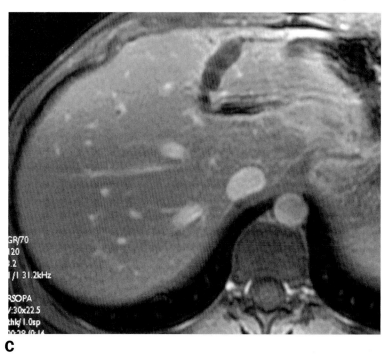

C

CASE 7.10

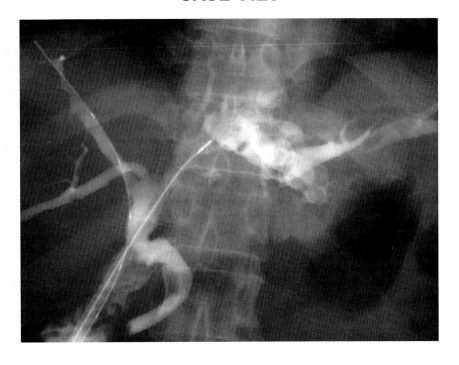

Findings

Case 7.9. A. T1-weighted MRI. There are two low-intensity tubular structures in the left lobe of the liver.
B. T2-weighted MRI. Low-intensity T2 structures appear to be present in two dilated left lobe bile ducts.
C. Gadolinium-enhanced MRI. Very low-intensity stones are visible within the dilated bile ducts.

Case 7.10. Percutaneous cholangiogram. The intrahepatic bile ducts within the left lobe of the liver are dilated and contain several filling defects. There is a stricture of the distal left hepatic ducts.

(From MacCarty RL. Inflammatory disorders of the biliary tract. In: Gore RM, Levine MS, editors. Textbook of gastrointestinal radiology. Vol 2. 2nd ed. Philadelphia: WB Saunders Company; 2000. p. 1375-94. By permission of the publisher.)

Differential Diagnosis

1. Cholangiocarcinoma
2. Oriental cholangiohepatitis
3. Benign biliary stricture—origin unknown

Diagnosis

Oriental cholangiohepatitis

Discussion

Oriental cholangiohepatitis is most common in Southeast Asia. The cause of the disease is not known, but associations with clonorchiasis, ascariasis, and nutritional deficiency have been suggested. Dilatation of intrahepatic and extrahepatic ducts containing pigmented stones and infected fluid is seen pathologically. The infection results in biliary strictures. Patients usually present with recurrent attacks of abdominal pain, fever, and jaundice. Localized intrahepatic segmental ductal stenosis with upstream dilatation may occur, especially in the lateral segment of the left lobe or posterior segment of the right hepatic lobe. Sonographic and CT findings include intrahepatic or extrahepatic duct stones, dilatation of the intrahepatic or extrahepatic ducts, increased periportal echogenicity, segmental lobar atrophy, and gallstones. Cholangiographic findings include bile duct stones, ductal dilatation and focal strictures, acute peripheral tapering, and decreased arborization of the intrahepatic bile ducts.

CASE 7.11

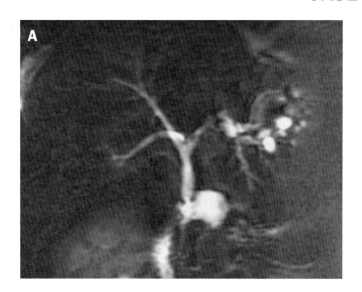

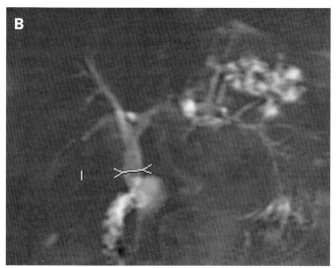

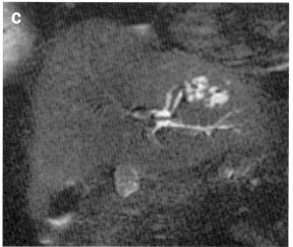

Findings

MRCP. **A** through **C.** The extrahepatic bile duct is mildly dilated to the level of a choledochoenterostomy. Several saccular fluid collections communicating with the biliary system are present in the lateral segment of the left hepatic lobe. Small filling defects are present within these fluid collections.

Differential Diagnosis

1. Caroli disease
2. Liver abscesses

Diagnosis

Liver abscesses due to bacterial cholangitis

Discussion

Abscesses can develop in the liver as a result of bacterial cholangitis, usually due to bile stasis or obstruction. Patients usually present with signs and symptoms of an infection and jaundice. *Escherichia coli* is the most common organism. The abscesses typically communicate with the biliary system. Treatment is focused on relieving the obstruction and administering antibiotics. Chronic cholangitis can result in bile duct strictures, attenuation of the peripheral bile ducts at cholangiography, and biliary cirrhosis.

Inflammatory Diseases of the Bile Ducts

		Case
Primary sclerosing cholangitis (PSC)	Band strictures (beaded appearance), segmental strictures, pruned-tree appearance, mural irregularity, and diverticular outpouchings. Increased risk of cholangiocarcinoma	7.1–7.5
Primary biliary cirrhosis	Autoimmune cholestatic disease involving small bile ducts. Cirrhosis results in crowding and deformity of bile ducts	7.6 and 7.7
Acquired immuno-deficiency syndrome cholangiopathy	Indistinguishable from PSC. PSC changes plus papillary stenosis highly suspicious	7.8
Oriental cholangiohepatitis	Focal strictures, intraductal stones, intrahepatic and extrahepatic duct dilatation, straight rigid intrahepatic ducts	7.9 and 7.10
Bacterial cholangitis	Ductal irregularity, strictures, small abscess cavities that communicate with bile ducts	7.11

CASE 7.12

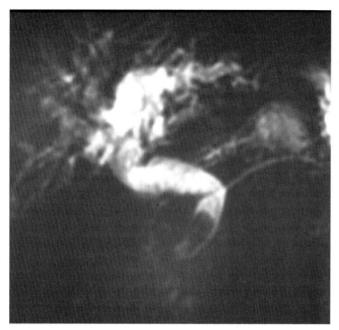

A

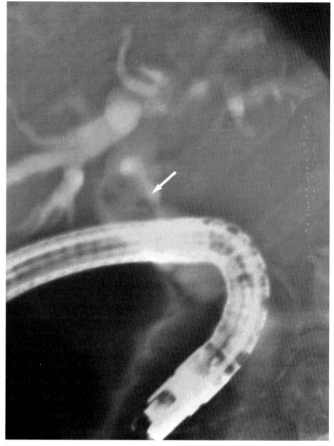

B

Findings

A. MRCP. The intrahepatic and extrahepatic bile ducts are dilated to the level of the distal common bile duct. There is a large filling defect within the distal common bile duct.

B. ERCP. The large filling defect is visible within the dilated common bile duct. The filling defect has moved into the proximal common bile duct (arrow).

Differential Diagnosis

Choledocholithiasis

Diagnosis

Choledocholithiasis

Discussion

Choledocholithiasis can develop de novo within the bile ducts or as calculi that have passed through the cystic duct from the gallbladder. Choledocholithiasis is found in 12% to 15% of patients undergoing cholecystectomy, but this rate increases with age, duct size, and chronicity of symptoms. Typical symptoms include biliary colic, jaundice, cholangitis, and pancreatitis. The correct imaging test to begin the evaluation depends on the clinical suspicion of choledocholithiasis. If the suspicion is high, ERCP usually is indicated so the calculus can be removed at the same time. MRCP is an excellent noninvasive approach for imaging the bile ducts and is indicated in patients less likely to require intervention.

CASE 7.13

A

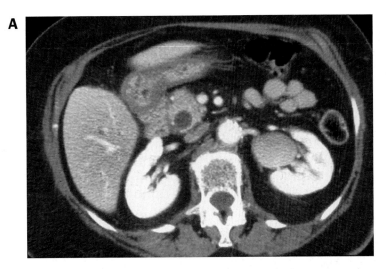

B

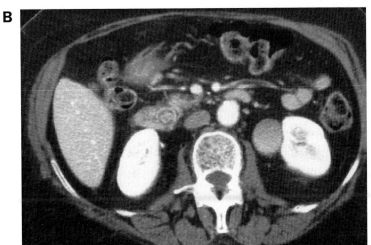

Findings
Contrast-enhanced CT. **A.** The intrapancreatic portion of the common bile duct is dilated. **B.** The distal common bile duct contains a filling defect. A rim of fluid attenuation is seen around the filling defect.

Differential Diagnosis
Choledocholithiasis

Diagnosis
Choledocholithiasis

Discussion
The composition of bile duct calculi can vary in the percentage of calcium bilirubinate, cholesterol, and pigment. Stones containing calcium are the easiest to recognize because of their high attenuation. Pure cholesterol stones are of low attenuation and very difficult to detect at CT. Most calculi are of mixed composition, and the vast majority can be recognized at CT, especially with proper CT technique. Two helpful findings have been described to represent the appearance of a calculus within the bile duct imaged in cross-section. The commonest finding is referred to as the target sign with a ring of water attenuation around the stone (as in this case). The crescent sign is a variant of the target sign with only a crescent of water attenuation surrounding the calculus.

CASE 7.14

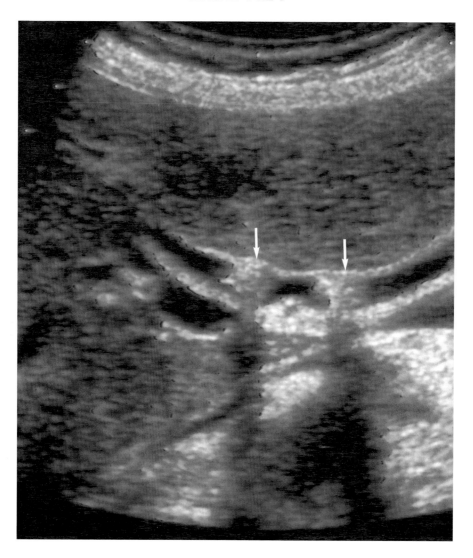

Findings

Sonogram. Longitudinal view of the common bile duct has two echogenic structures (arrows) in a dilated duct which have posterior acoustic shadowing.

Differential Diagnosis

Choledocholithiasis

Diagnosis

Choledocholithiasis

Discussion

Because ultrasonography is noninvasive, inexpensive, and readily available, it is usually the test of choice when patients present with biliary-related symptoms. The best sensitivities reported for detection of common bile duct stones by sonography are approximately 75%. A nondilated duct, nonshadowing stones, bowel gas, arterial calcifications, and cholecystectomy clips often make this diagnosis difficult. The markedly dilated duct, posterior shadowing of the stones, and location of the stones in the mid common bile duct make the diagnosis easy in this case. When clinical suspicion of choledocholithiasis is high but no stones are seen with sonography, MRCP or ERCP is often recommended for further evaluation.

CASE 7.15

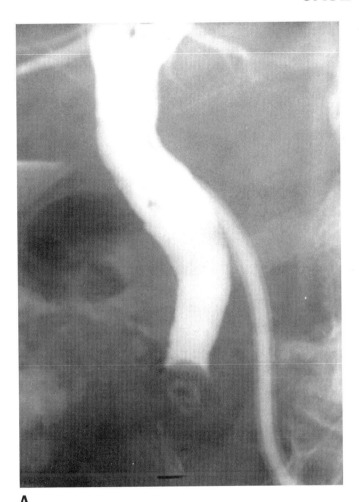

A

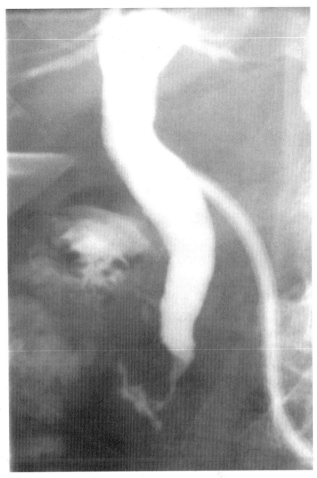

B

Findings

T-tube cholangiogram. **A.** A meniscus is formed from a filling defect in the distal common bile duct. **B.** The filling defect is no longer seen.

Differential Diagnosis

1. Passage of a common bile duct stone
2. Ampullary carcinoma
3. Pseudocalculus

Diagnosis

Pseudocalculus

Discussion

A pseudocalculus is an apparent filling defect within the ampullary segment of the common bile duct due to spasm of the sphincter of Oddi. With relaxation of the sphincter (which can be assisted with the use of intravenous glucagon or by waiting 10-15 minutes), the filling defect disappears and contrast material flows into the duodenum normally. A key finding distinguishing a real stone from a pseudocalculus is the presence of contrast outlining the inferior aspect of the filling defect of a true calculus. In this case, only the superior meniscus is present. It is important to be aware of this entity so that an interventional procedure is not performed needlessly.

CASE 7.16

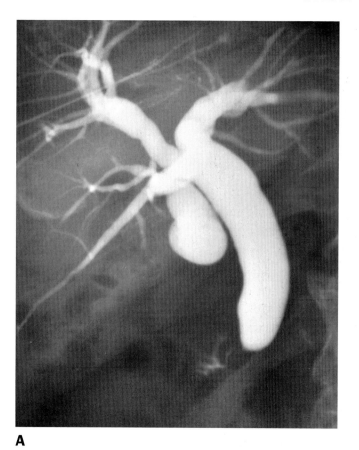

A

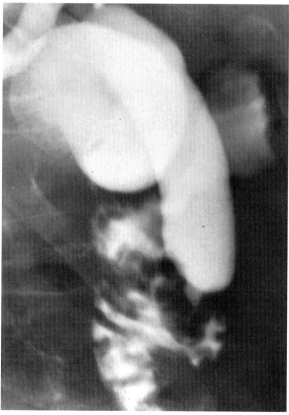

B

Findings
Transhepatic cholangiogram. **A** and **B.** There is moderate dilatation of the intrahepatic and extrahepatic bile ducts to the level of the papilla. There is a short segment of narrowing at the level of the papilla.

Differential Diagnosis
1. Spasm of the sphincter of Oddi
2. Papillary stenosis
3. Postcholecystectomy syndrome

Diagnosis
Papillary stenosis

Discussion
Papillary stenosis is an anatomical abnormality of the sphincter of Oddi with partial or complete narrowing of this segment of the duct. The finding is due to inflammation or fibrosis, usually caused by pancreatitis, choledocholithiasis, or surgical trauma. Papillary stenosis also is found in patients with acquired immunodeficiency syndrome-related cholangiopathy. Treatment usually is papillotomy performed at ERCP.

Spasm of the sphincter of Oddi (sphincter of Oddi dyskinesia) is a functional abnormality of the sphincter, which does not relax normally (case 7.15). The sphincter normally has alternating low and high muscular tone several times per minute. Patients with this disorder have increased baseline pressures of the sphincter or an increase in the amplitude and frequency of the phasic contractions. There is also a paradoxic increase in muscular tone to cholecystokinin. This diagnosis is usually made at manometry. Postcholecystectomy syndrome refers to spasm of the sphincter of Oddi in patients who have had a cholecystectomy and biliary-type pain.

CASE 7.17

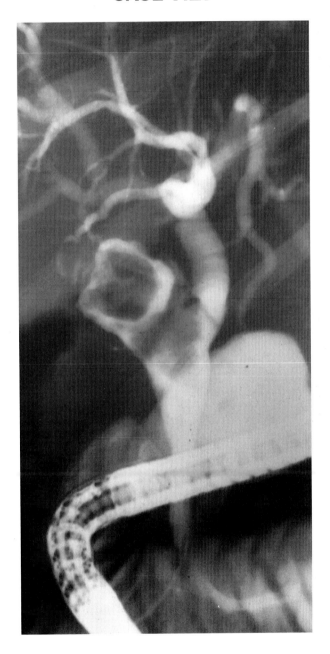

Findings

ERCP. There is a large filling defect within the cystic duct and secondary narrowing of the common hepatic duct.

Differential Diagnosis

Mirizzi syndrome

Diagnosis

Mirizzi syndrome

Discussion

Mirizzi syndrome is an inflammatory stricture of the common hepatic or common bile duct due to an impacted stone in the cystic duct or neck of the gallbladder. The biliary stricture can lead to stasis, obstruction, cholangitis, and jaundice. In chronic cases, secondary biliary cirrhosis can develop. ERCP is the best procedure for making this diagnosis, although findings at CT and sonography also can be diagnostic.

CASE 7.18

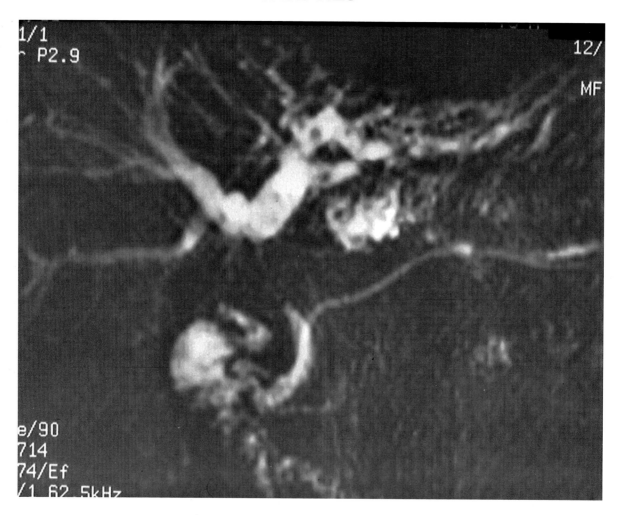

Findings

MRCP. The intrahepatic bile ducts are dilated and contain numerous small filling defects. The common hepatic duct is narrowed for a long segment, and the common bile duct and pancreatic duct are of normal caliber.

Differential Diagnosis

1. Extrinsic compression of the common hepatic duct by adenopathy
2. Mirizzi syndrome
3. Primary sclerosing cholangitis
4. Cholangiocarcinoma

Diagnosis

Extrinsic compression of the common hepatic duct by adenopathy (with intrahepatic bile duct stones)

Discussion

The differential possibilities for narrowing of the biliary system can be shortened by considering the location of the narrowing. Hilar lymphadenopathy is the commonest cause for narrowing of the common hepatic duct. Mirizzi syndrome should be considered if there are clinical symptoms of acute cholecystitis. Primary sclerosing cholangitis does not result in mass effect, but rather bile duct narrowing. Although cholangiocarcinoma can occur anywhere within the ducts, the confluence of the right and left ducts is a much more common location.

CASE 7.19

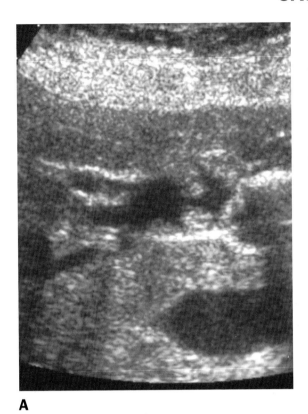

A

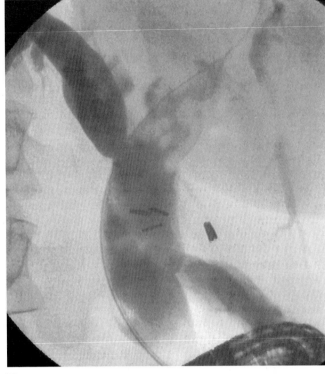

B

Findings

A. Sonogram. Several polypoid masses are present within the dilated extrahepatic duct.

B. ERCP. Multiple small polypoid filling defects are present in the extrahepatic and visualized intrahepatic bile ducts.

Differential Diagnosis

1. Intraductal mucous plugs
2. Intraductal calculi or sludge balls
3. Intraductal blood clots
4. Intraductal cholangiocarcinoma
5. Biliary papillomatosis

Diagnosis

Biliary papillomatosis

Discussion

Biliary papillomatosis is an extremely rare condition; fewer than 100 cases have been described in the English literature.

It is characterized by multiple and recurrent papillary adenomas in the biliary tract. The extrahepatic ducts and large intrahepatic ducts are most commonly involved. Patients usually present in their sixth or seventh decade with cholangitis or obstructive jaundice. Sonographic findings usually include multiple solid filling defects attached to the wall of a dilated extrahepatic duct. Differentiating biliary papillomatosis from other endoluminal masses (nonshadowing stones, sludge balls, mucous plugs, blood clots, or cholangiocarcinoma) is often extremely difficult. Final diagnosis still relies on histologic results.

Papillary adenomas can secrete mucin, and mucinous discharge from a dilated ampulla is a common finding at ERCP. Some of the elongated filling defects seen on ERCP likely are mucous plugs. Atypical and dysplastic changes often are present in biliary papillary adenomas, and transition to adenocarcinoma has been reported frequently. Because of this, surgical resection of the affected segment(s) or liver transplantation is the recommended therapy for this disease.

CASE 7.20

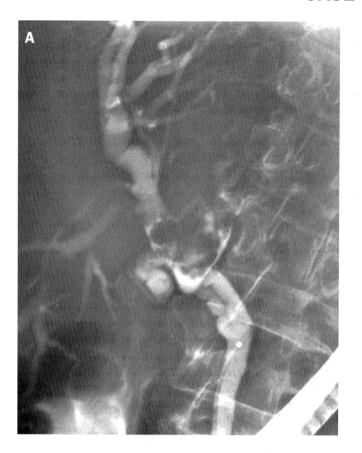

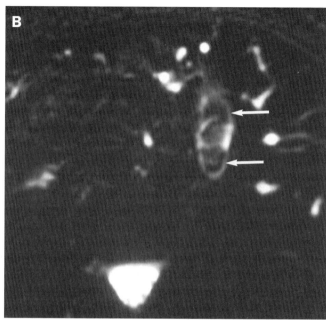

Findings

ERCP. **A.** There is a polypoid intraluminal filling defect within the common hepatic duct with extension into the left hepatic bile duct, which has an anomalous low insertion. The mass expands the duct. The left ductal system is poorly visualized.

B. Axial MRCP. The left hepatic bile duct is dilated and contains a polypoid filling defect (arrows). Multiple dilated proximal left intrahepatic bile ducts are visible.

Differential Diagnosis

1. Intraductal cholangiocarcinoma
2. Intraductal blood clot
3. Intraductal mucous plug
4. Intraductal calculi

Diagnosis

Intraductal cholangiocarcinoma

Discussion

Intraductal cholangiocarcinomas usually have a better prognosis than the scirrhous subtypes. These tumors arise within the bile ducts and grow as intraluminal masses. Many are well-differentiated adenocarcinomas and secrete mucin. In some cases, mucin obstructs the duct and obscures the primary tumor. Intraductal cholangiocarcinomas are analogous to intraductal papillary mucinous neoplasm of the pancreas. It is not always possible to differentiate blood clot and mucin from tumor—but either finding should raise suspicion of an underlying neoplasm. Calculi usually have rounded and multifaceted edges.

CASE 7.21

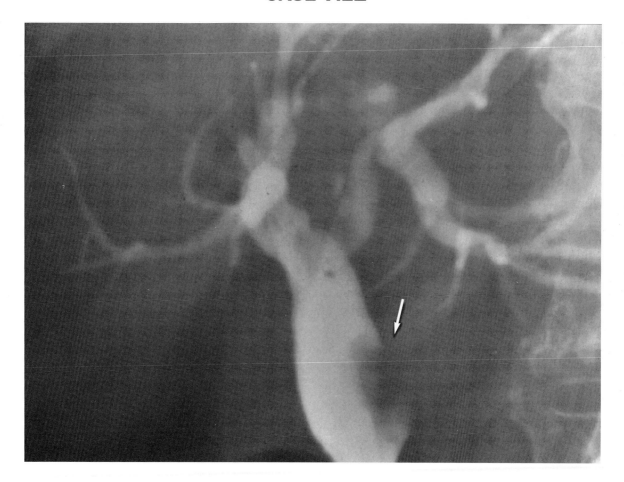

Findings

ERCP. There is a polypoid filling defect (arrow) in the extrahepatic bile duct. The common hepatic duct is moderately dilated.

Differential Diagnosis

1. Adenoma
2. Blood clot or mucous plug
3. Adherent debris or calculus
4. Cholangiocarcinoma

Diagnosis

Cholangiocarcinoma

Discussion

Cholangiocarcinoma arising in the common bile duct has the best prognosis. This filling defect is polypoid in appearance, whereas most cholangiocarcinomas are infiltrating. An adenoma could have a similar appearance. Stones usually are not adherent to the wall, and plugs of mucus are more elongated.

CASE 7.22

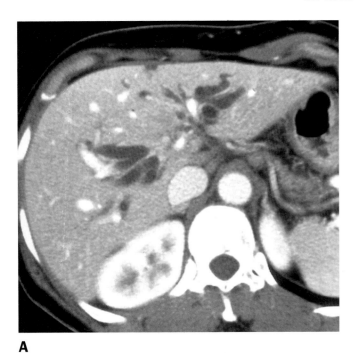

A

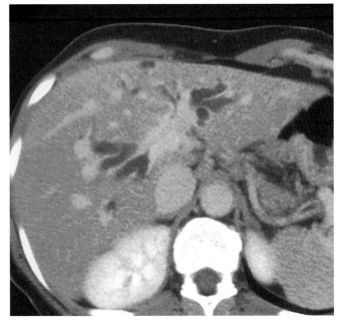

B

Findings

A. Contrast-enhanced CT. The bile ducts are dilated to the central portion of the liver without evidence of an obstructing mass.

B. Delayed enhanced CT. There is an enhancing mass at the level of the bifurcation of the left and right hepatic ducts with secondary obstruction of the bile ducts in both the right lobe and the left lobe of the liver.

Differential Diagnosis
1. Cholangiocarcinoma
2. Metastasis

Diagnosis
Cholangiocarcinoma (Klatskin type)

Discussion
Cholangiocarcinomas most commonly arise at the confluence of the right and left hepatic ducts. They are usually scirrhous carcinomas and often are referred to as Klatskin tumors. Most of the tumors are either hypoattenuating or isoattenuating compared with the liver during the arterial and portal venous phases of contrast enhancement. Scirrhous cholangiocarcinomas incite a desmoplastic reaction. The fibrotic nature of these tumors can be identified as the tumor enhances on delayed imaging (as in this case). The size of these lesions can vary from 2 to 10 cm in diameter. Although most are infiltrating along the course of the bile ducts, some present as more circumscribed polypoid masses. Tumors that are isoattenuating are the most difficult to identify. Their presence may be suspected by lobar atrophy of a hepatic segment, as a result of chronic biliary obstruction by the tumor. Metastasis to regional lymph nodes occurs in the portacaval and peripancreatic regions. Surgical resection in patients without metastases usually depends on the proximal extent of the tumor. Today, most surgeons do not consider an operation if the tumor extends proximal to the second-order biliary branches.

CASE 7.23

A

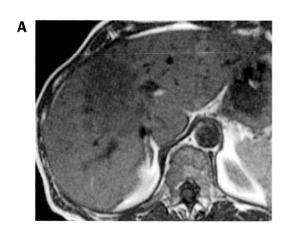

B

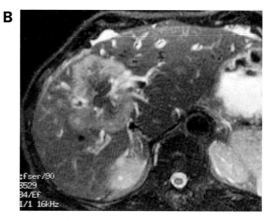

C

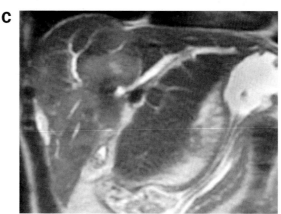

Findings

A. T1-weighted MRI. A large hypointense mass is located in the central portion of the liver.

B. T2-weighted MRI. The large mass is heterogeneous in signal intensity and causes obstruction of multiple intrahepatic bile ducts.

C. Coronal MRCP. The mass is slightly hyperintense compared with the liver. Multiple dilated bile ducts are obstructed by the mass.

Differential Diagnosis

1. Cholangiocarcinoma
2. Metastasis
3. Hepatocellular carcinoma

Diagnosis

Cholangiocarcinoma (Klatskin type)

Discussion

This is an example of the expansile form of cholangiocarcinoma occurring at the confluence of the right and left hepatic bile ducts. This large Klatskin tumor is well demarcated on the T2-weighted MRI examination. The excellent contrast resolution available at MRI makes identification of cholangiocarcinoma superior to either CT or sonography. MRCP is a helpful technique to display the biliary anatomy in a familiar coronal plane. T1-weighted images are particularly helpful to assess for extrahepatic metastases and adenopathy.

CASE 7.24

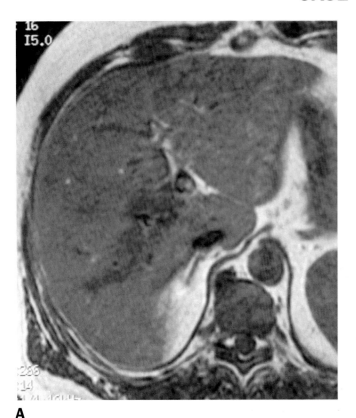

A

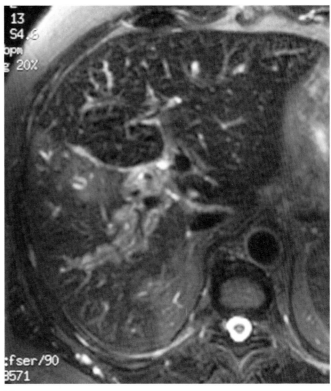

B

Findings

A. T1-weighted MRI. There is a linear region of abnormally low signal intensity in the region of the right posterior portal vein.

B. T2-weighted MRI. A linear region of nodular thickening of high signal intensity extends within the distribution of the right posterior portal triad.

Differential Diagnosis
1. Sclerosing cholangitis
2. Infiltrative cholangiocarcinoma
3. Ascending cholangitis

Diagnosis
Infiltrative cholangiocarcinoma

Discussion

Infiltrative cholangiocarcinoma can be very difficult to detect, and assessment of its full extent also can be difficult. MRI is the best imaging examination to visualize this tumor. Bile duct thickening can be found in patients with sclerosing cholangitis, but it is usually only a few millimeters in thickness. Marked bile duct thickening (as in this case) is nearly always associated with tumor from infiltrating cholangiocarcinoma. This tumor is seen to encase the portal vein and hepatic artery centrally, a feature that renders it unresectable.

CASE 7.25

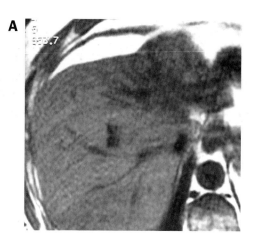

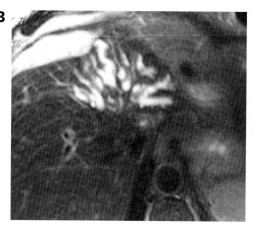

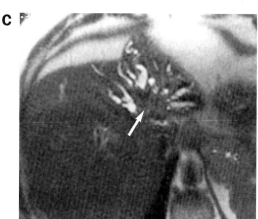

Findings

A. T1-weighted MRI. The left lobe of the liver is atrophic, and the signal intensity of this lobe is heterogeneous.

B. T2-weighted MRI. Multiple dilated bile ducts are seen within an atrophic left lobe. They converge to a central point.

C. T2-weighted MRI (different level than in **B**). The dilated left lobar ducts converge to a central mass of low signal intensity (arrow).

Differential Diagnosis

Cholangiocarcinoma

Diagnosis

Cholangiocarcinoma with lobar atrophy

Discussion

This case illustrates the typical findings of lobar atrophy in a patient with a slow-growing cholangiocarcinoma obstructing a lobar branch bile duct. The tumor is difficult to see because it is isointense or hypointense compared with the liver. The lesion can be at an advanced stage because its detection is often delayed without clinical symptoms. Surgical resection might be possible if the tumor does not involve the main portal vein and proper hepatic artery.

CASE 7.26

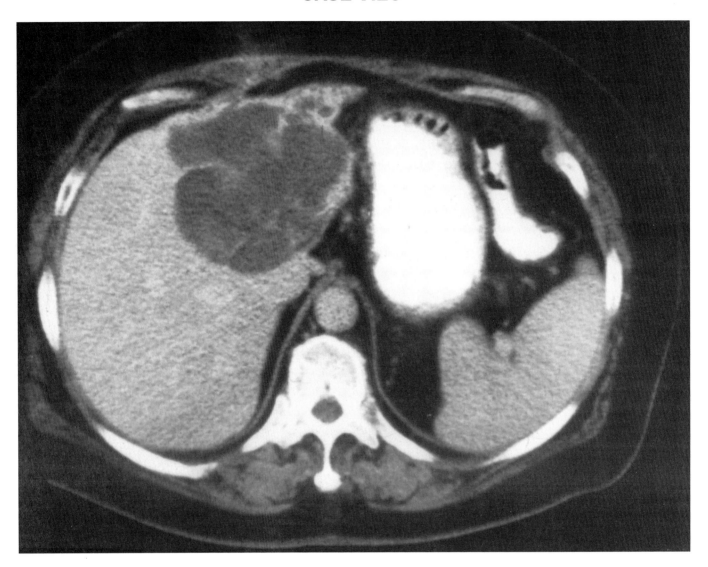

Findings
Contrast-enhanced CT. A large hypoattenuating mass is present in the left lobe of the liver. Two dilated bile ducts are present in the left hepatic lobe.

Differential Diagnosis
1. Metastases
2. Hepatocellular carcinoma
3. Cholangiocarcinoma
4. Biliary cystadenoma

Diagnosis
Intrahepatic cholangiocarcinoma

Discussion
Although cholangiocarcinomas are most commonly found at the confluence of the right and left biliary ducts, some arise in the peripheral ductal system. These tumors can become large because they do not always cause symptoms at an early stage. Upstream ductal dilatation usually is present, and, depending on the location of the tumor, there may be lobar atrophy from chronic biliary obstruction.

Hepatocellular carcinomas (cases 6.49 through 6.65) usually are hypervascular tumors, and biliary cystadenomas (case 6.47) predominantly are cystic and septated (although enhancing nodules can be seen with cystadenocarcinomas). A metastasis could be indistinguishable from this lesion.

Masses and Filling Defects of the Bile Ducts

		Case
Benign*		
Choledocholithiasis	Posterior shadowing echogenic foci in a dilated duct on sonography. Target or meniscus sign on CT. MRCP and ERCP are more sensitive	7.12–7.14
Pseudocalculus	Apparent filling defect due to spasm of sphincter of Oddi. Transient. Absent inferior meniscus	7.15
Papillary stenosis	Distal common bile duct stricture	7.16
Mirizzi syndrome	Inflammatory stricture of common duct caused by stone impacted in cystic duct	7.17
Extrinsic compression of common duct by adenopathy	Smooth narrowing of common hepatic duct	7.18
Biliary papillomatosis	Multiple solid filling defects attached to the wall of a dilated duct. High incidence of malignant transformation. Mucous filling defects often associated	7.19
Malignant		
Cholangiocarcinoma	Intraductal polypoid tumors have the best prognosis. Scirrhous or infiltrating tumors are the most common type. Confluence of right and left biliary ducts most common site (Klatskin tumor). Lobar atrophy. Large peripheral hypovascular mass	7.20–7.26

*Other benign biliary filling defects include sludge balls, mucous plugs, and blood clots.

CASE 7.27

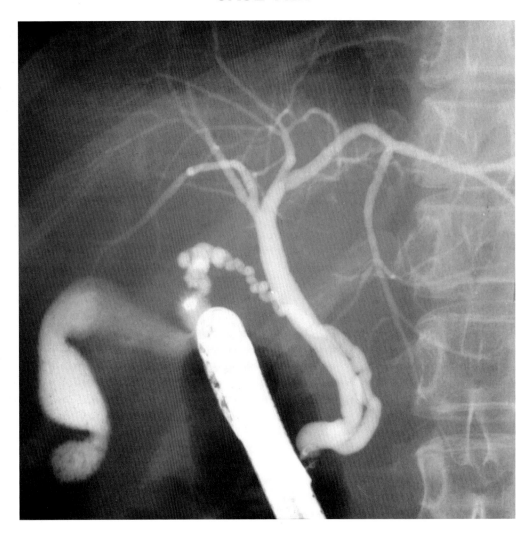

Findings
ERCP. There is a low insertion of the cystic duct to the common bile duct. The cholangiogram is otherwise unremarkable.

Differential Diagnosis
Low insertion of the cystic duct

Diagnosis
Low insertion of the cystic duct

Discussion
Anomalies of the biliary tract are relatively common. The commonest anomaly is an aberrant intrahepatic duct draining into a contralateral main or common hepatic duct.

For example, the bile duct draining the right anterior hepatic lobe can anomalously drain into the left main bile duct or common hepatic duct. Anomalies of the cystic duct also are relatively common (as in this case). Major cystic duct anomalies include the following:
1. Absence of the cystic duct with direct drainage of the gallbladder into the common hepatic duct
2. Low insertion (as in this case)
3. Long conjoined segment of the cystic duct with the common duct
4. Insertion into the right hepatic duct
5. Insertion at the level of bifurcation

These major cystic duct anomalies are illustrated on page 548, and common intrahepatic duct variations are illustrated on page 549.

CASE 7.28

A

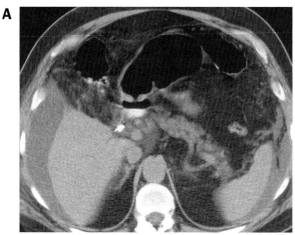

B

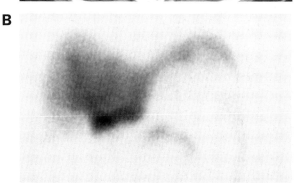

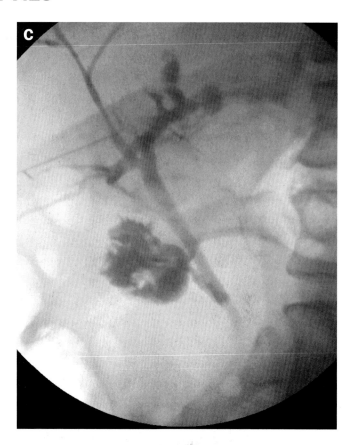

Findings

A. Unenhanced CT. Postoperative changes of cholecystectomy are present. There is a moderate amount of ascites in the visualized abdomen.

B. Hepatobiliary scintigram. One-hour hepatoiminodiacetic acid scan shows an abnormal collection of tracer in the post-cholecystectomy bed and additional tracer uptake outlining the peritoneal cavity. No definite tracer is seen to pass into the bowel.

C. Percutaneous transhepatic cholangiogram. There is leakage of contrast from the cystic duct stump. The common duct remains intact.

Differential Diagnosis
Biliary leak

Diagnosis
Biliary leak

Discussion
Ninety-five percent of biliary leaks are iatrogenic, and most arise as a result of complications of surgery to the biliary tree. Iatrogenic biliary injuries are more common with laparoscopic cholecystectomy than with open cholecystectomy. Extravasation of small quantities of bile is fairly common after cholecystectomy and usually is of little clinical significance. The most worrisome leaks are those in which bile ascites is present and no bile is seen to enter the small bowel on hepatoiminodiacetic acid scan. In these cases, prompt drainage is required to decrease morbidity. Percutaneous transhepatic cholangiography usually is required to determine the level of the ductal injury and to exclude ligation, laceration, or transection of the bile ducts. These major duct injuries ultimately require choledochojejunostomy or hepaticojejunostomy if clinically feasible.

CASE 7.29

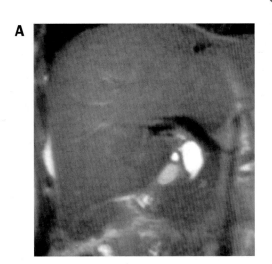

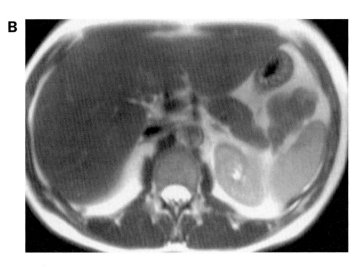

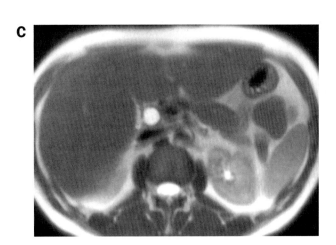

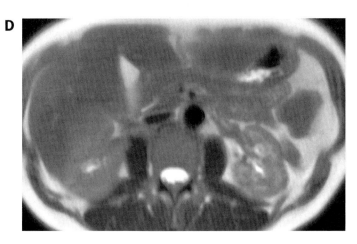

Findings
MRCP. **A.** Coronal image. **B** through **D.** Axial images. Fusiform focal dilatation of the common bile duct. The duct above and below this region (**B** and **D**) appears normal.

Differential Diagnosis
1. Choledochal cyst, type I
2. Biliary obstruction, cause undetermined

Diagnosis
Choledochal cyst, type I

Discussion
Choledochal cysts are congenital cystic dilatations of the bile ducts. The cause of choledochal cysts is not known, but it has been hypothesized that an anomalous connection between the pancreatic duct and the biliary system allows pancreatic secretions to weaken the wall of the duct with subsequent dilatation. The majority of cases are diagnosed in girls before the age of 10 years. There is an association between choledochal cysts and other biliary tract anomalies (especially biliary tract stenosis and atresia), congenital hepatic fibrosis, and medullary sponge kidney. Complications include rupture, stasis with cholangitis, stone formation, liver abscess, cirrhosis, and cholangiocarcinoma. The classification of choledochal cysts is based on the location of the cyst(s) within the biliary system, as shown in the figure on page 547.

CASE 7.30

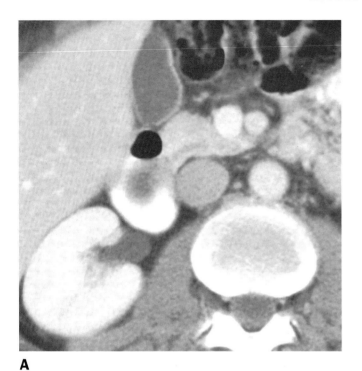

A

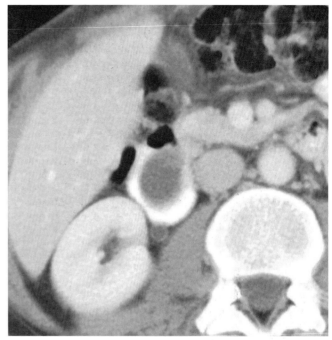

B

Findings

Contrast-enhanced CT. **A** and **B.** A water-attenuation mass arises from the region of the ampulla and fills most of the duodenal lumen.

Differential Diagnosis

Choledochocele

Diagnosis

Choledochocele (type III choledochal cyst)

Discussion

A choledochocele is a protrusion of a dilated intramural segment of the common bile duct into the duodenum. It is considered a type of choledochal cyst (type III). It has been referred to by several terms, including duodenal duplication cyst, diverticulum of the common bile duct, and enterogenous cyst of the duodenum. It is analogous to a ureterocele. Patients with a choledochocele usually complain of nausea, vomiting, and biliary colic. At cholangiography, a saclike dilatation of the common bile duct is seen. Because the dilated ductal segment is filled with bile (it also can contain sludge and stones), it will be water attenuation at CT.

CASE 7.31

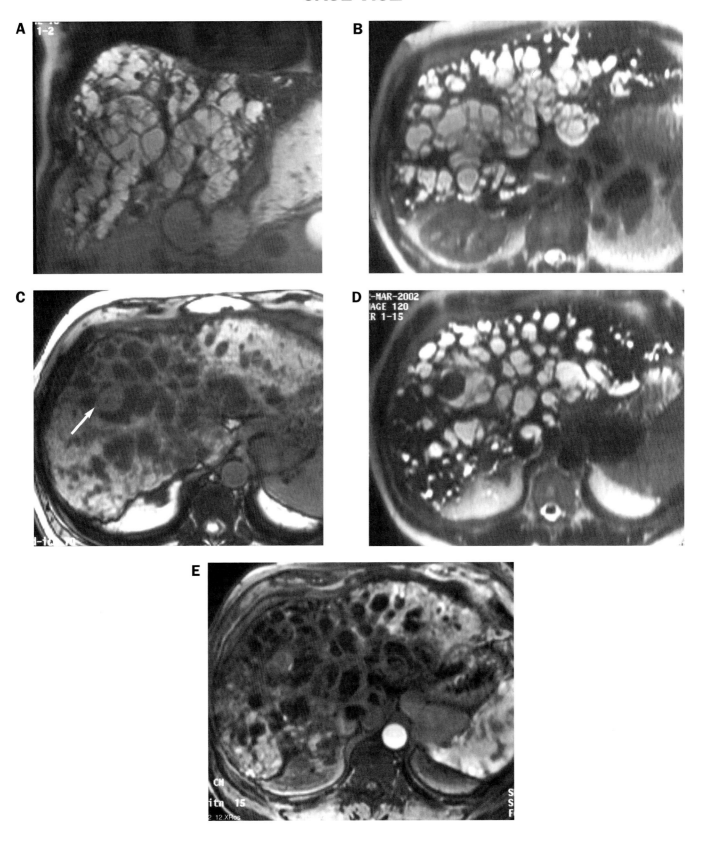

A

B

C

D

E

Findings

MRCP. **A** and **B.** Marked dilatation of a majority of the intrahepatic biliary system. Some normal-caliber ducts are visible.

C. T1-weighted MRI. Multiple dilated intrahepatic ducts. There is a focal mass within the right lobe of the liver (arrow).

D. T2-weighted MRI. The focal mass is of low signal intensity. The dilated ducts are of high signal intensity.

E. Dynamic contrast-enhanced MRI. The mass within the right lobe of the liver enhances heterogeneously during the early phases of contrast enhancement.

Differential Diagnosis

Caroli disease with complicating hepatocellular carcinoma

Diagnosis

Caroli disease with complicating hepatocellular carcinoma

Discussion

Complications of Caroli disease include stone formation, recurrent cholangitis, liver abscess, and hepatocellular carcinoma (as in this case). There is a 100-fold increase in the risk for development of hepatocellular carcinoma compared with the risk in the normal population.

CASE 7.32

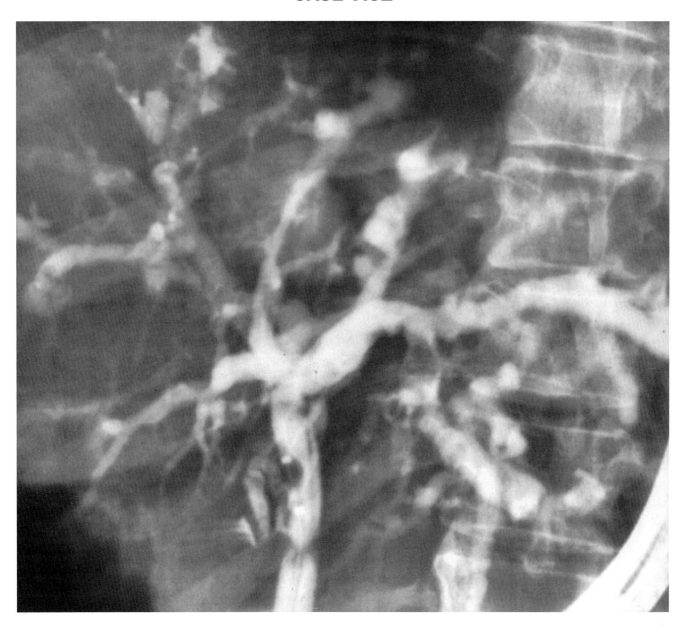

Findings
ERCP. Multiple cystic dilatations of the intrahepatic bile ducts are seen throughout the liver.

Differential Diagnosis
1. Caroli disease
2. Multiple biliary abscesses

Diagnosis
Caroli disease

Discussion
Caroli disease is a form of choledochal cystic disease with segmental saccular dilatation of the intrahepatic ducts and a normal-caliber extrahepatic duct (type V). Patients with Caroli disease usually present during adulthood with symptoms of cholangitis. There is an association between Caroli disease and renal tubular ectasia.

Miscellaneous Bile Duct Conditions

		Case
Cystic duct	Anomalies	7.27
	Many congenital variants	(see page 548)
Bile leak	Loculated or free fluid	7.28
	Usually requires cholangiography to define site of leak	
Choledochal cysts		
Type I	Fusiform	7.29
Type II	Diverticulum	
Type III	Choledochocele	7.30
Type IV	Intrahepatic and extrahepatic	
Type V	Caroli (intrahepatic)	7.31 and 7.32
		(see page 547)

CASE 7.33

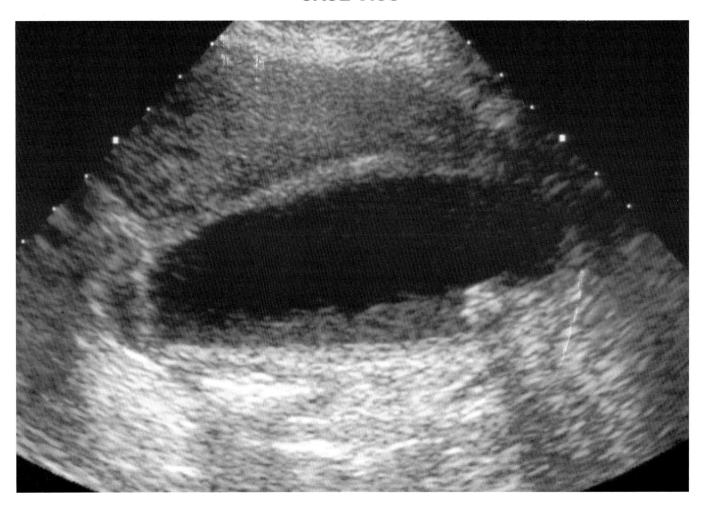

Findings
Sonogram. The gallbladder wall is thickened, and sludge and a stone within its lumen cast an acoustic shadow. There is a thin hypoechoic zone about the gallbladder.

Differential Diagnosis
Acute cholecystitis and cholelithiasis

Diagnosis
Acute cholecystitis and cholelithiasis

Discussion
There are many sonographic signs of acute cholecystitis, including cholelithiasis or sludge, intramural thickening with zones of lucency, distention of the gallbladder, sonographic Murphy sign, perihepatitis, and pericholecystic fluid. The most accurate sign is the combination of cholelithiasis, intramural edema, and maximal pain over the gallbladder (sonographic Murphy sign). Perihepatitis manifests as a zone of decreased hepatic echogenicity about the gallbladder (as in this case).

CASE 7.34

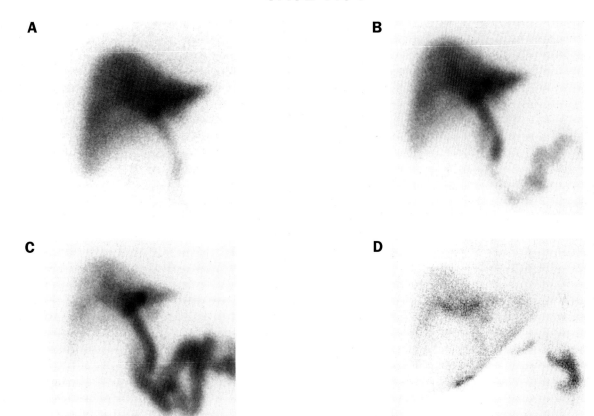

A **B**

C **D**

Findings
Cholescintigram. **A.** 10 minutes after injection.
Nonvisualization of the gallbladder. **B.** 20 minutes after
injection. Nonvisualization of the gallbladder. **C.** 60
minutes after injection. Nonvisualization of the gallbladder.
D. 4 hours after injection. Nonvisualization of the
gallbladder with increased uptake within the liver about
the gallbladder.

Differential Diagnosis
1. Acute cholecystitis
2. Chronic cholecystitis
3. Pancreatitis
4. Hyperalimentation

Diagnosis
Acute cholecystitis

Discussion
Cholescintigraphy usually is performed with technetium
99m-labeled iminodiacetic acid analogues. Today, diisopropyl-
iminodiacetic acid (DISIDA) and mebrofenin are the most
popular agents because they can be used in patients with
hyperbilirubinemia (up to a bilirubin value of 20 mg/dL).
The agent is taken up by the liver and excreted without
conjugation. Normally, the gallbladder contains tracer
uptake within 30 minutes after administration.
Nonvisualization of the gallbladder is suspicious for cystic
duct obstruction; however, some gallbladders are slow to
fill (distended gallbladders and those with bile stasis), and
delayed imaging is needed. False-positive studies are rare,
usually due to intermittent obstruction of the cystic duct
by a moving stone. False-negative results can be caused by
any of the conditions in the differential list above.

In the case shown here, despite delayed imaging, the
gallbladder never fills. The 4-hour image shows increased
uptake about the gallbladder due to the adjacent
inflammation (perihepatitis).

CASE 7.35

CASE 7.36

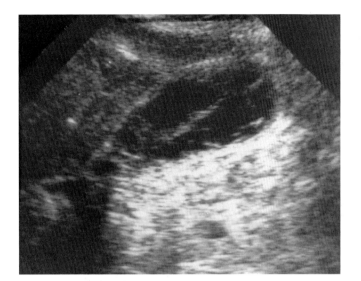

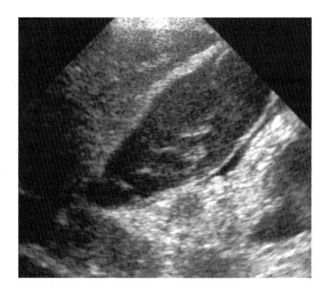

Findings

Case 7.35. Sonogram. The gallbladder wall is irregularly thickened, and there are several linear filling defects in the gallbladder lumen.

Case 7.36. Sonogram. The wall of the gallbladder is thickened, and there is a small amount of pericholecystic fluid. Echogenic debris fills the gallbladder lumen. Echogenic linear filling defects also are seen within the lumen.

Differential Diagnosis

Gangrenous cholecystitis

Diagnosis

Gangrenous cholecystitis

Discussion

Acute cholecystitis is caused by obstruction of the cystic duct by a calculus with secondary gallbladder distention, ischemia, wall edema, and transmural necrosis. Gangrenous cholecystitis is a designation used for severe gallbladder inflammation. At sonography, there is usually pronounced intramural edema or sloughing of the mucosa into the gallbladder lumen (as in these cases).

Gangrenous cholecystitis should be treated urgently to prevent gallbladder perforation and abscess from developing.

CASE 7.37

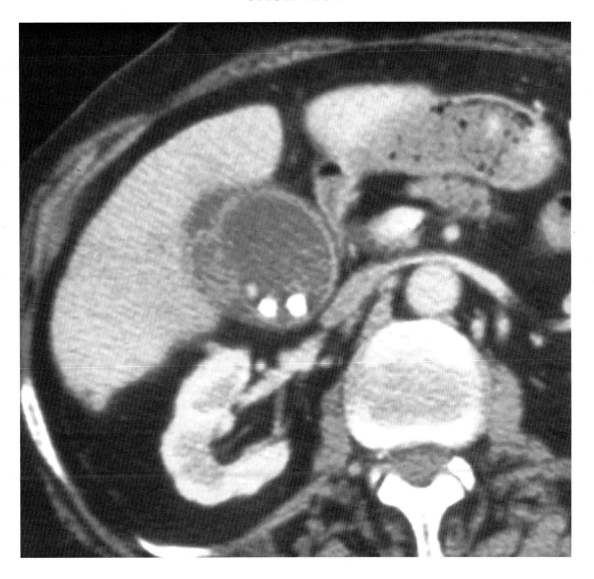

Findings
Contrast-enhanced CT. Cholelithiasis. The gallbladder wall is thickened, and there is a small pericholecystic fluid collection.

Differential Diagnosis
1. Gangrenous cholecystitis
2. Gallbladder carcinoma

Diagnosis
Gangrenous cholecystitis with pericholecystic fluid collection

Discussion
CT is usually not the primary imaging tool for the diagnosis of acute cholecystitis. It is optimally used when there are confusing findings either clinically or with sonography or cholescintigraphy or when complications of cholecystitis are suspected. The most common complication of cholecystitis is a pericholecystic fluid collection from perforation due to gangrenous cholecystitis. These fluid collections often are infected. Usually the wall of the gallbladder is of water attenuation (due to edema), and it may have a striated appearance. Attenuation changes can occur within the surrounding liver, and fluid may be identified in the posterior subhepatic space (Morrison pouch).

CASE 7.38   **CASE 7.39**

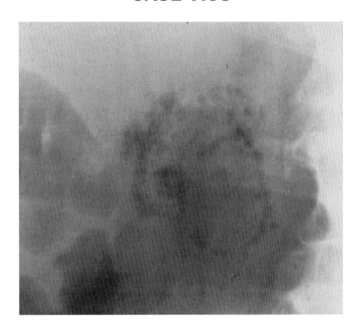   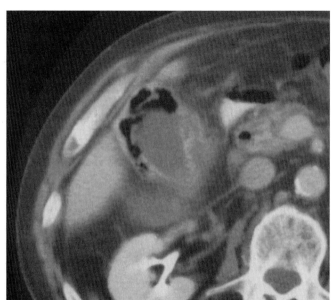

Findings

Case 7.38. Abdominal plain radiograph. There is a collection of extraluminal gas within the right upper quadrant. Gas is seen within the wall of the gallbladder and surrounding the gallbladder.

Case 7.39. Contrast-enhanced CT. The gallbladder wall is thickened, and gas can be seen within its wall. Prominent inflammatory changes and fluid are present in the pericholecystic region.

Differential Diagnosis

Emphysematous cholecystitis

Diagnosis

Emphysematous cholecystitis

Discussion

Emphysematous cholecystitis is a severe form of cholecystitis caused by a gas-forming organism. Up to 30% of patients have diabetes, and a large number are elderly. Ischemia of the gallbladder may be an underlying cause or contribute to the condition in a large percentage of cases. Infection with *Clostridium perfringens* often is present, producing the gas that is pathognomonic of this disease. The gas can reside within the wall or the lumen of the gallbladder or both. If gas is seen outside the lumen, it often indicates gallbladder perforation and a pericholecystic abscess. Cholelithiasis may or may not be present. The cystic duct is patent.

CASE 7.40

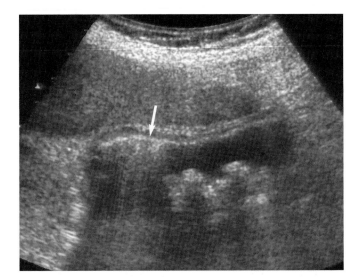

CASE 7.41

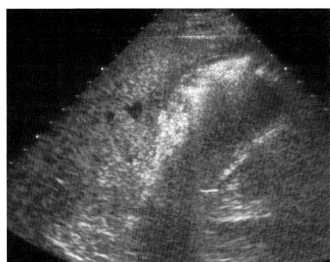

Findings

Case 7.40. Sonogram. The gallbladder wall is thickened. Dependently layering gallstones are present. A bright echogenic rim is seen along the nondependent wall of the gallbladder (arrow) with "dirty" posterior shadowing.

Case 7.41. Sonogram. Abnormal echogenicity is present along the anterior wall of the gallbladder with "dirty" posterior acoustic shadowing, making visualization of the gallbladder difficult. Hypoechogenicity is seen within the liver parenchyma adjacent to the abnormal gallbladder.

Differential Diagnosis

1. Emphysematous cholecystitis
2. Porcelain gallbladder

Diagnosis

Emphysematous cholecystitis

Discussion

Air within the wall of the gallbladder at sonography appears as echogenic foci that cause a "dirty" shadow. A porcelain gallbladder (case 7.46) with wall calcification should cast a "clean" shadow, or the gallbladder may be difficult to identify. If emphysematous cholecystitis is suspected, it is often helpful to confirm the finding with abdominal plain radiography or CT. The gas can extend from the wall into the gallbladder lumen and pericholecystic tissues.

CASE 7.42

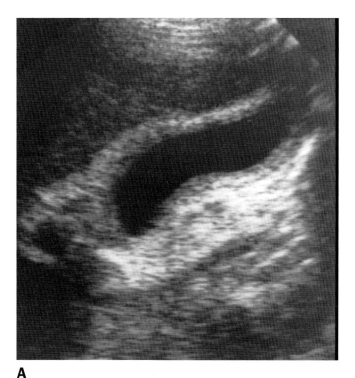

A

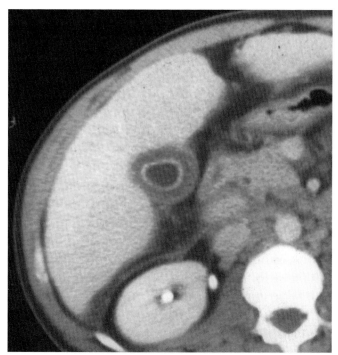

B

Findings
A. Sonogram. The wall of the gallbladder is thickened. No calculi are present.

B. Contrast-enhanced CT. The gallbladder wall is thickened, and the mucosa is hyperenhancing. No calculi are present.

Differential Diagnosis
1. Chronic cholecystitis
2. Acalculous cholecystitis
3. Various metabolic disturbances

Diagnosis
Acalculous cholecystitis

Discussion
Acalculous cholecystitis refers to acute inflammatory changes of the gallbladder without stones. The actual cause of the disease is unclear; however, vascular insufficiency of the gallbladder is a likely cause. Clinical settings associated with acalculous cholecystitis include hyperalimentation, trauma, prolonged care in an intensive care unit, infectious colitis, vascular disease of any cause, and an immunocompromised host. Sonography, CT, or cholescintigraphy can suggest the diagnosis by confirming either inflammatory changes in the wall of the gallbladder or occlusion of the cystic duct. At sonography, the gallbladder is thickened and has focal or striated sonolucency. Intramural wall edema and perihepatitis can be seen at CT. Nonfilling of the gallbladder is found at cholescintigraphy.

CASE 7.43

A
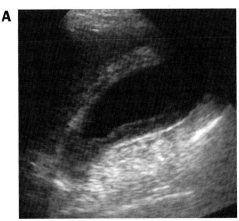

B
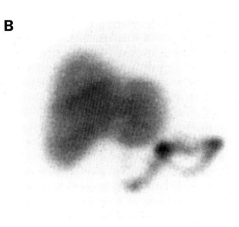

C
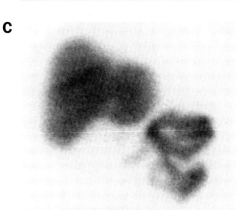

D
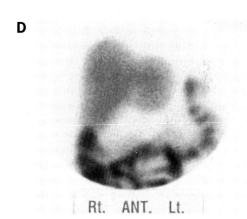

Rt. ANT. Lt.

Findings

A. Gallbladder sonogram. The gallbladder contains dependently layering echogenic debris (sludge), and the wall of the gallbladder is thickened. No stones are visible.

B through **D.** Cholescintigram. Nonfilling of the gallbladder on the 30-minute (**B**), 60-minute (**C**), and 4-hour (**D**) delayed images.

Differential Diagnosis
1. Acalculous cholecystitis
2. Chronic cholecystitis

Diagnosis
Acalculous cholecystitis

Discussion

The diagnosis of acalculous cholecystitis can be difficult. Patients at greatest risk include patients in the intensive care unit requiring narcotics, those receiving hyperalimentation, and those in whom the blood supply to the gallbladder could be jeopardized (hypotension, vasculitis, severe atherosclerosis). Many of these patients have been fasting, and a distended gallbladder containing sludge will be present. It is unclear which imaging method is best for diagnosing this disorder. At sonography, findings of an inflamed gallbladder (thickened wall with striations, pericholecystic fluid, and a positive sonographic Murphy sign) without calculi are most helpful. Nonfilling of the gallbladder at cholescintigraphy is the primary finding. If the gallbladder has not filled at 60 minutes, morphine often is given to constrict the sphincter of Oddi and direct bile flow into the cystic duct. Alternatively, delayed imaging can be extended to 4 hours, as in this case. Nonfilling of the gallbladder at this point is consistent with cholecystitis.

CASE 7.44

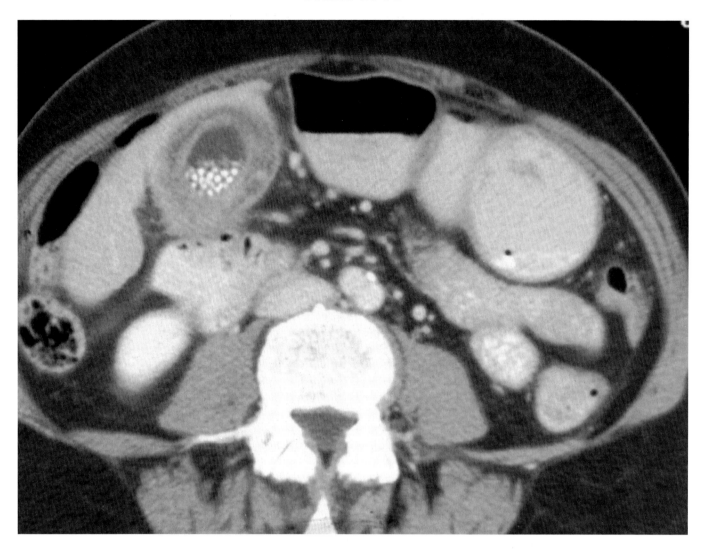

Findings

Contrast-enhanced CT. The wall of the gallbladder is markedly thickened and heterogeneous in attenuation. Multiple gallstones are present.

Differential Diagnosis
1. Acute cholecystitis
2. Chronic cholecystitis
3. Adenomyomatosis

Diagnosis
Chronic cholecystitis

Discussion

It may be difficult to differentiate acute from chronic cholecystitis radiographically. In both cases the wall of the gallbladder is thickened and cholelithiasis usually is visible. Symptomatic evaluation usually differentiates acute disease from chronic disease. Chronic disease is associated with a history of multiple episodes of abdominal pain without the presence of acute symptoms and signs that include fever and leukocytosis.

CASE 7.45

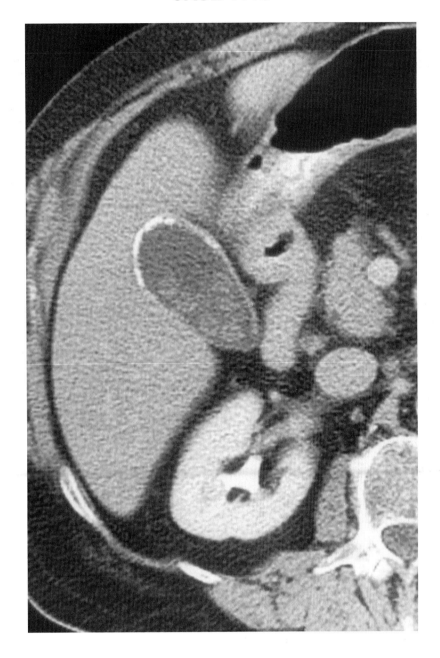

Findings
Contrast-enhanced CT. The wall of the gallbladder is calcified and contains calculi.

Differential Diagnosis
Porcelain gallbladder with cholelithiasis

Diagnosis
Porcelain gallbladder with cholelithiasis

Discussion
Porcelain gallbladder refers to calcification of the wall of the gallbladder. The calcification can be either linear or punctate. This gallbladder wall calcification develops as a result of a chronically obstructed cystic duct and changes of chronic cholecystitis. The importance of this condition is an increased risk of gallbladder carcinoma (case 7.58). In fact, in 25% of patients with porcelain gallbladder, gallbladder carcinoma develops without cholecystectomy.

CASE 7.46

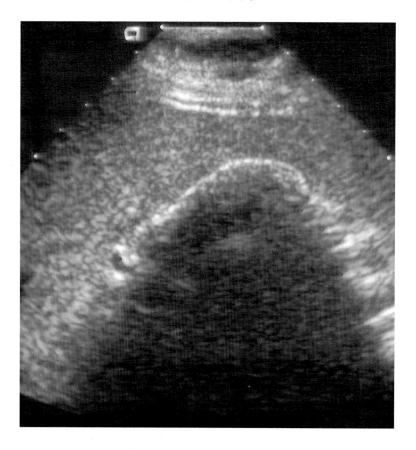

Findings

Sonogram. A thin echogenic arc (representing the anterior wall of the gallbladder) is present with complete "clean" shadowing of the remainder of the gallbladder lumen and back wall.

Differential Diagnosis

1. Porcelain gallbladder
2. Gallstones (wall-echo-shadow complex)
3. Emphysematous cholecystitis

Diagnosis

Porcelain gallbladder

Discussion

Dystrophic calcification within the wall of an obstructed and chronically inflamed gallbladder produces a brittle wall and has led to the term *porcelain gallbladder*. The condition is associated with gallstones in more than 90% of cases. Stone disease often can be difficult to identify sonographically (as in this case) because of acoustic shadowing from the calcified gallbladder wall.

Porcelain gallbladder should be able to be differentiated clinically and sonographically from emphysematous cholecystitis (cases 7.40 and 7.41). The air within the gallbladder wall or lumen produces a "dirty" posterior shadow. The wall-echo-shadow triad of a gallbladder filled with stones (case 7.49) should give two echogenic lines separated by a thin line of sonolucency. "Clean" posterior shadowing should be seen posterior to the deep echogenic arc (gallstones). Unless there are medical contraindications, prophylactic cholecystectomy is recommended in patients with a porcelain gallbladder because of an increased risk of gallbladder carcinoma.

CASE 7.47

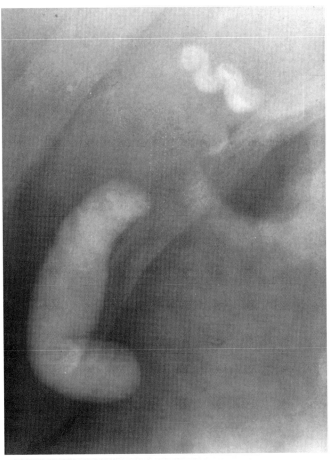

A

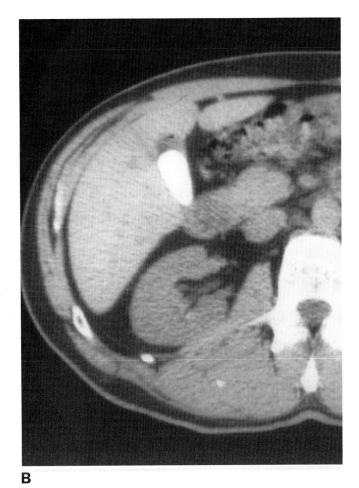

B

Findings
A. Abdominal plain radiograph. The gallbladder and cystic duct are opaque and contain multiple stones.

B. Unenhanced CT. High-attenuation material fills the gallbladder.

Differential Diagnosis
1. Milk of calcium bile
2. Vicarious excretion of contrast material
3. Prior ERCP with cholelithiasis

Diagnosis
Milk of calcium bile

Discussion
Milk of calcium bile is calcium carbonate, calcium phosphate, or calcium bilirubinate that is highly concentrated within the gallbladder because of cystic duct obstruction and chronic gallbladder inflammation. Because it is dense enough to detect on plain radiography, it is referred to as milk of calcium bile or the limy bile syndrome.

Inflammatory Diseases of the Gallbladder

		Case
Acute cholecystitis	Due to cystic duct obstruction. Thickened gallbladder wall, cholelithiasis, and positive sonographic Murphy sign. Nonfilling at cholescintigraphy	7.33 and 7.34
Gangrenous cholecystitis	Severe inflammation of the gallbladder with sloughing of mucosa into the lumen. High risk of perforation or pericholecystic abscess	7.35–7.37
Emphysematous cholecystitis	Acute cholecystitis with gas in wall of gallbladder or lumen or both. Gas produced by *Clostridium perfringens*. More common in diabetics. High risk of perforation. Patent cystic duct	7.38–7.41
Acalculous cholecystitis	Same findings as acute cholecystitis without cholelithiasis. Patent cystic duct	7.42 and 7.43
Chronic cholecystitis	Similar to acute cholecystitis. No fevers or leukocytosis. Porcelain gallbladder. Milk of calcium bile. Chronic cystic duct obstruction	7.44–7.47

CASE 7.48

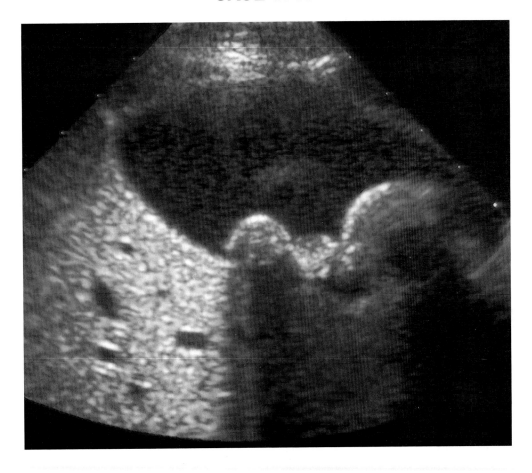

Findings

Sonogram. Rounded echogenic filling defects are present dependently within the gallbladder with associated posterior acoustic shadowing. The gallbladder appears otherwise normal.

Differential Diagnosis

Gallstones

Diagnosis

Gallstones

Discussion

Gallstones are common and found in approximately 8% of the general population. They are 4 times more common in women. The vast majority of patients with gallstones are asymptomatic. The most common symptom is biliary colic. The pain usually ends when a stone dislodges from the gallbladder neck or passes through the cystic duct. Impacted stones in the cystic duct can lead to acute cholecystitis. Ultrasonography is extremely useful for the detection of gallstones; reported sensitivity is 95% and specificity approaches 100%.

Gallstones can be differentiated from sludge balls (case 7.51) because gallstones should exhibit posterior acoustic shadowing. Detection of gallstones sometimes is challenging in a collapsed gallbladder, and right upper quadrant ultrasonography should be performed with the patient in a fasting state. Because the majority of patients with gallstones remain asymptomatic, only symptomatic patients require surgical intervention.

CASE 7.49

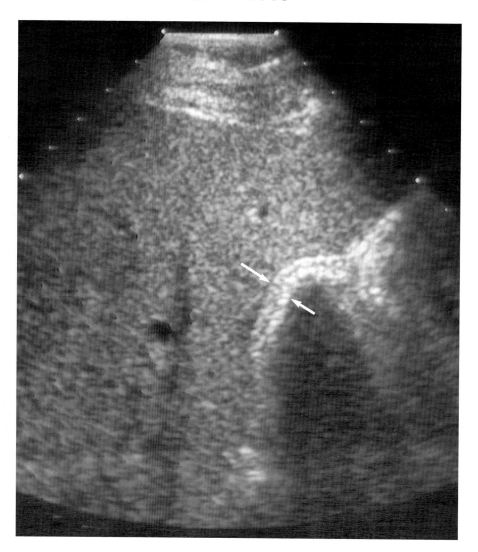

Findings

Sonogram. Two curved echogenic lines (arrows) are separated by a thin hypoechoic space. Acoustic shadowing is seen behind the deeper echogenic line.

Differential Diagnosis

1. Gallstones (wall-echo-shadow triad)
2. Porcelain gallbladder
3. Emphysematous cholecystitis

Diagnosis

Gallstones (wall-echo-shadow triad)

Discussion

A gallbladder filled with stones often results in the sonographic appearance referred to as the wall-echo-shadow triad. The superficial echogenic arc represents the gallbladder wall, and the deeper echogenic arc with "clean" posterior acoustic shadowing represents the gallstones. The thin hypoechoic line between the two echogenic arcs represents fluid within the gallbladder lumen.

The wall-echo-shadow triad caused by gallstones usually can be differentiated from the single thin echogenic line with "clean" posterior acoustic shadowing seen with a porcelain gallbladder (case 7.46) or the "dirty" posterior acoustic shadowing seen in emphysematous cholecystitis (cases 7.40 and 7.41).

CASE 7.50

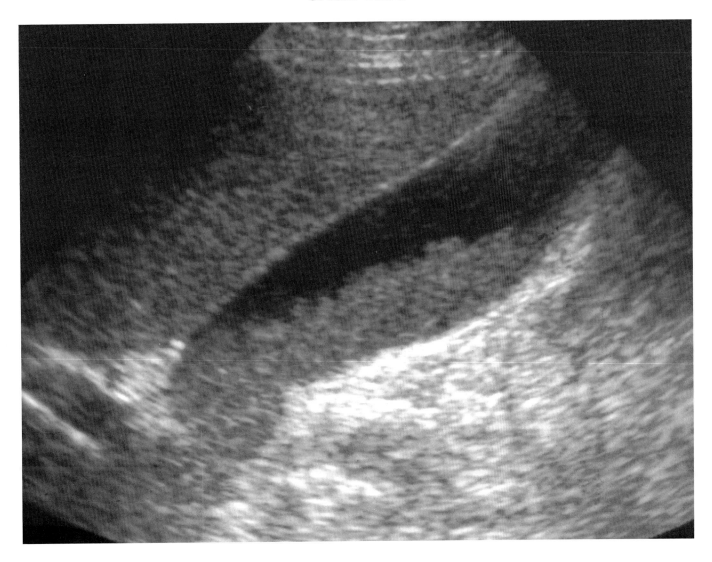

Findings
Sonogram. Longitudinal view of the gallbladder shows dependent layering low-level echogenic material within the gallbladder with no posterior acoustic shadowing.

Differential Diagnosis
Gallbladder sludge

Diagnosis
Gallbladder sludge

Discussion
Gallbladder sludge is concentrated, echogenic bile containing particulate material composed of cholesterol crystals and calcium bilirubinate granules. Sludge usually layers dependently within the gallbladder. It should not result in posterior acoustic shadowing unless stones also are present. Sludge most commonly results from bile stasis and is frequent in patients who undergo prolonged fasting or hyperalimentation. It also occurs in patients with biliary obstruction. Gallbladder sludge may be a precursor to stone formation, but in most cases it disappears without forming stones.

CASE 7.51

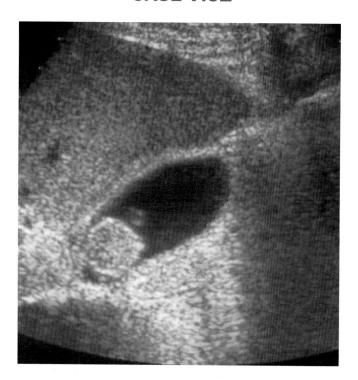

CASE 7.52

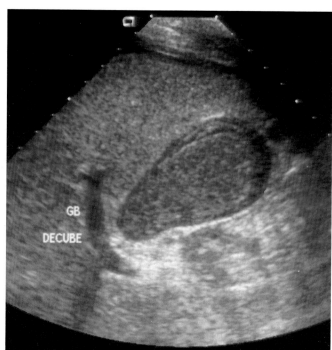

Findings

Case 7.51. Sonogram. A rounded echogenic mass is present near the neck of the gallbladder. This mass was mobile within the gallbladder with repositioning of the patient.

Case 7.52. Sonogram. A large mixed-echogenicity mass nearly fills the gallbladder lumen.

Differential Diagnosis
1. Tumefactive sludge (sludge balls)
2. Gallbladder carcinoma
3. Gallbladder metastases

Diagnosis
Tumefactive sludge

Discussion
Tumefactive sludge is a ball of sludge and can be mistaken for tumor without careful sonographic evaluation. Lack of shadowing distinguishes sludge balls from gallstones. Mobility within the gallbladder and lack of internal blood flow allow differentiation of sludge balls from polyps and tumors.

CASE 7.53

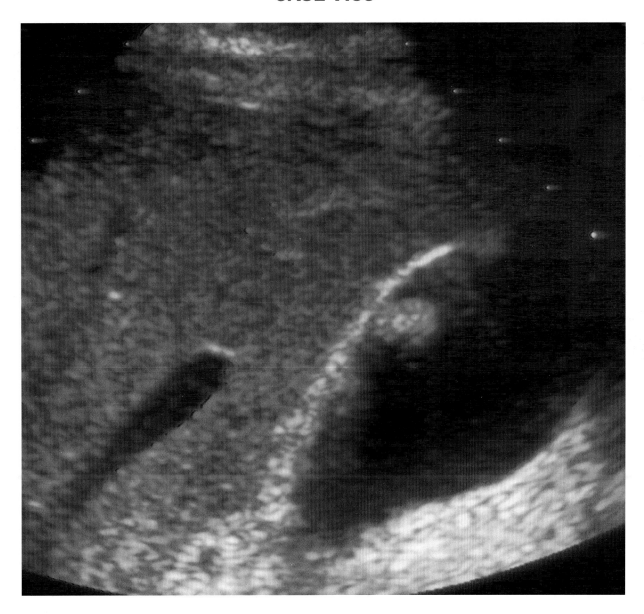

Findings

Sonogram. A solitary nonshadowing filling defect is present within the gallbladder.

Differential Diagnosis

1. Cholesterol polyp
2. Adenoma
3. Metastasis

Diagnosis

Cholesterol polyp

Discussion

Cholesterol polyps of the gallbladder are classified as a form of cholesterolosis. Cholesterolosis is a condition of unknown origin in which cholesterol is deposited within the lamina propria of the gallbladder. Cholesterol polyps are the commonest type of gallbladder polyp. Because they usually are multiple and small (<10 mm), it is common to detect only the largest at sonography. Gallstones shadow and move, whereas cholesterol polyps do not shadow and are nonmobile.

CASE 7.54

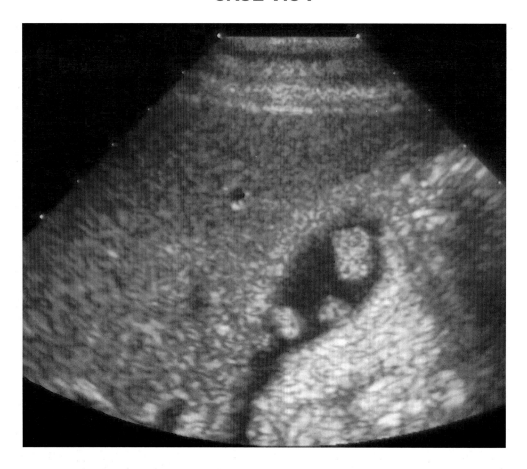

Findings

Sonogram. Several nonshadowing filling defects are present within the gallbladder lumen, arising from the gallbladder wall.

Differential Diagnosis

1. Cholesterol polyps
2. Gallbladder adenomas

Diagnosis

Cholesterol polyps

Discussion

Most polyps of the gallbladder are cholesterol polyps. These types of polyps are a form of cholesterolosis. Cholesterol polyps usually are pedunculated with a single layer of epithelium covering a core of cholesterol-filled cells. There are no known clinical sequelae to this finding. At sonography, these polyps can be distinguished from calculi by the absence of an acoustic shadow and attachment to the gallbladder wall. Adenomatous polyps are usually solitary filling defects and are much less common than cholesterol polyps. Polyps larger than 1 cm may be malignant. In most cases, when a gallbladder polyp larger than 1 cm is identified, the gallbladder is surgically removed to exclude malignancy.

Multiple polypoid intraluminal masses resembling polyps also can be seen in patients with metastatic melanoma (case 7.62). Detection of gallbladder polyps should be viewed with suspicion in patients with a history of melanoma. Usually other evidence of metastases is present.

CASE 7.55

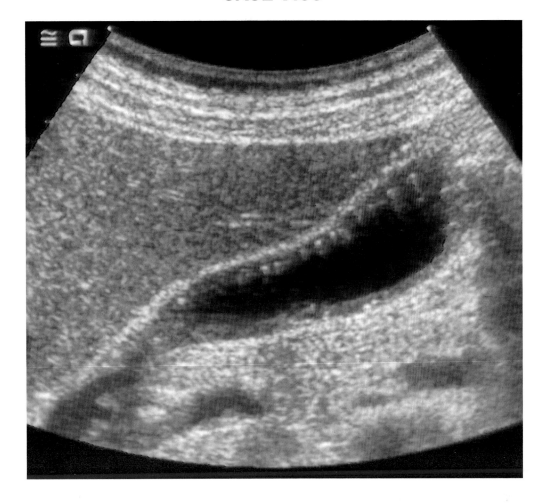

Findings
Sonogram. The gallbladder wall is diffusely thickened. There are echogenic foci within the nondependent wall with associated comet-tail artifacts that project into the lumen.

Differential Diagnosis
1. Adenomyomatosis (diffuse)
2. Acute cholecystitis
3. Chronic cholecystitis

Diagnosis
Adenomyomatosis (diffuse)

Discussion
Adenomyomatosis usually affects only a segment of the gallbladder (cases 7.56 and 7.57). Diffuse involvement can resemble either acute or chronic cholecystitis. The finding of echogenic foci within the thickened wall with the comet-tail ring-down artifact is highly suggestive of adenomyomatosis. The cause of this condition is unknown.

In the past, adenomyomatosis was classified as one of the hyperplastic cholecystoses—a nonneoplastic, noninflammatory gallbladder abnormality. The term "hyperplastic cholecystoses" is not used widely today. Adenomyomatosis refers to convoluted infoldings of the normal gallbladder mucosa (Rokitansky-Aschoff sinuses) with associated smooth muscle proliferation. There is secondary wall thickening that can be diffuse or segmental. Diffuse involvement can resemble either acute or chronic cholecystitis. The finding of echogenic foci within the thickened gallbladder wall with associated comet-tail artifact is highly suggestive of adenomyomatosis. The comet-tail reverberation artifacts are due to precipitated cholesterol crystals trapped within the Rokitansky-Aschoff sinuses.

CASE 7.56

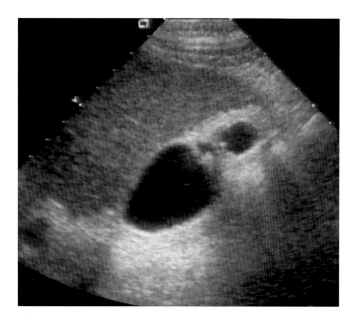

CASE 7.57

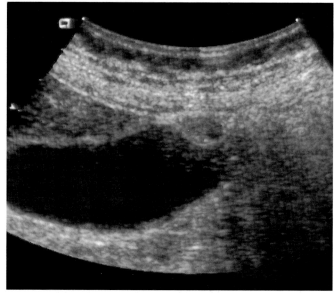

Findings

Case 7.56. Sonogram. There is marked annular thickening of the gallbladder wall at the fundus with a thick septation that causes near complete segmentation of the gallbladder.

Case 7.57. Sonogram. Focal masslike thickening of the wall of the gallbladder is present near the fundus.

Differential Diagnosis
1. Focal adenomyomatosis
2. Gallbladder carcinoma

Diagnosis
Focal adenomyomatosis

Discussion

Focal adenomyomatosis is characterized by hyperplasia of the mucosa and smooth muscle with secondary gallbladder wall thickening. Mucosal herniations into the muscular layer, called Rokitansky-Aschoff sinuses, often contain precipitated cholesterol crystals. Adenomyomatosis is usually focal in the fundus but may be diffuse throughout the gallbladder (case 7.55). These two cases show two common sonographic appearances of focal adenomyomatosis. Segmental involvement can narrow and distort the gallbladder lumen (case 7.56) or cause a filling defect in the fundus (case 7.57). Differentiation of focal adenomyomatosis from gallbladder carcinoma sometimes is difficult. Echogenic foci within the focal gallbladder wall thickening with comet-tail artifacts are due to precipitated cholesterol crystals within the Rokitansky-Aschoff sinuses and are nearly always pathognomonic for adenomyomatosis. This condition has no malignant potential. The cause of adenomyomatosis is unknown.

CASE 7.58

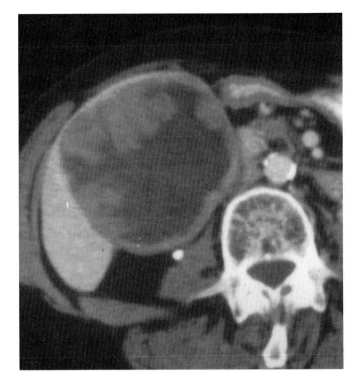

CASE 7.59

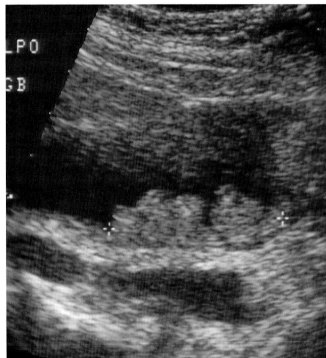

Findings

Case 7.58. Contrast-enhanced CT. The gallbladder is distended, and there is a polypoid mass within the lumen of the gallbladder arising from its wall.

Case 7.59. Sonogram. A 4-cm polypoid mass is present along the dependent wall of the gallbladder.

Differential Diagnosis
Gallbladder carcinoma (polypoid)

Diagnosis
Gallbladder carcinoma (polypoid)

Discussion

Although the commonest manifestation of a gallbladder carcinoma is an infiltrating mass arising from the gallbladder fossa and extending into the liver (cases 7.60 and 7.61), approximately one-quarter of gallbladder carcinomas appear as polypoid masses. These usually are well-differentiated tumors that are more likely to be resected for cure because of their well-circumscribed growth pattern.

The ability to demonstrate blood flow within polypoid gallbladder masses on sonography allows differentiation of gallbladder polyps (or carcinoma) from tumefactive sludge (cases 7.51 and 7.52).

CASE 7.60

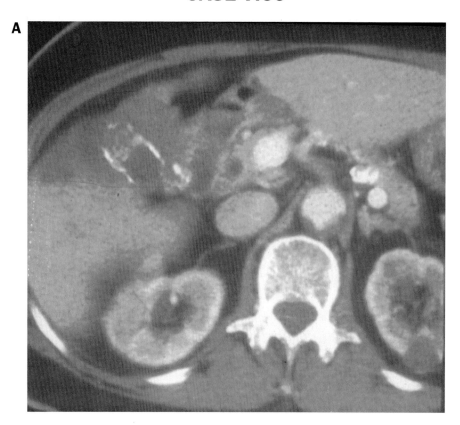

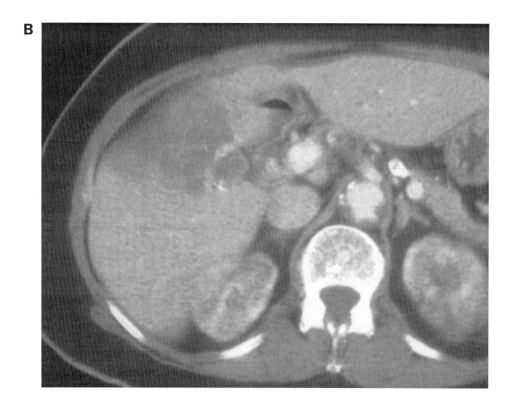

CASE 7.61

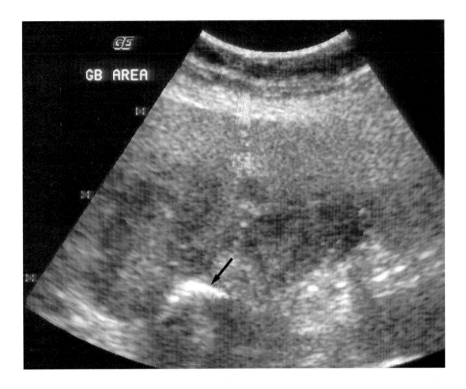

Findings

Case 7.60. Contrast-enhanced CT. **A** and **B.** A contracted, peripherally calcified (porcelain) gallbladder is present within a poorly defined hypoattenuating liver mass.

Case 7.61. Sonogram. A large, poorly defined hypoechoic mass is present in the gallbladder fossa with extension into the adjacent liver. A posteriorly shadowing gallstone (arrow) is seen along the inferior aspect of the obliterated gallbladder lumen.

Differential Diagnosis

1. Gallbladder carcinoma
2. Hepatocellular carcinoma
3. Complicated cholecystitis
4. Metastases to the gallbladder

Diagnosis

Gallbladder carcinoma

Discussion

Gallbladder carcinoma usually arises as a result of chronic cholecystitis. Most patients have gallstones, and porcelain gallbladder (caused by chronic cholecystitis) is a known risk factor. In the United States, the majority of patients are elderly women. There are two morphologic tumor types: scirrhous and polypoid. The scirrhous form infiltrates the liver from the gallbladder, and the polypoid form (cases 7.58 and 7.59) grows into and eventually fills the gallbladder lumen. The prognosis from this disease is poor, in that 85% of patients die within the first year.

Three main presentations are found at cross-sectional imaging studies. These include a gallbladder fossa mass (most common), polypoid mass, or mural thickening (least common). When a nonspecific-appearing liver mass is discovered, the finding of stones or a porcelain gallbladder (as in these cases) is helpful for suggesting the correct diagnosis. These tumors can spread by various routes. Spread into the adjacent liver is most common, and often the tumor can spread locally into the porta hepatis and cause biliary obstruction. Regional lymphadenopathy, hematogenous spread into the liver, and biliary invasion also can occur.

CASE 7.62

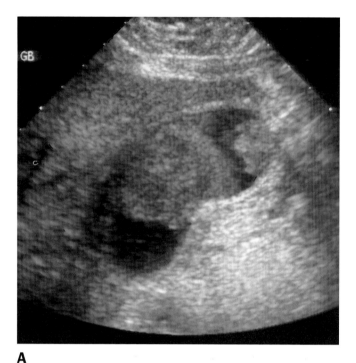

A

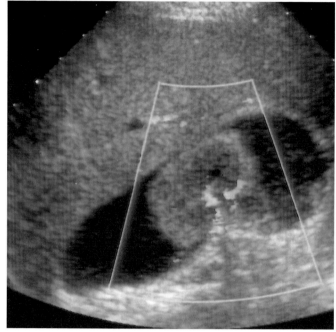

B

Findings

A. Sonogram. Two large polypoid masses are present within the gallbladder.

B. Color-Doppler sonogram. Blood flow is easily demonstrated within the largest polypoid mass.

Differential Diagnosis
1. Gallbladder carcinoma
2. Gallbladder polyps (adenomas)
3. Gallbladder metastases

Diagnosis
Gallbladder metastases (melanoma)

Discussion
Metastatic disease to the gallbladder is uncommon. The most common tumor to metastasize to the gallbladder is melanoma (less commonly gastric and pancreatic carcinoma). Gallbladder polyps in patients with a history of melanoma should be viewed with suspicion. However, patients with melanoma metastatic to the gallbladder usually have other evidence of metastatic disease elsewhere in the abdomen. This same sonographic appearance can be seen with gallbladder adenomas or gallbladder carcinoma. However, gallbladder adenomas are almost always solitary.

Masses and Filling Defects of the Gallbladder

		Case
Benign		
Gallstones	Stones are mobile with posterior acoustic shadowing. Gallbladder filled with stones results in wall-echo-shadow triad	7.48 and 7.49
Sludge	Dependently layering low-level echogenic material with no posterior acoustic shadowing	7.50
Tumefactive sludge	Sludge balls that can resemble polypoid tumors. Should be mobile and have no internal blood flow	7.51 and 7.52
Gallbladder polyps	Usually less than 1 cm. Most commonly cholesterol polyps. Nonmobile and no posterior acoustic shadowing. Internal blood flow sometimes is seen in larger polyps	7.53 and 7.54
Adenomyomatosis	Convoluted infoldings of gallbladder mucosa with smooth muscle proliferation. Gallbladder wall thickening and echogenic foci with ring-down artifact representing cholesterol crystals trapped within the Rokitansky-Aschoff sinuses. Focal adenomyomatosis can appear masslike	7.55–7.57
Malignant		
Gallbladder carcinoma	Polypoid form presents as a polypoid mass in gallbladder lumen. Scirrhous form infiltrates the liver from the gallbladder	7.58–7.61
Metastasis	Indistinguishable radiographically from a benign polyp or gallbladder carcinoma. Melanoma common	7.62

CASE 7.63

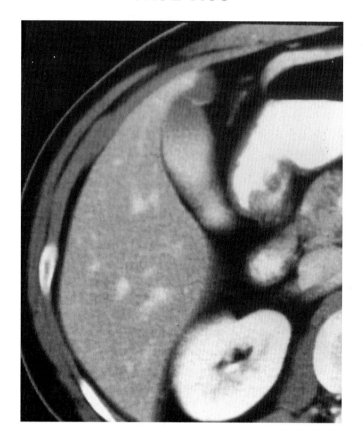

CASE 7.64

A

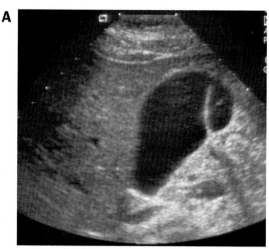

B

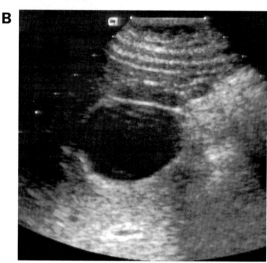

Findings
Case 7.63. Contrast-enhanced CT. High-attenuation material is present within the gallbladder lumen. Near the tip of the gallbladder fundus is a region of focal narrowing.

Case 7.64. Sonogram. **A** and **B.** Longitudinal (**A**) and transverse (**B**) views of the gallbladder show a thin infolding of the gallbladder wall near the fundus.

Differential Diagnosis
1. Phrygian cap of the gallbladder
2. Circumferential adenomyomatosis

Diagnosis
Phrygian cap of the gallbladder

Discussion
A phrygian cap is a congenital infolding of the gallbladder wall that does not have any know clinical sequela. It is most likely to be confused with focal adenomyomatosis of the gallbladder (cases 7.56 and 7.57), in which there is localized, circumferential narrowing of the lumen of the gallbladder caused by a septum or annular thickening of the gallbladder wall. These two conditions can be distinguished because a phrygian cap is always located in the gallbladder fundus and is composed of a thin membrane of tissue, whereas adenomyomatosis is thicker and can be located anywhere in the gallbladder.

CASE 7.65

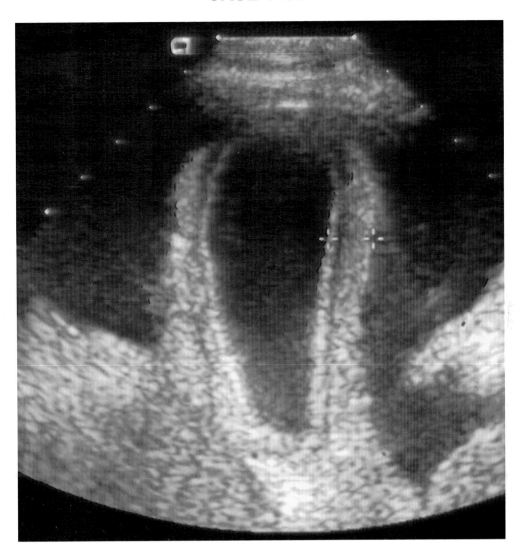

Findings

Sonogram. The gallbladder wall is markedly thickened. A large amount of ascites is present around the gallbladder.

Differential Diagnosis

1. Cholecystitis
2. Adenomyomatosis
3. Hepatitis
4. Cirrhosis
5. Portal hypertension
6. Hypoproteinemia
7. Heart failure
8. Lymphatic obstruction
9. Renal failure
10. Pancreatitis

Diagnosis

Diffuse gallbladder wall thickening (due to ascites, cirrhosis, and portal hypertension)

Discussion

Diffuse gallbladder wall thickening is present when the wall is 3 mm or more in diameter. The wall usually is uniformly echogenic without evidence of intramural edema (linear zones of sonolucency). As a solitary finding it has little specificity and must be viewed in context with other clinical findings. The most common cause of a thick gallbladder wall on sonography is a nondistended gallbladder (usually due to the patient having a recent meal). Abnormal gallbladder wall thickening can, therefore, not be confidently diagnosed unless the gallbladder is well distended.

CASE 7.66

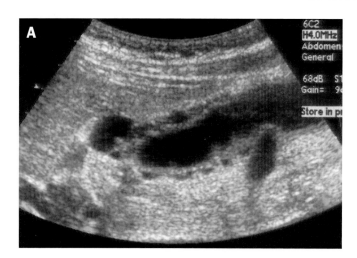

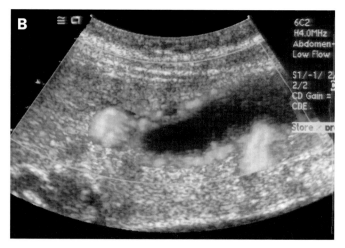

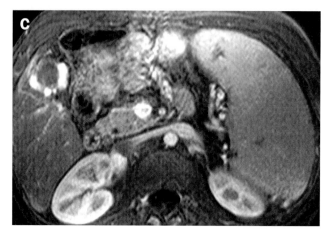

Findings

A. Sonogram. Cystic thickening of the gallbladder wall is seen on this gray-scale image.

B. Color-Doppler sonogram. The cystic spaces within the gallbladder wall represent vessels.

C. MRI. This post-gadolinium image demonstrates large collateral vessels around the gallbladder in the right upper quadrant. Incidentally noted is splenomegaly, also consistent with changes of portal venous hypertension.

Differential Diagnosis
Gallbladder varices

Diagnosis
Gallbladder varices

Discussion
Gallbladder varices are a rare cause of gallbladder wall thickening, which can be diagnosed easily with the use of color Doppler sonography. They develop in patients with portal hypertension, particularly in those with chronic portal vein thrombosis. Gallbladder varices are almost always asymptomatic. In rare instances, they may result in life-threatening hemobilia or rupture of the gallbladder.

Miscellaneous Gallbladder Conditions

		Case
Phrygian cap	Thin membrane in gallbladder fundus	7.63 and 7.64
Wall thickening	Nonspecific: ascites, cirrhosis, portal venous hypertension	7.65
Gallbladder varices	Collateral vessels around gallbladder, usually with portal venous hypertension	7.66

DIFFERENTIAL DIAGNOSES

Bile Duct Obstruction

Benign

Choledocholithiasis

Sludge balls, mucous plugs, blood
clots

Mirizzi syndrome (edema from
cystic duct stone)

Benign stricture

Surgery or intervention

Passed stone

Pancreatitis

Trauma

Cholangitis (infectious,
primary sclerosing
cholangitis, Oriental
cholangiohepatitis, acquired
immunodeficiency
syndrome)

Sphincter of Oddi spasm

Biliary papillomatosis

Malignant

Cholangiocarcinoma

Pancreatic carcinoma

Ampullary, duodenal carcinoma

Invasive gallbladder carcinoma

Adenopathy (benign and
malignant)

Diffuse Gallbladder Wall Thickening (≥3 mm)

Biliary

Acute cholecystitis

Chronic cholecystitis

Adenomyomatosis

Primary sclerosing cholangitis

Nonbiliary

Nonfasting gallbladder

Hepatitis, cirrhosis

Portal hypertension, ascites

Hypoproteinemia

Heart failure

Pancreatitis

Lymphatic obstruction

Gallbladder varices

Gallbladder Masses and Filling Defects

Stones

Tumefactive sludge (sludge balls)

Polyps (cholesterol, adenomatous)

Adenomyomatosis

Gallbladder carcinoma

Gallbladder metastases

Acoustic Shadowing From Gallbladder Fossa

Gallstones (wall-echo-shadow triad)

Porcelain gallbladder (clean shadow)

Emphysematous cholecystitis (dirty
shadow from wall)

Intraluminal gas (dirty shadow,
usually due to interventional
procedure)

CHOLEDOCHAL CYSTS

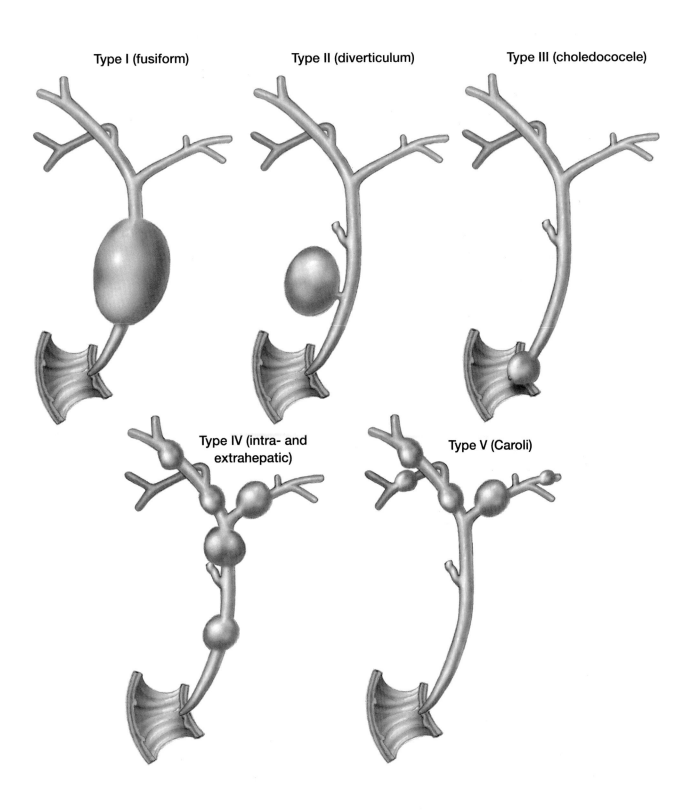

Type I (fusiform)

Type II (diverticulum)

Type III (choledococele)

Type IV (intra- and extrahepatic)

Type V (Caroli)

CYSTIC DUCT ANOMALIES

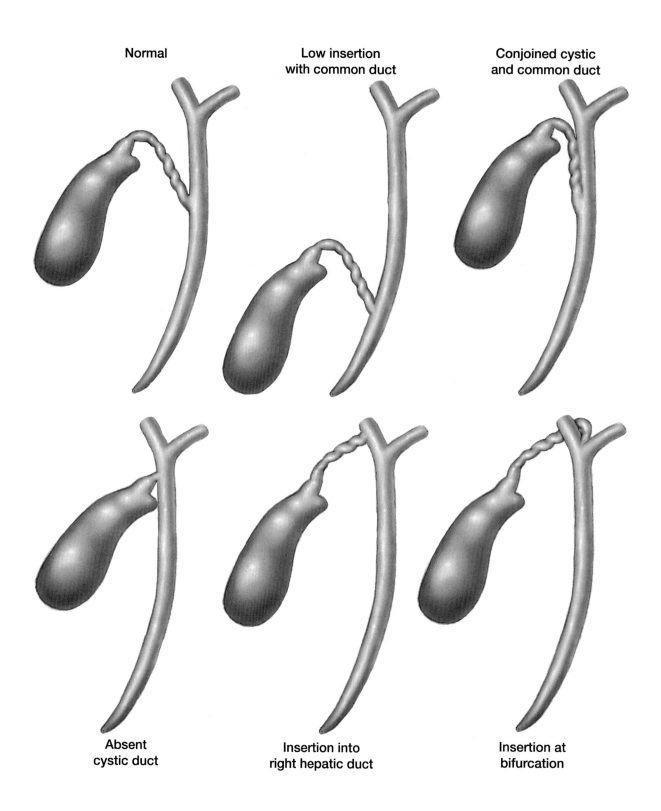

Normal

Low insertion
with common duct

Conjoined cystic
and common duct

Absent
cystic duct

Insertion into
right hepatic duct

Insertion at
bifurcation

INTRAHEPATIC DUCT VARIATIONS

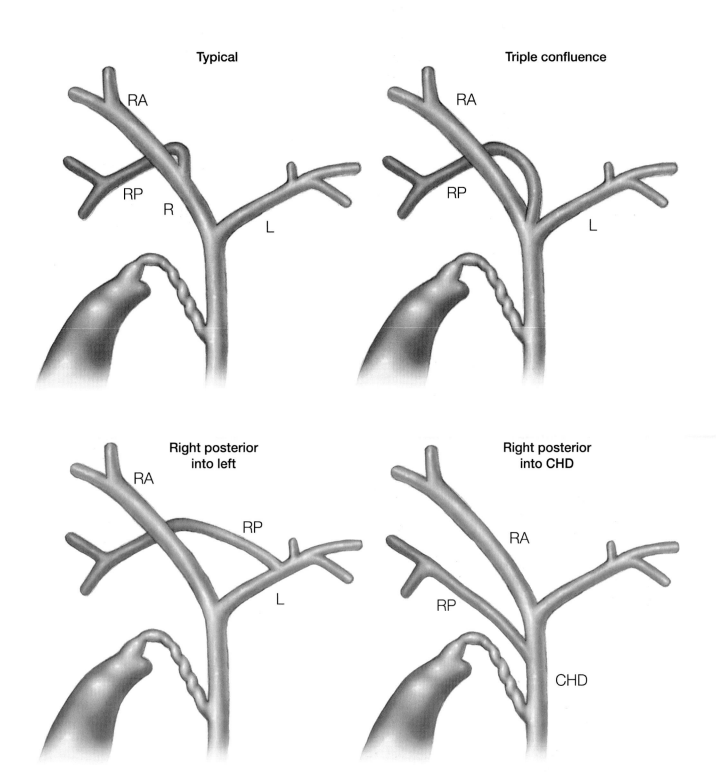

Typical

Triple confluence

Right posterior
into left

Right posterior
into CHD

BILE DUCT CONDITIONS

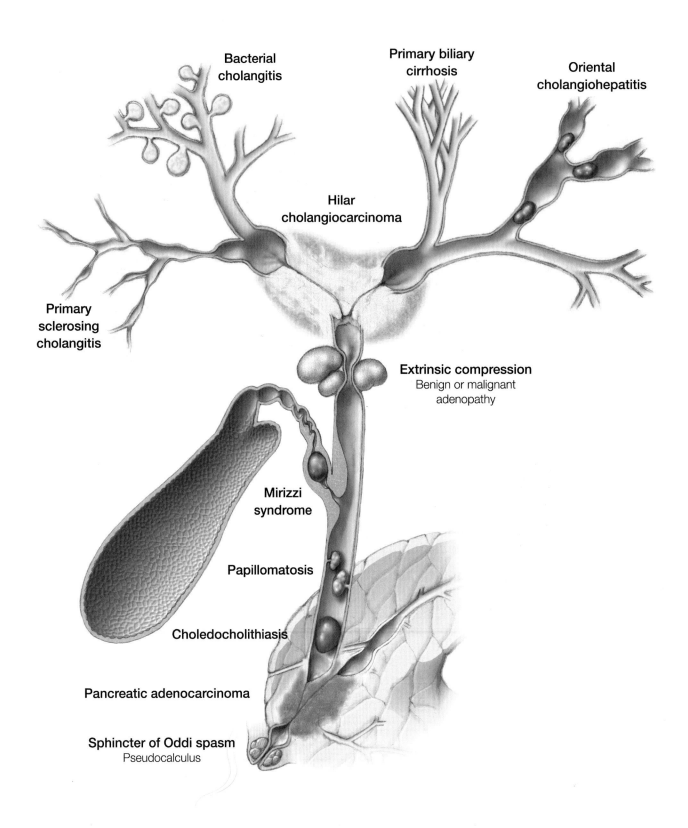

GALLBLADDER MASSES

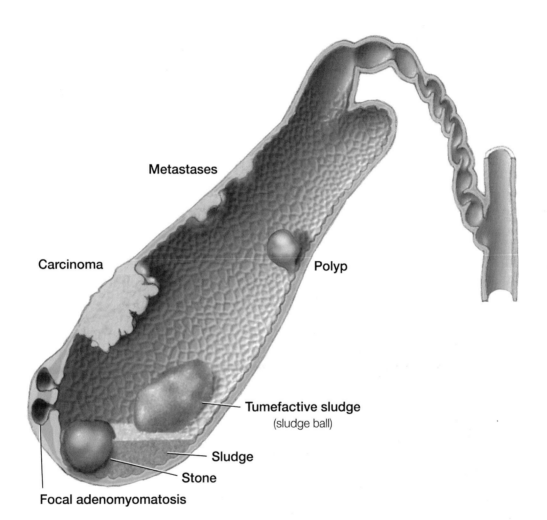

Metastases

Carcinoma

Polyp

Tumefactive sludge
(sludge ball)

Sludge

Stone

Focal adenomyomatosis

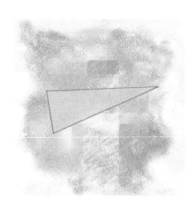

CHAPTER 8

PANCREAS

CASE 8.1

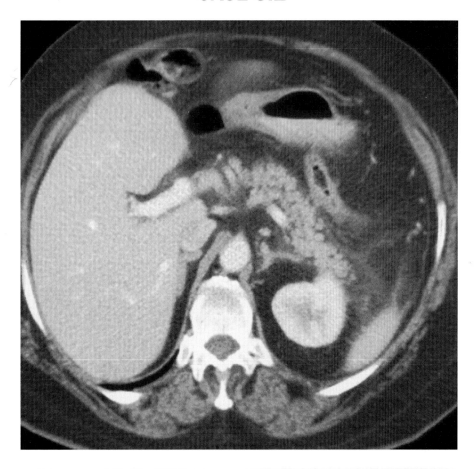

Findings

Contrast-enhanced CT. Peripancreatic stranding and an effusion are present about the tail of the pancreas. The pancreas is homogeneously perfused.

Differential Diagnosis

Acute pancreatitis

Diagnosis

Acute pancreatitis

Discussion

Acute pancreatitis usually is caused by either alcoholism or biliary tract disease (gallstones). In approximately one-fourth of patients, the cause of pancreatitis is never established. Pancreas divisum (cases 8.66–8.68) has also been implicated as a cause of acute pancreatitis due to functional obstruction of the pancreatic duct at the accessory papilla of Santorini. Other, less common causes include drugs, hypercalcemia, hyperlipidemia, viral infections, endotoxins, trauma, and others. Symptoms include abdominal pain, nausea, vomiting, and distention. Serum amylase and lipase levels are increased in about 80% of patients with acute pancreatitis. The absolute values of the enzymes do not necessarily correlate with the severity of disease.

The CT appearance of acute pancreatitis usually takes two forms: diffuse glandular enlargement or a normal-sized gland with a peripancreatic effusion (as in this case). Focal pancreatitis (case 8.4) is less common. The gland can be normal-appearing in mild pancreatitis. The staging system reported by Balthazar and colleagues can be helpful to estimate the severity of disease. Grade A refers to a normal-appearing pancreas. Progressively increasing grades of severe pancreatitis are B) focal or diffuse enlargement, C) intrinsic pancreatic abnormality with inflammatory changes in the peripancreatic tissues, D) a fluid collection or phlegmon, and E) two or more large phlegmonous collections or peripancreatic gas.

CASE 8.2

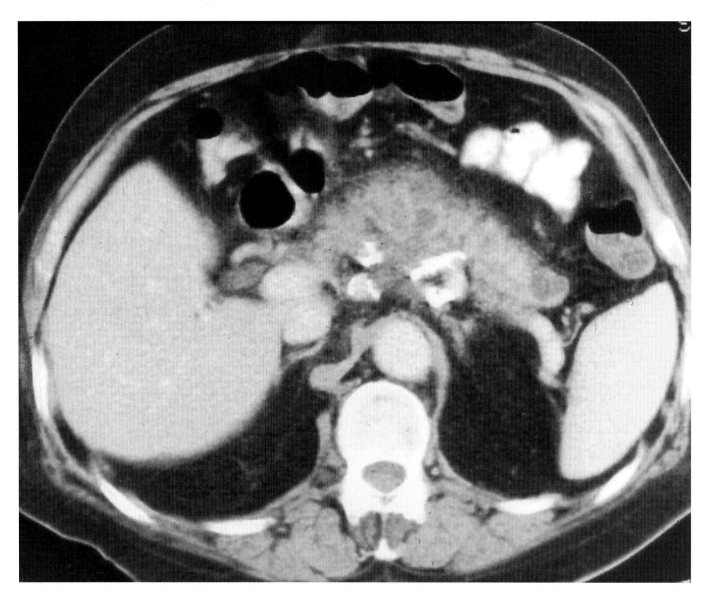

Findings
Contrast-enhanced CT. The pancreas is diffusely enlarged. There are several intrapancreatic fluid collections. A small peripancreatic effusion is present.

Differential Diagnosis
Acute pancreatitis

Diagnosis
Acute pancreatitis

Discussion
This case shows findings of severe acute pancreatitis with the presence of two or more intrapancreatic fluid collections (grade E, Balthazar criteria). Patients with severe acute pancreatitis usually have a protracted clinical illness and have higher incidences of pancreatic abscess and dying of complications of their illness.

CASE 8.3

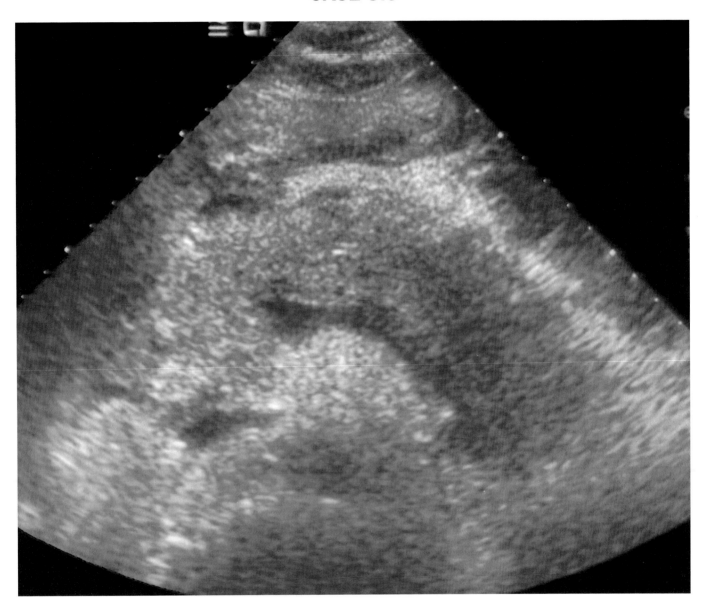

Findings
Sonogram. Diffuse enlargement and decreased echogenicity of the pancreas with a small amount of peripancreatic fluid.

Differential Diagnosis
Acute pancreatitis

Diagnosis
Acute pancreatitis

Discussion
Findings of diffuse acute pancreatitis include enlargement of the gland, hypoechogenicity relative to the liver, and peripancreatic fluid. These sonographic findings usually are seen only in moderate or severe acute pancreatitis. The pancreas often has a normal sonographic appearance in mild cases of pancreatitis. One of the major roles of sonography in patients with acute pancreatitis is to assess for stone disease in the biliary system as a possible cause for the pancreatitis. Differentiation between necrotic and nonnecrotic pancreatitis is not possible with sonography.

CASE 8.4

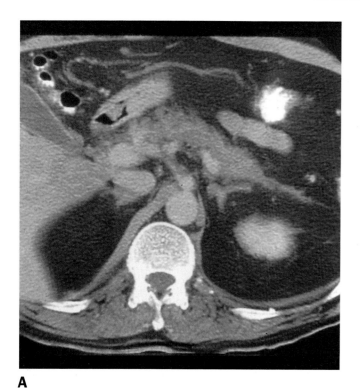

A

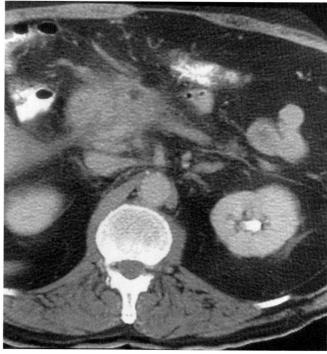

B

Findings

Contrast-enhanced CT. **A** and **B**. Focal enlargement of the pancreatic head. The body and tail of the pancreas are of normal size. There is blurring of the tissue planes about the mass in the head of the gland. Soft tissue thickening and stranding are present in the left anterior pararenal space.

Differential Diagnosis

1. Focal pancreatitis
2. Ductal adenocarcinoma
3. Islet cell tumor

Diagnosis

Focal pancreatitis

Discussion

Focal pancreatitis occurs in less than 20% of patients with acute pancreatitis. Usually the pancreatic head is involved. Often the disease is mild and due to choledocholithiasis. As in this case, other common findings of acute pancreatitis are present, including loss of discrete planes between the mass and the retroperitoneal fat and peripancreatic soft tissue stranding.

CASE 8.5

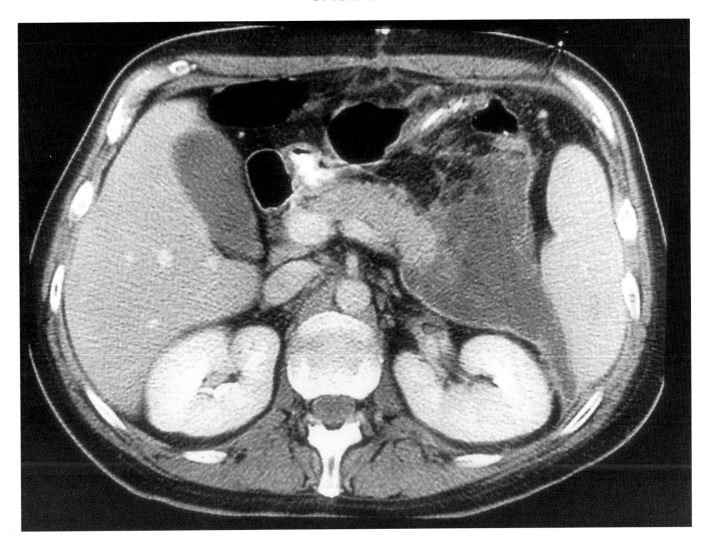

Findings
Contrast-enhanced CT. A large fluid collection is present in the region of the pancreatic tail. There is no perfusion of the pancreatic tail.

Differential Diagnosis
Acute pancreatitis with pancreatic necrosis

Diagnosis
Acute pancreatitis with pancreatic necrosis

Discussion
Pancreatic necrosis should be excluded in each patient with acute pancreatitis. The absence of perfusion of a segment(s) of the pancreas is diagnostic for pancreatic parenchymal necrosis. This is the most severe stage of pancreatic inflammation and is associated with the highest morbidity and mortality rates. Common complications associated with pancreatic necrosis include infection, pseudoaneurysm formation, splenic and portal vein thrombosis, biliary obstruction, and many systemic problems.

CASE 8.6

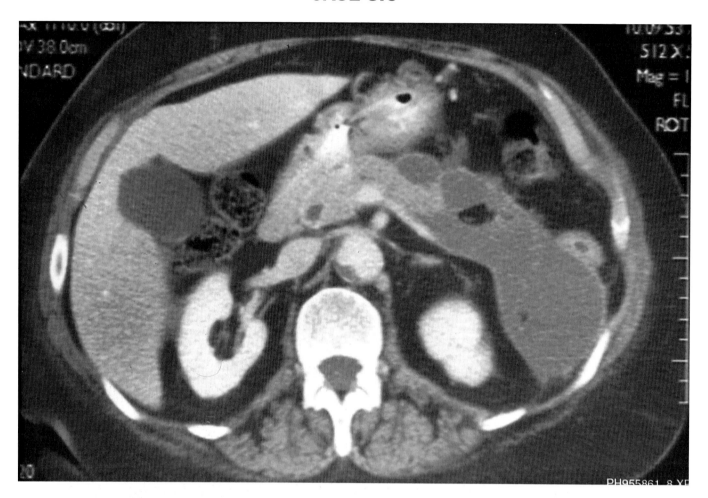

Findings

Contrast-enhanced CT. A large fluid collection is present in the region of the body and tail of the pancreas. The fluid collection is well demarcated and contains fat. The pancreas is normal in size and enhancement (tail seen on more cephalad images).

Differential Diagnosis

Acute pancreatitis with a pseudocyst

Diagnosis

Acute pancreatitis with a pseudocyst

Discussion

Fluid collections can be identified in about half of all patients with acute pancreatitis. Most fluid collections are absorbed within 2 to 3 weeks. These are referred to as peripancreatic fluid collections. Fluid collections that last more than 6 weeks are referred to as pseudocysts and usually have a thick fibrous wall. These collections usually indicate a persistent communication with the pancreatic duct. They tend to remain the same size but can enlarge over time. Pseudocysts can compress adjacent organs and cause obstruction or pain. Because of the potential for complications (pancreatic peritonitis, abscess, pseudoaneurysm formation and rupture), pseudocysts more than 4 cm in diameter are usually drained, even if asymptomatic.

CASE 8.7

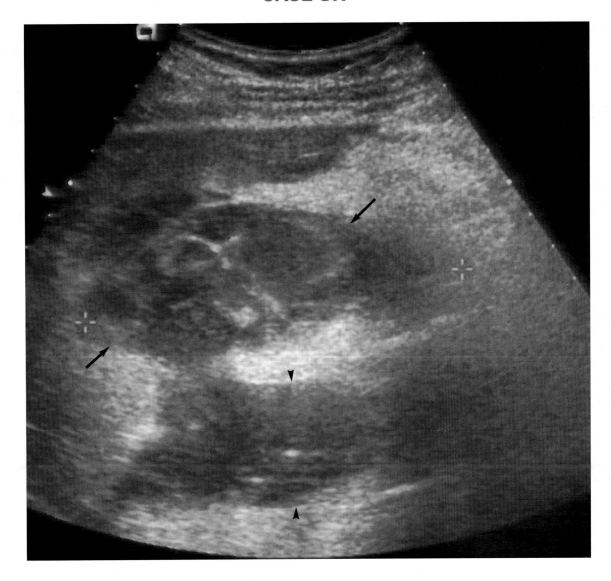

Findings

Transverse sonogram. Diffuse enlargement and decreased echogenicity of the pancreas (arrowheads) is present. A large, mixed echogenicity fluid collection (arrows) is located anterior to the pancreas, which contains echogenic debris.

Differential Diagnosis

Acute pancreatitis (with associated complicated peripancreatic fluid collection)

Diagnosis

Acute pancreatitis (with infected peripancreatic fluid collection)

Discussion

Sonography is often a valuable tool to determine the nature of a peripancreatic fluid collection or pseudocyst. Complicated peripancreatic fluid collections or pseudocysts containing hemorrhagic or infected fluid often exhibit homogeneous fluid attenuation on CT. Sonography easily shows the complexity of this peripancreatic fluid collection in the setting of acute pancreatitis. On sonography-guided aspiration in this case, infected fluid was found.

CASE 8.8

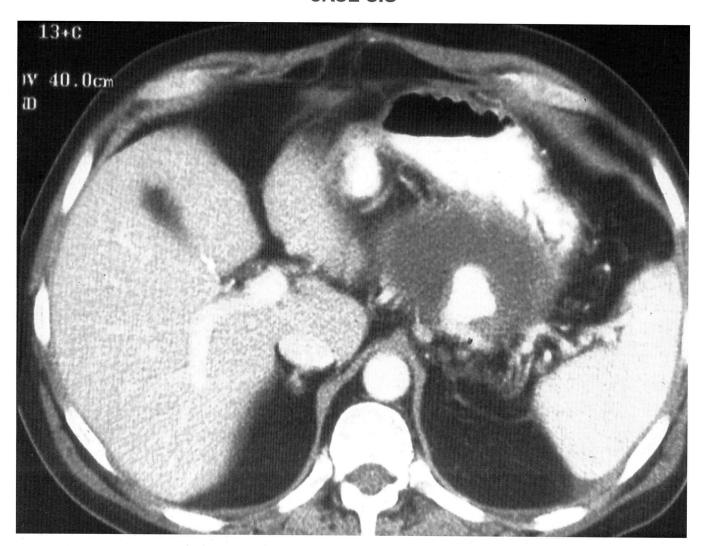

Findings

Contrast-enhanced CT. A large fluid collection is present in the lesser sac. An irregular collection of contrast enhancement is present within the fluid collection.

Differential Diagnosis

1. Pancreatic pseudocyst
2. Pancreatic fluid collection with pseudoaneurysm

Diagnosis

Pancreatic fluid collection with pseudoaneurysm

Discussion

Pancreatitis can lead to weakening of the walls of the vessels that come into contact with the pancreatic enzymes produced during an episode of acute pancreatitis. As the wall weakens, a pseudoaneurysm can develop. Ruptured pseudoaneurysms bleed into the retroperitoneum, bowel lumen, or peritoneal space. This is usually a sudden and catastrophic event with a high mortality rate. Recognition of the pseudoaneurysm and surgical or endovascular repair or embolization are critical to preventing life-threatening hemorrhage.

CASE 8.9

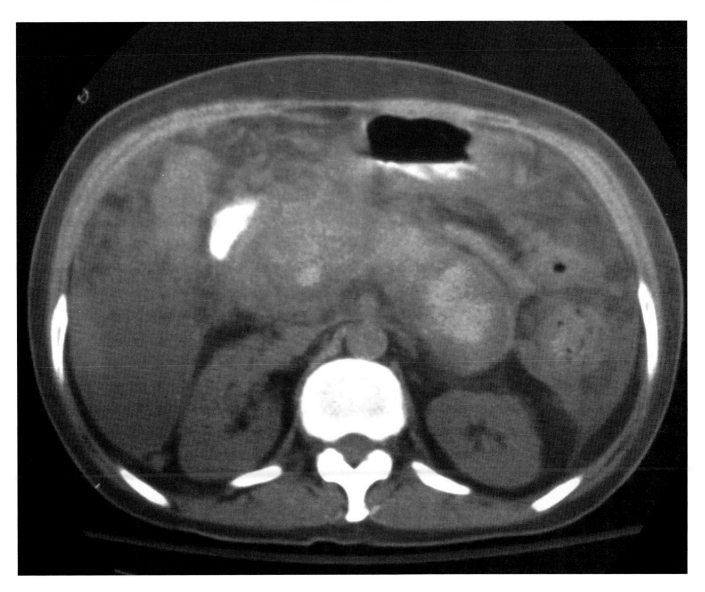

Findings
Unenhanced CT. The pancreas is enlarged and contains multiple regions of high attenuation. Peripancreatic, mesenteric, and abdominal fluid also is present.

Differential Diagnosis
Hemorrhagic pancreatitis

Diagnosis
Hemorrhagic pancreatitis

Discussion
Pancreatic hemorrhage is an uncommon finding in patients with pancreatitis. The inflammatory changes can cause erosion of the pancreatic vessels, pseudoaneurysm formation, and eventually retroperitoneal hemorrhage. High-attenuation fluid on unenhanced CT is key to the diagnosis of pancreatic hemorrhage. If patients are unstable from blood loss, emergency angiography with embolization of the bleeding vessel may be required. Usually, pancreatic necrosis also is present.

CASE 8.10

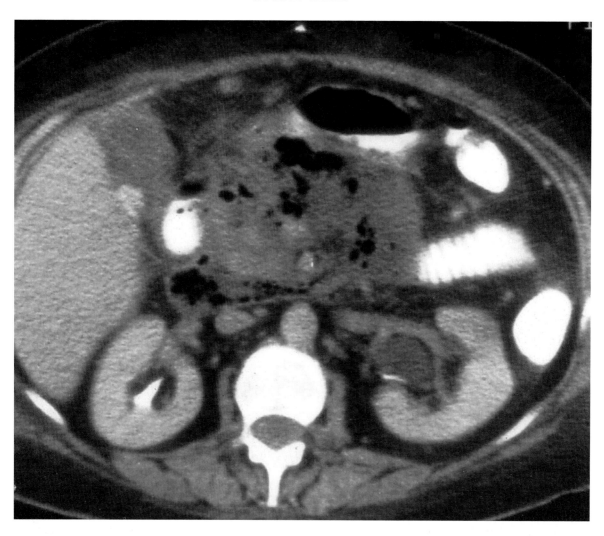

Findings
Contrast-enhanced CT. Fluid and gas are present within the lesser sac.

Differential Diagnosis
Pancreatic abscess

Diagnosis
Pancreatic abscess

Discussion
Pancreatic abscess usually develops as a complication of pancreatic necrosis. Pancreatic pseudocysts also can become infected. These can develop from a few days to several weeks after the onset of acute pancreatitis. Systemic signs of infection and sepsis usually are present, although occult presentations can occur. Most abscesses present only as an abnormal fluid collection. Poorly defined fluid collections that are present 2 to 4 weeks after the onset of pancreatitis are highly suspicious for an abscess. In suspicious cases, percutaneous aspiration of the fluid for microbiologic assessment is required. About 20% of abscesses contain gas (as in this case), a feature making the diagnosis much more likely. Recognition of an abscess is important, because untreated it has a high mortality rate.

CASE 8.11

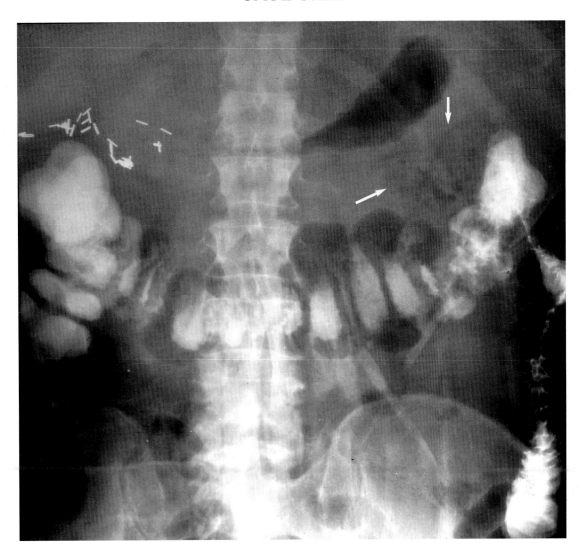

Findings
Single-contrast barium enema. Separation of the stomach and colon with an abnormal gas collection in the region of the lesser sac (arrows). The left transverse and upper descending colon is narrowed. Multiple surgical clips in the right upper quadrant.

Differential Diagnosis
Pancreatic abscess with inflammatory narrowing of the colon (colon cutoff sign)

Diagnosis
Pancreatic abscess with inflammatory narrowing of the colon (colon cutoff sign)

Discussion
Pancreatic abscess containing gas can be recognized on abdominal radiographs. Gas located between the colon and the stomach is usually extraluminal and within the lesser sac. A pancreatic abscess without gas is usually not visible on an abdominal radiograph. Pancreatic inflammatory fluid preferentially occupies the left anterior pararenal space. Inflammatory fluid in this location often bathes the colon and causes colonic spasm. Persistent spasm causes partial colonic obstruction with gaseous dilatation of the colon proximal to the splenic flexure. This constellation of events is radiographically referred to as the "colon cutoff sign." It may be the only clue to the presence of pancreatitis on an abdominal radiograph.

CASE 8.12

CASE 8.13

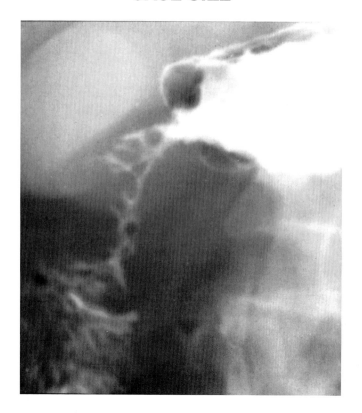

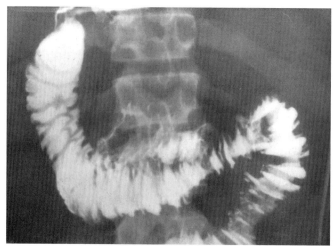

Findings

Case 8.12. UGI. Marked narrowing of the proximal duodenum. The mucosa through this narrowed region is intact.

Case 8.13. UGI. Widening of the duodenal C loop and thickening of the folds of the proximal small bowel.

Differential Diagnosis

1. Acute pancreatitis
2. Pancreatic mass
3. Pancreatic abscess

Diagnosis

Acute pancreatitis

Discussion

Acute pancreatitis can cause various upper gastrointestinal abnormalities. Enlargement of the duodenal C loop is most common and can be due to pancreatic enlargement or peripancreatic fluid collections. Narrowing of the duodenal lumen usually is due to severe spasm and can result in gastric outlet obstruction. Occasionally, the inflammation can be long-lasting and result in a duodenal stricture. If the pancreatic effusion is large enough, the inflammatory changes can extend beyond the lesser sac and involve the small bowel mesentery. Thickening of the folds in the proximal small bowel often is associated with extension of the peripancreatic effusion into the small bowel mesentery and with pancreatic ascites.

CASE 8.14

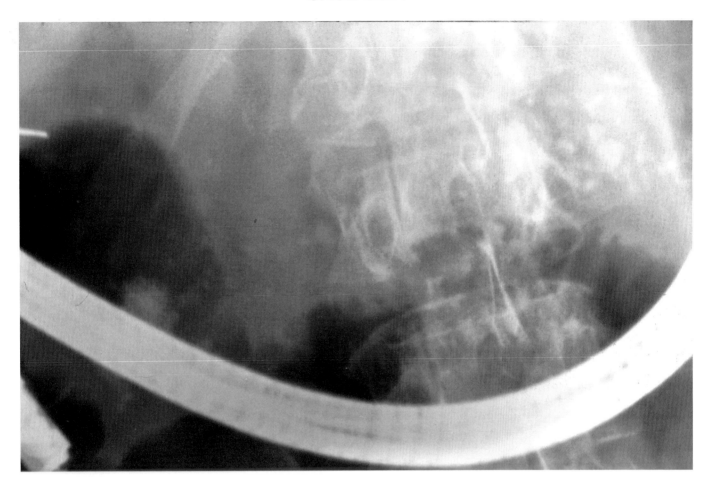

Findings

Abdominal radiograph. Multiple calcifications in the upper abdomen are located in the region of the pancreas.

Differential Diagnosis

Chronic pancreatitis

Diagnosis

Chronic pancreatitis

Discussion

Chronic pancreatitis is characterized by irreversible morphologic and functional pancreatic damage. Most cases are due to alcoholism. Hyperlipidemia, hyperparathyroidism, trauma, and pancreas divisum have been associated with this condition. Pain, weight loss, diabetes, and malabsorption are found clinically. The calcifications in chronic pancreas are ductal in location, usually small and irregular in shape. The presence of pancreatic ductal calcifications is pathognomonic of chronic pancreatitis.

CASE 8.15

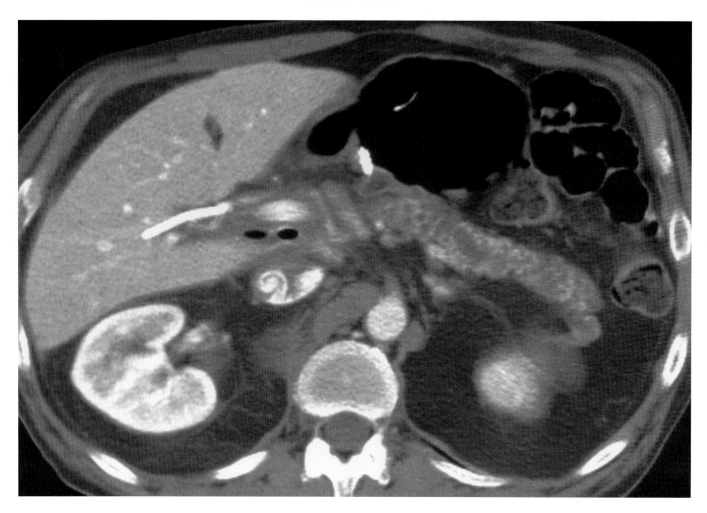

Findings
Contrast-enhanced CT. The pancreas is atrophic. Main and side branch ductal dilatation is present. A biliary stent and cystgastrostomy tube are present.

Differential Diagnosis
1. Chronic pancreatitis
2. Intraductal pancreatic mucinous neoplasm
3. Pancreatic ductal obstruction—cause undetermined

Diagnosis
Chronic pancreatitis

Discussion
The CT diagnosis of chronic pancreatitis depends on assessment of the pancreatic parenchyma and pancreatic duct and the presence of calculi. The pancreatic parenchyma can vary from enlarged to normal to atrophic. An atrophic gland is a helpful finding when present. Pancreatic ductal dilatation and dilatation of its side branches are characteristic of chronic pancreatitis. Ductal dilatation should be continuous to the ampulla. It is important to see ductal dilatation throughout the gland to exclude an obstructing neoplasm. Approximately half of patients with chronic pancreatitis have ductal calcifications. Calculi are the most reliable finding for the disease. It may be difficult to differentiate intraductal pancreatic mucinous neoplasm (IPMN) from ductal changes in chronic pancreatitis. Generally, ductal dilatation is the predominant finding with IPMN, whereas parenchymal atrophy dominates with chronic pancreatitis. In equivocal cases, ERCP is recommended.

CASE 8.16

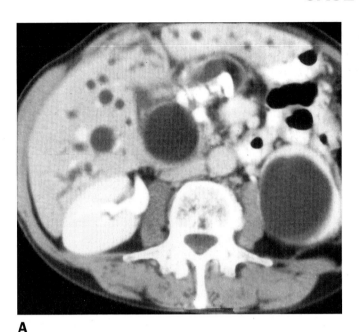

A

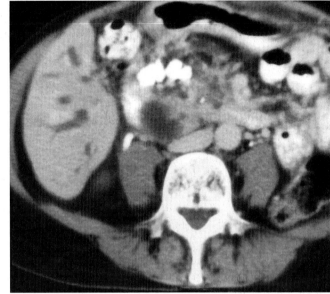

B

Findings

Contrast-enhanced CT. **A** and **B.** Dilatation of the biliary and main pancreatic ducts. There are coarse calcifications within the pancreatic duct. Benign left renal cyst.

Differential Diagnosis

1. Chronic pancreatitis (with benign stricture)
2. Chronic pancreatitis (with ductal adenocarcinoma)

Diagnosis

Chronic pancreatitis (with associated benign biliary duct stricture)

Discussion

Pancreatic ductal calcifications are the most helpful finding to suggest the diagnosis of chronic pancreatitis. The calculi are often small and irregular in shape. They can be coarse in appearance (as in this case). Those associated with familial pancreatitis and cystic fibrosis are usually the largest stones. Dilatation of the biliary tree raises the possibility of a mass in the region of the pancreatic head or distal common bile duct. A careful search for a mass should be performed. Biliary strictures can occur from changes of chronic pancreatitis (as in this case). Pancreatic cancers develop in 2% to 3% of patients with chronic pancreatitis; therefore, a change in the imaging findings or clinical symptoms should prompt a careful search for tumor.

CASE 8.17

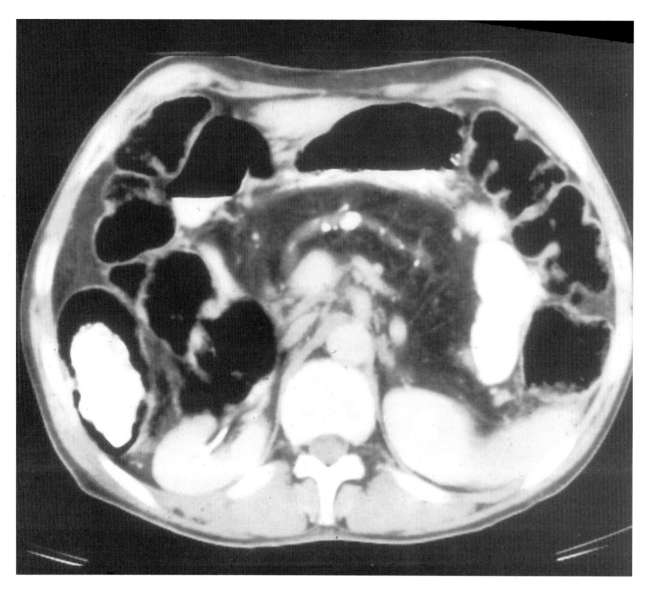

Findings
Contrast-enhanced CT. Fatty replacement of the pancreas. Several calculi are visible within the main pancreatic duct.

Differential Diagnosis
1. Chronic pancreatitis
2. Cystic fibrosis

Diagnosis
Chronic pancreatitis with fatty replacement of the pancreas

Discussion
Fatty replacement of the pancreas most often is found in patients with chronic pancreatitis, obesity, diabetes, or cystic fibrosis. It also can occur sporadically without definite cause. Pancreatic insufficiency may or may not accompany fatty replacement. Pancreatic insufficiency usually indicates loss of more than 90% of functioning pancreatic tissue. Diabetes and malabsorption are the main symptoms of pancreatic insufficiency. This patient had chronic pancreatitis. Pancreatic ductal calcifications led to ductal obstruction and secondary pancreatic parenchymal fatty replacement.

CASE 8.18

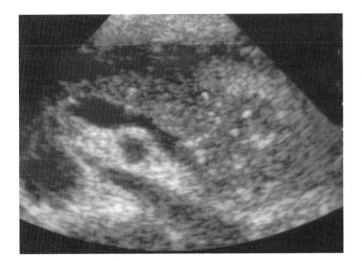

CASE 8.19

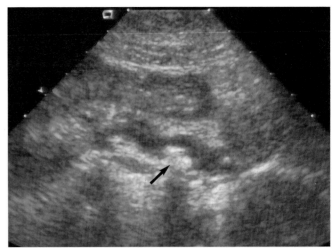

Findings

Case 8.18. Sonogram. The pancreatic gland is generous in size with decreased echogenicity and multiple echogenic foci in the visualized body and tail of the pancreas.

Case 8.19. Sonogram. The main pancreatic duct is significantly dilated and contains a large posteriorly shadowing stone (arrow). There is diffuse atrophy of the visualized pancreatic gland.

Differential Diagnosis

Chronic pancreatitis

Diagnosis

Chronic pancreatitis

Discussion

Each of these two cases has a classic sonographic appearance of chronic pancreatitis. Case 8.18 has multiple tiny echogenic foci (calculi) scattered in the visualized pancreatic parenchyma. Shadowing may or may not be visible depending on the size of the calcifications. These tiny calcifications are in an intraductal location, but side branch ducts are generally not visible at sonography. The size and echotexture of the pancreas can vary in chronic pancreatitis. Although nonspecific, the enlargement and relative hypoechogenicity of the visualized pancreas in case 8.18 favor some degree of acute inflammation. The pancreas tends to be atrophic in cases of chronic pancreatitis without associated acute inflammation. When calcifications migrate from side branches into the main pancreatic duct, or when calcifications form primarily in the main duct, an appearance such as that in case 8.19 may be seen. Chronic main duct obstruction by stones often results in an irregular or beaded dilatation of the duct and associated atrophy of the pancreatic gland.

CASE 8.20

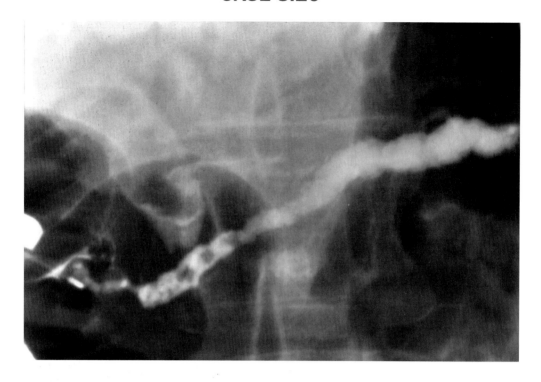

CASE 8.21

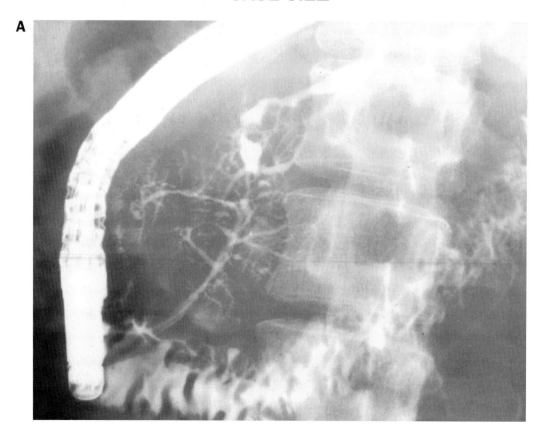

CASE 8.21 (continued)

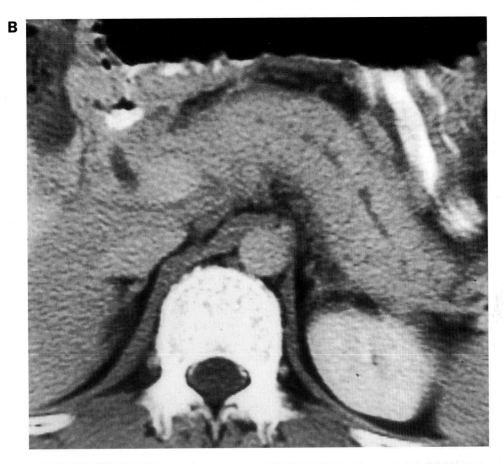

B

Findings

Case 8.20. ERCP. The main pancreatic duct is irregularly dilated and contains several filling defects in the region of the pancreatic head.

Case 8.21. A. ERCP. The pancreatic duct in the head of the pancreas is irregular in contour. Side branch ducts are variable in shape—dilated, irregular in contour, and beaded. Within the body and tail of the pancreas, the duct is dilated and irregular in contour.

B. Contrast-enhanced CT. The main pancreatic duct is mildly dilated and is irregular and beaded in contour.

Differential Diagnosis

Chronic pancreatitis

Diagnosis

Chronic pancreatitis

Discussion

ERCP and MRCP are the most helpful techniques to make the diagnosis of chronic pancreatitis. Typical changes include ductal dilatation, ductal contour irregularity, and clubbing and stenosis of the side branches. Filling defects within the ducts are usually calculi. Advanced changes of chronic pancreatitis lead to a chain-of-lakes or beaded appearance of the side branches.

CASE 8.22

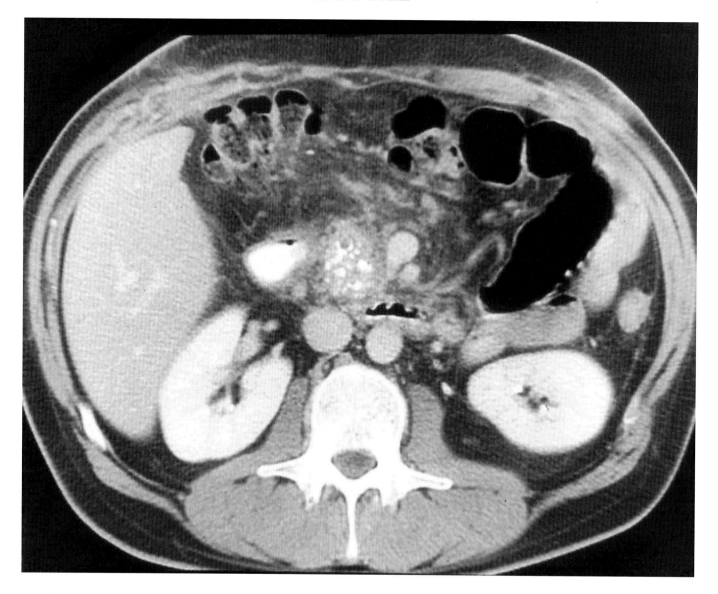

Findings

Contrast-enhanced CT. Multiple calcifications are present within the pancreatic head. There is mild soft tissue stranding within the peripancreatic tissues.

Differential Diagnosis

1. Chronic pancreatitis
2. Familial pancreatitis

Diagnosis

Familial pancreatitis

Discussion

Familial pancreatitis is a term used to encompass two types of disease: 1) a familial occurrence of pancreatitis in kindreds with hyperlipidemia, hyperparathyroidism, cystic fibrosis, and cholelithiasis and 2) an autosomal dominant inherited syndrome referred to as hereditary pancreatitis. Patients with the latter type have an early age at onset of pancreatitis (often during childhood), pain, disability, and common complications including pancreatic insufficiency, pseudocyst formation, and an increased incidence of pancreatic carcinoma. Calcifications usually are large within dilated pancreatic ducts.

CASE 8.23

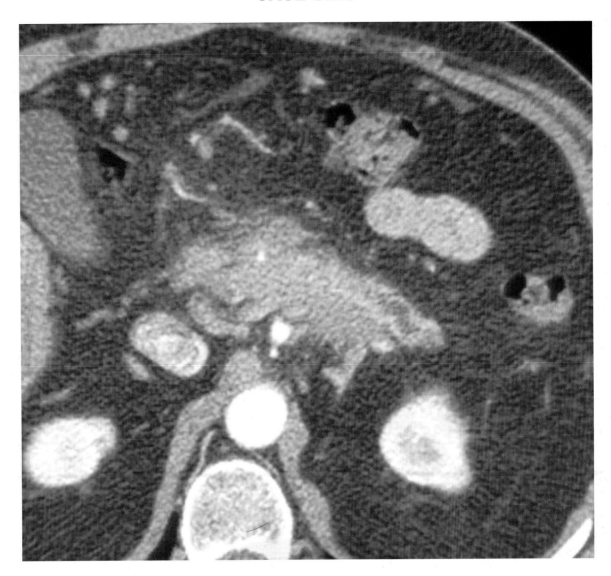

Findings

Contrast-enhanced CT. The body of the pancreas is enlarged and of low attenuation. The duct in the pancreatic tail is dilated to the level of the mass. Soft tissue stranding is present about the pancreas.

Differential Diagnosis

1. Acute pancreatitis
2. Autoimmune pancreatitis
3. Ductal adenocarcinoma

Diagnosis

Autoimmune pancreatitis

Discussion

Autoimmune pancreatitis is a subtype of pancreatitis that can be associated with both acute and chronic changes to the pancreas. It usually affects older persons (mean age, 60 years). Clinical symptoms in these patients are usually much less severe than in those with usual pancreatitis. Patients usually have increased IgG levels. Associated conditions often include Sjögren syndrome, primary sclerosing cholangitis, and systemic lupus erythematosus. Imaging studies usually show diffuse or focal enlargement of the pancreas with pancreatic ductal narrowing. Oral corticosteroid therapy usually is effective for treating this condition.

Inflammatory Diseases of the Pancreas

		Case
Acute diffuse pancreatitis	Diffuse enlargement or peripancreatic effusion. Soft tissue stranding	8.1–8.3
Acute focal pancreatitis	Segmental mass and fluid and soft tissue stranding	8.4
Necrotizing pancreatitis	Nonenhancement of a segment after intravenous contrast. Hemorrhage in some cases	8.5
Complications of acute pancreatitis	Complications include pseudocysts, abscesses, pseudoaneurysms, splenic or portal vein thrombosis, hemorrhage	8.6–8.13
Chronic pancreatitis	Ductal calcifications. Ductal dilatation. Parenchymal atrophy	8.14–8.21
Familial pancreatitis	Positive family history. Early onset. Ductal dilatation with coarse calcifications	8.22
Autoimmune pancreatitis	Older persons. Associated autoimmune disorders. Mild symptoms	8.23

CASE 8.24

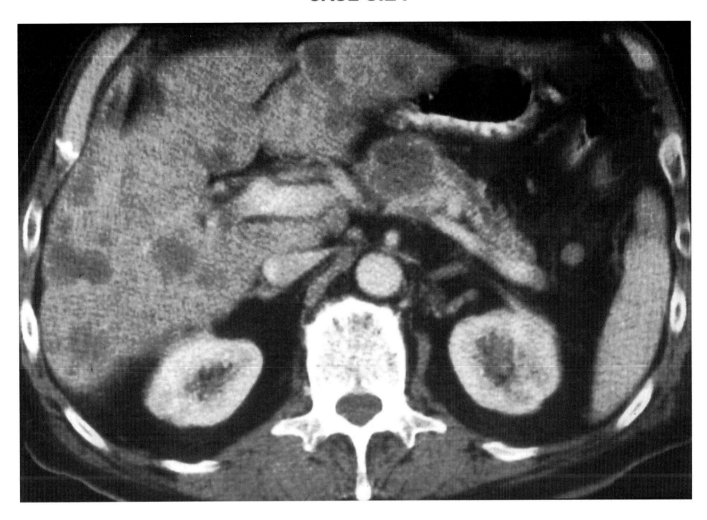

Findings

Contrast-enhanced CT. A large hypoattenuating mass is present in the body of the pancreas. The pancreatic duct in the region of the tail is dilated. Multiple hepatic metastases are present.

Differential Diagnosis

Ductal adenocarcinoma

Diagnosis

Ductal adenocarcinoma

Discussion

Pancreatic ductal adenocarcinoma is the fifth most common cause of death from cancer in the United States (less common than lung, colon, breast, and prostate). Despite imaging advances, there has been no improvement in the mortality from this disease. This is likely due to these tumors being discovered after they have already metastasized and to their rapid growth characteristics. Radiologists have an important role in the detection of this tumor (to explain symptoms) and in the staging of disease extent.

Most ductal cancers are hypoattenuating, but small tumors may be detectable only if they alter the texture of the pancreatic parenchyma or obstruct the main pancreatic duct. Staging is based on assessment of local disease extent, vascular encasement, lymphatic or peritoneal spread, and hepatic metastases. In this case, the typical features of a nonresectable ductal cancer are present: a large mass obstructing the pancreatic duct, and hepatic metastases.

CASE 8.25

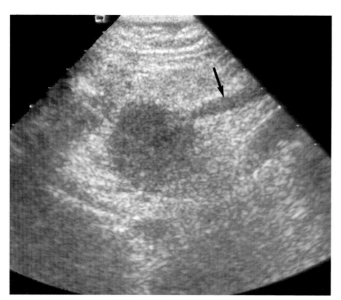

A

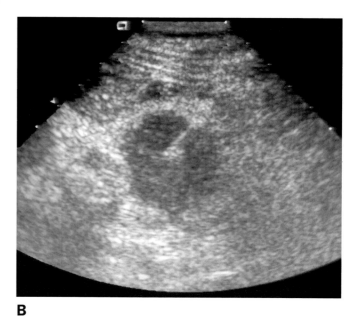

B

Findings

Sonogram. **A.** Transverse view of the pancreas shows a
large hypoechoic mass in the head of the pancreas with
marked dilatation of the main pancreatic duct to the level
of this mass (arrow). **B.** A biopsy needle is visualized
within the pancreatic mass.

Differential Diagnosis

Ductal adenocarcinoma

Diagnosis

Ductal adenocarcinoma

Discussion

The most common sonographic appearance of pancreatic
carcinoma is a poorly defined hypoechoic mass with
associated pancreatic duct dilatation. The biliary ducts
also are often dilated if the tumor is in the head of the
pancreas. This associated ductal dilatation is less common
in other solid hypoechoic pancreatic masses, which include
islet cell tumors, metastases, lymphoma, or focal pancreatitis.
Although Doppler ultrasonography can be useful for
determining vascular involvement of the tumor, contrast-
enhanced CT is considered a better staging tool. When
clinically indicated, percutaneous ultrasonography-guided
biopsy often is used to obtain a tissue diagnosis. Advantages
of sonography-guided biopsy over CT-guided biopsy
include the ability to displace overlying bowel loops
with transducer compression and real-time visualization
of peripancreatic vessels during the biopsy.

CASE 8.26

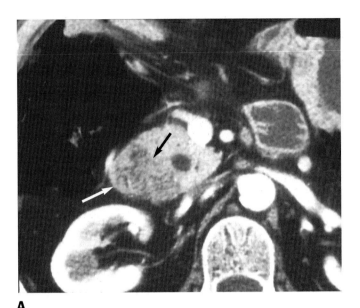

A

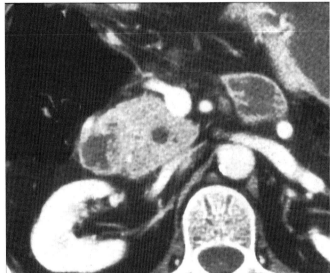

B

Findings

Contrast-enhanced CT. **A.** Pancreatic phase of contrast enhancement. A hypoattenuating region is present within the head of the pancreas (arrows). **B.** Portal venous phase of contrast enhancement. The pancreatic head is nearly isoattenuating. The duodenum is seen lateral to the pancreatic head.

Differential Diagnosis

1. Ductal adenocarcinoma
2. Focal pancreatitis

Diagnosis

Ductal adenocarcinoma

Discussion

Recent CT technology with multidetector scanners allows rapid acquisition of image data during multiple different phases of contrast enhancement. Hypovascular masses (such as ductal adenocarcinoma) usually are optimally identified during the pancreatic phase of contrast enhancement. Tissue contrast between the enhancing pancreatic parenchyma and a hypoattenuating mass is usually maximal. In most patients, this occurs approximately 45 seconds after initiation of contrast material administration. Portal venous phase imaging is useful for the detection of hepatic metastases and regional lymphadenopathy. In patients with a suspected pancreatic carcinoma, dual-phase imaging (pancreatic and portal venous phases) is recommended.

CASE 8.27

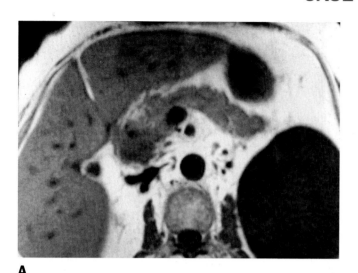

A

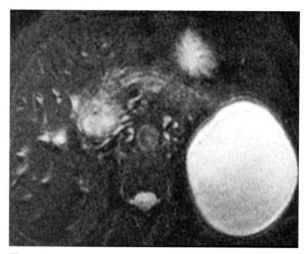

B

Findings

A. T1-weighted MRI. A hypointense mass is present within the head of the pancreas.

B. T2-weighted MRI. The mass is hyperintense. The tumor does not extend beyond the pancreas. A large benign cyst is present in the upper pole of the left kidney.

Differential Diagnosis

1. Ductal adenocarcinoma
2. Islet cell tumor
3. Pancreatic metastases
4. Focal pancreatitis

Diagnosis

Ductal adenocarcinoma

Discussion

Although CT remains the primary imaging method for assessment of the pancreas, MRI can be used if patients have renal insufficiency or iodine allergies and cannot receive intravenous contrast material. Pancreatic cancers are hypointense on T1-weighted images and hyperintense on T2-weighted images. Small tumors are best depicted on T1-weighted images with use of fat saturation. With this technique, the pancreas appears hyperintense compared with the hypointense mass. Dynamic imaging after intravenous administration of gadolinium also can be used to identify a hypoenhancing mass. Findings at dynamic imaging mimic those found at CT.

CASE 8.28

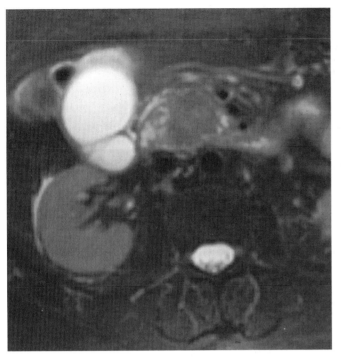

A

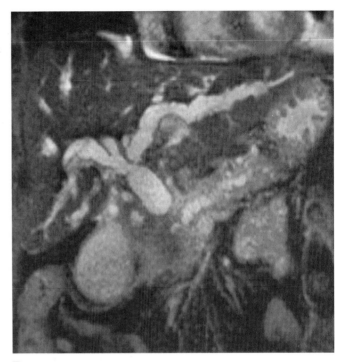

B

Findings

A. Contrast-enhanced MRI. A solid mass is located within the pancreatic head.

B. MRCP. Dilatation of both the biliary system and the pancreatic duct to the level of the pancreatic head. A hypointense mass is present in the pancreatic head.

Differential Diagnosis

1. Ductal adenocarcinoma
2. Focal pancreatitis

Diagnosis

Ductal adenocarcinoma (double duct sign)

Discussion

Secondary findings can be helpful for the detection of small pancreatic tumors. Secondary findings include ductal dilatation proximal to the tumor (this includes dilatation of both the biliary and the pancreatic ducts if the tumor is located in the pancreatic head—as in this case), vascular encasement, hepatic metastases, regional lymphadenopathy, peritoneal carcinomatosis, and ascites.

CASE 8.29

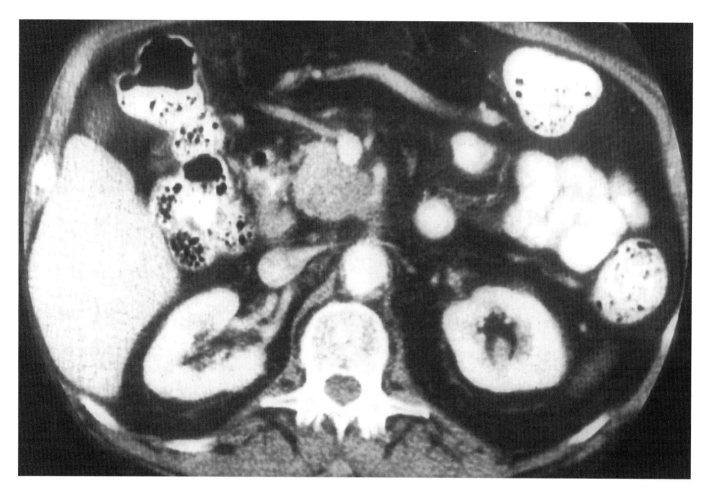

Findings
Contrast-enhanced CT. The uncinate process of the pancreas is enlarged, rounded, and hypoattenuating. Soft tissue extends from the uncinate process to the superior mesenteric artery and obliterates the fat plane about the artery.

Differential Diagnosis
Ductal adenocarcinoma

Diagnosis
Ductal adenocarcinoma

Discussion
The uncinate process is normally triangular, located posterior to the superior mesenteric vein. It is normally isoattenuating with the remainder of the pancreas. Rounding of the uncinate process should prompt consideration of a mass. The additional findings of a change in attenuation compared with the remainder of the gland and extension of the process to encase the superior mesenteric artery are typical of a carcinoma.

CASE 8.30

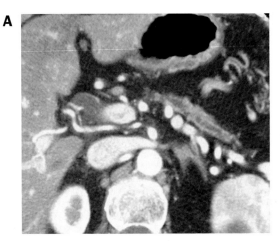

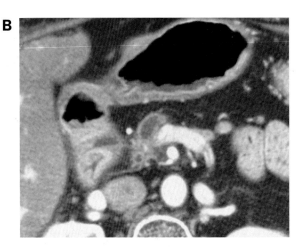

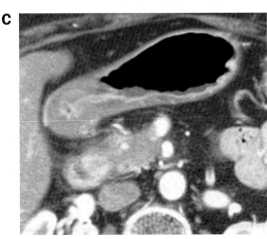

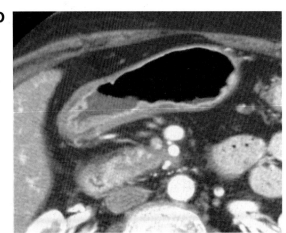

Findings

Contrast-enhanced CT. **A** through **D.** The pancreatic duct in the region of the tail of the pancreas is dilated, and the pancreatic parenchyma is atrophic. The duct ends in the region of the pancreatic head. The texture of the slightly hypoattenuating obstructing mass is homogeneous soft tissue. Soft tissue extends and encases the superior mesenteric artery and deforms the superior mesenteric vein.

Differential Diagnosis

Ductal adenocarcinoma

Diagnosis

Ductal adenocarcinoma

Discussion

Not all pancreatic cancers are hypoattenuating at CT.

Some are isoattenuating with the pancreatic parenchyma. Detection can be difficult if the mass is small and does not alter the contour of the normal pancreas. Identification of the site of the obstructed pancreatic duct is a key finding in localizing the mass. In some cases, the mass alters the normal pancreatic parenchymal texture, often appearing more solid and homogeneous than the normal gland. Atrophy of the parenchyma upstream from the mass usually indicates chronicity of the obstruction.

Another clue to the presence of tumor in this case is tumor extension into the fat about the superior mesenteric artery and vein. Normally there is always a cuff of fat around the artery. The superior mesenteric vein (SMV) is normally in contact with the neck of the pancreas without a surrounding fatty cuff. The SMV is normally either round or elliptical. In this case, the vein is deformed by the adjacent mass, indicating venous invasion.

CASE 8.31

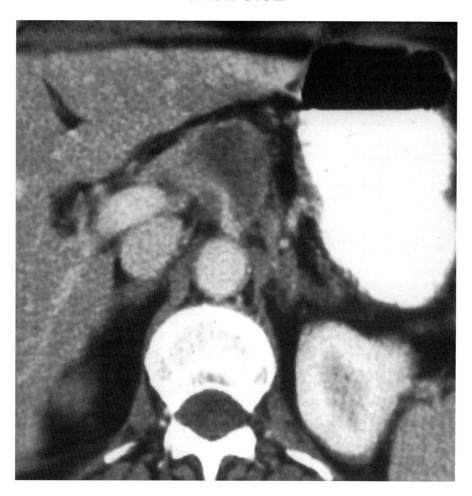

Findings
Contrast-enhanced CT. There is a large hypoattenuating mass in the body of the pancreas. The mass extends posteriorly and encases the superior mesenteric artery.

Differential Diagnosis
Ductal adenocarcinoma

Diagnosis
Ductal adenocarcinoma, nonresectable

Discussion
A key growth characteristic of ductal cancers is the proclivity to encase vascular structures and invade perineural structures. Vascular encasement is a major cause of nonresectability. Perineural invasion is the major reason that patients experience back pain with these tumors. In this case, the tumor is not resectable because of encasement of the superior mesenteric artery.

Nonresectability occurs when any of the following exist:

Arterial invasion: usually the superior mesenteric artery or celiac axis

Venous invasion: limited involvement of the superior mesenteric vein (SMV) or junction of the SMV and portal vein usually is considered resectable and reconstructable. More extensive venous involvement may not be resectable (depending on local surgical views), except in selected specialty centers

Regional lymphadenopathy with metastatic tumor: Today, sampling of enlarged nodes with endoscopic ultrasonography-performed biopsy is common preoperatively

Distant metastases: most common to liver, peritoneum, and lungs

CASE 8.32

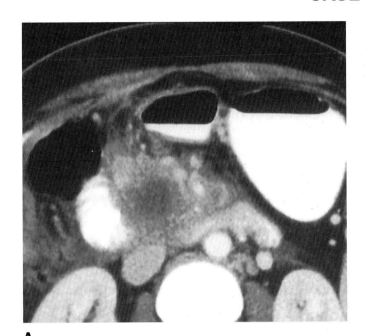

A

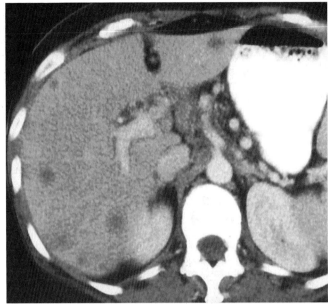

B

Findings

Contrast-enhanced CT. **A.** There is a large hypoattenuating mass in the region of the pancreatic head. The superior mesenteric vein is occluded. The superior mesenteric artery is encased, and there is mass effect on the medial aspect of the duodenum. **B.** Multiple hepatic metastases and periportal lymphadenopathy are visible.

Differential Diagnosis

Nonresectable ductal adenocarcinoma

Diagnosis

Nonresectable ductal adenocarcinoma

Discussion

Nonresectability usually is determined on the basis of vascular invasion by the tumor (superior mesenteric artery encasement, extensive involvement or occlusion of the superior mesenteric vein, or splenic vein occlusion), regional lymphadenopathy, and hepatic metastases or peritoneal metastases. In this case, vascular, lymphatic, and hepatic criteria are met, and thus the tumor is nonresectable. Radiographic staging is highly beneficial, because patients with advanced disease can be spared unnecessary operation.

CASE 8.33

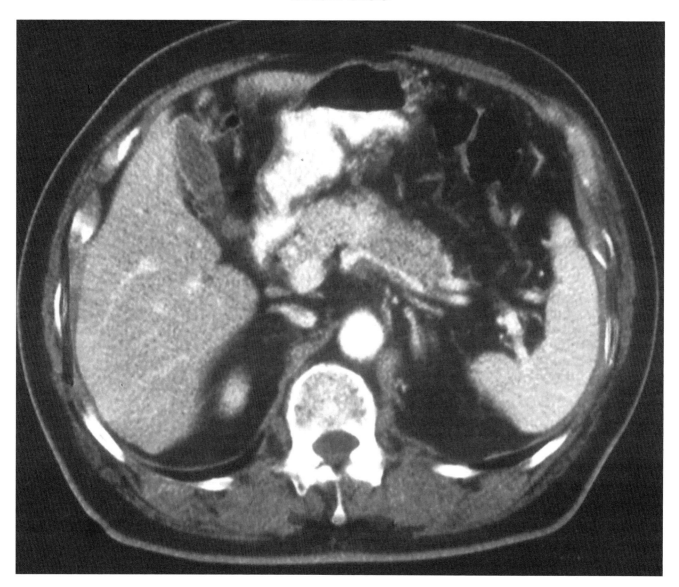

Findings

Contrast-enhanced CT. A large hypoattenuating region is present in the body and tail of the pancreas. The splenic vein is narrowed and encased by soft tissue.

Differential Diagnosis

1. Ductal adenocarcinoma
2. Focal pancreatitis

Diagnosis

Ductal adenocarcinoma

Discussion

Pancreatic tumors may not deform the contour of the gland (as in this case). Detection usually depends on a difference in enhancement between the tumor and the pancreatic parenchyma. Texture differences between the normal parenchyma that may contain fatty marbling and a solid tumor also may be a clue to the presence of a mass.

Encasement of the splenic artery and vein without involvement of the celiac axis or superior mesenteric artery usually requires a distal pancreatectomy and splenectomy. In such cases, multiple upper abdominal collaterals often are visible.

CASE 8.34

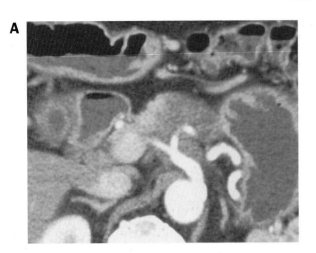

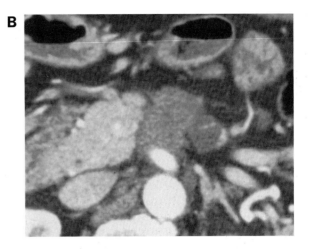

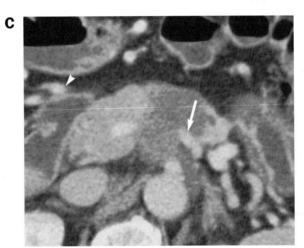

Findings

A and **B.** Contrast-enhanced CT (pancreatic phase). An infiltrating low-attenuation mass is present in the body of the pancreas and encases the celiac axis and superior mesenteric artery.

C. Contrast-enhanced CT (portal venous phase). The low-attenuation pancreatic mass has occluded the splenic vein (arrow), and multiple associated collateral vessels are seen in the upper abdomen (arrowhead).

Differential Diagnosis

Ductal adenocarcinoma

Diagnosis

Ductal adenocarcinoma (nonresectable)

Discussion

Pancreatic ductal adenocarcinomas arising in the body or tail of the gland often result in splenic vein occlusion. Multiple collateral vessels in the upper abdomen in a patient with pancreatic adenocarcinoma are highly suggestive of tumor-related venous occlusion and should prompt a careful evaluation of the portal, splenic, and mesenteric veins. Dual-phase pancreatic imaging clearly shows the arterial encasement and venous occlusion in this case, which renders this pancreatic adenocarcinoma nonresectable.

CASE 8.35

A
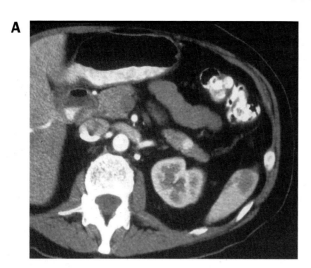

B
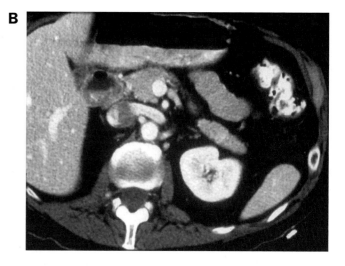

Findings

Contrast-enhanced CT. Biphasic arterial (**A**) and portal venous (**B**) phases of enhancement. During the arterial phase of contrast enhancement, there is a small hypervascular mass within the pancreatic tail. The mass is isoattenuating with the remainder of the pancreas during the portal venous phase.

Differential Diagnosis

1. Islet cell tumor
2. Hypervascular metastasis

Diagnosis

Islet cell tumor, insulinoma

Discussion

Islet cell tumors of the pancreas are rare pancreatic neoplasms. It is important to try to differentiate them from ductal tumors because their prognosis and treatment are different. Islet cell tumors are slow-growing neoplasms; more than 60% of patients are alive 10 years after the initial diagnosis. This contrasts with ductal tumors, with which there are very few 5-year survivors.

Islet cell tumors usually can be differentiated from ductal tumors by their vascularity, propensity to calcify, and their lack of vascular encasement. Islet cell tumors usually are hypervascular neoplasms and enhance briskly during the early phases of contrast enhancement. Because these tumors are slow-growing, calcification can be found in many

of them. Calcification is highly unusual among ductal tumors. Malignant islet cell tumors metastasize to regional lymph nodes and the liver, as is the case with ductal tumors, but vascular encasement and neural invasion are rare.

Clinically, islet cell tumors can be classified as hyperfunctioning or nonhyperfunctioning. The hyperfunctioning tumors are most commonly insulinomas and gastrinomas. Other unusual hyperfunctioning tumors include glucagonomas, somatostatinomas, and others producing a mixture of hormones. These tumors usually are recognized because of the clinical syndrome associated with hormone overproduction. Imaging is used to localize the tumor that is known to be present. Nonhyperfunctioning islet cell tumors are not associated with a clinical syndrome and usually are discovered incidentally or as a result of nonspecific clinical symptoms. Because of the lack of symptoms prompting early investigation, these tumors often are larger and many have metastasized at the time of diagnosis.

The patient described here had an insulinoma, the commonest hyperfunctioning tumor. These tumors are benign, solitary, and less than 2 cm in diameter in 90% of patients. This case illustrates the importance of scanning during the arterial phase of contrast enhancement to detect these hypervascular tumors at CT. Sonography, especially intraoperative sonography, is useful for the detection of these tumors. Reports also exist of successful detection with MRI.

CASE 8.36

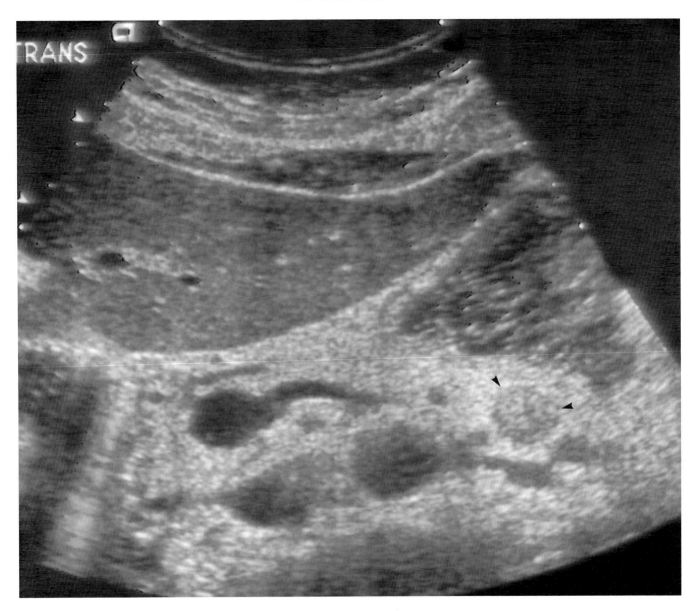

Findings

Sonogram. Transverse view of the pancreas with water in the stomach (arrowheads) shows a single, well-defined, hypoechoic mass in the tail of the pancreas.

Differential Diagnosis

1. Islet cell tumor
2. Other hypoechoic pancreatic mass

Diagnosis

Islet cell tumor, insulinoma

Discussion

This case shows the importance of having the patient drink water before a sonographic examination for pancreatic islet cell tumor. The insulinoma in this case is easily visualized in the tail of the pancreas deep to the fluid-filled stomach. Visualization of the distal body and tail of the pancreas is often impossible if the stomach is gas-filled. Insulinomas most often are hypoechoic compared with the pancreas.

CASE 8.37

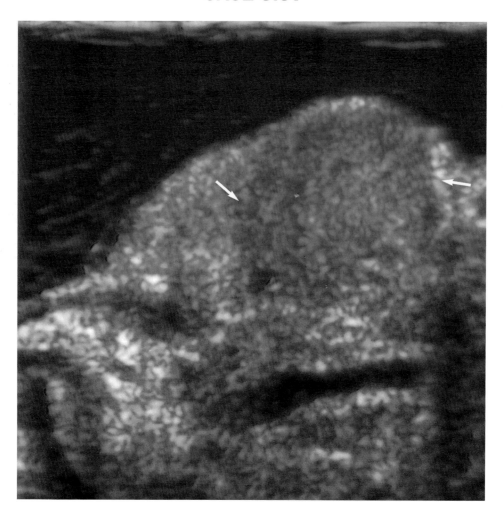

Findings

Intraoperative sonogram. A well-defined hypoechoic mass (arrows) is present in the head of the pancreas anterior to the main pancreatic duct.

Differential Diagnosis

1. Islet cell tumor
2. Ductal adenocarcinoma

Diagnosis

Islet cell tumor, insulinoma

Discussion

Intraoperative sonography is very sensitive for detecting insulinomas. Studies have shown a near 100% sensitivity for detection of insulinomas with the combination of intraoperative ultrasonography and palpation of the gland. In addition to detection of pancreatic tumors, intraoperative ultrasonography is a valuable tool for evaluating the relationship of the tumor to the pancreatic duct. When an adequate margin of normal pancreatic tissue is present between the mass and the pancreatic duct, an enucleation procedure is performed. Without an adequate margin, a partial pancreatectomy is performed. Intraoperative ultrasonography also is used commonly after tumor enucleation to assess for damage to the pancreatic duct. A normal dilated pancreatic duct after intravenous administration of secretin is highly suggestive of an intact duct.

CASE 8.38

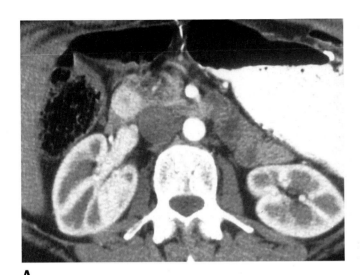

A

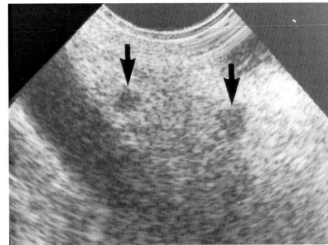

B

Findings

A. Contrast-enhanced CT (arterial phase). An enhancing mass is present in the region of the duodenum.

B. Intraoperative sonogram. Two tiny hypoechoic masses are present in the pancreas (arrows).

Differential Diagnosis

1. Hypervascular metastases
2. Duodenal gastrointestinal stromal tumor
3. Islet cell tumors

Diagnosis

Islet cell tumors, multiple gastrinomas

Discussion

Gastrinomas arise outside the pancreas in about half of all patients and can be multiple. These tumors usually are confined to a region known as the gastrinoma triangle—defined by corners at the ampulla of Vater, junction of the cystic duct and common bile duct, and the junction of the neck and body of the pancreas. The tumors vary in size from 1 to 20 mm in diameter. Some gastrinomas arise within lymph nodes in the gastrinoma triangle. Although the tumor visualized at CT in this patient is large, the additional small millimeter-sized tumors visualized at sonography are very challenging to detect.

About half of all gastrinomas arise in patients with multiple endocrine neoplasia type 1. These tumors tend to be multiple and small. They are less aggressive than those occurring sporadically.

CASE 8.39

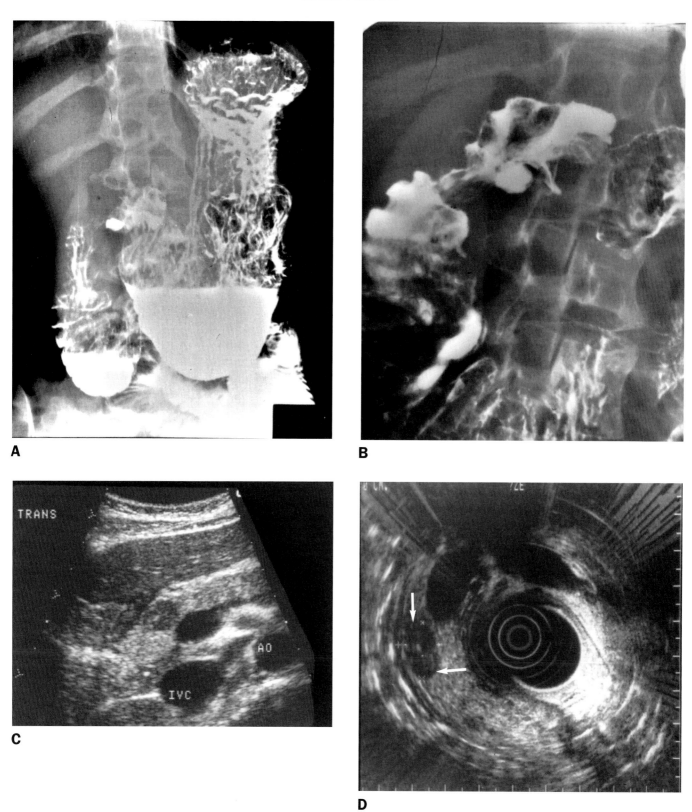

A

B

C

D

Findings

Double-contrast UGI. **A** and **B.** There is an excess amount of fluid in the stomach, which contains multiple thickened folds. There is an ulcer in the duodenal bulb. The duodenum is dilated and contains excess fluid.

C. Transverse sonogram of the pancreas. There is a 1-cm hypoechoic mass within the neck of the pancreas. AO, aorta; IVC, inferior vena cava.

D. Endoscopic sonogram. A 1-cm hypoechoic mass (arrows) in the neck of the pancreas is confirmed.

Differential Diagnosis

Islet cell tumor, gastrinoma

Diagnosis

Islet cell tumor, gastrinoma

Discussion

Gastrinomas are responsible for the Zollinger-Ellison syndrome. Affected patients have overproduction of gastrin and excess stomach acid with subsequent thickening of the folds of the stomach, gastritis, duodenitis, peptic ulcer disease, and esophagitis. Although ulcerations can be found anywhere in the stomach or duodenum, the duodenal bulb is the commonest location. Nearly three-fourths of gastrinomas are malignant. These tumors can be multiple, and many occur in an extrapancreatic location (usually within the gastric antrum or proximal duodenum). Most are less than 2 cm in diameter. Because of their small size, multiplicity, and extrapancreatic location, they are difficult to detect with standard cross-sectional imaging tools. These tumors usually have a high concentration of somatostatin receptors, and the majority can be detected with octreotide scintigraphy.

CASE 8.40

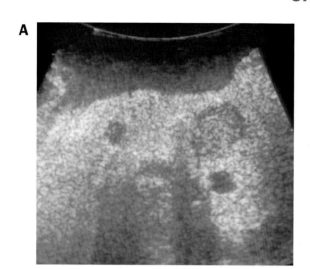

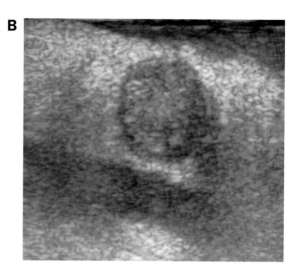

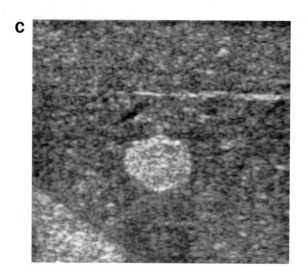

Findings

Intraoperative sonogram. **A.** Three well-defined
hypoechoic masses are present in the body and tail of
the pancreas. **B.** This coned-down view of one of these
pancreatic lesions with a higher-frequency transducer
more clearly shows the tumor anterior to the splenic vein.
C. A well-defined hyperechoic mass is present in the liver
with mild associated posterior acoustic shadowing.

Differential Diagnosis

Metastatic islet cell neoplasm

Diagnosis

Metastatic islet cell tumors, metastatic gastrinoma

Discussion

Intraoperative ultrasonography is extremely sensitive for
the evaluation of islet cell tumors. Islet cell tumors usually
present as small, well-defined hypoechoic lesions. Unlike
the primary tumors, metastatic islet cell lesions tend to be
echogenic. The echogenic liver lesion in this case was
metastatic gastrinoma. Echogenic hepatic lesions in the
setting of islet cell neoplasm should be considered metastases
until proved otherwise. The posterior acoustic shadowing
behind the echogenic hepatic lesion (in this case) should
be another clue that this does not likely represent a cavernous
hemangioma.

CASE 8.41

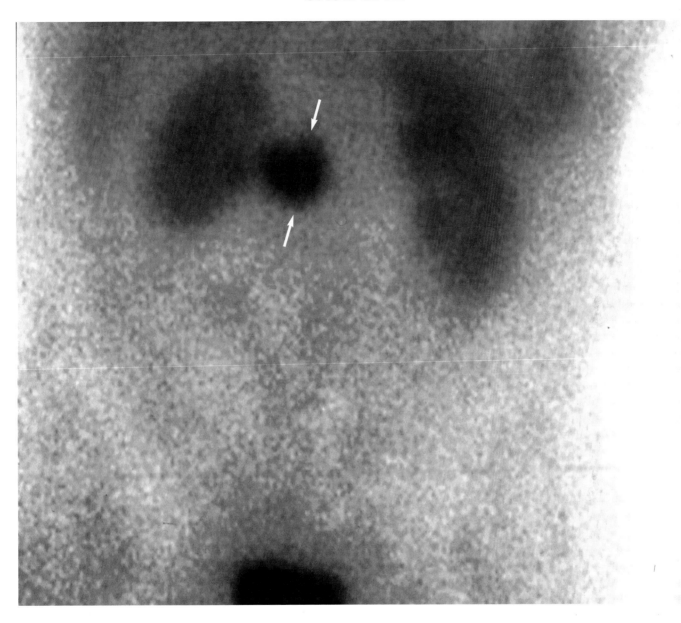

Findings
Indium-111-diethylenetriamine pentaacetic acid-octreotide scintigram. Abnormal uptake in the region of the pancreatic head (arrows).

Differential Diagnosis
Islet cell tumor

Diagnosis
Islet cell tumor: gastrinoma

Discussion
Octreotide scintigraphy is helpful for the diagnosis of gastrinomas because of the high concentration of somatostatin receptors within these tumors. This is a highly useful test to localize the gastrinoma in patients with Zollinger-Ellison syndrome. Other neuroendocrine tumors also have a high affinity for octreotide.

Hyperfunctioning Islet Cell Tumors

Type	Key clinical symptoms
Insulinoma	Hypoglycemia: sweating, trembling, palpitations, nervousness
Gastrinoma	Abdominal pain, diarrhea, vomiting, hematemesis, melena, weight loss
Glucagonoma	Necrolytic erythema migrans, diarrhea, diabetes, glossitis
Vipoma	WDHA syndrome: watery diarrhea, hypokalemia, achlorhydria
Somatostatinoma	Diarrhea, steatorrhea, weight loss

CASE 8.42

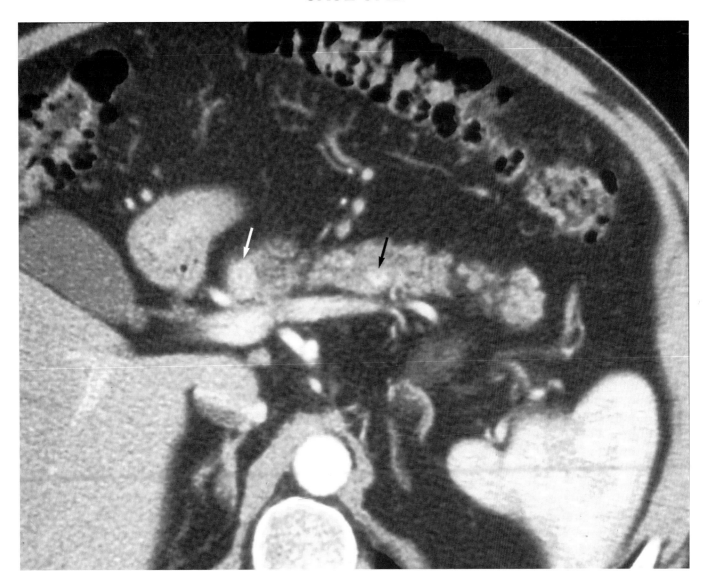

Findings
Contrast-enhanced CT. There are two small hyperenhancing masses within the body of the pancreas (arrows).

Differential Diagnosis
Multiple endocrine neoplasia type 1 with multiple islet cell tumors

Diagnosis
Multiple endocrine neoplasia type 1 with multiple islet cell tumors

Discussion
Patients with multiple endocrine neoplasia type 1 have an inherited disorder of tumors arising in the pancreas (multiple islet cell tumors), parathyroid gland, and pituitary gland. Islet tumors behave differently from those arising sporadically. They are usually small, multiple, and biologically less aggressive. The small size of the tumors makes complete detection very difficult, even with intraoperative sonography.

CASE 8.43

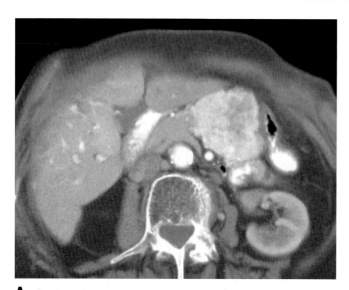

A

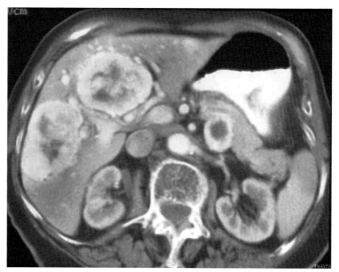

B

Findings
Contrast-enhanced CT. **A** and **B.** A hyperenhancing mass is in the body of the pancreas. An enlarged peripancreatic lymph node is present posterior to the pancreatic body, and two larger, but similar-appearing masses, are present in the liver.

Differential Diagnosis
1. Islet cell tumor with metastases
2. Metastases to the pancreas and liver (primary unknown)

Diagnosis
Islet cell tumor with metastases—nonhyperfunctioning

Discussion
Nonhyperfunctioning islet cell tumors are not associated with a clinical syndrome and often present with nonspecific abdominal complaints. Usually a large mass is detected in the pancreas. It can be distinguished from ductal cancer because of its hyperenhancement, lack of vascular encasement, and propensity to calcify. Treatment usually is symptomatic. Large tumors that do not respond to symptomatic therapy may be treated with embolization as a nonoperative approach to debulking these large masses.

CASE 8.44

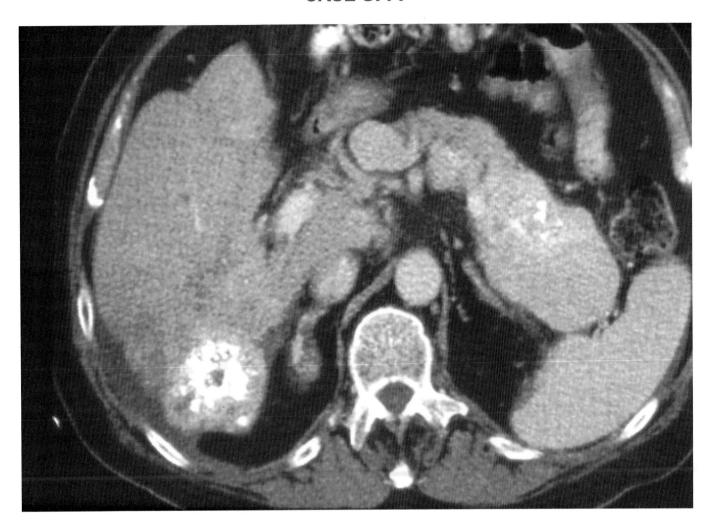

Findings

Contrast-enhanced CT (portal venous phase). There is a large mass in the body and tail of the pancreas. The mass contains calcification and enhances similarly to the spleen. A calcified mass also is present in the right lobe of the liver.

Differential Diagnosis

Nonhyperfunctioning calcified islet cell carcinoma

Diagnosis

Nonhyperfunctioning calcified islet cell carcinoma

Discussion

This case exemplifies the typical nonhyperfunctioning pancreatic islet cell tumor. Its large size and calcification without vascular encasement are characteristic of the tumor. Liver metastases also can calcify, indicating the slow growth of these lesions. The calcification usually is coarse and dystrophic in appearance.

CASE 8.45

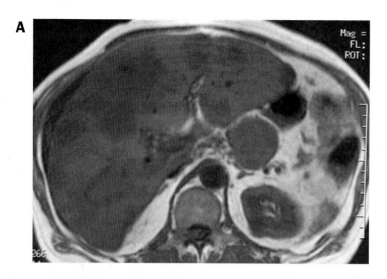

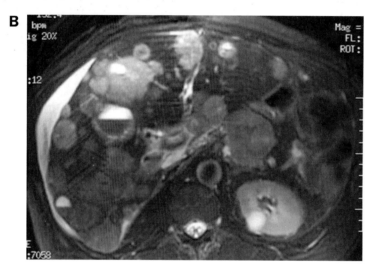

Findings

Abdominal MRI. **A.** T1-weighted MRI. A 4-cm mass is present in the body of the pancreas. There are multiple hepatic metastases. **B.** T2-weighted MRI shows multiple hyperintense masses that correspond to those seen on the T1-weighted image. The masses in the liver are of variable intensity. Some contain a fluid-fluid layer. Ascites.

Differential Diagnosis

1. Islet cell carcinoma with hepatic metastases
2. Neuroendocrine metastases to liver and pancreas

Diagnosis

Islet cell carcinoma with hepatic metastases

Discussion

This case is a typical example of a malignant nonhyper-functioning islet cell tumor at MRI. MRI is useful to follow patients with this tumor because in many cases oral and intravenous contrast material are not necessary for assessing the size and progression of the lesions. In addition, because these hepatic lesions can become isoattenuating at CT, MRI is an optimal technique for completely evaluating the full extent of the tumors. The fluid-fluid layers in the hepatic metastases are commonly seen in hypervascular metastases, especially neuroendocrine metastases (islet cell, carcinoid, pheochromocytoma).

CASE 8.46

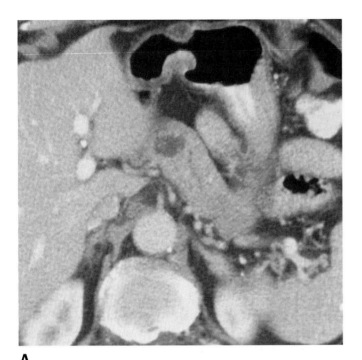

A

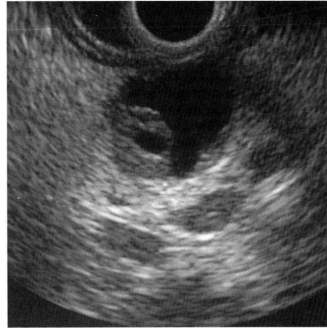

B

Findings

A. Contrast-enhanced CT. A cystic mass is present in the body of the pancreas. The pancreatic duct proximal to the mass is mildly dilated.

B. Endoscopic sonogram. The mass is predominantly cystic but contains a mural nodule.

Differential Diagnosis

1. Ductal adenocarcinoma
2. Cystic metastases to the pancreas
3. Cystic islet cell tumor
4. Mucinous cystic neoplasm of the pancreas

Diagnosis

Cystic islet cell tumor

Discussion

Islet cell tumors usually are solid lesions. Large tumors often undergo central necrosis and calcification but retain a rim of hyperenhancing tissue. Rarely, islet cell tumors appear cystic (water density) without evidence of hyperenhancement (as in this case). The sonogram reveals the complex (containing a septation and nodule) cystic nature of the mass. According to standard CT criteria, this most likely would have been a ductal adenocarcinoma or cystic mucinous neoplasm. If the patient had a clinical syndrome associated with an islet cell tumor, then the radiologist should be suspicious that this is a cystic islet cell variant. The sonographic appearance of this mass is most consistent with a mucinous cystic neoplasm.

Features of Ductal Adenocarcinoma and Islet Cell Tumors

Feature	Ductal	Islet cell
Size	≤4 cm	0.5 mm-10 cm
Vascularity	Hypovascular	Hypervascular
Vascular encasement	Common	Rare
Calcification	Rare	Common
Ductal dilatation	Common	Possible (mass effect)

CASE 8.47

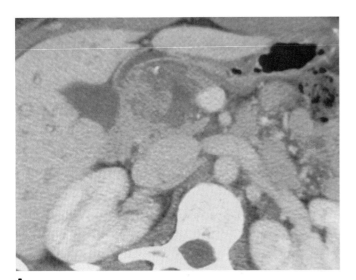

A

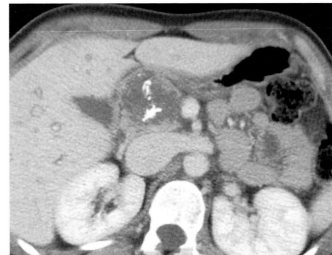

B

Findings

Contrast-enhanced CT. **A** and **B**. A mixed solid and cystic mass is present in the head of the pancreas. The inferior portion of this mass is predominantly cystic and contains coarse calcifications centrally.

Differential Diagnosis

1. Mucinous cystadenocarcinoma
2. Serous cystadenoma, atypical
3. Solid and papillary epithelial neoplasm
4. Islet cell tumor

Diagnosis

Solid and papillary epithelial neoplasm

Discussion

Solid and papillary epithelial neoplasms are rare tumors found almost exclusively in young women. These tumors can be predominantly cystic or solid or a combination of both. Intratumoral calcification is common, as in this case. The tumor usually is curable with surgical resection.

CASE 8.48

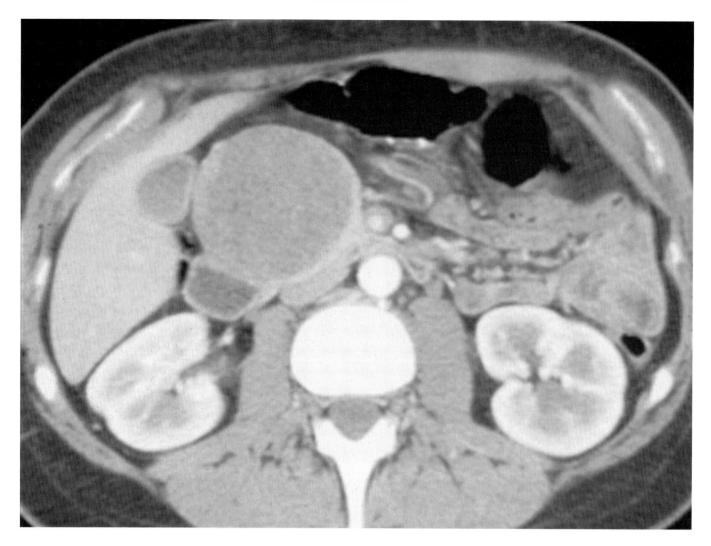

Findings
Contrast-enhanced CT. A large, well-circumscribed, low-attenuation mass is present in the head of the pancreas. A rim of solid soft tissue is present near its periphery.

Differential Diagnosis
1. Mucinous cystadenocarcinoma
2. Serous cystadenoma, atypical
3. Solid and papillary epithelial neoplasm
4. Metastasis

Diagnosis
Solid and papillary epithelial neoplasm

Discussion
This rare tumor can resemble other, more common pancreatic tumors. The key to recognizing this tumor is a consistent history. It is most commonly found in young (average age, 24 years) females, often those of African descent. The tumor usually is curable with resection. At CT, it can be predominantly cystic or solid or a mixture. Intratumoral calcification occurs often. The cystic regions often are due to hemorrhage within the mass. At MRI, regions of high signal can be seen on the T1-weighted image.

CASE 8.49

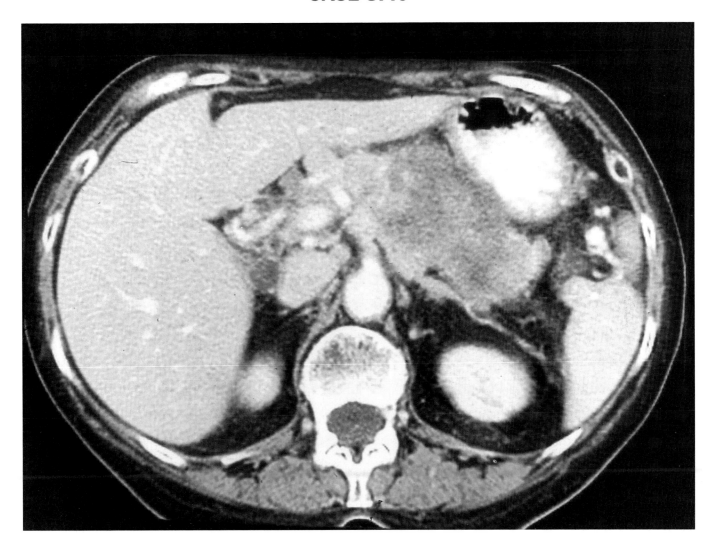

Findings

Contrast-enhanced CT. A large mixed-attenuation mass is present in the body of the pancreas. Enlarged lymph nodes are present about the celiac axis.

Differential Diagnosis

1. Ductal adenocarcinoma
2. Islet cell carcinoma
3. Acinar cell carcinoma

Diagnosis

Acinar cell carcinoma

Discussion

Acinar cell carcinoma is a rare pancreatic tumor. It usually is identified at an advanced stage in older men. No specific symptoms are associated with this tumor, but occasionally patients present with metastatic fat necrosis due to the systemic release of lipase by the tumor. It usually presents as a larger tumor than ductal cancers and may be more encapsulated (less desmoplastic response compared with ductal cancer).

CASE 8.50

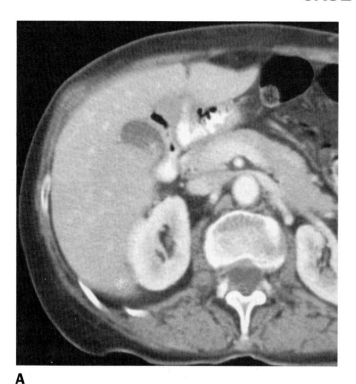

A

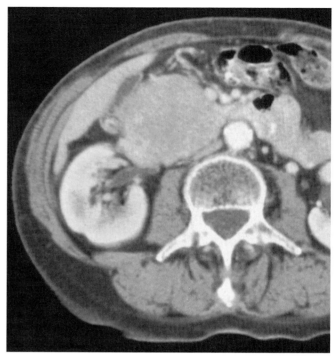

B

Findings
Contrast-enhanced CT. **A** and **B.** A 6-cm mass is present in the head and uncinate process of the pancreas. The mass is well circumscribed with mild homogeneous enhancement and no associated vascular encasement or pancreatic or biliary duct dilatation.

Differential Diagnosis
1. Atypical ductal adenocarcinoma
2. Atypical islet cell tumor
3. Lymphoma
4. Acinar cell carcinoma
5. Metastasis

Diagnosis
Primary pancreatic lymphoma

Discussion
Non-Hodgkin lymphoma of the pancreas is rare and constitutes less than 1% of all pancreatic tumors. The pancreas is more commonly involved as a component of widespread lymphatic disease rather than as the primary location of tumor.

Several features of the mass in this case are extremely atypical for the more common solid pancreatic tumors, including ductal adenocarcinoma and islet cell tumor. The well-defined nature of the tumor, lack of encasement of adjacent vascular structures, and lack of pancreatic duct and biliary duct obstruction should be strong evidence that this is unlikely to be a ductal adenocarcinoma. Nonhyperfunctioning islet cell tumors (case 8.43) can be large but usually have heterogeneous hyperenhancement. Cystic components and tumoral calcification are common. In contrast, pancreatic lymphomas usually present as large, mildly enhancing homogeneous masses. Lymphadenopathy or splenomegaly (not seen in this case) also favors the diagnosis of pancreatic lymphoma. Biopsy usually is necessary to make the diagnosis. Pancreatic non-Hodgkin lymphoma generally is treated with chemotherapy with or without radiation.

CASE 8.51

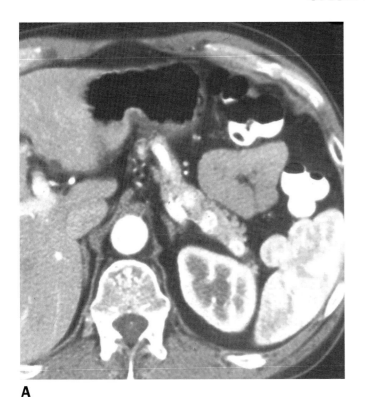

A

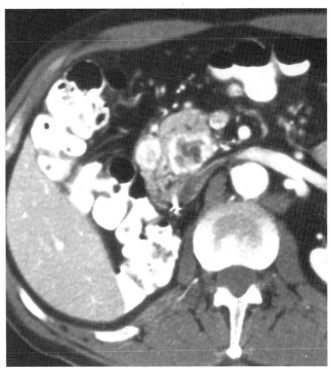

B

Findings

Contrast-enhanced CT (pancreatic phase of enhancement).
A and **B.** Multiple hyperenhancing masses are present
throughout the pancreas. The patient has had a right
nephrectomy.

Differential Diagnosis

1. Pancreatic metastases
2. Multiple islet cell tumors

Diagnosis

Pancreatic metastases, renal adenocarcinoma primary

Discussion

The pancreas is an uncommon location for metastases,
with the exception of renal adenocarcinoma and melanoma,
which have a propensity to spread to this organ. Other
tumors such as lung cancer and various soft tissue sarcomas
also can spread to the pancreas.

CASE 8.52

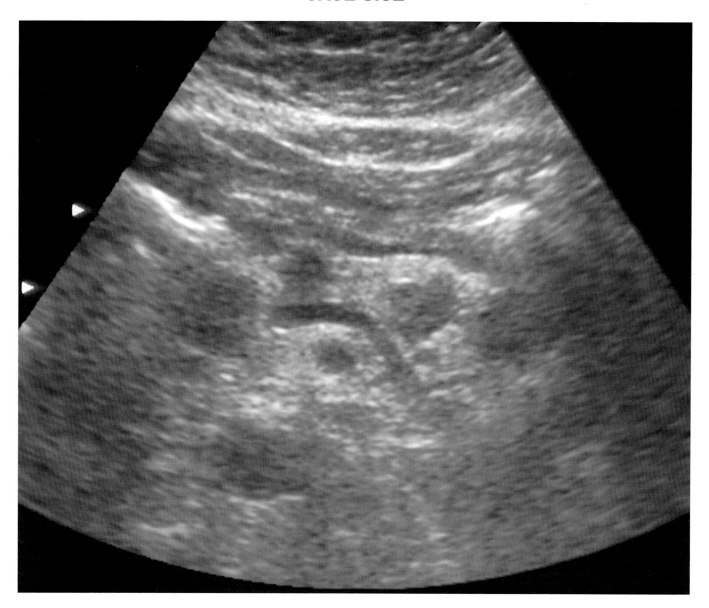

Findings
Sonogram. Transverse view of the pancreas shows four hypoechoic masses.

Differential Diagnosis
1. Islet cell tumors
2. Metastases
3. Lymphoma

Diagnosis
Pancreatic metastases, melanoma primary

Discussion
Pancreatic metastases are rare and found in only 3% of autopsies in patients with proven malignancy. Melanoma (as in this case) and metastatic renal adenocarcinoma have a propensity to involve the pancreas. However, other evidence of metastatic disease usually is present in addition to the pancreatic metastases. Pancreatic non-Hodgkin lymphoma also can present as multiple hypoechoic pancreatic masses. Concomitant intra-abdominal lymphadenopathy often is present.

Solid Masses of the Pancreas

		Case
Ductal adenocarcinoma	Hypoattenuating mass. Ductal obstruction. Vascular encasement	8.24–8.34
Islet cell tumor	Hyperenhancing mass. Calcification. No vascular encasement. Clinical syndrome helpful	8.35–8.46
Solid and papillary epithelial neoplasm	Solid and cystic mass. Calcification common. Young women	8.47 and 8.48
Acinar cell carcinoma	Hypoenhancing mass. Usually larger than ductal adenocarcinoma. Older men. Fat necrosis	8.49
Lymphoma	Large, well-defined, homogeneous, mildly enhancing mass. Bulky lymphadenopathy or splenomegaly	8.50
Metastases	Renal carcinoma most common, hypervascular	8.51 and 8.52
Focal pancreatitis	Isoattenuating or hypoattenuating mass. Peripancreatic inflammatory changes. Clinical correlation important	8.4

CASE 8.53

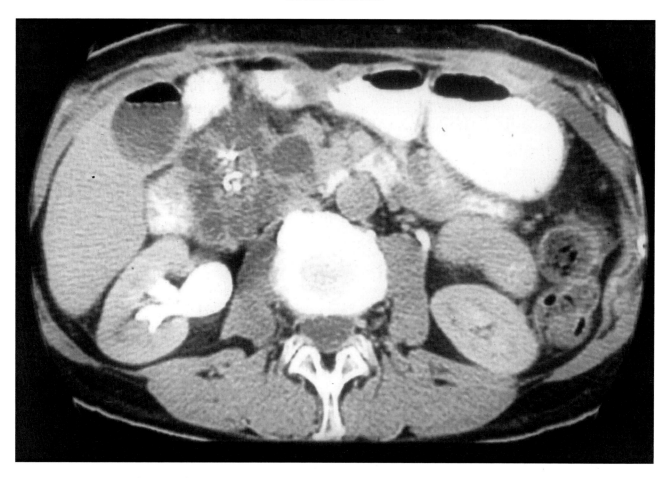

Findings
Contrast-enhanced CT. A large mass is present within the pancreatic head. The mass contains multiple small cysts and septal calcifications.

Differential Diagnosis
Serous cystadenoma

Diagnosis
Serous cystadenoma

Discussion
Cystic masses of the pancreas are classified as either serous cystadenomas or mucinous cystic neoplasms. With few exceptions, serous cystadenomas are benign tumors that do not require resection unless symptomatic. Mucinous cystic neoplasms are considered premalignant (mucinous cystadenoma) or malignant (mucinous cystadenocarcinoma).

Differentiation of these tumors can be important because the treatment is potentially different (serous tumors can be observed; mucinous tumors are removed whenever possible). Differentiation of these tumors is not always possible, but some general rules can be helpful. Serous tumors have a honeycombed appearance, containing many (≥ 6) small (<2 cm) cysts. Occasionally, larger cysts are present in a serous tumor, but the majority of the cysts should be small. Mucinous tumors isolated from the main pancreatic duct usually have a few (<6) large (≥ 2 cm) cysts. Both types of tumors can contain calcification(s). Septal calcification is typical of a serous tumor. A central scar is sometimes found with a serous tumor.

In this patient, the typical features of a serous tumor are present. The mass contains multiple small cysts. A few of the cysts are large, but the majority are less than 2 cm. Septal calcification is present.

CASE 8.54

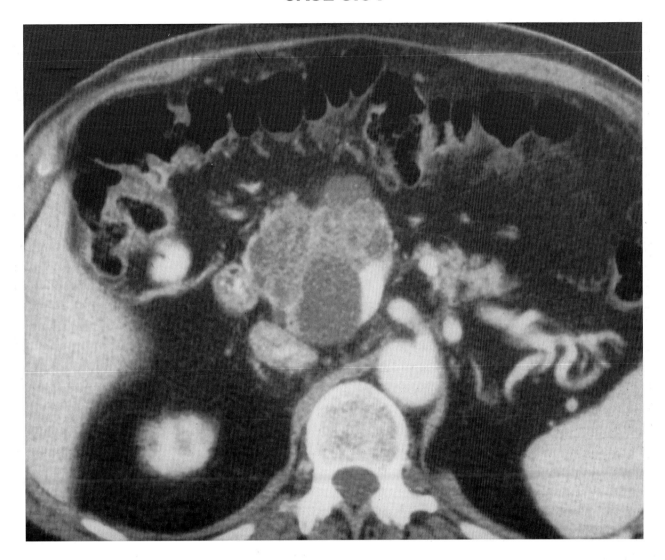

Findings

Contrast-enhanced CT. There is a large cystic mass in the pancreatic head. The mass contains both small and large cysts. A central region appears solid.

Differential Diagnosis

1. Serous cystadenoma
2. Mucinous cystic neoplasm
3. Cystic—indeterminate neoplasm

Diagnosis

Cystic—indeterminate neoplasm (serous cystadenoma pathologically)

Discussion

Some cystic neoplasms appear with features of both serous and mucinous subtypes. In this case the tumor contains both small and large cysts. These types of tumors probably are best classified as a cystic—indeterminate mass. Further evaluation with biopsy can be helpful. Core biopsy of the septations can be diagnostic. Other centers analyze the cyst aspirate for levels of CA19-9. The level of serum CA19-9 is not increased in benign mucinous lesions; however, it is increased in both malignant and inflammatory conditions (pancreatic pseudocyst). As a result, we do not routinely measure it in aspirated cyst fluid. Our experience has shown that the majority of these indeterminate lesions are serous cystadenomas.

CASE 8.55

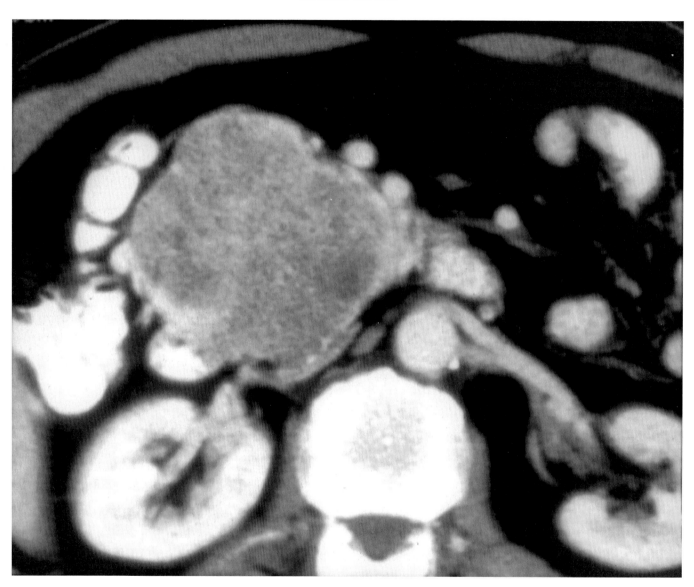

Findings
Contrast-enhanced CT. There is a low-attenuation mass in the pancreatic head. The mass is well circumscribed. A few cysts are identifiable within the mass.

Differential Diagnosis
1. Serous cystadenoma
2. Mucinous cystic neoplasm

Diagnosis
Serous cystadenoma

Discussion
Serous cystadenomas can contain cysts that are so small they approach or are below the spatial resolution of the CT scanner. The mass may appear to be predominantly solid. In this case, a few cysts are definitely detectable. The low attenuation of the mass is a clue to its cystic nature. The innumerable enhancing septations make the mass appear pseudosolid. These lesions also can appear solid at sonography because of the many acoustic interfaces present within the mass. MRI is useful for proving the cystic nature of the mass. These lesions will be of very high intensity on T2-weighted images.

CASE 8.56

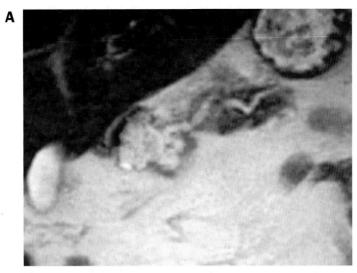

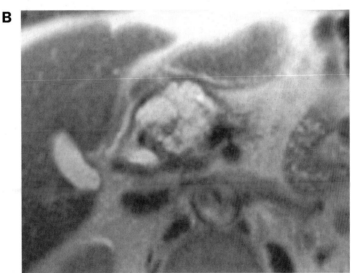

Findings

Pancreatic MRI without intravenous contrast enhancement.
A and **B**. There is a 4-cm mass in the pancreatic head with
pancreatic ductal dilatation proximal to the mass. The
mass is of very high signal intensity on T2-weighted images
(**A** and **B**). The contour is lobulated (**A**), and the mass
appears septated (**B**).

Differential Diagnosis

Serous cystadenoma

Diagnosis

Serous cystadenoma

Discussion

Pancreatic masses that are indeterminate at CT and
sonography can sometimes be better characterized at MRI.
Serous tumors, because of their cystic nature, are of high
signal intensity on T2-weighted images (and of low signal
on T1-weighted images). These tumors are well
circumscribed. If the many septations that divide the tumor
into a honeycomb appearance or a central scar can be
identified (as in this case), a serous cystadenoma is suggested.

CASE 8.57

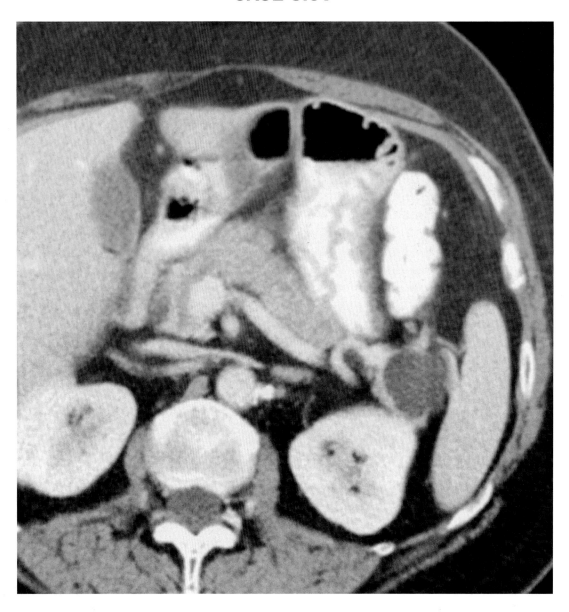

Findings
Contrast-enhanced CT. A 4-cm cystic mass bulges within the tail of the pancreas. The mass is slightly lobulated but appears unilocular without septations.

Differential Diagnosis
1. Mucinous cystic neoplasm
2. Pseudocyst

Diagnosis
Mucinous cystadenoma

Discussion
Mucinous tumors isolated from the pancreatic duct usually have a few cysts (<6) that are 2 cm or more in diameter. This mass resembles a pseudocyst. Historical context is important, because patients with a recent episode of pancreatitis probably should have their mass followed, because it most likely represents a pseudocyst. Patients without a history of pancreatitis most likely have a mucinous tumor. Findings of thick septations and mural nodules are worrisome for a mucinous cystadenocarcinoma.

CASE 8.58

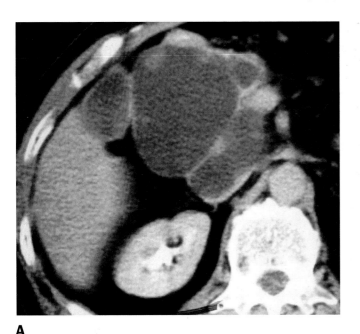

A

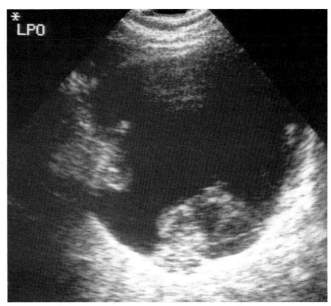

B

Findings

A. Contrast-enhanced CT. There is a large cystic mass in the pancreatic head. The mass contains a few loculations and multiple enhancing nodules.

B. Transabdominal sonogram. A large cystic mass contains multiple mural nodules.

Differential Diagnosis

1. Mucinous cystic neoplasm
2. Metastasis

Diagnosis

Mucinous cystadenocarcinoma

Discussion

This case illustrates typical features of a mucinous tumor with a few large cystic spaces. The mural nodules are a worrisome finding for malignancy.

CASE 8.59

A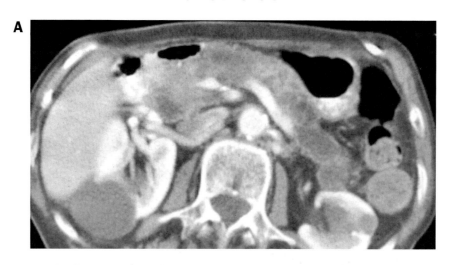

B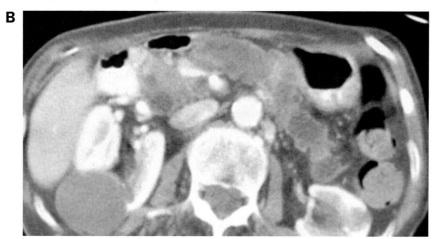

Findings

Contrast-enhanced CT. **A** and **B.** The main pancreatic duct is massively dilated throughout the pancreas.

Differential Diagnosis

1. Duodenal carcinoma
2. Ampullary neoplasm
3. Ductal adenocarcinoma
4. Intraductal pancreatic mucinous neoplasm
5. Chronic pancreatitis

Diagnosis

Intraductal pancreatic mucinous neoplasm

Discussion

Mucinous tumors develop in isolation from the pancreatic duct or they arise within the main pancreatic duct or its side branches. Intraductal tumors are slow-growing tumors and can be multicentric. As a well-differentiated neoplasm, they usually produce mucin that dilates the involved ducts. The small villous tumors may be detectable as frondlike enhancing filling defects within the dilated pancreatic duct. Chronic obstruction can lead to pancreatic parenchymal atrophy. Rarely, the mucin calcifies. The pathognomonic finding is the presence of mucin emanating from the papilla of Vater at ERCP.

Neoplastic obstruction of the duct usually is associated with a mass. Ductal dilatation in chronic pancreatitis is usually less severe and often associated with multiple ductal calcifications.

CASE 8.60

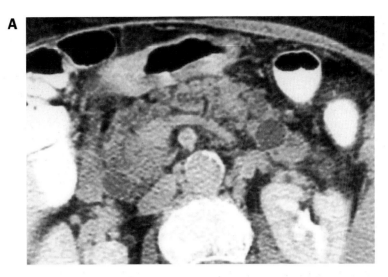

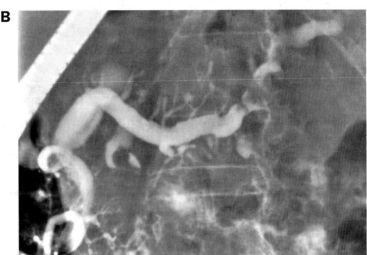

Findings

A. Contrast-enhanced CT. There are several cystic masses within the pancreas.

B. ERCP. The main and side branches of the pancreatic duct are dilated. There is a filling defect within the main pancreatic duct in the pancreatic tail.

Differential Diagnosis

1. Intraductal pancreatic mucinous neoplasm
2. Chronic pancreatitis

Diagnosis

Intraductal pancreatic mucinous neoplasm

Discussion

ERCP remains the standard for the diagnosis of intraductal pancreatic mucinous neoplasm. Pancreatic ductal dilatation with filling defect(s) is the main radiographic finding. Mucin flowing from the papilla of Vater is pathognomonic at ERCP. It is usually impossible to differentiate the ductal filling defects as mucin or tumor. At CT, the intraductal mucin can mimic solid tissue attenuation (as in this case). This case illustrates the occasional difficulty in recognizing the continuously dilated pancreatic duct. In patients with equivocal CT findings, ERCP is recommended.

CASE 8.61

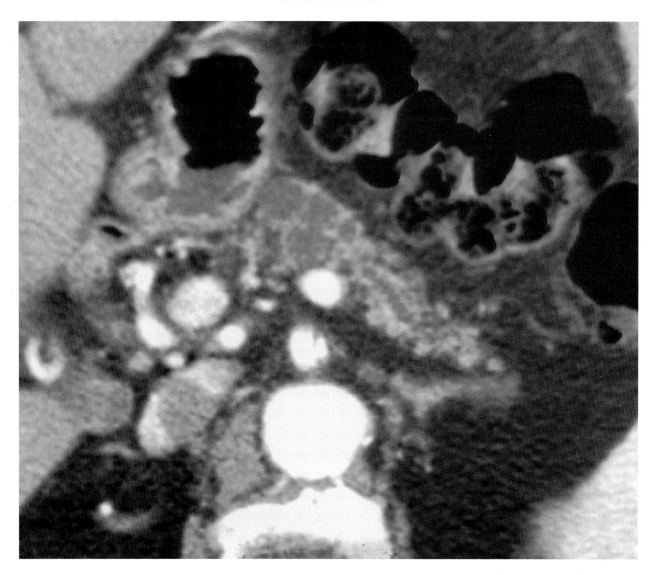

Findings
Contrast-enhanced CT. There is a multicystic mass arising from the body of the pancreas. Mild pancreatic ductal dilatation is present proximal to the mass.

Differential Diagnosis
1. Serous cystadenoma
2. Intraductal pancreatic mucinous neoplasm, side branch variant

Diagnosis
Intraductal pancreatic mucinous neoplasm, side branch variant

Discussion
Mucinous neoplasms arising in the pancreatic side branch ducts can be difficult to diagnose with cross-sectional imaging techniques. In many cases, they have a unilocular or multilocular appearance similar to serous or mucinous cystic tumors. ERCP is the best test to make a definitive diagnosis. MRCP also might be helpful. Identification of a dilated side branch duct, with or without a filling defect, is typical of intraductal pancreatic mucinous neoplasm arising in a side branch. Ductal dilatation due to mass effect, or as a consequence of excess mucin production, can occur. Some authors have referred to these branch duct neoplasms as "ductectatic" mucinous cystadenomas.

CASE 8.62

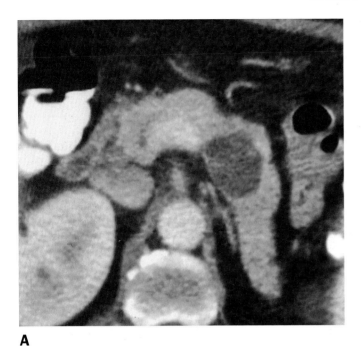

A

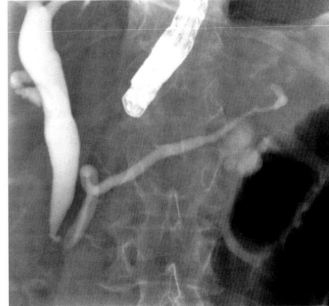

B

Findings

A. Contrast-enhanced CT. There is a 2.5-cm cystic mass within the body of the pancreas. The mass contains enhancing tissue.

B. ERCP. A cyst fills with contrast material from a pancreatic duct side branch within the pancreatic body.

Differential Diagnosis

1. Intraductal pancreatic mucinous neoplasm arising from a pancreatic duct side branch
2. Pseudocyst

Diagnosis

Intraductal pancreatic mucinous neoplasm arising from a pancreatic duct side branch

Discussion

At CT or MRCP, it is often very difficult to determine definitively whether the cystic mass communicates with the pancreatic ductal system. ERCP is the best technique for this question. All mucinous cystic neoplasms have similar histologic features and biologic behavior. Treatment is also similar for all of these tumors, in that surgical excision is preferred, if possible. In this case, the main pancreatic duct appears normal but there is filling of a mass from a pancreatic side branch. The nodular enhancing tissue within the mass at CT suggests its neoplastic nature.

Mucinous Cystic Neoplasms: Subtypes

Location relative to pancreatic duct	Appearance
Isolated from pancreatic duct	Few large cysts; mural nodules and thick septations in cystadenocarcinoma
Arising within main pancreatic duct	Dilated main pancreatic duct, enhancing filling defects in pancreatic duct, mucin from papilla of Vater
Arising within pancreatic duct side branches	Dilated side branches can resemble mucinous or serous subtype, with or without main duct dilatation

Features of Serous and Mucinous Cystic Pancreatic Tumors

Feature	Serous cystadenoma	Mucinous cystadenoma
No. of cysts	≥ 6	<6
Size of majority of cysts, cm	<2	≥ 2
Calcification	Septal	Dystrophic
Metastases	No	Possible
Mural nodules	No	Cystadenocarcinoma
Central scar	Yes	No

CASE 8.63

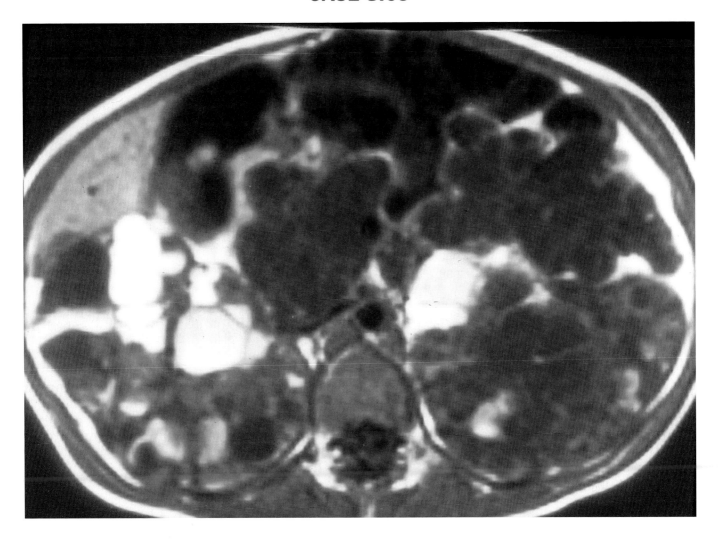

Findings

T1-weighted MRI. Diffuse cystic changes throughout both kidneys and the pancreas. Many of the cysts in the kidneys are of high signal intensity.

Differential Diagnosis

1. Polycystic renal disease
2. von Hippel-Lindau disease

Diagnosis

Polycystic renal disease

Discussion

Adult polycystic kidney disease is an autosomal dominant disease affecting more than 600,000 Americans and an estimated 12.5 million people worldwide. The disease causes multiple cysts on each kidney which enlarge and multiply over time. Kidneys progressively increase in size and, ultimately, renal failure occurs.

One-third of patients have cysts within their liver, and a smaller percentage have pancreatic cysts. Cysts developing in the pancreas and liver do not usually impair organ function.

CASE 8.64

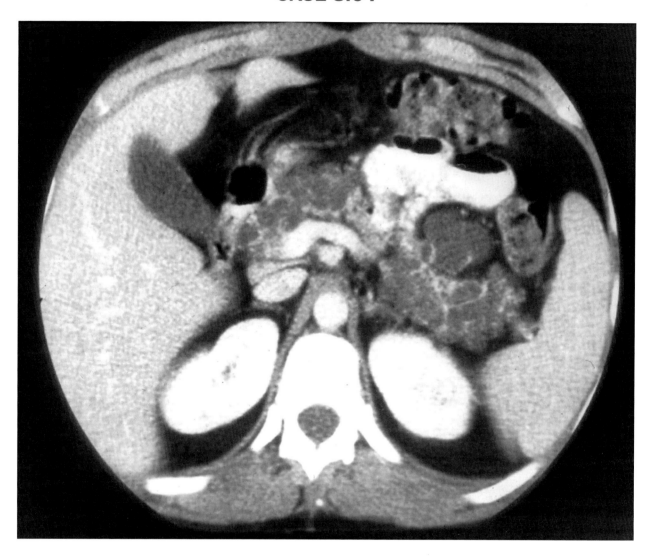

Findings
Contrast-enhanced CT. The pancreas is replaced with innumerable tiny cysts.

Differential Diagnosis
1. Polycystic kidney disease
2. von Hippel-Lindau disease

Diagnosis
von Hippel-Lindau disease

Discussion
Von Hippel-Lindau disease is an autosomal dominant multisystem inherited disorder. The commonest manifestations include retinal, cerebellar, spinal, and medullary hemangioblastomas, renal cysts and carcinoma, pancreatic cysts, pheochromocytoma, and papillary cystadenoma of the epididymis. Patients also have an increased incidence of serous cystadenomas and islet cell tumors of the pancreas.

The onset of the disease occurs in early adulthood; retinal cancers develop at an average age of 25 years, cerebellar cancers at 30 years, and renal cancers at 37 years. In families with a high incidence of pheochromocytomas, adrenal tumors usually develop initially. Death usually occurs from hemangioblastomas or renal adenocarcinomas.

The patient in this case has the typical findings of diffuse pancreatic cytosis found in von Hippel-Lindau disease.

Cystic Masses of the Pancreas

		Case
Serous cystadenoma	≥6 cysts. <2 cm for majority of cysts. Honeycombed, central scar. Septal calcifications	8.53–8.56
Mucinous cystadenoma or cystadenocarcinoma	<6 cysts total. Majority ≥2 cm in diameter. Mural nodules and thick septations favor cystadenocarcinoma	8.57 and 8.58
Intraductal pancreatic mucinous neoplasm	May arise in main duct or side branch ducts	8.59–8.62
Solid and papillary epithelial neoplasm	Can be predominantly cystic or solid or a combination. Calcification common. Young African women	8.48
Cystic islet cell tumor	Unusual presentation, resembles mucinous tumor. Usually retains rim of hyperenhancing tissue. Clinical syndrome helpful	8.46
Polycystic renal disease	Disease obvious with renal cysts. Pancreatic cysts in 20%	8.63
von Hippel-Lindau disease	Pancreatic cystosis, islet cell, serous cystadenoma. Renal adenocarcinoma. Pheochromocytoma. Retinal or cerebellar hemangioblastomas	8.64
Pseudocyst	Fluid collection >6 weeks after acute pancreatitis. Persistent communication with pancreatic duct. Fibrous wall	8.6
Abscess	Poorly defined fluid collection that may contain gas	8.10

CASE 8.65

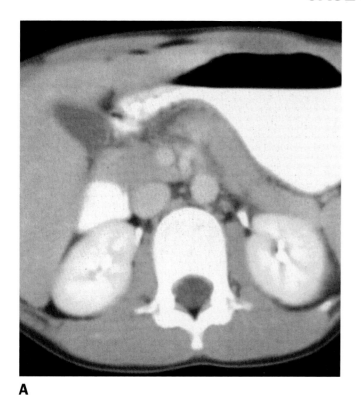

A

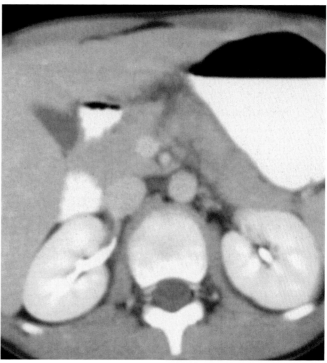

B

Findings

Contrast-enhanced CT. **A** and **B**. There is a linear low-attenuation defect between the head and body of the pancreas with a small amount of peripancreatic fluid.

Differential Diagnosis

1. Pancreatic laceration or transection
2. Pancreatitis with pseudocyst

Diagnosis

Pancreatic transection

Discussion

Pancreatic trauma is usually due to gunshot wounds, direct blows to the abdomen, or high-speed automobile accidents.

The boy in this case injured his abdomen by falling on the handlebars of his bicycle. The mortality from these injuries approaches 20% and is nearly always associated with other abdominal injuries. Symptoms can be minor, but typically the symptoms mimic acute pancreatitis.

CT is usually used to make the diagnosis. Imaging features may mimic acute pancreatitis with diffuse or focal gland enlargement and soft tissue stranding and thickening. Occasionally, a hyperdense mass due to a hematoma is detected near the laceration. A low-attenuation defect within the gland is good evidence for a laceration. Lacerations most often occur between the neck and body of the gland. These changes can be subtle, and good CT technique with intravenous contrast material and thin collimation is important for optimal detection.

CASE 8.66

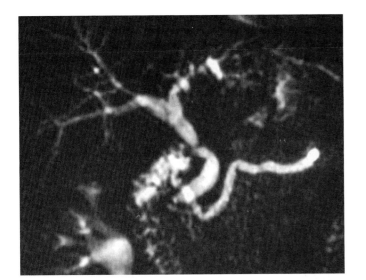

CASE 8.67

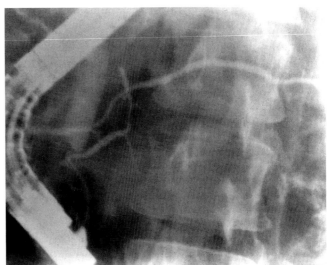

Findings

Case 8.67. MRCP. The pancreatic duct is uniformly dilated and empties via the accessory papilla into the duodenum.

Case 8.68. ERCP. Both the dorsal and the ventral pancreatic ducts have been filled. There is no communication between these ducts.

Differential Diagnosis

Pancreas divisum

Diagnosis

Pancreas divisum

Discussion

Pancreas divisum is a congenital anomaly of the pancreas in which the embryologic dorsal and ventral portions of the pancreas fail to fuse completely. As a result, the dorsal pancreatic enlage (drained by the duct of Santorini) does not communicate with the ventral pancreas (drained by the duct of Wirsung). The duct of Santorini empties via the accessory papillae (as in this case). The duct of Wirsung empties into the major papilla. Some authorities believe that patients with pancreas divisum have a higher incidence of pancreatitis because the main pancreatic duct does not empty normally.

CASE 8.68

A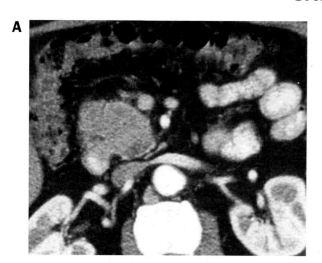

B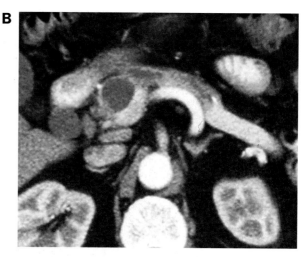

C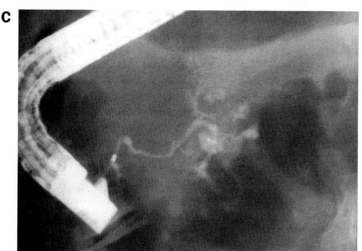

Findings

Contrast-enhanced CT. **A.** The head of the pancreas is generous in size but of normal homogeneous attenuation. **B.** The pancreatic duct in the body of the pancreas is dilated to the level of a well-defined fluid collection.

C. ERCP. Only the duct of the ventral pancreas is opacified with injection of the major papilla.

Differential Diagnosis

1. Pancreas divisum with an obstructing pseudocyst
2. Pancreas divisum with a mucinous cystic neoplasm

Diagnosis

Pancreas divisum with an obstructing pseudocyst

Discussion

Pancreas divisum is believed to predispose to acute pancreatitis because the body and tail of the pancreas must drain by the smaller accessory papilla. The relative obstruction predisposes to pancreatitis. In this patient, a well-defined pseudocyst (the sequela of prior acute pancreatitis) is present in the body of the pancreas. The mass effect from the pseudocyst causes dilatation of the duct in the body and tail of the pancreas. ERCP is diagnostic of pancreas divisum with opacification of the small, rapidly arborizing ventral pancreatic duct. Although a mucinous cystic neoplasm could have this appearance, it is much less likely with pancreas divisum.

CASE 8.69

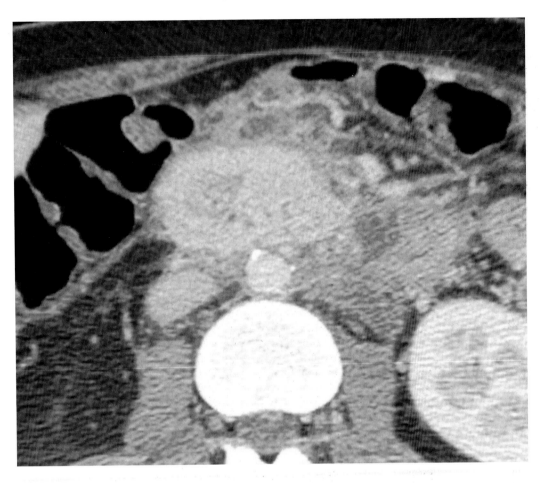

Findings

Contrast-enhanced CT. The pancreatic head is enlarged and contains a central region of low attenuation. Fluid and soft tissue stranding are present within the peripancreatic soft tissues.

Differential Diagnosis

1. Acute pancreatitis
2. Annular pancreas with pancreatitis

Diagnosis

Annular pancreas with acute pancreatitis

Discussion

Annular pancreas is a congenital anomaly. Two theories exist about the abnormal embryologic development of the pancreas. One theory postulates that the ventral pancreas fails to atrophy, thereby encircling the duodenum. The other theory states that the ventral pancreas becomes adherent to the duodenum and is stretched around it as it rotates into normal position. About half of patients present with this abnormality as neonates, whereas the other half present during adulthood. Symptoms are due to duodenal obstruction. Adult patients and older children remain asymptomatic until the duodenal lumen is critically narrowed from either peptic ulcer disease (25%-50%) or pancreatitis (15%-30%). A gastrojejunostomy usually is performed to relieve the obstruction.

ERCP is usually the definitive test, showing the ventral pancreatic duct encircling the duodenum with a normal duct in the body and tail of the gland. In this case, the enhancing pancreatic tissue can be seen to encircle the duodenum (the low-attenuation region within the pancreas). The duodenal nature of the low-attenuation region was confirmed by tracing it on consecutive slices.

CASE 8.70

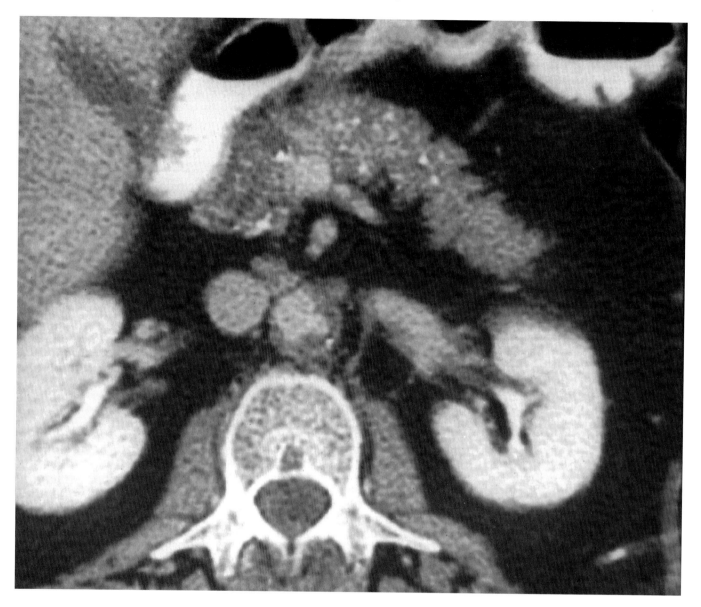

Findings
Contrast-enhanced CT. Multiple tiny calcifications are present throughout the pancreas.

Differential Diagnosis
1. Histoplasmosis
2. Sarcoidosis
3. Chronic pancreatitis

Diagnosis
Sarcoidosis

Discussion
Sarcoidosis involving the abdomen is an unusual finding. Abnormalities in the abdomen may or may not be associated with changes in the chest typical of sarcoidosis. Abdominal findings include hepatosplenomegaly, lymphadenopathy, and calcifications in the liver, spleen, and pancreas. Other granulomatous diseases could present in a similar fashion. These findings are unusual for chronic pancreatitis because the calcifications are not intraductal and are not associated with ductal dilatation.

Miscellaneous Pancreatic Conditions

		Case
Transection	Resembles acute pancreatitis with history of abdominal trauma	8.65
Pancreas divisum	Rapid arborization of the ventral pancreatic duct with injection of the major papilla. Dorsal duct fills from minor papilla. Perhaps predisposes to pancreatitis	8.66–8.68
Annular pancreas	Pancreatic tissue or duct encircles the duodenum	3.37 and 8.69
Sarcoidosis	Scattered nonductal calcifications	8.70

DIFFERENTIAL DIAGNOSES

Solid Pancreatic Masses

Ductal adenocarcinoma
Islet cell tumor
Solid and papillary epithelial
  neoplasm
Acinar cell carcinoma
Metastases
Lymphoma

Cystic Pancreatic Masses

Pseudocyst
Serous cystadenoma
Mucinous cystadenoma or
  cystadenocarcinoma
Intraductal pancreatic mucinous
  neoplasm
Solid and papillary epithelial
  neoplasm
Cystic islet cell tumor
Polycystic kidney disease
Von Hippel-Lindau disease
Abscess

Pancreatic Calcifications

Chronic pancreatitis
Islet cell tumor
Serous cystadenoma
Mucinous cystic neoplasm
Solid and papillary epithelial
  neoplasm
Granulomatous infection

SOLID PANCREATIC MASSES

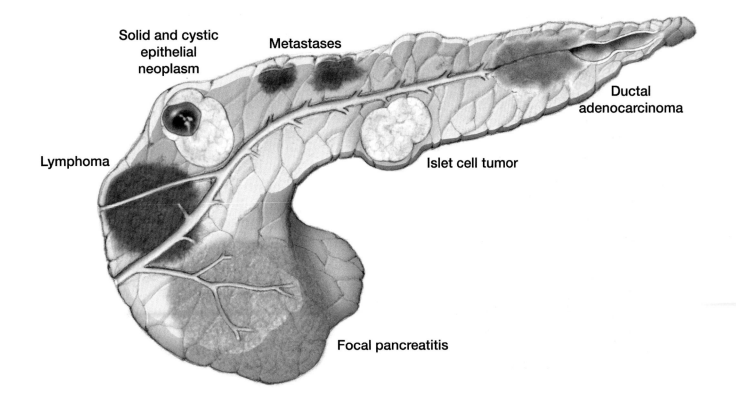

Solid and cystic
epithelial
neoplasm

Metastases

Ductal
adenocarcinoma

Lymphoma

Islet cell tumor

Focal pancreatitis

CYSTIC PANCREATIC MASSES

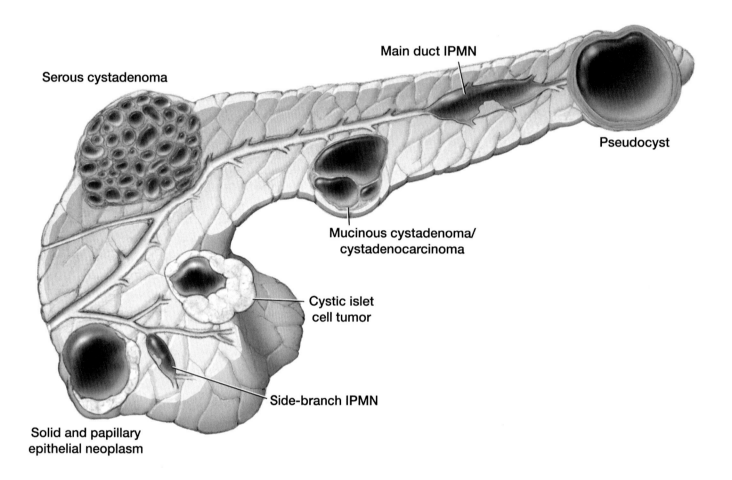

IPMN, intraductal pancreatic mucinous neoplasm.

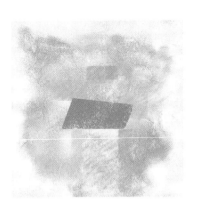

CHAPTER 9

SPLEEN

CASE 9.1

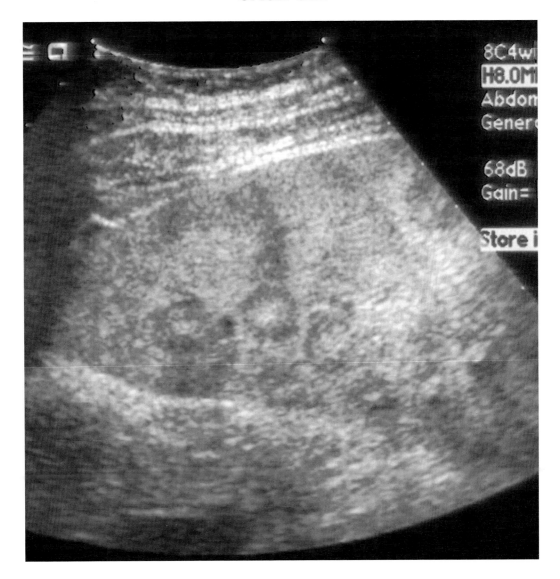

Findings

Sonogram of the spleen. Multiple target lesions are present throughout the spleen.

Differential Diagnosis

1. Metastases
2. Lymphoma
3. *Candida* microabscesses
4. Mycobacterial infection

Diagnosis

Candida microabscesses

Discussion

Fungal infections involving the liver and spleen usually develop in immunocompromised persons receiving chemotherapy. These infections can be difficult to detect with imaging studies because of their small size. In 50% of blood cultures, results are negative. In these cases, biopsy and histologic confirmation of infection may be necessary.

The typical target or bull's-eye lesion at sonography is an echogenic center surrounded by a hypoechoic band. As the lesions heal, they often become homogeneously hypoechoic. Most lesions are 5 to 10 mm in diameter. The finding of similar-appearing lesions in the liver or kidneys is helpful to suggest *Candida* infection.

CASE 9.2

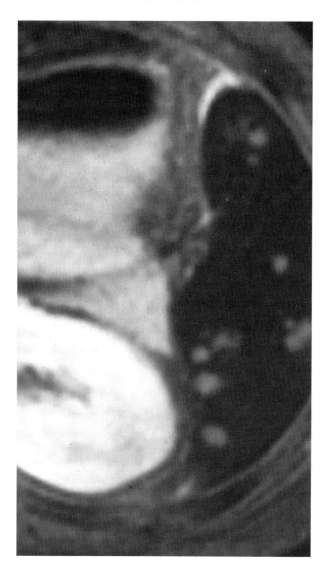

Findings

T2-weighted unenhanced MRI. The spleen is of abnormally low signal intensity. There are multiple tiny high-intensity masses throughout.

Differential Diagnosis

1. Metastases
2. Lymphoma
3. *Candida* microabscesses
4. Mycobacterial infection

Diagnosis

Candida microabscesses and hemosiderosis

Discussion

In patients with suspected *Candida* microabscesses and a negative abdominal sonogram, MRI can be helpful to assess for these tiny abscesses. This patient had received multiple transfusions for a hematopoietic malignancy, and hemosiderosis (secondary hemochromatosis) had developed. Excess iron from transfusions is accumulated in the reticuloendothelial system and lowers the splenic signal. Suppression of the normal splenic signal increases contrast and visibility of the high-signal microabscesses.

CASE 9.3

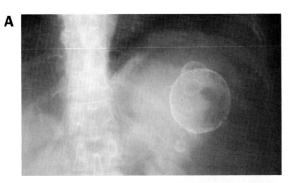

A

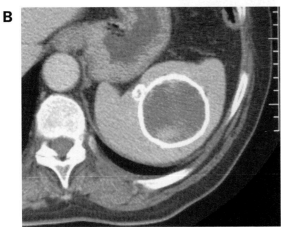

B

CASE 9.4

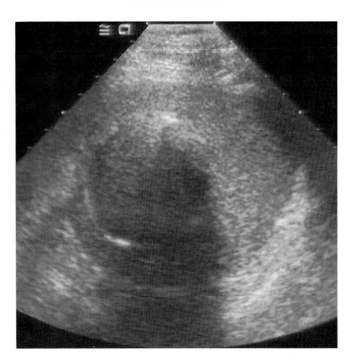

Findings

Case 9.3. A. Abdominal radiograph. Several peripherally calcified masses of variable size are present in the spleen.

B. Contrast-enhanced CT. The peripherally calcified masses contain water-attenuation fluid.

Case 9.4. Splenic sonogram. A large mass is present in the spleen. The rim of the mass is hyperechoic, and there is a strong acoustic shadow from the rim indicating calcification.

Differential Diagnosis
1. Echinococcal cysts
2. Traumatic splenic cyst
3. Intrasplenic aneurysm
4. Metastases

Diagnosis
Echinococcal cysts

Discussion

Splenic involvement in patients with echinococcal disease is unusual—occurring in less than 2% of patients with this disease. Liver, lung, bone, and brain are more commonly involved. Splenic involvement usually is due to systemic dissemination or intraperitoneal spread. *Echinococcus granulosus* is the most common form to affect the spleen, with sharply defined cysts and daughter cysts. *Echinococcus multilocularis* presents with tiny cystic masses that have the appearance of an invasive malignancy. Liver cysts usually are present if splenic cysts exist.

Sonographic findings include anechoic splenic cysts with or without daughter cysts. Calcification of the wall (as in this case) is helpful. Occasionally the abnormality presents as a solid mass. CT is helpful for showing a cyst with subtle wall calcification. The interior attenuation of the cyst may be higher than water because of the presence of hydatid sand and inflammatory cells.

Positive radiographic findings, clinical suspicion in patients from an endemic area, and positive serologic tests are most helpful for making the diagnosis.

CASE 9.5

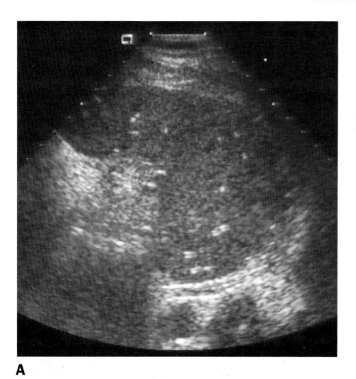

A

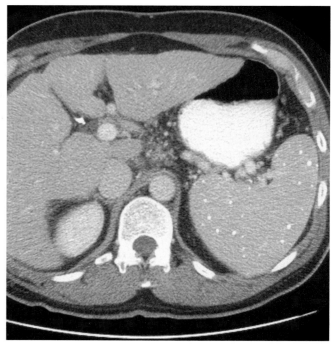

B

Findings

A. Abdominal sonogram. Multiple tiny hyperechoic masses are present throughout the spleen.

B. Contrast-enhanced CT. Multiple tiny calcifications are present in the spleen.

Differential Diagnosis
1. Healed granulomatous infection
2. *Candida* microabscesses
3. Extrapulmonary *Pneumocystis* infection
4. Treated lymphoma
5. Treated metastases

Diagnosis
Healed granulomatous infection, histoplasmosis

Discussion
Multiple calcified granulomas in the spleen are common, and they are usually the sequelae of healed infection from prior histoplasmosis. Radiographically similar findings can be found in patients with healed tuberculosis, *Mycobacterium avium-intracellulare*, and sarcoidosis and patients who have had infection with *Pneumocystis carinii*. Multiple punctate calcifications could develop in patients who have had successful treatment for lymphoma and metastases with splenic involvement.

CASE 9.6

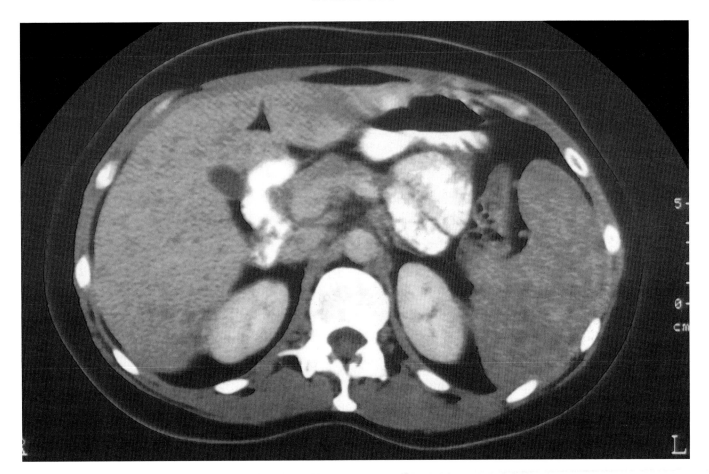

Findings

Contrast-enhanced CT (delayed). Multiple hypoattenuating masses are present throughout the spleen and liver.

Differential Diagnosis

1. Metastases
2. Lymphoma
3. Candidiasis
4. Mycobacterial infection
5. Granulomatous infection

Diagnosis

Granulomatous infection, sarcoidosis

Discussion

Sarcoidosis is a disease of unknown cause that usually affects the lung and mediastinum. Abdominal sarcoidosis is unusual; when it occurs, it can affect the solid organs of the abdomen and lymph nodes. Although pulmonary involvement is often present concurrently, it is not required. Sarcoid can present in various ways, with hepatosplenomegaly, multiple low-attenuation filling defects within the solid organs (as in this case), diffuse calcifications, or lymphadenopathy.

Inflammatory Diseases of the Spleen

		Case
Candidiasis	Multiple tiny low-attenuation splenic lesions. Target appearance on sonography. Liver also usually involved. Immunosuppressed patients	9.1 and 9.2
Echinococcal cysts	Peripherally calcified cyst and daughter cysts. Liver disease usually present when spleen is involved. Usually from endemic area	9.3 and 9.4
Healed granulomatous infection, histoplasmosis	Multiple tiny calcified splenic granulomas. Calcified granulomas in the lungs and calcified hilar and mediastinal nodes often present	9.5
Sarcoidosis	Multiple tiny hypoattenuating splenic lesions. Chronic changes can result in calcified splenic granulomas. Adenopathy may be present	9.6

CASE 9.7

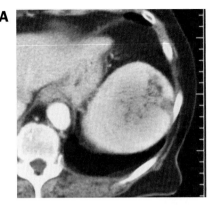

A

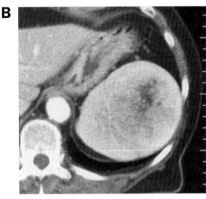

B

CASE 9.8

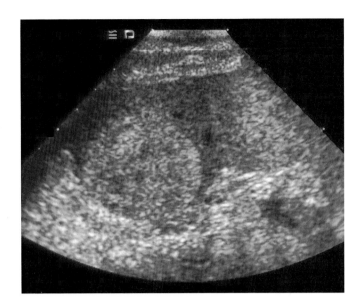

Findings

Case 9.7. Contrast-enhanced CT. **A** and **B.** A large, well-defined, solitary hyperenhancing mass is present in the spleen. Several hypoattenuating regions are present within the mass.

Case 9.8. Abdominal sonogram. A solitary, moderately heterogeneous echogenic mass is present within the spleen.

Differential Diagnosis

1. Metastases
2. Lymphoma
3. Hemangioma
4. Hamartoma

Diagnosis

Hemangioma

Discussion

Hemangiomas of the spleen have many of the same characteristics as hemangiomas within the liver. They are the most common benign tumor to affect the spleen. They are usually incidental findings. Pathologically, splenic hemangiomas are similar, with endothelium-lined vascular spaces of various sizes. Kasabach-Merritt syndrome may occur with large hemangiomas—with findings of anemia, infarction, high-output congestive heart failure, thrombocytopenia, and coagulopathy.

Although hemangiomas may enhance after intravenous contrast material in a pattern similar to that of hepatic hemangiomas, our experience is that this occurs in a minority of cases. In most instances, a heterogeneously enhancing mass is discovered which has nonspecific imaging characteristics. In these cases, comparison with prior films or follow-up imaging to assess for growth can be helpful. The sonographic appearance of hemangiomas is also similar to that found in the liver. These lesions are usually echogenic, but they may appear more complex. If necessary, percutaneous biopsy can be performed safely.

CASE 9.9

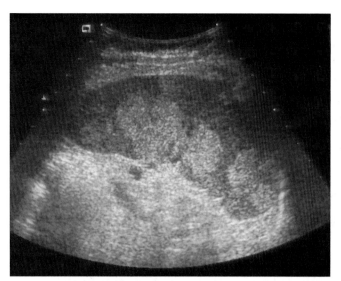

A

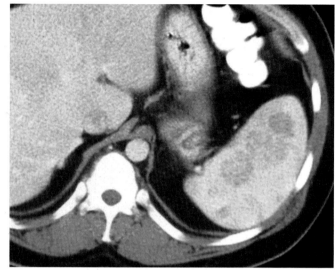

B

Findings

A. Abdominal sonogram. Multiple homogeneous echogenic masses are present throughout the spleen.

B. Contrast-enhanced CT. Several masses are present in the spleen. Some of these masses contain globular enhancement.

Differential Diagnosis

1. Hemangiomas
2. Metastases
3. Lymphoma

Diagnosis

Multiple hemangiomas

Discussion

Hemangiomas are usually solitary but can be multiple. Splenic hemangiomas can be part of generalized angiomatosis (Klippel-Trénaunay-Weber syndrome) or associated with the Kasabach-Merritt syndrome. They also have been reported to be associated with portal venous hypertension.

CASE 9.10

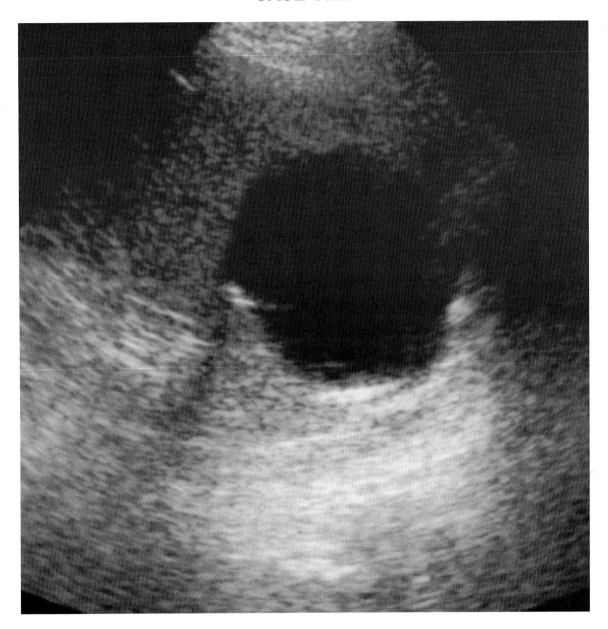

Findings
Abdominal sonogram. A well-defined anechoic mass with posterior acoustic enhancement is present within the spleen. The mass contains a dependent septation.

Differential Diagnosis
Benign splenic cyst

Diagnosis
Benign splenic cyst

Discussion
Splenic cysts are usually anechoic structures with well-defined walls and increased through-transmission at sonography. Intracystic debris due to hemorrhage can be seen within these lesions. Septations (trabeculation) are seen in up to one-third of cysts.

CASE 9.11

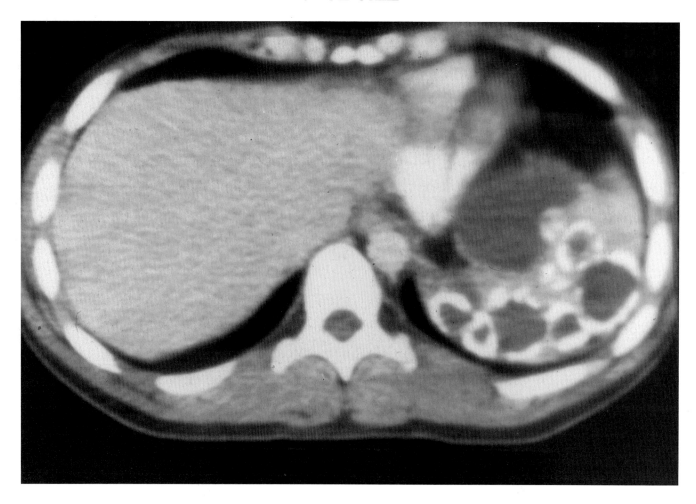

Findings
Contrast-enhanced CT. Multiple peripherally calcified cysts are present throughout the spleen.

Differential Diagnosis
1. Epidermoid cyst
2. Parasitic cyst
3. Secondary cyst

Diagnosis
Epidermoid cysts

Discussion
Splenic cysts are divided pathologically into either true (with a cellular lining) or false (without a cellular lining) cysts. True cysts that are not parasitic in origin often are referred to as epidermoid cysts. They are believed to arise from an embryonic inclusion of the surface mesothelium in the developing spleen. False cysts have a smooth fibrous lining and are believed to arise from prior splenic trauma, infarction, or infection. It can be difficult to distinguish the two types of cysts radiologically. Peripheral calcification (as in this case) can be seen with either type of cyst. Parasitic cysts usually are echinococcal in origin.

CT findings of a well-defined, water-attenuation mass without enhancement are typical. Peripheral septations can occur and sometimes are referred to as trabeculation. Some authorities believe that these are more commonly found in true cysts.

CASE 9.12

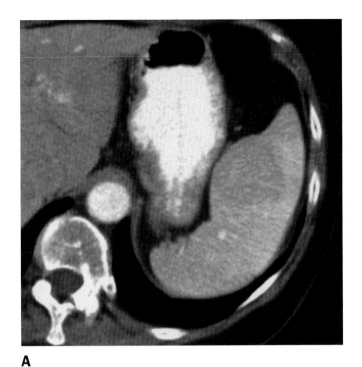

A

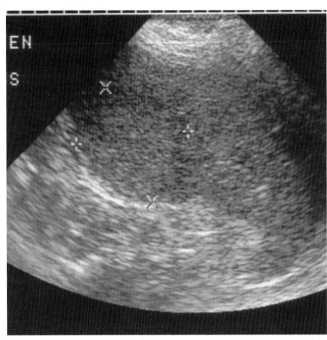

B

Findings

A. Contrast-enhanced CT. A large, homogeneously enhancing mass is present in the spleen. The attenuation of the mass is slightly lower than that of the spleen.

B. Abdominal sonogram. A poorly circumscribed mass is present in the spleen. The mass is similar in echotexture to the normal spleen.

Differential Diagnosis

1. Metastases
2. Lymphoma
3. Hemangioma
4. Hamartoma

Diagnosis

Hamartoma

Discussion

Hamartomas of the spleen are benign tumors composed of normal cellular elements in abnormal quantity, degree of differentiation, cellular arrangement, or a combination of all three features. Pathologically, they are classified into three types: red pulp (vascular), white pulp (lymphomatous), or mixed. They are usually solid tumors without encapsulation. Clinically they may be asymptomatic, or they may be associated with hypersplenism (anemia, thrombocytopenia, pancytopenia).

At sonography they usually appear homogeneously echogenic, but they may contain cystic spaces. The appearance at CT is variable—usually presenting as a hypoattenuating or isoattenuating mass. Large lesions can have scars, cystic regions, and calcification.

CASE 9.13

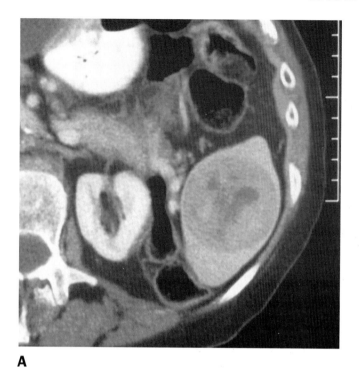

A

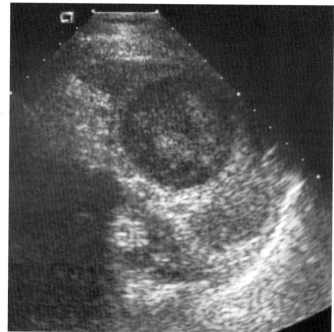

B

Findings

A. Contrast-enhanced CT. A well-circumscribed, heterogeneously enhancing mass is present in the spleen.

B. Abdominal sonogram. The mass is of heterogeneous echotexture and its borders are well defined.

Differential Diagnosis

1. Lymphoma
2. Metastases
3. Hemangioma
4. Histoplasmosis
5. Tuberculosis
6. Inflammatory pseudotumor

Diagnosis

Inflammatory pseudotumor

Discussion

Inflammatory pseudotumor is a rare entity composed of a localized area of inflammatory and fibroblastic cells surrounding regions of hemorrhage and necrosis. These lesions usually are discovered incidentally. The radiographic appearance is nonspecific, except that the mass is usually well defined and heterogeneous internally. Calcification may be present. Occasionally, a central stellate scar is present.

CASE 9.14

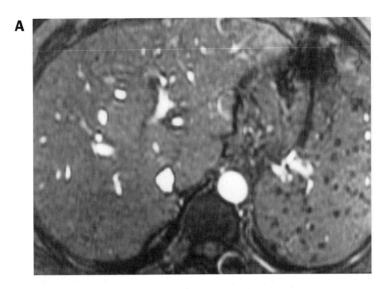

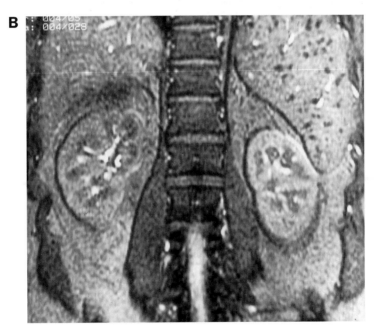

Findings
A and **B.** MRI of the abdomen (gradient echo). Multiple low-attenuation nodules are present throughout the spleen.

Differential Diagnosis
Siderotic nodules (Gamna-Gandy bodies)

Diagnosis
Siderotic nodules (Gamna-Gandy bodies)

Discussion
In patients with cirrhosis and portal venous hypertension, small nodules (3-8 mm in diameter) can develop within the spleen from prior organized hemorrhage. The deposited hemosiderin explains the findings that are best appreciated on gradient echo pulse sequences. Approximately 10% of patients with portal venous hypertension have these nodules. They can occur within a normal or enlarged spleen. The siderotic nodules have no clinical significance themselves, except to indicate the presence of portal venous hypertension.

CASE 9.15

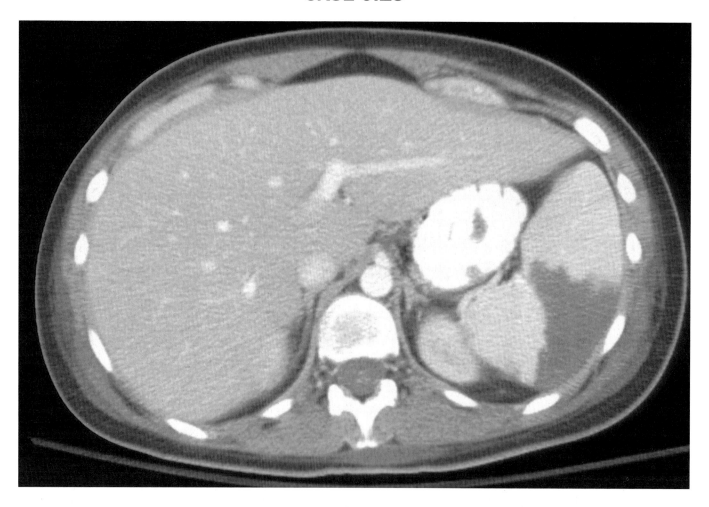

Findings
Contrast-enhanced CT. There is a wedge-shaped low-attenuation defect within the spleen.

Differential Diagnosis
Splenic infarction

Diagnosis
Splenic infarction

Discussion
Splenic infarction usually is caused by emboli (most commonly in older persons) or thrombi (due to an underlying hematologic disorder). Patients usually present with sudden pain in the left upper quadrant. Infarction results in a weakened area of the spleen which can rupture and tissue that is prone to infection. Close observation and follow-up for one of these complications usually are recommended.

Although this case illustrates the most classic findings of splenic infarction with a wedge-shaped peripheral defect, infarction can present as a heterogeneous mass that may be indistinguishable from a neoplasm. If the clinical history is not revealing, a biopsy may be necessary.

CASE 9.16

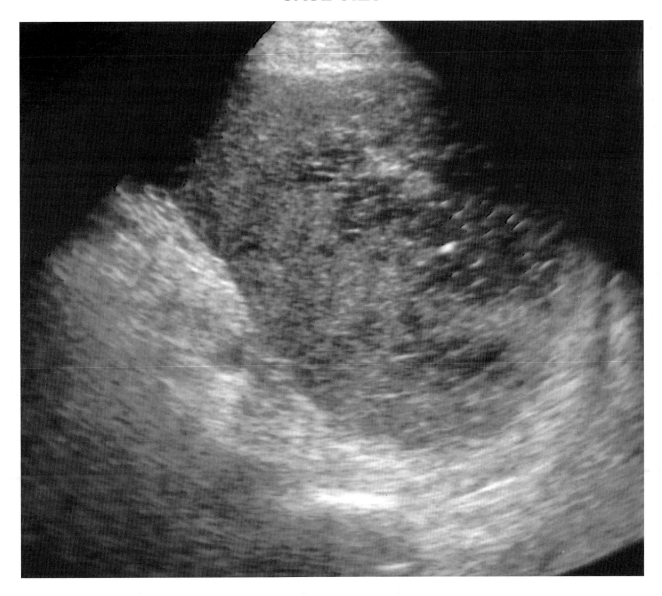

Findings

Abdominal sonogram. Several hypoechoic regions are present within the spleen.

Differential Diagnosis

1. Lymphoma
2. Metastases
3. Infarction
4. Abscess

Diagnosis

Splenic infarction

Discussion

The appearance of a splenic infarct at sonography depends on its age. Acutely, splenic infarction appears as a poorly delineated hypoechoic region(s). A wedge-shaped abnormality may be present. Aging infarcts become better marginated and echogenic, with focal atrophy and scarring.

This case illustrates several hypoechoic regions, some with poor and some with good delineation. The larger region contains some central hyperechoic islands within it—likely representing evolution of a healing infarct.

CASE 9.17

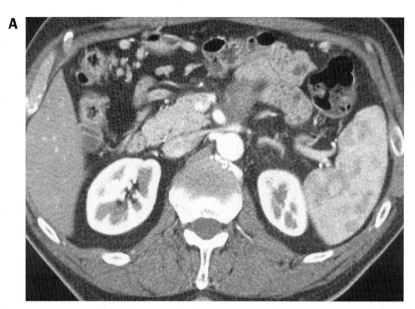

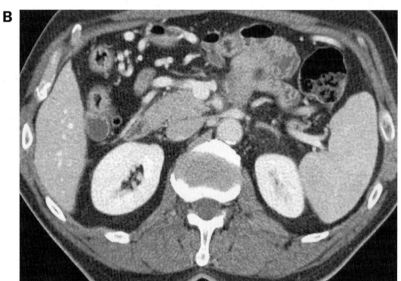

Findings

Contrast-enhanced CT. **A.** Arterial phase of contrast enhancement shows multiple regions of hypoattenuation throughout the spleen. **B.** Portal venous phase of contrast enhancement shows a normal homogeneous spleen.

Differential Diagnosis

Splenic pseudomass

Diagnosis

Splenic pseudomass

Discussion

Enhancement of the spleen is often heterogeneous during the early phases of contrast enhancement because of variable rates of flow through the red pulp. This finding should not be considered an abnormality unless it persists into the later portal venous phase of enhancement. Generally, a homogeneous splenic blush should be seen within 2 minutes after bolus injection of contrast material.

CASE 9.18

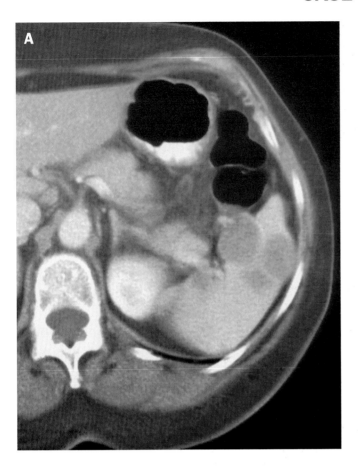

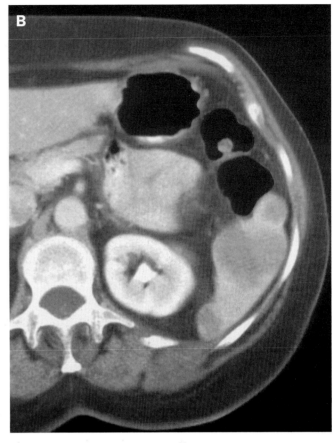

Findings
A and **B.** Contrast-enhanced CT. Several well-defined hypoattenuating masses are present within the spleen.

Differential Diagnosis
1. Metastases
2. Lymphoma
3. Multiple hemangiomas
4. Multiple benign cysts

Diagnosis
Lymphoma

Discussion
Lymphoma is the commonest malignant tumor to affect the spleen. Splenic involvement occurs in approximately one-third of patients with lymphoma (either Hodgkin or non-Hodgkin). Current imaging techniques are not optimal for detecting the disease. Splenomegaly is one of the most common findings in patients with lymphoma. However, the presence of an enlarged spleen does not necessarily indicate lymphomatous involvement, especially in patients with bone marrow involvement and splenomegaly due to extramedullary hematopoiesis. As a result, splenectomy is often necessary to detect splenic involvement. Splenomegaly also is unreliable in Hodgkin disease because one-third of patients with splenic involvement have a normal-sized spleen, and one-third of patients with splenomegaly do not have splenic involvement.

Splenic lymphoma occurs in four major patterns: homogeneous enlargement, miliary involvement, multiple masses, and a solitary large mass. The accuracy of CT for detecting lymphoma is approximately 60%. Regional and systemic adenopathy can be helpful for suggesting lymphoma. Splenic infarction can be seen in patients with splenic lymphoma, with the characteristic peripheral, wedge-shaped regions of hypoattenuation.

CASE 9.19

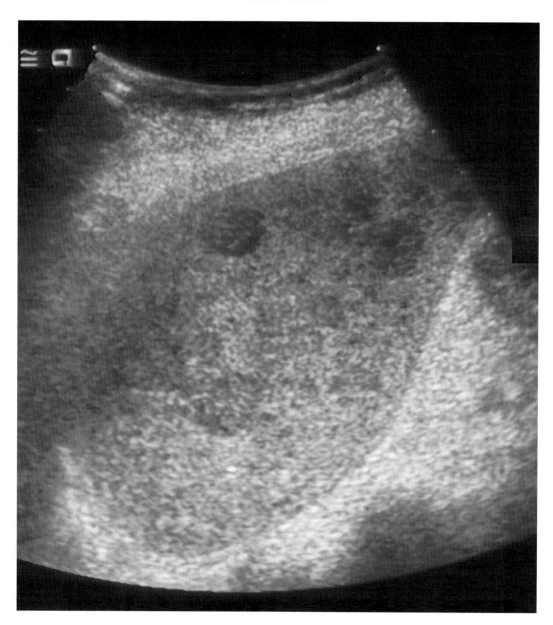

Findings

Abdominal sonogram. The spleen is enlarged and contains multiple hypoechoic masses.

Differential Diagnosis

1. Metastases
2. Lymphoma

Diagnosis

Lymphoma

Discussion

Lymphoma usually presents as a diffuse or focal (small nodular lesions or large lesions) hypoechoic pattern. Low-grade disease usually presents with the diffuse or small nodular pattern, whereas high-grade disease usually presents with large masses. Detection of adenopathy elsewhere in the abdomen also can be helpful for suggesting the diagnosis.

CASE 9.20

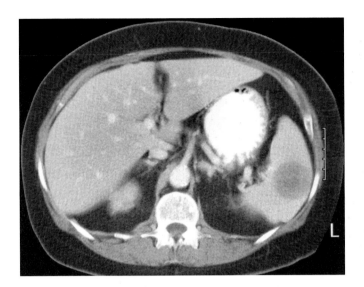

CASE 9.21

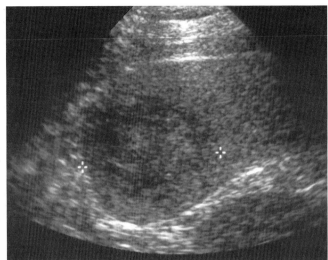

Findings

Case 9.20. Contrast-enhanced CT. A well-defined focal mass is present within the spleen.

Case 9.21. Abdominal sonogram. A solid mass in the spleen contains heterogeneous echotexture (slightly hypoechoic compared with the remainder of the spleen).

Differential Diagnosis
1. Metastases
2. Lymphoma
3. Hamartoma

Diagnosis
Metastases (melanoma primary)

Discussion

Metastasis to the spleen usually occurs by hematogenous arterial seeding. Venous seeding can occur in patients with portal venous hypertension. The spleen is a relatively uncommon site for metastasis, occurring in less than 10% of patients at autopsy. The commonest primary tumors to metastasize to the spleen include melanoma, breast, ovary, and lung.

Metastases can have a widely variable appearance, ranging from cystic to heterogeneous to solid masses. Some will be well defined and others infiltrative. The keys for detection are to identify regions of hypoattenuation at CT (or hypoechoic or hyperechoic regions at sonography) and to correlate these findings with the clinical history of a malignancy. Patients with melanoma metastases can have lesions with cystic necrosis and fluid visualized centrally or a sonographic halo around the circumference of the mass.

Masses of the Spleen

		Case
Benign		
Hemangioma	Most common benign tumor of spleen. May have peripheral globular enhancement and hyperechoic appearance, as in liver. Frequently atypical in appearance	9.7–9.9
Splenic cyst	True cysts (epidermoid cysts) have a cellular lining. False cysts (due to trauma, infection, or infarction) have only a fibrous lining. Anechoic with posterior acoustic enhancement. Thin peripheral calcification in both true and false splenic cysts	9.10 and 9.11
Hamartoma	Benign tumor with disorganized normal cellular elements. Solid tumor with variable echogenicity and enhancement	9.12
Inflammatory pseudotumor	Rare, well-defined mass surrounding hemorrhage and necrosis. Occasional central stellate scar	9.13
Siderotic nodules (Gamna-Gandy bodies)	Tiny benign siderotic nodules in the spleen in 10% of patients with portal hypertension. Best seen as multiple tiny splenic nodules on gradient echo MRI	9.14
Infarct	Classically wedge-shaped, peripheral, low-attenuation, hypoechoic lesion. Can appear masslike	9.15 and 9.16
Pseudomass	Heterogeneous enhancement of spleen on early phases. Abnormalities should resolve on portal venous phase	9.17
Candidiasis	Multiple tiny low-attenuation splenic lesions. Target appearance on sonography. Liver also usually involved. Immunosuppressed patients	9.1 and 9.2
Echinococcal cysts	Peripherally calcified cyst and daughter cysts. Liver disease usually present when spleen is involved. Usually from endemic area	9.3 and 9.4
Sarcoidosis	Multiple tiny hypoattenuating splenic lesions. Adenopathy may be present	9.6
Malignant		
Lymphoma	Commonest malignant tumor of spleen. Solitary or multiple masses. Adenopathy common	9.18 and 9.19
Metastases	Uncommon site for metastases. Most commonly melanoma, breast, ovary, and lung	9.20 and 9.21

CASE 9.22

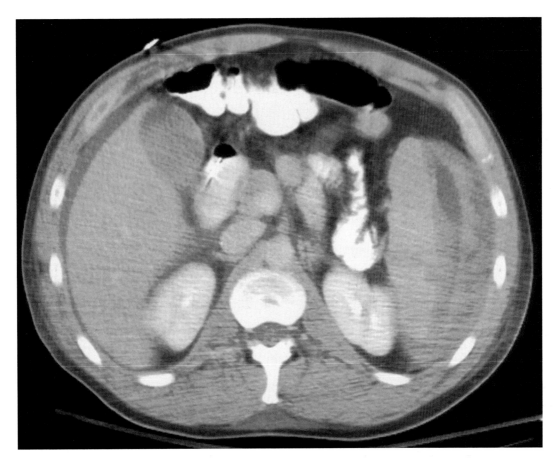

Findings
Contrast-enhanced CT. A mixed-attenuation mass is present within a subcapsular location about the lateral aspect of the spleen.

Differential Diagnosis
Subcapsular splenic hematoma

Diagnosis
Subcapsular splenic hematoma

Discussion
The spleen is the most commonly injured organ after blunt abdominal trauma, constituting 25% of solid-organ injuries. Physical complaints and findings of splenic injury after blunt trauma include left upper quadrant pain, referred left shoulder pain, hypotension, and shock. Diagnostic peritoneal lavage may be used in the emergency department to assess for hemoperitoneum in the unstable patient. The presence of hemoperitoneum has a high association with splenic injury. In stable patients, contrast-enhanced CT is the preferred method to assess for splenic injuries.

Splenic injuries can be classified at CT as 1) subcapsular or intrasplenic hematomas, 2) lacerations, 3) fractures, or 4) vascular pedicle injuries. Intrasplenic hematomas usually appear as a hypoattenuating focal mass. Aging hematomas at unenhanced CT may appear isoattenuating. Subcapsular hematomas (as in this case) appear as a crescent of fluid or mixed attenuation collections. Small subcapsular collections can be difficult to differentiate from perisplenic fluid. Lacerations are low-attenuation linear abnormalities that do not cross the spleen entirely. Fractures extend entirely through the spleen and may result in devascularized fragments. They are found most commonly in the splenic poles. Vascular pedicle injuries usually result in severe bleeding and hemodynamic instability. Patients usually are taken to the operating room for emergency repair.

CASE 9.23

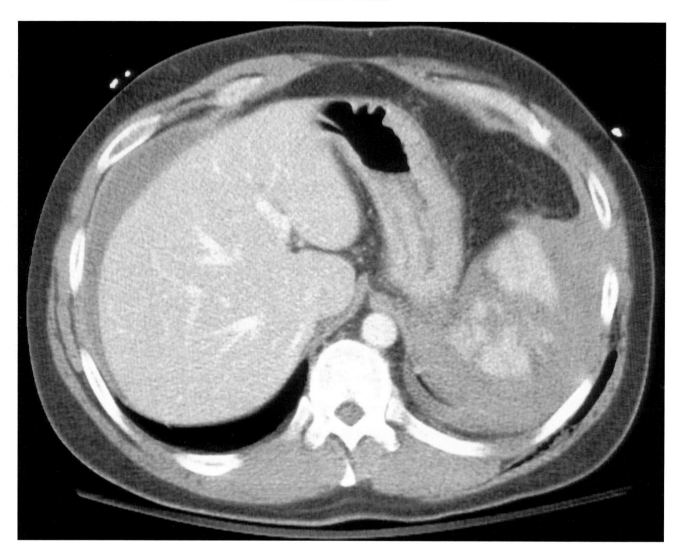

Findings

Contrast-enhanced CT. Multiple linear abnormalities divide the spleen into multiple small pieces. There is fluid about the spleen and a left pleural effusion.

Differential Diagnosis

Multiple splenic lacerations

Diagnosis

Multiple splenic lacerations (shattered spleen)

Discussion

A shattered spleen is a severe splenic injury with a high incidence of vascular pedicle injuries. Because of the dual blood supply to the spleen by way of the splenic artery and the short gastric arteries, this condition may result in nonenhancement of the lower polar spleen with upper pole perfusion by way of the short gastric arteries. In some cases, lacerations can be subtle findings. The findings of perisplenic fluid (clot) and thickening of the anterior pararenal fascia and the lateral conal fascia can be useful indicators of a splenic injury.

Several grading systems exist for classifying splenic injuries; none have been adopted for standard care and reporting.

CASE 9.24

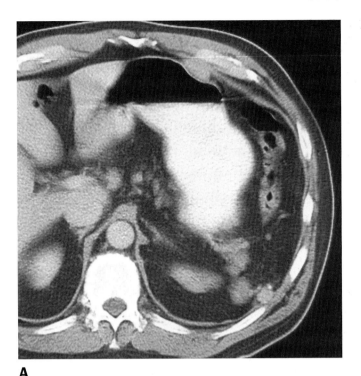

A

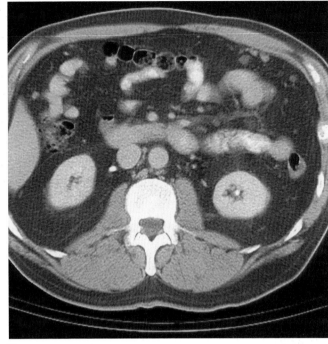

B

Findings
Contrast-enhanced CT. **A** and **B**. Several soft tissue attenuation nodules are present in the splenic bed. Soft tissue nodules also are present in the region of the omentum.

Differential Diagnosis
1. Metastases
2. Splenosis

Diagnosis
Splenosis

Discussion
Splenosis refers to autotransplantation of splenic tissue. Splenic trauma is the most common cause, with seeding of splenic tissue throughout the peritoneal cavity, where it can grow if blood supply is established. Splenosis also has been reported within the pleural space, retroperitoneum, pericardium, lung, and subcutaneous tissues. One-fourth to two-thirds of splenic injuries result in splenosis. The condition usually is asymptomatic, but it can be confused with other peritoneal conditions, including metastases, mesothelioma, or endometriosis. A history of splenic trauma is often key for suggesting the diagnosis.

Splenules discovered at CT usually are round or oval with homogeneous enhancement after intravenous contrast administration. Nuclear scintigraphy is usually the best test for making this diagnosis.

CASE 9.25

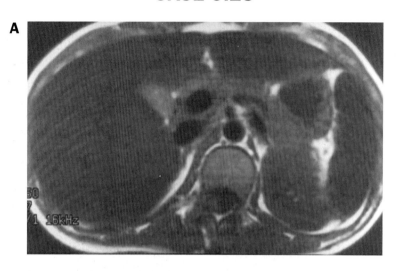

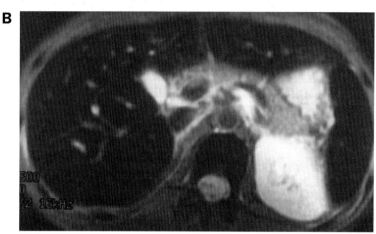

Findings

MRI of the abdomen. **A.** T1-weighted. **B.** T2-weighted. The liver, spleen, and bone marrow are of abnormally low signal intensity. The pancreas is of normal signal.

Differential Diagnosis

1. Secondary hemochromatosis
2. Primary hemochromatosis

Diagnosis

Secondary hemochromatosis

Discussion

Secondary hemochromatosis is a condition of excess iron deposition within the reticulo-endothelial system, usually due to blood transfusions or rhabdomyolysis. It should be distinguished from primary hemochromatosis, in which there is abnormal iron absorption and deposition and subsequent cellular damage within the liver, heart, and pancreas. Secondary hemochromatosis has little clinical significance, whereas primary hemochromatosis requires treatment to prevent organ damage.

Secondary hemochromatosis is most easily recognized at MRI on gradient echo or T2-weighted pulse sequences. There is abnormally low signal within the liver, spleen, and bone marrow (as in this case). The pancreas is of normal signal. At CT, the liver and spleen are hyperattenuating (usually Hounsfield units are in excess of 100). Primary hemochromatosis has iron deposition (and low MRI signal) in the liver, pancreas, and heart. Involvement of the pancreas is the easiest key finding for differentiating primary from secondary hemochromatosis.

CASE 9.26

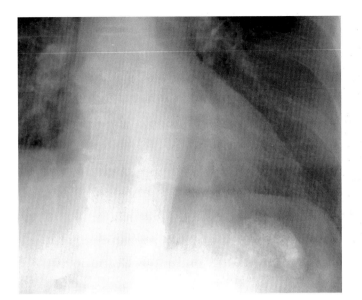

CASE 9.27

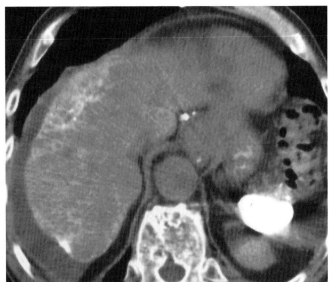

Findings

Case 9.26. Abdominal radiograph. The spleen is abnormally dense, and there is a suggestion of hyperdense nodules in the upper abdomen.

Case 9.27. Unenhanced CT. The spleen is hyperattenuating. There are hyperattenuating lymph nodes in the gastrohepatic ligament. The liver is of heterogeneous attenuation.

Differential Diagnosis

1. Thorium dioxide exposure
2. Autosplenectomy from sickle cell disease

Diagnosis

Thorium dioxide exposure

Discussion

Both of these patients had prior thorium dioxide administration. Thorium dioxide was previously used as an intravascular contrast agent. Thorium 232 is an alpha emitter with a very long half-life which accumulates within the reticuloendothelial system. Uptake of the agent occurs in the spleen, liver, and lymph nodes. Splenic changes include fibrosis and atrophy. The radiation associated with this agent predisposes patients to angiosarcoma, hepatocellular carcinoma, and cholangiocarcinomas.

At CT, the most common finding is hyperattenuating spleen and liver. Filling defects or heterogeneous attenuation within the liver or spleen should prompt investigation for a complicating neoplasm. Patients with sickle cell disease would not be expected to have changes in the liver or lymph nodes.

CASE 9.28

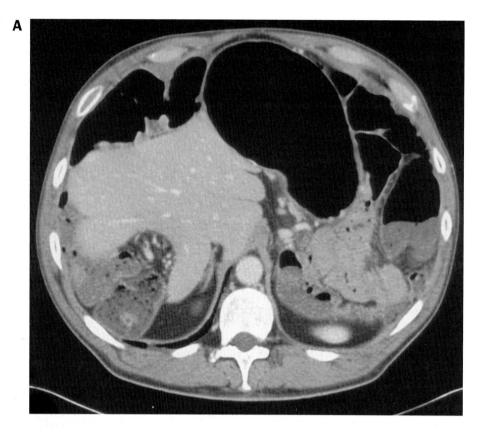

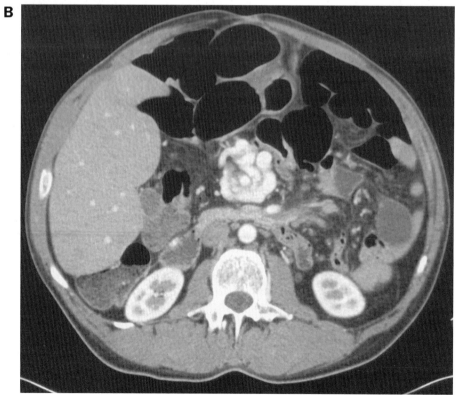

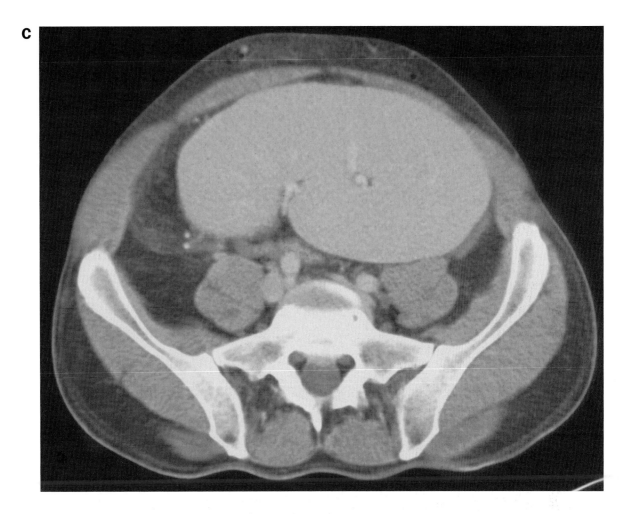

C

Findings
A through **C.** Contrast-enhanced CT. The spleen is not present in the left upper quadrant, but it is visible in the pelvis. The mesenteric vasculature has a whorled appearance.

Differential Diagnosis
Wandering spleen

Diagnosis
Wandering spleen

Discussion
A wandering spleen is the result of splenic ligamentous laxity, likely due to abnormal embryologic fusion of the posterior mesogastrium or to lack of formation of the normal splenorenal and gastrosplenic ligaments. Because of its hypermobility, the spleen can move to abnormal locations within the peritoneal cavity. Usually a mass is discovered in an otherwise asymptomatic patient. Occasionally, vascular torsion of the splenic pedicle can result in splenic congestion or infarction. Torsion can be chronic and intermittent.

Radiographic findings at CT show an abnormal location or change in splenic shape. Patients with infarction have the typical features of an infarct(s) with a portion of or the entire spleen hypoperfused. Treatment in symptomatic patients usually is operative splenopexy. Splenectomy is reserved only for patients with infarction.

CASE 9.29

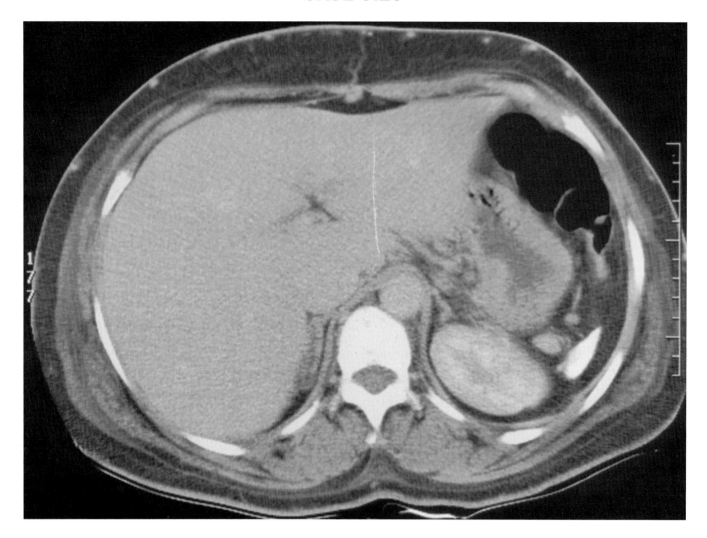

Findings
Contrast-enhanced CT. The spleen is shrunken and calcified.

Differential Diagnosis
1. Autosplenectomy from sickle cell disease
2. Thorium dioxide exposure

Diagnosis
Autosplenectomy from sickle cell disease

Discussion
Sickle cell anemia (disease) results from homozygous inheritance of the hemoglobin 5-producing gene and affects 1 in 500 African Americans. Sickle cell trait (heterozygous form) is found in 1 in 10 African Americans. Abnormal hemoglobin 5 can result in rigid, crescentic, or sickle-shaped erythrocytes. This can lead to hemolysis and vascular occlusion(s). In patients with homozygous sickle cell disease, splenic infarctions can lead to loss of function, gradual decrease in size, and ultimately fibrosis and calcification (autosplenectomy). Loss of splenic function results in an increased susceptibility to aggressive infections.

Autosplenectomy in sickle cell disease appears as a small, densely calcified spleen on CT or plain radiography. The calcified spleen may be as small as 1 cm. Technetium-99m liver-spleen scans show no splenic uptake. Thorium dioxide exposure can result in a similar appearance of the spleen. However, liver and lymph node calcification also is often present with thorium dioxide exposure. Clinical history usually easily differentiates these two disease processes.

Miscellaneous Splenic Conditions

		Case
Subcapsular hematoma	Crescent-shaped, nonenhancing fluid collection in a subcapsular location	9.22
Shattered spleen	Multiple fracture lines traverse spleen. Associated perisplenic stranding and fluid	9.23
Splenosis	Solitary or multiple nodules, usually left upper quadrant, variable size. Enhancement mimics spleen	9.24
Hemochromatosis	Primary, may not affect spleen. Secondary, spleen always affected	9.25
	Secondary, low MRI signal diffusely in spleen, marrow, and liver. Pancreas usually spared	
Thorium dioxide exposure	Dense, atrophic spleen, regional high-density lymph nodes. Liver also usually affected	9.26 and 9.27
Wandering spleen	Soft tissue mass with enhancement similar to spleen. Spleen not present in usual fossa. Can undergo torsion	9.28
Autosplenectomy	Dense, atrophic spleen. History of sickle cell disease	9.29

DIFFERENTIAL DIAGNOSES

Solid Masses

Benign
   Hemangioma
   Hamartoma
   Inflammatory pseudotumor
   Splenic infarct

Malignant
   Lymphoma
   Metastasis
   Angiosarcoma

Cystic Masses

True cyst (epidermoid cyst)
False cyst (posttraumatic cyst)
Echinococcal cyst
Bacterial abscess
Cystic metastasis

Multiple Small (<1 cm) Lesions

Fungal microabscesses (*Candida*, histoplasmosis)
Multiple bacterial abscesses
Lymphoma
Sarcoidosis
Gamna-Gandy bodies
Metastases
Pseudotumors (early phase of contrast enhancement)

SPLENIC MASSES

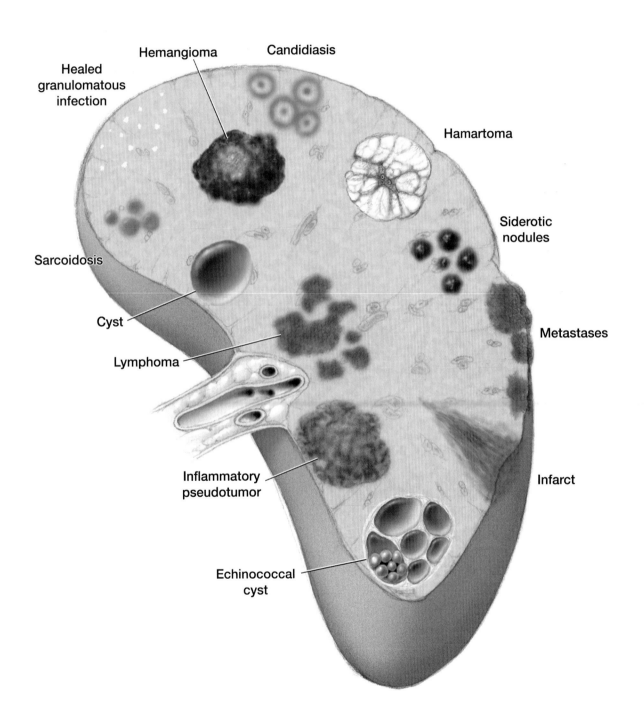

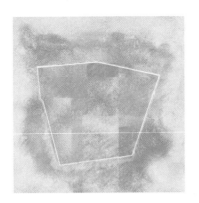

CHAPTER 10
PERITONEUM AND MESENTERY

CASE 10.1

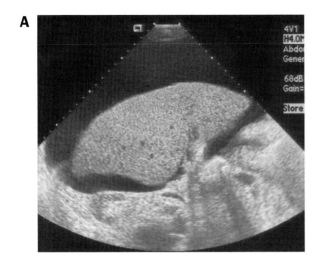

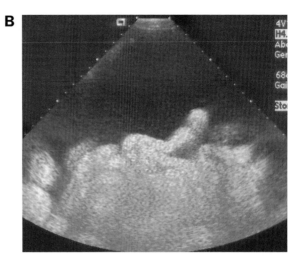

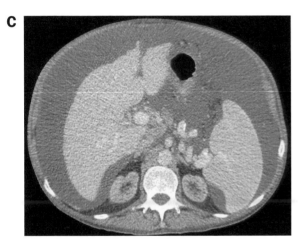

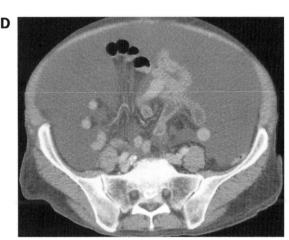

Findings

Sonogram. **A** and **B.** A large amount of anechoic fluid surrounds the liver and bowel loops in the right lower quadrant.

Contrast-enhanced CT. **C** and **D.** A large amount of fluid is present in the peritoneal cavity. The liver has a cirrhotic configuration, and the spleen is enlarged.

Differential Diagnosis

Simple ascites

Diagnosis

Simple ascites

Discussion

In the vast majority of cases, ascites is a transudate and due to cirrhosis and portal hypertension. Cardiac failure and peritoneal carcinomatosis are other common causes of ascites. Rarely, ascites is due to blood, bile, chyle, pus, or urine. Paracentesis is a safe, easy, and cost-effective method to determine the cause of ascites. Ascites due to cirrhosis and portal hypertension usually can be treated medically. Refractory ascites may require frequent large-volume paracenteses, a transjugular intrahepatic portacaval shunt, or a portosystemic surgical shunt.

Small amounts of ascites often accumulate in the hepatorenal recess (Morrison pouch) or pelvic cul-de-sac. Large amounts of ascites, as in this case, result in medial displacement of bowel loops. Uncomplicated ascites should be anechoic on sonography.

CASE 10.2

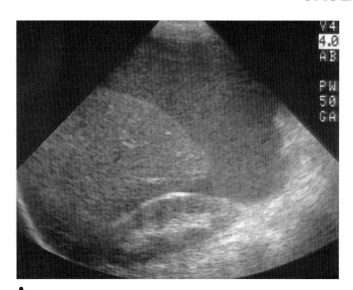

A

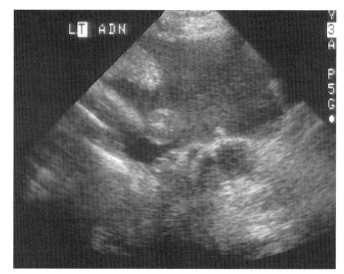

B

Findings

Sonogram. **A** and **B.** A large amount of ascites is present around the liver and bowel. The ascites contains diffuse low-level echoes.

Differential Diagnosis

1. Complicated ascites
2. Simple ascites

Diagnosis

Complicated ascites (spontaneous bacterial peritonitis)

Discussion

Simple transudative ascites due to portal hypertension and cardiac failure usually is sonolucent. Ascites complicated by hemorrhage, infection, or malignancy often contains floating debris or septations. The complicated ascites in this case was due to infection (peritonitis). Spontaneous bacterial peritonitis (SBP) occurs almost exclusively in patients with cirrhosis. This spontaneous infection is thought to develop from translocation of any organism (most common in *Escherichia coli*) from the gut, into the mesenteric lymph nodes, and finally into the ascites. Patients usually present with fever and an increased leukocyte count. SBP can be deadly, but less than 5% of patients die if appropriate antibiotics are administered in a timely fashion.

CASE 10.3

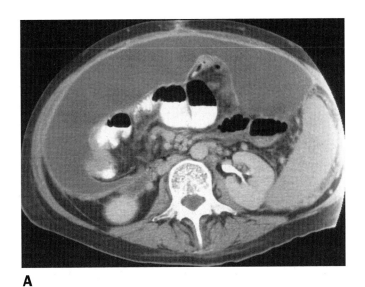

A

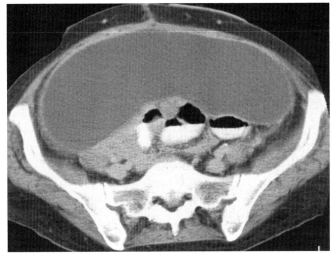

B

Findings

Contrast-enhanced CT. **A** and **B**. A large fluid collection is present in the anterior peritoneal cavity. The fluid is loculated and does not extend around the spleen or into the left paracolic gutter. The fluid collection has a thick, enhancing rind.

Differential Diagnosis

1. Intraperitoneal abscess
2. Simple ascites

Diagnosis

Intraperitoneal abscess

Discussion

Intraperitoneal abscesses usually develop from contaminated material related to perforation of a viscus (e.g., perforated gastric or duodenal ulcer, appendicitis, diverticulitis, biliary disease) or as a result of direct contamination during operation. The most common organisms found in intraperitoneal abscesses are *Escherichia coli, Streptococcus, Staphylococcus,* or *Klebsiella* or a mixture of these organisms. Patients almost always present with pain, fever, and an increased leukocyte count.

A loculated fluid collection with an enhancing rind is strongly suggestive of an abscess. Bubbles of gas within the loculated fluid collection (approximately 30% of cases) are even more specific for an abscess. Abscesses usually contain multiple septations and complicated fluid with low-level echoes on sonography. Depending on the cause of the abscess, ultrasonography- or CT-guided percutaneous drainage or surgery is the primary treatment, in addition to intravenous antibiotics.

Findings in this case that point away from simple ascites are the loculated nature of the fluid, the way the fluid compresses the bowel posteriorly rather than displacing it medially (case 10.1), and the thick, enhancing rind around the fluid.

CASE 10.4

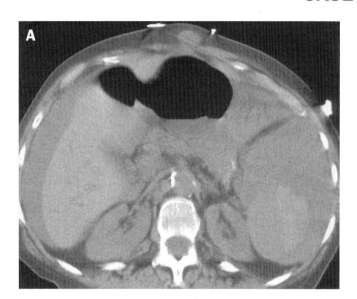

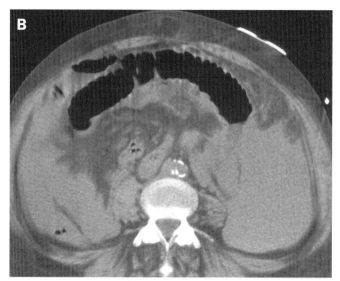

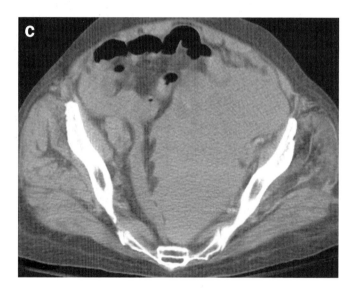

Findings

Unenhanced CT. **A** through **C.** High-density material is present around the lateral inferior tip of the spleen. Moderate amount of slightly high-density ascites throughout the peritoneal cavity.

Differential Diagnosis

1. Hemoperitoneum
2. Simple ascites

Diagnosis

Hemoperitoneum

Discussion

The attenuation of peritoneal fluid often gives a clue to its composition. Simple transudative ascites usually has attenuation values between −10 and +10 Hounsfield units (HU). Exudative ascites usually is more than +15 HU. Blood in the peritoneal cavity usually is about +45 HU. High-density blood implies that the bleed is recent. Layering blood of different ages (different attenuations) often also is present in hemoperitoneum. The peritoneal blood in this case was due to a laceration of the inferior aspect of the spleen during a motor vehicle accident.

CASE 10.5

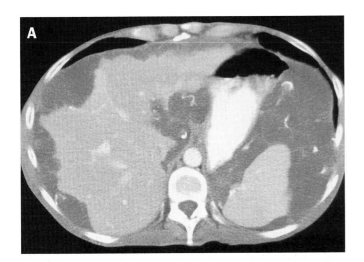

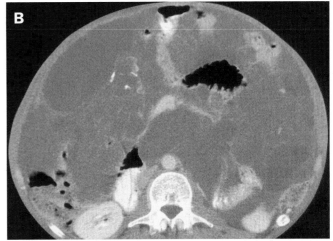

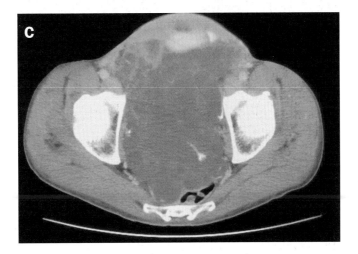

Findings

Contrast-enhanced CT. **A** through **C.** The peritoneal cavity is filled with low-density masses. The ascites contains numerous calcific arcs and rings and internal septations and results in a scalloped contour along the liver and spleen.

Differential Diagnosis

1. Pseudomyxoma peritonei
2. Simple ascites

Diagnosis

Pseudomyxoma peritonei

Discussion

Pseudomyxoma peritonei refers to a gelatinous (mucinous) ascites that occurs as a result of a ruptured appendiceal mucocele or intraperitoneal spread of mucinous tumor, including mucinous adenocarcinomas of the ovary, appendix, colon, and, rarely, the pancreas. Pseudomyxoma peritonei can be differentiated from simple ascites on CT by the scalloped appearance of the liver margin, caused by the mass effect of the mucinous implants. High-attenuation septa and punctate or ringlike calcifications often are present within mucinous ascites in large-volume disease, as in this case. When large-volume disease is present, the source of the pseudomyxoma peritonei often is difficult to determine. This patient had pseudomyxoma peritonei due to an appendiceal mucinous cystadenocarcinoma.

CASE 10.6

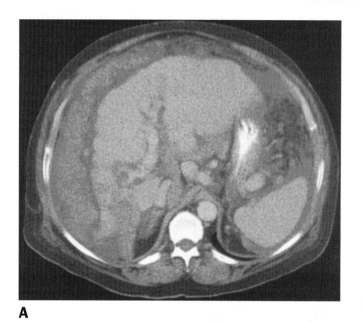

A

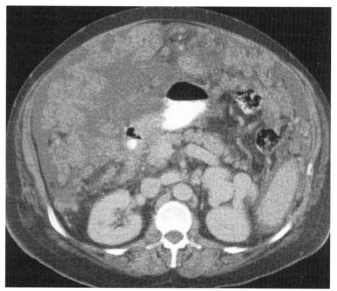

B

Findings

Contrast-enhanced CT. **A** and **B.** Enhancing nodules are seen along the peritoneal surfaces with marked nodular thickening of the omentum. A small amount of associated ascites also is present.

Differential Diagnosis

1. Peritoneal carcinomatosis
2. Malignant mesothelioma
3. Tuberculous peritonitis

Diagnosis

Peritoneal carcinomatosis (with omental caking)

Discussion

Peritoneal carcinomatosis (metastasis) most commonly is caused by ovarian, colon, stomach, or pancreatic carcinoma. The natural flow of ascites in the peritoneal cavity determines the location of malignant peritoneal seeding. The most common sites of peritoneal carcinomatosis are the pelvic cul-de-sac, the right paracolic gutter, the root of the mesentery at the ileocecal junction, and the sigmoid mesocolon (case 10.7).

The omental surface is also a common location for tumor seeding. Eventually, the omental fat can become completely replaced by tumor, resulting in a thick, confluent, soft tissue mass, often referred to as "omental caking." Omental caking of tumor displaces the bowel posteriorly away from the anterior abdominal wall, as in this case. Peritoneal malignant mesothelioma and tuberculous peritonitis could give a similar CT appearance, including the omental caking.

CASE 10.7

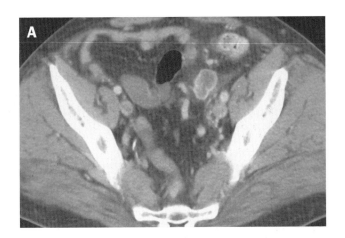

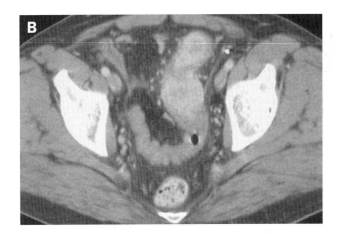

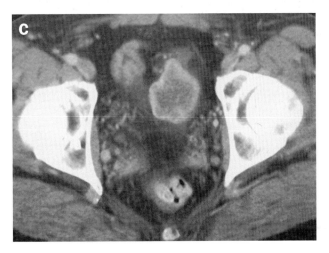

Findings

Contrast-enhanced CT. **A** through **C.** Several peripherally enhancing, centrally necrotic masses are present along the sigmoid mesentery and sigmoid colon.

Differential Diagnosis

1. Colon carcinoma
2. Invasive peritoneal metastases
3. Primary peritoneal tumor
4. Peritoneal abscesses (diverticulitis)

Diagnosis

Invasive peritoneal metastases

Discussion

Peritoneal metastases may occur through direct invasion of the adjacent peritoneal reflections by tumor involving a contiguous abdominal organ. This is most common with primary tumors of the pancreas, liver, gallbladder, or stomach. Alternatively, peritoneal metastases may occur by intraperitoneal seeding of tumor cells, which spread according to pathways of ascitic flow. The most common sites of peritoneal carcinomatosis are the pelvic cul-de-sac, paracolic gutters, and the sigmoid mesocolon (as in this case). The most common tumors to spread in the peritoneum by seeding are ovarian and gastrointestinal tumors. The peritoneal metastases in this case were from a primary renal cell carcinoma. The patient presented with gastrointestinal bleeding due to invasion of the peritoneal metastases into the sigmoid colon. Clinical history is important in this case to determine the likely diagnosis. Other peritoneal tumors or even a complicated perisigmoid abscess due to diverticulosis could give a similar CT appearance.

CASE 10.8

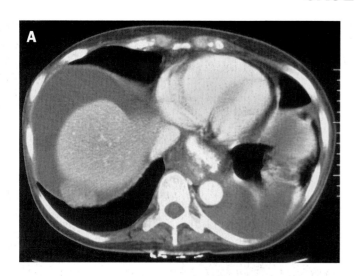

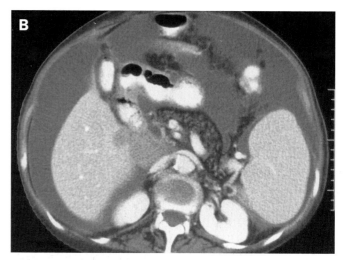

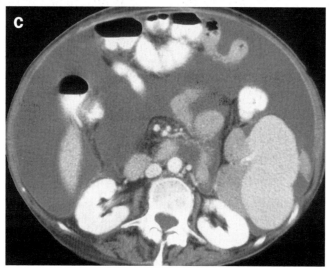

Findings

Contrast-enhanced CT. **A** through **C**. Multiple enhancing soft tissue masses are present along the peritoneum adjacent to the liver and spleen and in the mesentery. A large amount of ascites also is seen.

Differential Diagnosis

1. Peritoneal metastases
2. Primary peritoneal mesothelioma

Diagnosis

Primary peritoneal mesothelioma

Discussion

Mesothelioma is a rare neoplasm affecting the pleura (75% of cases) and peritoneum (25% of cases). Most peritoneal mesotheliomas are malignant and occur in male patients with an initial asbestos exposure 30 to 40 years before development of tumor. Widespread progression of malignant cells on peritoneal surfaces results in copious fluid production (ascites). Because of the great variability in the histologic appearance of mesothelioma cells, the diagnosis often is difficult for pathologists. Laparotomy with extensive tissue sampling often is necessary to make the diagnosis. Treatment consists of a combination of surgery, chemotherapy, and radiation. Peritoneal metastases could give an identical radiographic appearance.

CASE 10.9

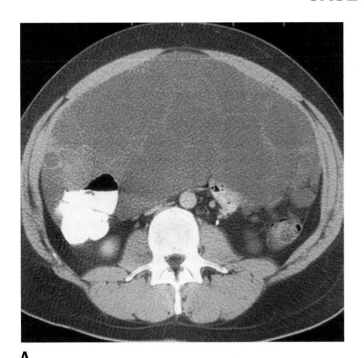

A

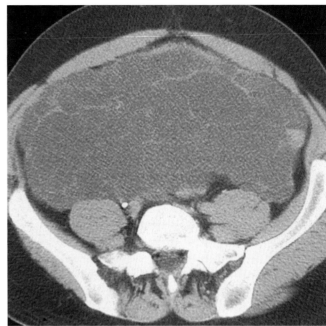

B

Findings

Contrast-enhanced CT. **A** and **B.** A huge low-attenuation peritoneal mass is present, containing multiple thin, enhancing septae.

Differential Diagnosis

1. Pseudomyxoma peritonei
2. Malignant peritoneal mesothelioma
3. Cystic peritoneal mesothelioma
4. Tuberous peritonitis
5. Abdominal lymphangioma

Diagnosis

Cystic peritoneal mesothelioma

Discussion

Cystic peritoneal mesothelioma is a very rare benign neoplasm arising from the mesothelial cells of the peritoneum. Unlike malignant peritoneal mesothelioma, benign cystic peritoneal mesothelioma is not associated with prior asbestos exposure and occurs mainly in young women (mean age at presentation, 37 years). Cystic peritoneal mesothelioma appears as a low-attenuation (on CT) or anechoic (on ultrasonography) multiloculated cystic mass filling the peritoneal cavity. Treatment of cystic peritoneal mesothelioma is surgical resection. Because adherence of the neoplasm makes complete removal of the tumor difficult, additional operations often are necessary. Despite this problem, the prognosis in patients with cystic peritoneal mesothelioma is good.

CASE 10.10

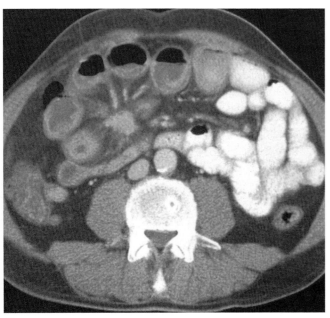

A

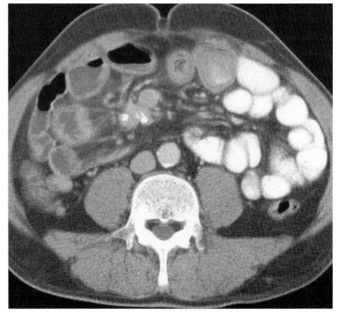

B

Findings

Contrast-enhanced CT. **A** and **B**. A spiculated soft tissue mass with associated calcification is present in the mesentery. There is thickening of an adjacent loop of ileum.

Differential Diagnosis

1. Carcinoid tumor
2. Retractile mesenteritis
3. Desmoid tumor
4. Metastases

Diagnosis

Carcinoid tumor

Discussion

Carcinoid tumor is the most common primary tumor of the small bowel and arises from enterochromaffin cells of Kulchitsky in the crypts of Lieberkühn. The primary small bowel tumors are usually small (<1.5 cm). Growth of these tumors into the mesentery induces an intense fibrotic reaction resulting in the so-called sunburst appearance on CT. Calcification is found in 70% of these foci of mesenteric carcinoid tumor. The triad of a calcified mesenteric mass, radiating strands, and adjacent bowel wall thickening or mass is highly suggestive of carcinoid tumor. Retractile mesenteritis can have a similar CT appearance. Desmoid tumors usually occur in Gardner syndrome after total colectomy. Metastases rarely incite a similar desmoplastic reaction.

CASE 10.11

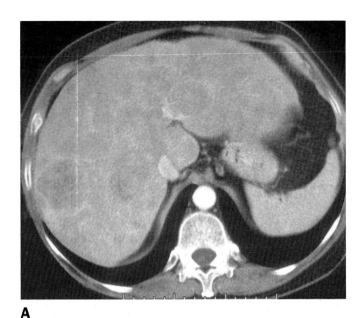

A

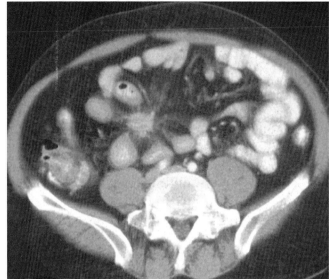

B

Findings

Contrast-enhanced CT. **A.** Multiple low-attenuation masses with peripheral enhancement are present in the liver. **B.** A low-attenuation mesenteric mass is present with radiating strands.

Differential Diagnosis

1. Carcinoid tumor
2. Metastases

Diagnosis

Metastatic carcinoid tumor

Discussion

Ninety percent of small bowel carcinoid tumors occur in the ileum. Extension of tumor into the adjacent mesentery with serotonin production induces a typical desmoplastic response. The radiating strands (sunburst appearance) of mesenteric carcinoid represent thickening along the neurovascular bundles and result in mesenteric retraction around the tumor. Mesenteric metastases from other tumors rarely cause this desmoplastic response. In addition, peritoneal or mesenteric metastases from other primary tumors usually are multiple, as opposed to the solitary lesion of carcinoid. Surgical resection of mesenteric carcinoid is performed to prevent complications of obstruction and ischemia. Because of vascular encasement around the tumor, segmental resection of the adjacent small bowel often is necessary. A primary carcinoid tumor, which may be small and multicentric, frequently is found in the resected intestinal specimen. Symptoms attributable to the carcinoid syndrome usually are found only in patients with hepatic metastases. Patients with hepatic metastases can have tricuspid valve insufficiency due to direct release of serotonin into the hepatic veins.

CASE 10.12

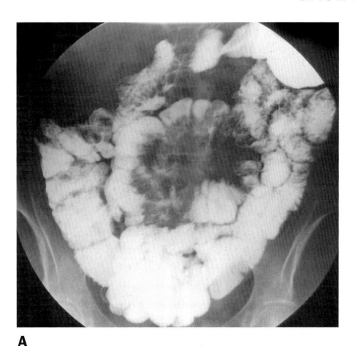

A

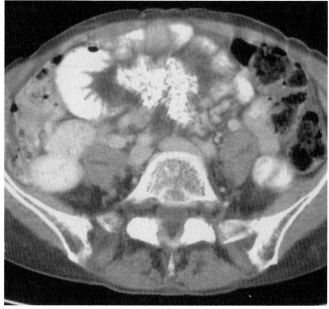

B

Findings

A. Small bowel follow-through. A mass within the small bowel mesentery displaces multiple small bowel loops.

B. Contrast-enhanced CT. A large, poorly defined calcified mesenteric mass displaces small bowel loops.

Differential Diagnosis
1. Carcinoid tumor
2. Retractile mesenteritis
3. Retained foreign body

Diagnosis
Retractile mesenteritis

Discussion

Retractile mesenteritis is a disease of unknown cause. It has been given various names (panniculitis, mesenteric lipodystrophy, sclerosing mesenteritis, or retractile mesenteritis) depending on the predominant histologic features of inflammatory cells, fat necrosis, or fibrosis. A mesenteric mass of variable size usually is present, although panniculitis may initially present with mesenteric soft tissue stranding without a mass. Dense calcification of the mass is common. Secondary tethering of the bowel and obstruction can occur. Occasionally, vascular encasement and bowel ischemia can develop. Differentiation of this process from a carcinoid tumor may not always be possible. Spokewheel thickening of the mesentery and associated bowel wall thickening usually are features of a carcinoid tumor. A radiographically invisible retained foreign body also could cause inflammatory changes in the mesentery, mimicking retractile mesenteritis.

CASE 10.13

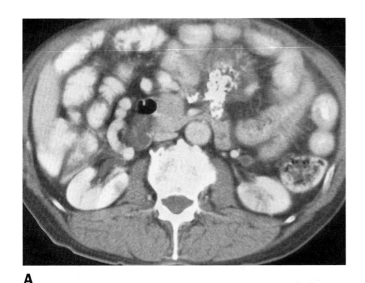

A

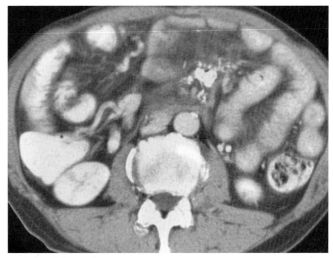

B

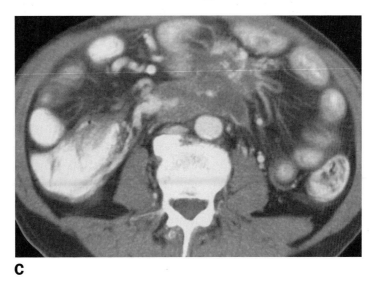

C

Findings

Contrast-enhanced CT. **A** through **C.** An ill-defined low-attenuation mass is present in the small bowel mesentery. The mass has a large amount of calcification and tethers adjacent bowel loops.

Differential Diagnosis

1. Retractile mesenteritis
2. Carcinoid tumor

Diagnosis

Retractile mesenteritis

Discussion

Retractile mesenteritis is a benign idiopathic disorder due to fibrous evolution of mesenteric panniculitis. Men in their fifth and sixth decades of life most commonly are affected. The most common appearance at CT is a solitary, ill-defined mass at the root of the small bowel mesentery with marked associated calcification. Tethering of adjacent bowel loops and vascular encasement also are frequent. Differentiation of retractile mesenteritis from a mesenteric carcinoid metastasis (cases 10.10 and 10.11) is not always possible. A mesenteric mass this large would be unusual for a carcinoid tumor. In addition, large carcinoids are nearly always associated with liver metastases.

CASE 10.14

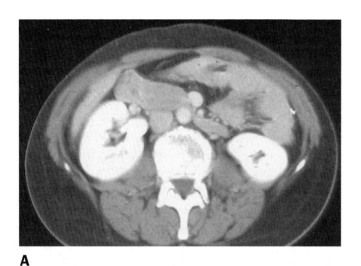

A

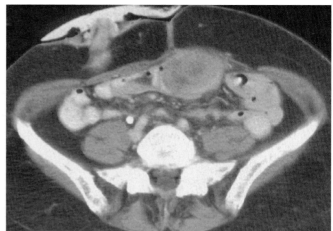

B

Findings

Contrast-enhanced CT. **A** and **B.** A mass is present in the mesentery in the left upper abdomen, and a second, larger, mixed-attenuation mass is in the anterior peritoneum. Postoperative changes of total colectomy with ileostomy in the right lower quadrant.

Differential Diagnosis

1. Metastases
2. Desmoid tumors (Gardner syndrome)

Diagnosis

Desmoid tumors (Gardner syndrome)

Discussion

Gardner syndrome is a variant of familial adenomatous polyposis syndrome with associated bone and skin abnormalities, mesenchymal tumors, and desmoids. The tubulovillous adenomas in the colon usually are evident by age 20 years, and colorectal cancer develops in nearly all patients without total proctocolectomy.

Desmoid tumors are benign fibrous neoplasms that usually occur in patients with Gardner syndrome after total colectomy. Desmoids can occur within the mesentery or in the abdominal wall and are multiple in 75% of cases. Although benign, these tumors often are locally aggressive and frequently recur. Because of this, surgery usually is reserved for life-threatening complications, including obstruction, infected fistula formation, or hemorrhage. Operation often results in the development of larger, more aggressive desmoid tumors and the increased possibility of complication.

CASE 10.15

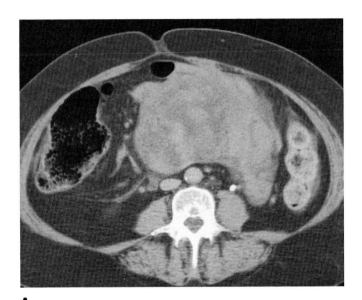

A

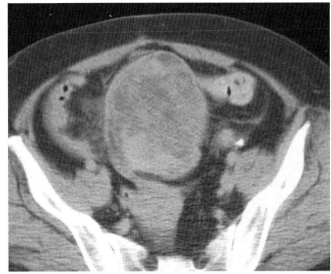

B

Findings

Contrast-enhanced CT. **A** and **B.** A very large mixed-attenuation mass is present in the mesentery of the lower abdomen.

Differential Diagnosis

1. Lymphoma
2. Metastatic adenopathy
3. Desmoid
4. Other primary mesenchymal mesenteric tumor

Diagnosis

Gastrointestinal stromal tumor

Discussion

Primary neoplasms of the mesentery are extremely rare (approximately 1 case per 250,000 population) and are usually of mesenchymal origin. Most of these tumors are large when detected because of the large potential space in which they can grow. Approximately two-thirds of these primary mesenteric tumors are benign, and the most common primary mesenteric tumor is the desmoid tumor (case 10.14). Desmoid tumors occur in approximately 25% of patients with Gardner syndrome. Other benign primary mesenteric tumors include lipomas, benign gastrointestinal tumors (GISTs), hemangiomas, and neurofibromas. The malignant primary mesenteric tumors include hemangiopericytomas, fibrosarcomas, liposarcomas, and malignant GISTs. These tumors usually are treated with surgical resection. Mesenteric lymphoma (case 10.16) is far more common than primary mesenteric tumors, but the mixed-attenuation nature of this mass and the lack of visualized retroperitoneal adenopathy are unusual in lymphoma.

CASE 10.16

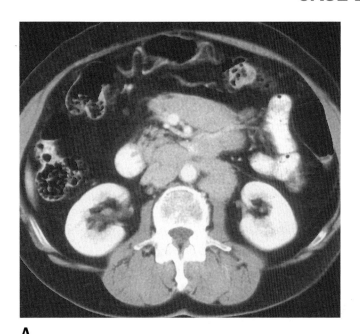

A

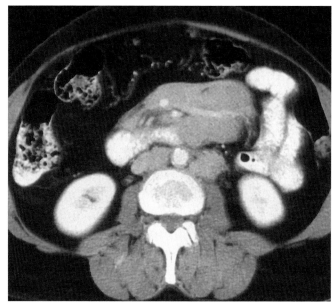

B

Findings
Contrast-enhanced CT. **A** and **B.** A large confluent soft tissue mesenteric mass encases branches of the superior mesenteric artery and vein. Retroperitoneal adenopathy also is present.

Differential Diagnosis
1. Mesenteric lymphoma
2. Metastatic lymphadenopathy

Diagnosis
Mesenteric non-Hodgkin lymphoma

Discussion
Lymphomatous involvement of the mesentery occurs in 5% of cases of Hodgkin lymphoma and in up to 50% of cases of non-Hodgkin lymphoma. The classic appearance of mesenteric lymphoma is seen in this case, with a lobulated confluent soft tissue mass encasing the superior mesenteric vessels, creating the sandwich or hamburger sign. Concomitant retroperitoneal adenopathy, inguinal adenopathy, and splenomegaly often are present in cases of mesenteric lymphoma. Nodal lymphomatous disease in the abdomen often responds well to chemotherapy. Other causes of mesenteric lymphadenopathy include metastatic disease, infectious or reactive adenopathy, and granulomatous disease.

CASE 10.17

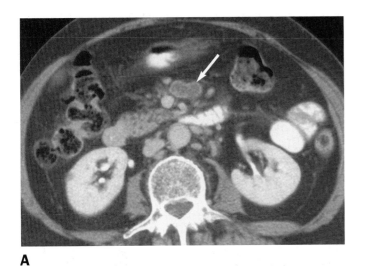

A

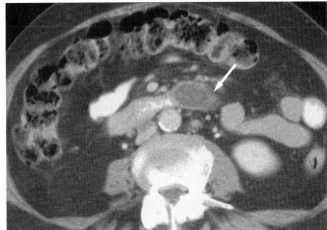

B

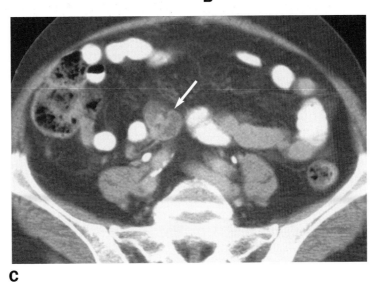

C

Findings
Contrast-enhanced CT. **A** through **C.** Enlarged low-attenuation, peripherally enhancing lymph nodes are present in the mesentery (arrows).

Differential Diagnosis
1. Treated lymphoma
2. Infectious lymphadenopathy
3. Necrotic metastatic lymphadenopathy
4. Whipple disease

Diagnosis
Treated lymphoma

Discussion
Low-attenuation lymphadenopathy is a fairly frequent finding in treated lymphoma and generally is seen when the nodes are decreasing in size and there has been a favorable response to chemotherapy. Low-attenuation mesenteric lymphadenopathy also can be due to infection—most commonly fungal (histoplasmosis) or mycobacterial (*Mycobacterium avium-intracellulare* and tuberculosis). Mycobacterial infection (case 10.18) is an important diagnostic consideration in patients who are positive for human immunodeficiency virus and have low-attenuation mesenteric adenopathy. Patients with Whipple disease can present with low-attenuation mesenteric adenopathy. These patients usually have a clinical history of malabsorption.

CASE 10.18

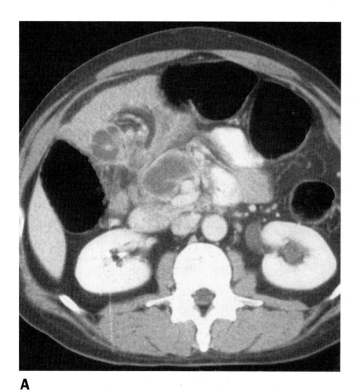

A

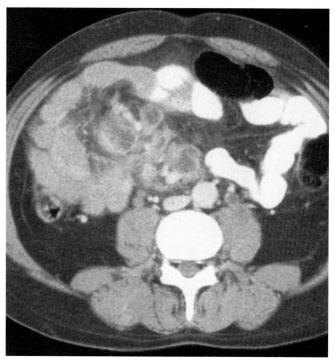

B

Findings

Contrast-enhanced CT. **A** and **B**. Multiple enlarged, peripherally enhancing, low-attenuation lymph nodes are present in the mesentery.

Differential Diagnosis

1. Lymphoma
2. Necrotic nodal metastasis
3. Infectious lymphadenopathy (*Mycobacterium avium-intracellulare*, tuberculosis)
4. Whipple disease

Diagnosis

Mycobacterium avium-intracellulare

Discussion

Ultrasonography-guided biopsy of the mesenteric lymphadenopathy in this patient who was positive for immunodeficiency virus (HIV) showed caseating granulomas. Special stains were positive for *Mycobacterium avium-intracellulare* (MAI). Differentiating common causes of extensive mesenteric and retroperitoneal lymphadenopathy can be difficult in a patient with HIV. However, the presence of central low-attenuating areas within the adenopathy is strongly suggestive of mycobacterial infection (tuberculosis or MAI). Approximately 65% of patients with HIV and lymphadenopathy due to mycobacterial infection have low-attenuation areas within the enlarged nodes, whereas only 2% of patients with HIV and adenopathy due to lymphoma or Kaposi sarcoma have centrally necrotic nodes.

The most common mycobacterial infection in patients with low-attenuating enlarged lymph nodes is tuberculosis, accounting for approximately 90% of cases. Radiologic differentiation of tuberculosis from MAI is difficult; however, focal hepatic or splenic abnormalities are more common in tuberculosis, as is peritoneal involvement (including ascites, peritoneal thickening, and omental infiltration).

CASE 10.19

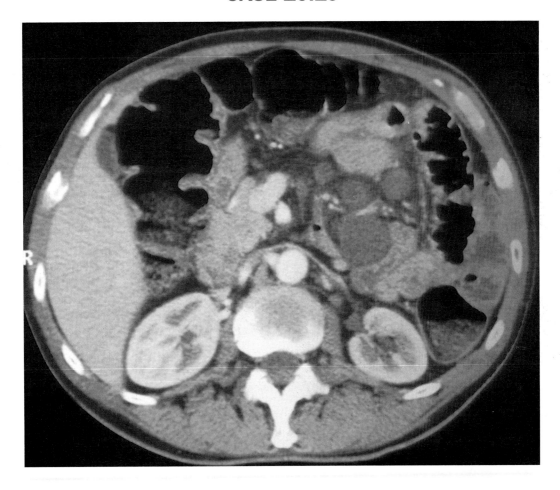

Findings

Contrast-enhanced CT. Several rounded cystic masses are present in the mesentery.

Differential Diagnosis

1. Treated lymphoma
2. Necrotic metastases
3. Mycobacterial infection
4. Whipple disease
5. Cavitary mesenteric lymph node syndrome

Diagnosis

Cavitary mesenteric lymph node syndrome

Discussion

Cavitary mesenteric lymph node syndrome (CMLNS) is an uncommon and poorly understood complication of celiac disease. On CT, CMLNS presents as multiple cystic masses in the mesentery, ranging in size from 2 to 7 cm. Diagnosis can be made by percutaneous aspiration or surgical excision. The benign cystic nodes of CMLNS contain chylous fluid surrounded by a thin rim of fibrous tissue. Because patients with celiac disease have an increased risk of malignancies (specifically lymphoma), tissue diagnosis is required for proper management. Mycobacterial infection also should be excluded when cystic mesenteric adenopathy is identified. The diagnosis of CMLNS in a patient with celiac disease is associated with a poor prognosis. Patients are at increased risk of intestinal hemorrhage and sepsis. Medical treatment includes institution of a strict gluten-free diet, corticosteroids, and infectious prophylaxis—all with variable effectiveness.

CASE 10.20

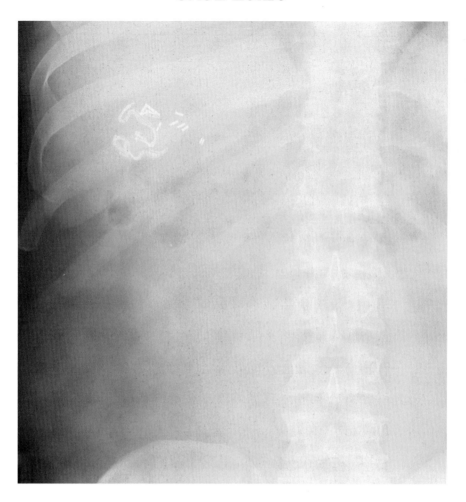

Findings
Abdominal radiograph. A serpiginous radiopaque filament is seen in the right upper quadrant adjacent to surgical clips.

Differential Diagnosis
Retained surgical sponge

Diagnosis
Retained surgical sponge

Discussion
Retained surgical sponges are reported in approximately 1 in 1,000 operations. Surgeons and operating teams rely on the practice of sponge and instrument counts to prevent retained surgical materials, but this obviously is not foolproof. The nonabsorbable cotton matrix of a surgical sponge can elicit two types of reactions within the peritoneal cavity. One is a fibrinous response, which results in a foreign body granuloma. The other is an exudative response, which leads to abscess formation. A sinus tract or fistula tract also may develop as an attempt by the body to extrude the foreign body either externally or into a hollow viscus.

The mortality rate associated with a retained surgical sponge is 10% to 35%. Expeditious removal of a retained sponge is recommended, and laparoscopic retrieval often is possible, especially if discovered early. Given the high associated morbidity and mortality rates, a familiarity with the x-ray and CT appearance of sponges and other surgical instruments is important when interpreting postoperative films. Modern surgical sponges usually are marked with radiopaque filaments, as in this case, and are easily visible on x-ray examination.

CASE 10.21

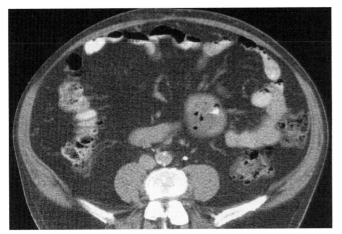

A

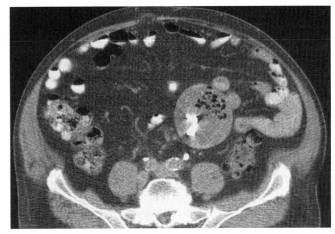

B

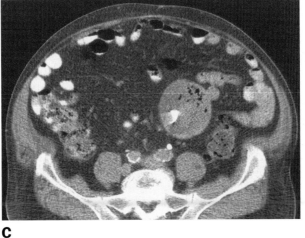

C

Findings
CT with oral contrast. **A** through **C**. A well-defined spherical mass is present in the left lower quadrant, which contains fluid, air, and a wavy high-attenuation structure centrally.

Differential Diagnosis
1. Abscess due to retained surgical sponge
2. Necrotic or infected mesenteric tumor

Diagnosis
Peritoneal abscess due to retained surgical sponge (gossypiboma)

Discussion
A surgical sponge in the peritoneal cavity and the masslike inflammatory reaction around the sponge sometimes are referred to as a gossypiboma. This case shows the exudative response to a retained surgical sponge, which has led to abscess formation. At CT, a gossypiboma usually presents as a well-circumscribed, low-attenuation peritoneal mass, which often has a spongiform gas pattern centrally as a result of gas trapped in the mesh of the sponge. Surgical sponges also usually contain a radiopaque filament, which has a serpiginous or wavy appearance, as in this case. Visualization of air-fluid levels and a well-defined enhancing rim favor abscess formation. At surgery, 20 mL of pus was present in the cavity around this retained surgical sponge. Other complications associated with gossypiboma include sinus tracts or fistula tracts to the skin or into a hollow viscus.

CASE 10.22

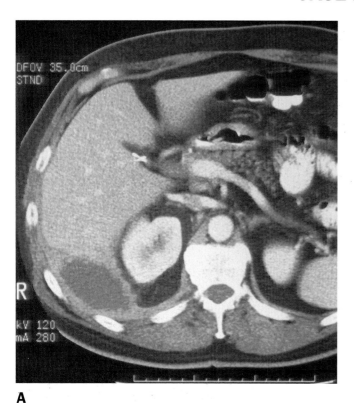

A

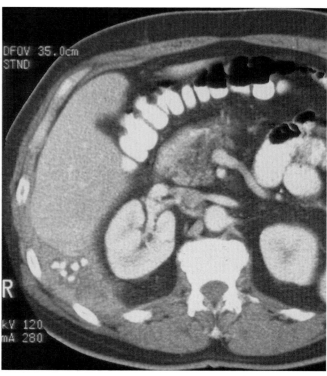

B

Findings
Contrast-enhanced CT. **A** and **B.** A peripherally enhancing fluid collection is present in the subhepatic space, which contains several small, rounded calcific densities. Cholecystectomy.

Differential Diagnosis
1. Abscess
2. Necrotic tumor

Diagnosis
Subhepatic abscess due to spilled gallstones

Discussion
Spillage of gallstones into the peritoneal cavity is more common with laparoscopic than open surgery and occurs in 5% to 30% of laparoscopic cholecystectomies. Spillage of stones usually occurs during dissection of the gallbladder off the liver bed, tearing with grasping forceps, or extraction of the gallbladder through one of the port sites. Complications related to spilled gallstones are rare and are thought to occur in only approximately 1 in 1,000 patients. The exact reason some spilled stones result in abscess formation is unknown. However, infective complications are thought to be more common when the stones are spilled along with infected bile and with bilirubinate stones, because they often contain viable bacteria. Abscesses due to spilled stones usually occur in the subdiaphragmatic or hepatorenal recesses (as in this case), but spilled stones and their infective complications can occur anywhere in the peritoneal cavity. Patients usually present with abscesses due to spilled gallstones from as early as 1 month to as long as 20 years after a cholecystectomy; the peak incidence is around 4 months. These patients often present without a fever and with a normal leukocyte count. These abscesses usually are treated with percutaneous drainage, and laparotomy commonly is reserved for cases in which percutaneous drainage fails.

CASE 10.23

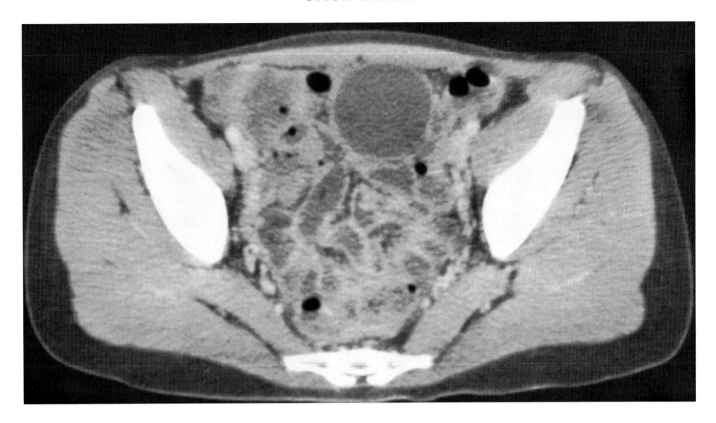

Findings

Contrast-enhanced CT. A thin-walled, rounded, fluid-density mass is present in the mesentery of the lower abdomen.

Differential Diagnosis

1. Enteric duplication cyst
2. Mesenteric cyst
3. Ovarian cyst
4. Lymphangioma

Diagnosis

Mesenteric cyst

Discussion

Mesenteric cysts are rare, usually asymptomatic benign abdominal tumors that often are detected incidentally during physical or radiologic examination. These cysts most commonly are diagnosed in patients in their 40s but also may affect young children. They are thought to develop from benign proliferations of ectopic lymphatics that lack communication to the normal lymphatic system. They can range in size from a few millimeters to 40 cm in diameter. These cysts most commonly are located in the ileal mesentery and can be unilocular or multilocular and contain chylous, serous, or, rarely, hemorrhagic fluid. Surgical enucleation is recommended to prevent possible complications of volvulus, obstruction, or, more rarely, infection or hemorrhage. Imaging differentiation of a mesenteric cyst from other cystic abdominal masses often is extremely difficult.

Fluid and Masses of the Peritoneum and Mesentery

		Case
Simple ascites	Anechoic. Transudate most commonly caused by cirrhosis and portal hypertension	10.1
Complicated ascites	Low-level echoes (caused by floating debris) and septations in the ascites. Common causes include infection, hemorrhage, and malignancy	10.2
Peritoneal abscess	Peripherally enhancing fluid collection with bubbles of gas. Caused by perforation of a viscus or surgery	10.3
Hemoperitoneum	Blood in peritoneum is usually around +45 Hounsfield units. Layering of blood products of different ages is common	10.4
Pseudomyxoma peritonei	Mucinous tumor (adenocarcinoma). Caused by ruptured appendiceal mucocele, ovary or colon cancer. Scalloped liver surface, calcifications, and enhancing septations	10.5
Peritoneal carcinomatosis	Multiple nodular peritoneal tumor implants and ascites. Omental caking common. Most commonly caused by ovarian or gastrointestinal primary tumors	10.6 and 10.7
Malignant peritoneal mesothelioma	Multiple peritoneal tumor implants and associated ascites. Usually occurs in men 30-40 years after asbestos exposure	10.8
Cystic peritoneal mesothelioma	Multiloculated low-attenuation peritoneal mass. Benign tumor in young women with no prior asbestos exposure	10.9
Carcinoid	Mesenteric invasion of tumor causes desmoplastic reaction, giving a sunburst appearance at CT. Hypervascular liver metastases are common	10.10 and 10.11

Fluid and Masses of the Peritoneum and Mesentery (continued)

		Case
Retractile mesenteritis	Idiopathic disease. Infiltrating mesenteric soft tissue mass, often with large amount of associated calcification and tethering of adjacent bowel loops	10.12 and 10.13
Desmoid tumor	Benign fibrous neoplasm of mesentery or abdominal wall. Most common in patients with Gardner syndrome after colectomy	10.14
Mesenteric gastro-intestinal stromal tumor	Rare malignant primary mesenteric tumor. Usually large, solitary, mixed-attenuation tumor	10.15
Lymphoma	Bulky, confluent mesenteric adenopathy around the mesenteric vessels creates sandwich or hamburger sign. Treated lymphoma can be low attenuation	10.16 and 10.17
Mycobacterial mesenteric adenopathy	Low-attenuation mesenteric adenopathy. Tuberculosis and *Mycobacterium avium-intracellulare* common in patients positive for human immunodeficiency vius	10.18
Cavitary mesenteric lymph node syndrome	Cystic mesenteric masses in patients with celiac disease	10.19
Gossypiboma	Retained sponge and host response. Can result in abscess formation. Usually contains a wavy metallic filament	10.20 and 10.21
Subhepatic abscess due to spilled gallstones	Rare complication of laparoscopic cholecystectomy. More common when spilled with infected bile or with bilirubinate stones	10.22
Mesenteric cyst	Rounded, fluid-attenuation mesenteric mass. Can result in obstruction or volvulus	10.23

CASE 10.24

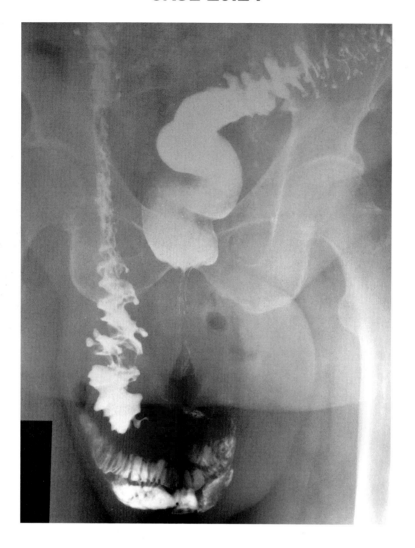

Findings

Single-contrast barium enema. The cecum and loops of distal small bowel are located in the scrotum.

Differential Diagnosis

Inguinal hernia (indirect)

Diagnosis

Inguinal hernia (indirect)

Discussion

Abdominal hernias can be characterized as *external* (extending beyond the normal contours of the abdomen or pelvis), *internal* (protrusion of a viscus through a peritoneal or mesenteric defect with an intact abdominal cavity), or *diaphragmatic*. Almost 75% of external hernias occur in the groin, the great majority of these being inguinal hernias.

Indirect inguinal hernias are the most common type, and the hernia sac and contents protrude into the inguinal canal and emerge at the external ring. This type of hernia is more common in males and often extends into the scrotum. The indirect inguinal hernia sac passes lateral to the inferior epigastric vessels. Less common direct inguinal hernias (case 10.25) protrude directly through a weak area in the abdominal wall medial to the inferior epigastric vessels. Direct inguinal hernias should not extend into the scrotum. Left-sided inguinal hernias can involve the sigmoid colon, whereas right-sided hernias can contain the cecum and small bowel (as in this case).

CASE 10.25

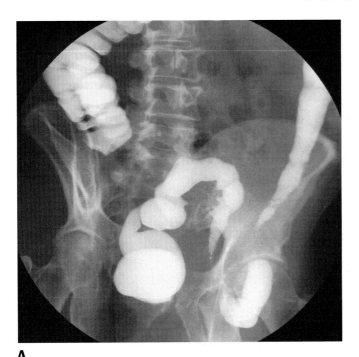

A

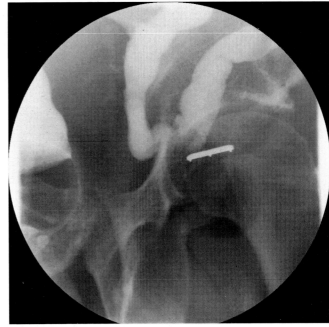

B

Findings
Single-contrast barium enema. **A.** A loop of sigmoid colon extends into the left groin beyond the normal contours of the pelvic cavity. **B.** This protruded loop of bowel could be easily pushed back into the pelvis with a compression device.

Differential Diagnosis
1. Inguinal hernia (direct)
2. Inguinal hernia (indirect)
3. Femoral hernia

Diagnosis
Inguinal hernia (direct)

Discussion
Direct inguinal hernias are less common than indirect inguinal hernias and usually occur in men. A direct inguinal hernia results from protrusion of abdominal contents through a weakening in the lower abdominal wall medial to the inferior epigastric vessels. These hernias usually have a fairly wide opening and rarely become incarcerated. Incarcerated hernias are hernias that cannot be manually reduced. Complications of incarcerated hernias include obstruction and bowel strangulation and ischemia. Surgery is indicated to avoid these possible complications.

The hernia in this case is unlikely to be an indirect inguinal hernia (case 10.24) because it does not follow the course of the inguinal canal and does not extend into the scrotum. Femoral hernias (cases 10.26 and 10.27) are uncommon in men, and the necks of these hernias usually are much smaller given the small potential space along the femoral vessels.

CASE 10.26

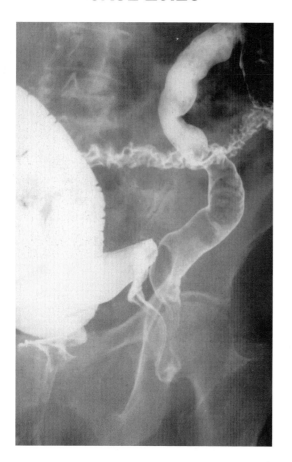

CASE 10.27

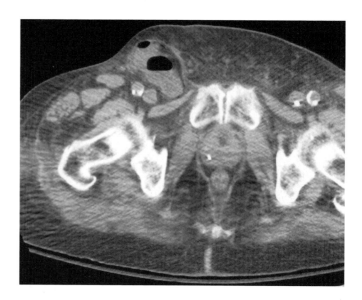

Findings

Case 10.26. Single-contrast barium enema. A loop of sigmoid colon is present within a hernia sac in the left inguinal region.

Case 10.27. Unenhanced CT. A loop of slightly dilated small bowel is present within a hernia sac just medial to the right femoral vein.

Differential Diagnosis
1. Inguinal hernia
2. Femoral hernia

Diagnosis
Femoral hernia

Discussion

At operation, femoral hernias were found and repaired in both of these cases. Femoral hernias are 3 times more common in women and constitute one-third of groin hernias in women. These hernias tend to be smaller than inguinal hernias, and the neck of the hernia always remains below the inguinal ligament and lateral to the pubic tubercle. On CT, the hernia can be seen to lie immediately medial to the femoral vein. Femoral hernias are often difficult to diagnose clinically because they tend to be small and have a deep location along the femoral vessels. Correct diagnosis is important because a femoral hernia is 10 times more prone to incarceration and strangulation than the more common inguinal hernia.

A Richter hernia refers to entrapment of one wall of the bowel in the orifice of the hernia. This is commonly found in older women with a femoral hernia. This type of hernia rarely causes obstruction, but it may result in ischemia of the trapped bowel wall.

CASE 10.28

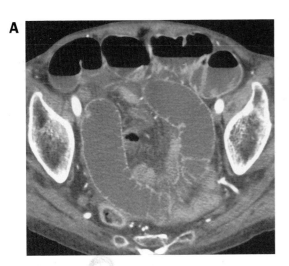

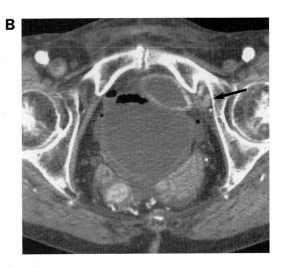

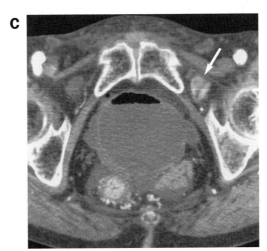

Findings

CT enterography. **A.** Multiple loops of dilated small bowel are present in the lower abdomen.

B and **C.** A compressed loop of bowel (arrows) extends through the left obturator foramen into a position between the left pectineus and obturator externus muscles.

Differential Diagnosis

Incarcerated obturator hernia

Diagnosis

Incarcerated obturator hernia

Discussion

Obturator hernias are most commonly found in elderly women (female:male ratio, 6:1). Patients typically present with symptoms of bowel obstruction and pain radiating down the medial thigh caused by compression of the obturator nerve as it exits the obturator canal. The obturator canal is situated in the anterosuperior aspect of the obturator foramen and contains the obturator artery, vein, and nerve. This canal is approximately 1 cm in diameter and 2 to 3 cm long. Although rare, recognition of an obturator hernia on CT is important because strangulated obturator hernias are associated with the highest mortality rate of all hernias.

Other pelvic wall hernias include sciatic and perineal hernias. The figure on page 717 shows the locations of pelvic wall and groin hernias.

CASE 10.29

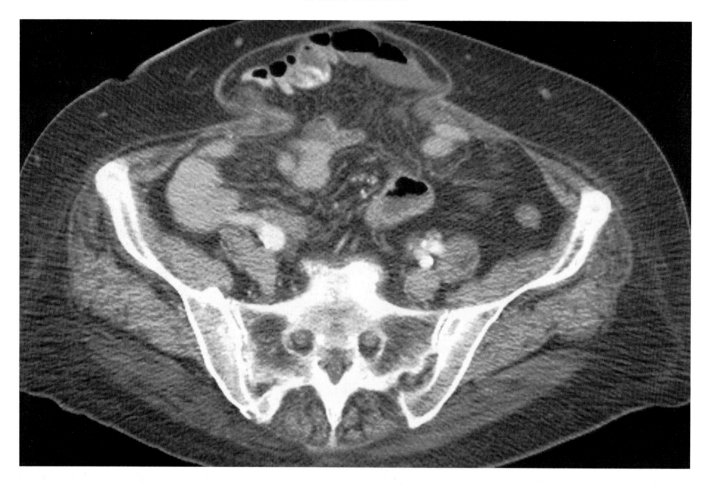

Findings
Contrast-enhanced CT. A large midline hernia contains several loops of normal-caliber small bowel.

Differential Diagnosis
Ventral (incisional) hernia

Diagnosis
Ventral (incisional) hernia

Discussion
Ventral hernias include herniations through areas of relative weakness in the musculature of the anterior or lateral abdominal wall. The majority occur in the midline, bulging through the linea alba, separating the rectus abdominus muscles. Ventral hernias frequently occur along prior surgical incisions, laparoscopy port sites, or stab wounds. Incarceration (trapping) of bowel loops in a ventral hernia may lead to infarction and require emergency surgery. Ventral hernias that have a wide opening, such as this one, are less likely to result in obstructive or ischemic complications than those with narrow openings.

CASE 10.30

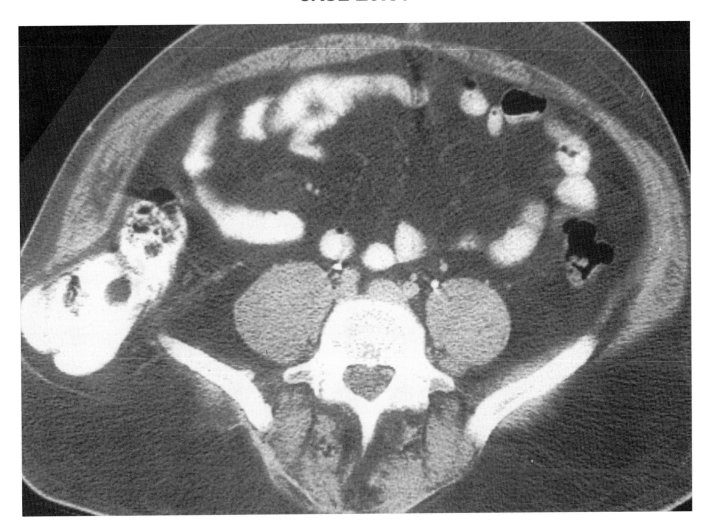

Findings
Contrast-enhanced CT. The cecum has herniated through an abdominal wall defect just posterior to the internal and external oblique muscles.

Differential Diagnosis
Lateral ventral hernia

Diagnosis
Lateral ventral hernia

Discussion
Lateral ventral hernias can occur spontaneously but commonly are located at sites of prior surgery (e.g., nephrectomy, cholecystectomy) or prior stab wound.

CASE 10.31

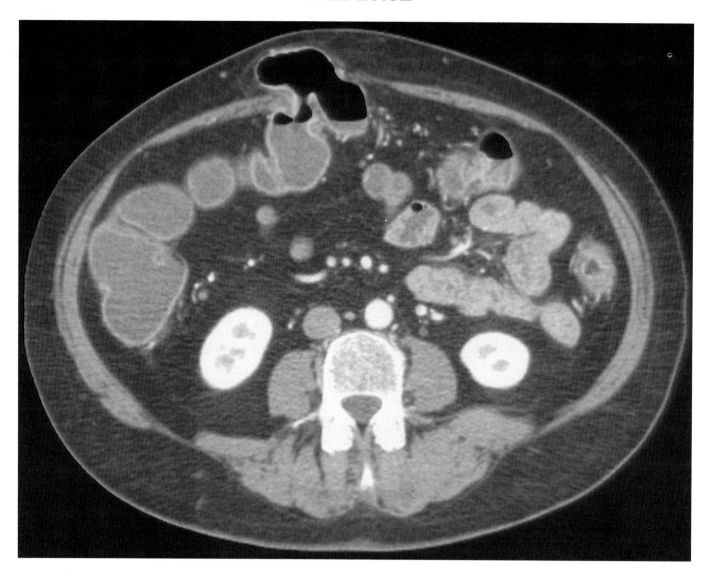

Findings
Contrast-enhanced CT. There is a defect in the anterior abdominal wall, near the midline. A portion of the wall of the colon has herniated through the defect.

Differential Diagnosis
Richter hernia

Diagnosis
Richter hernia

Discussion
A Richter hernia (also known as Richter-Littre or parietal hernia) involves only a portion of the circumference of a bowel loop. It usually does not affect the passage of bowel contents. Therefore, there is usually no obstruction, but strangulation of the affected portion of the bowel wall can occur.

CASE 10.32

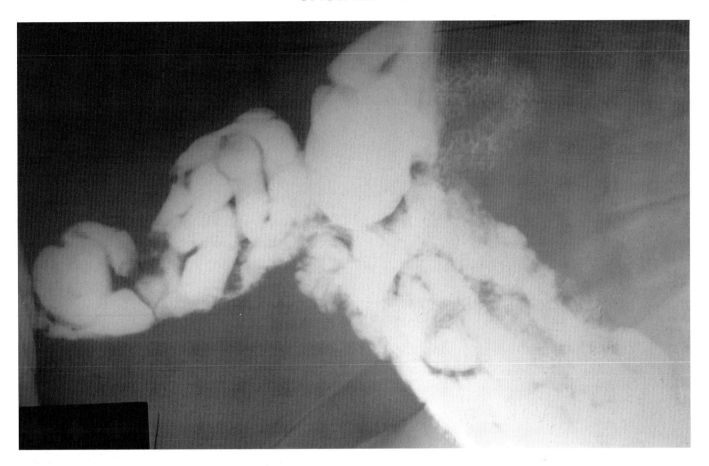

Findings
Small bowel follow-through. An ileostomy is shown on this lateral abdominal radiograph. Several small bowel loops have herniated through the abdominal wall defect into a parastomal location.

Differential Diagnosis
1. Parastomal hernia
2. Ventral hernia, midline

Diagnosis
Parastomal hernia

Discussion
Parastomal hernias often are found after an operation involving ileostomy or colostomy. The diagnosis may not be obvious when the patient is examined in the supine or prone position. A lateral radiograph with the ostomy tract in profile usually is helpful for displaying the anatomy. Often the diagnosis of a hernia is clinically apparent, but a radiographic examination can be helpful for determining the size of the hernia and its contents and to evaluate for obstruction.

CASE 10.33

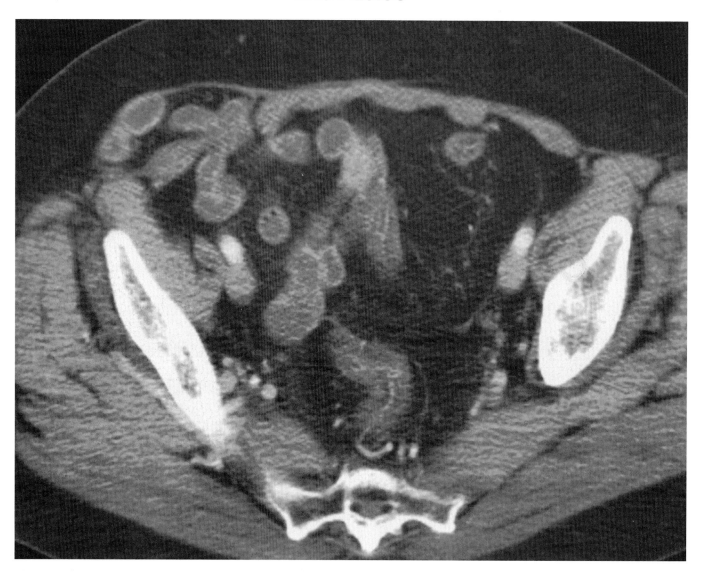

Findings
Contrast-enhanced CT. A herniated loop of bowel is seen entering the subcutaneous space lateral to the rectus abdominus muscle.

Differential Diagnosis
1. Spigelian hernia
2. Inguinal hernia

Diagnosis
Spigelian hernia

Discussion
A spigelian hernia is a type of external hernia in which the abdominal wall defect arises along the linea semilunaris, a connective tissue structure that runs from the costal cartilages to the symphysis pubis, just lateral to the rectus abdominus muscle. These hernias most often occur as a result of increased intra-abdominal pressure (e.g., in heavy laborers, patients with chronic obstructive lung disease, those with urinary or gastric retention, and in multiparous women).

Indirect inguinal hernias are located lateral to the epigastric vessels and follow the path of the spermatic cord.

CASE 10.34

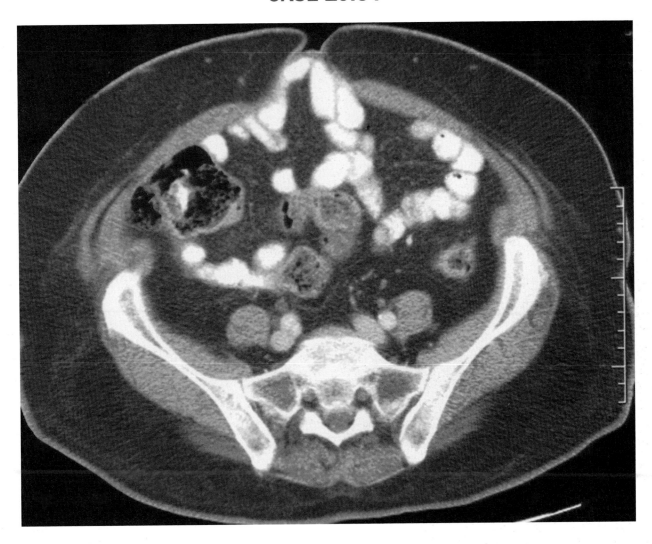

Findings
Contrast-enhanced CT. A "knuckle" of normal-caliber small bowel bulges from the peritoneum adjacent to the umbilicus.

Differential Diagnosis
1. Umbilical hernia
2. Ventral hernia

Diagnosis
Umbilical hernia

Discussion
Umbilical hernias due to a patent umbilical ring are common in infants and children. Incarceration of umbilical hernias in children is extremely rare. Treatment is usually observation because 95% of umbilical hernias close on their own by age 5 years.

Umbilical hernias in adults occur predominantly in patients with increased abdominal pressure, including women after pregnancy and patients with ascites or chronic bowel distention. An incarcerated umbilical hernia should be suspected when a patient presents with intestinal obstruction and paraumbilical pain, even if an obvious bulge cannot be palpated. A ventral hernia could give a similar CT appearance. Identifying a focal hernia at the umbilicus allows the correct diagnosis.

CASE 10.35

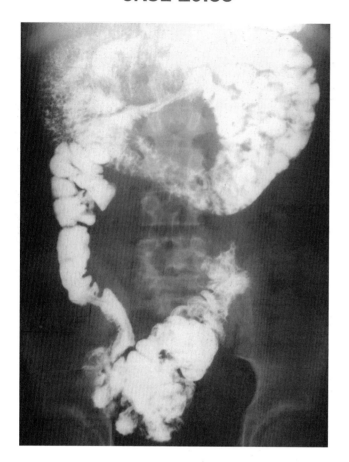

CASE 10.36

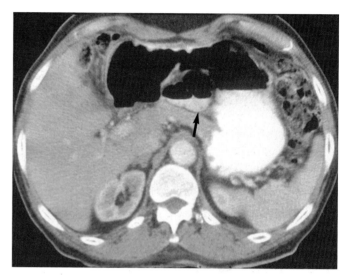

Findings

Case 10.35. Small bowel follow-through. Most of the small bowel is located in the upper abdomen and appears to be confined within a saclike structure.

Case 10.36. Contrast-enhanced CT. A loop of bowel (arrow) is located between the stomach and the body of the pancreas.

Differential Diagnosis

1. Paraduodenal hernia
2. Foramen of Winslow hernia

Diagnosis

Paraduodenal hernia

Discussion

Paraduodenal hernias are the most frequent type of internal hernias, making up approximately 50% of internal hernias. Most occur as a congenital anomaly of intestinal rotation and peritoneal attachment. Paraduodenal hernias usually (75%) occur on the left as a result of bowel herniating through a peritoneal reflection created by the inferior mesenteric artery. Bowel resides lateral to the ascending limb (fourth portion) of the duodenum. Less commonly (25%), paraduodenal hernias occur on the right through the fossa beneath the superior mesenteric artery. Radiographically, a mass of small bowel loops usually is located in the left upper quadrant, appearing to be encapsulated within a sac. Stasis of intraluminal barium and bowel dilatation may be present.

Foramen of Winslow internal hernias displace the stomach and duodenum to the left and the stomach anteriorly. A foramen of Winslow hernia could have this CT appearance. In addition to paraduodenal and foramen of Winslow hernias, transmesenteric, pericecal, intersigmoid, and mesocolic internal hernias also can occur. The figure on page 718 shows the possible locations for internal hernias.

CASE 10.37

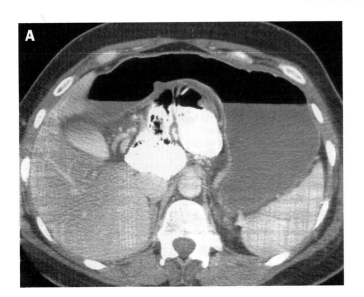

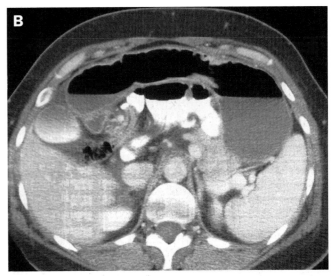

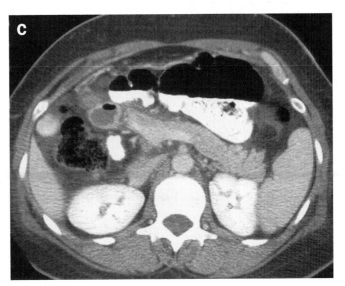

Findings

Contrast-enhanced CT. A through C. The contrast-enhanced cecum is located in an aberrant position in the lesser sac, positioned between the stomach, liver, and pancreas.

Differential Diagnosis

1. Foramen of Winslow hernia
2. Paraduodenal hernia

Diagnosis

Foramen of Winslow hernia

Discussion

Approximately 10% of all internal hernias occur as a result of protrusion of viscera into the lesser sac through the foramen of Winslow. The small bowel is involved in 70% of cases and the cecum and ascending colon in 30% of cases. A predisposing factor is excessive mobility of intestinal loops due to a long mesentery. Patients often present with acute pain and obstruction after an episode of sudden increased abdominal pressure (e.g., childbirth, weight lifting).

CASE 10.38

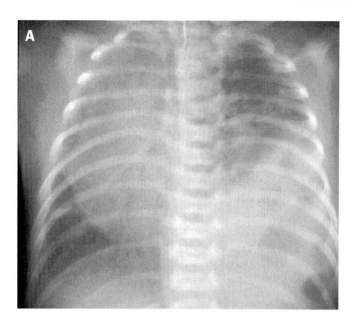

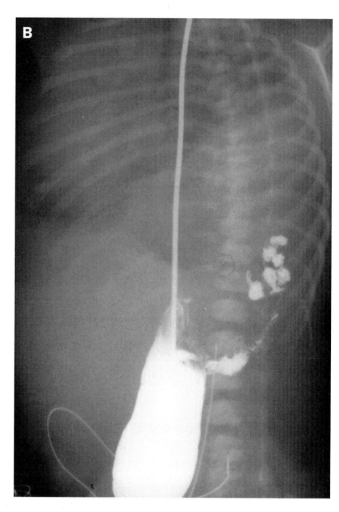

Findings

A. Chest radiograph. Opacification of the left lower lung is present, which contains several gas collections within it. The cardiothymic silhouette is displaced to the right.

B. Small bowel follow-through. Contrast material has been instilled into the stomach through a nasogastric tube. Small bowel loops are seen to enter the left thorax, traversing a posteriorly located diaphragmatic defect.

Differential Diagnosis

1. Bochdalek hernia
2. Traumatic diaphragmatic hernia

Diagnosis

Bochdalek hernia

Discussion

Symptomatic Bochdalek hernias are most common in infants. They occur as a result of incomplete closure of the pleuroperitoneal canal. The defect is always posterior and usually on the left. If the defect is large, nearly all of the abdominal contents can reside in the thorax. This can result in pulmonary developmental abnormalities and an associated high infant mortality rate. Traumatic hernias through the diaphragm usually follow a major traumatic event. They may not be detected immediately, and patients may present with pain or bowel obstruction years later.

CASE 10.39

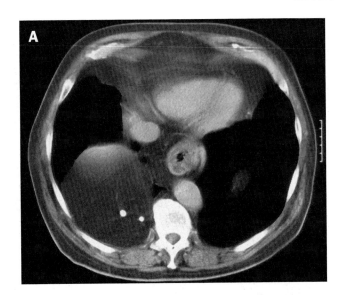

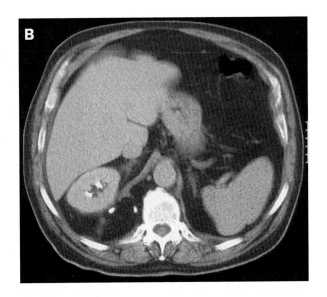

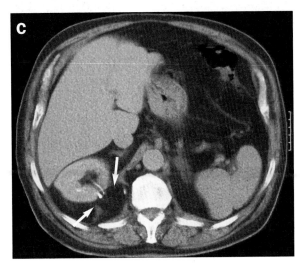

Findings

Contrast-enhanced CT (delayed images). **A** through **C.** There is a defect in the diaphragm posteriorly on the right (arrows), and peritoneal fat and a loop of proximal ureter have herniated into the right thoracic cavity. Sliding hiatal hernia.

Differential Diagnosis

Right-sided Bochdalek hernia

Diagnosis

Right-sided Bochdalek hernia

Discussion

Asymptomatic Bochdalek hernias in adults are more common than previously thought and have been reported to occur in approximately 0.2% of adults. Most of these posterior diaphragmatic hernias are discovered incidentally during CT or MRI. Bochdalek hernias are always located posteriorly and are usually on the left (70% of cases), unlike this case. Asymptomatic Bochdalek hernias usually contain only fat. Controversy remains as to whether these small asymptomatic Bochdalek hernias need to be treated surgically. When bowel or solid organs are present within the hernia, surgery is usually performed to prevent infarction or other complications.

CASE 10.40

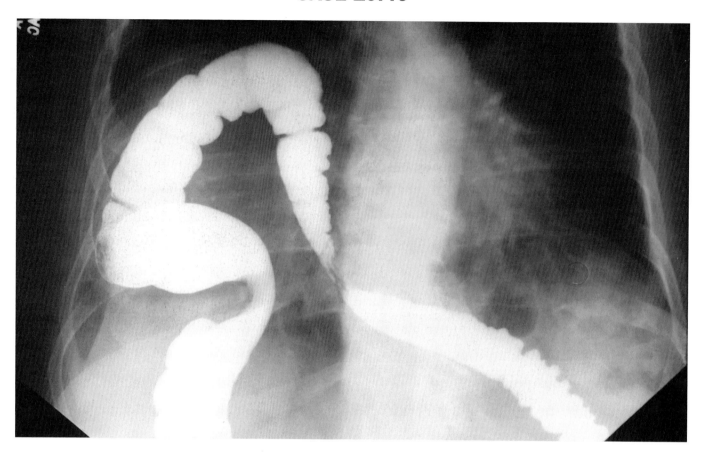

Findings
Single-contrast barium enema. A large segment of transverse colon has herniated into the thorax through a defect in the anterior portion of the diaphragm.

Differential Diagnosis
1. Morgagni hernia
2. Traumatic diaphragmatic hernia

Diagnosis
Morgagni hernia

Discussion
Morgagni hernias are less common than Bochdalek hernias. These hernias occur as a result of a midline defect in which the right and left pleuroperitoneal folds do not join. The substernal region is always affected, usually near the midline. The omentum often herniates into the thorax, but liver and colon also can be present.

CASE 10.41

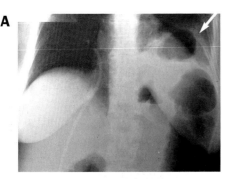

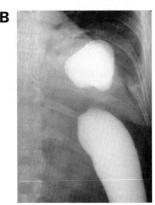

CASE 10.42

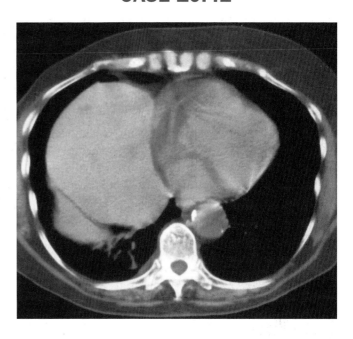

Findings

Case 10.41. A. Abdominal radiograph. There is a loculated collection of gas in the left upper abdomen (arrow), either in a subdiaphragmatic or intrathoracic location.

B. Single-contrast barium enema. The questionable gas collection is the splenic flexure of the colon, which has herniated through a small diaphragmatic defect. The colonic lumen is narrowed as it passes through the diaphragm, and barium could not be advanced into the more proximal colon, indicating obstruction.

Case 10.42. Unenhanced CT. The liver has herniated through the diaphragm and lies within the right thoracic cavity adjacent to the heart.

Differential Diagnosis
1. Traumatic diaphragmatic hernia
2. Morgagni diaphragmatic hernia

Diagnosis
Traumatic diaphragmatic hernia

Discussion

Traumatic abdominal hernia is a relatively rare condition due to either blunt external trauma or penetrating wounds. Occasionally, iatrogenic hernias may develop after subdiaphragmatic surgical procedures. The majority of diaphragmatic tears occur on the left, perhaps due to the protective effect of the liver on the right. The stomach is the organ most likely to herniate, followed by colon, small bowel, spleen, and omentum. Complications of obstruction and strangulation occur in the majority of patients if surgical correction is not performed. These complications are associated with a high mortality rate.

Hernias

		Case
External		
Indirect inguinal	Most common external hernia. Protrusion lateral to inferior epigastric vessels and into inguinal canal. Most common in men, with extension into scrotum	10.24
Direct inguinal	Protrusion medial to inferior epigastric vessels. Most common in men, but should not extend into scrotum	10.25
Femoral	Much more common in women. Herniation medial to femoral vein. High risk of incarceration	10.26 and 10.27
Obturator	Rare hernia usually occurring in elderly women. Protrusion through obturator canal. High morbidity and mortality	10.28
Ventral (incisional)	Most common midline. Common at sites of prior surgery	10.29–10.32
Spigelian	Protrusion lateral to rectus abdominus muscle	10.33
Umbilical	Protrusion through umbilical ring. Usually resolves spontaneously in infants	10.34
Internal		
Paraduodenal	Most common internal hernia. 75% occur on the left	10.35 and 10.36
Foramen of Winslow	Herniation into the lesser sac	10.37
Diaphragmatic		
Esophageal hiatus	Very common diaphragmatic hernia. Sliding or paraesophageal type	1.64 and 1.65
Bochdalek	Most common congenital diaphragmatic hernia. Always located posteriorly, usually on the left	10.38 and 10.39
Morgagni	Located anteriorly on the right	10.40
Traumatic	More common on the left. Follows blunt trauma or penetrating wound	10.41 and 10.42

CASE 10.43

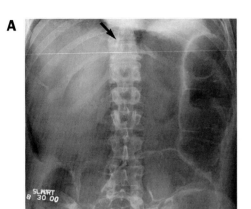

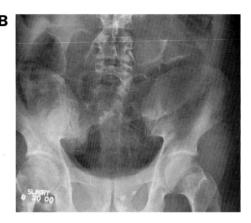

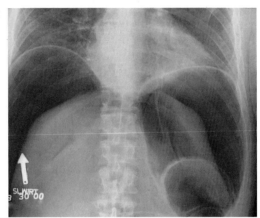

Findings

A and **B.** Supine abdominal radiograph. Air outlines the peritoneal cavity and liver. Gas is on both sides of the colonic wall and outlines the falciform ligament (arrow). **C.** Upright abdominal radiograph. A large amount of air is present beneath both domes of the diaphragm.

Differential Diagnosis

Pneumoperitoneum

Diagnosis

Pneumoperitoneum

Discussion

Pneumoperitoneum can be caused by recent surgery, bowel perforation, trauma, or peritoneal infection with gas-producing organisms. In a nonsurgical patient, the presence of free intraperitoneal air is highly suggestive of bowel perforation, most commonly caused by a perforated gastric or duodenal ulcer. Postoperative pneumoperitoneum usually resolves in 4 to 5 days. Pneumoperitoneum after this time or an increase in the amount of free intraperitoneal air on serial examinations is highly suggestive of a bowel leak.

Pneumoperitoneum is best visualized on upright films as air beneath the hemidiaphragms. Left lateral decubitus views can be helpful in critically ill patients who are unable to have upright views. Signs of pneumoperitoneum on supine plain films include 1) Rigler sign, gas on both sides of the bowel wall; 2) football sign, gas outlining the entire peritoneal cavity; 3) gas outlining the falciform ligament; and 4) an amorphous gas density over the liver, which can indicate free air positioned between the anterior abdominal wall and liver. All of these findings can be seen on the supine films in this case. Lung windows often are helpful for identifying small amounts of free intraperitoneal air at CT, which can be confused with intraluminal gas. This patient had pneumoperitoneum due to an iatrogenic colonic perforation during colonoscopy.

CASE 10.44

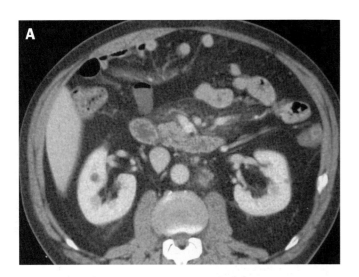

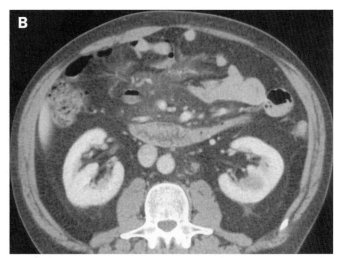

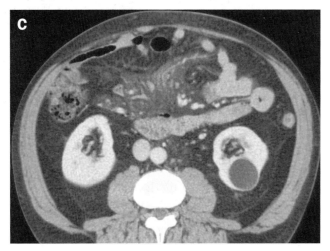

Findings

Contrast-enhanced CT. **A** through **C**. Mild, diffuse, high-attenuation stranding is present in the mesenteric fat.

Differential Diagnosis

1. Lymphoma
2. Mesenteric panniculitis
3. Mesenteric edema

Diagnosis

Misty mesentery (due to lymphoma)

Discussion

A wispy area of increased attenuation within the mesentery, often referred to as "misty mesentery," is a nonspecific finding at CT which can be due to fluid, inflammatory cells, fibrosis, or tumor in the mesenteric fat. The most common causes of mesenteric edema include heart failure, portal hypertension, hypoalbuminemia, and mesenteric arterial or venous thrombosis. Inflammatory processes such as pancreatitis, inflammatory bowel disease, and diverticulitis can result in a misty mesentery. Neoplasms (most commonly non-Hodgkin lymphoma) also can give this appearance. Finally, idiopathic causes such as retractile mesenteritis (mesenteric panniculitis) may result in a misty mesentery. Differentiation between these causes of a misty mesentery is often difficult, but the possibilities may be narrowed down by clinical history and follow-up imaging.

CASE 10.45

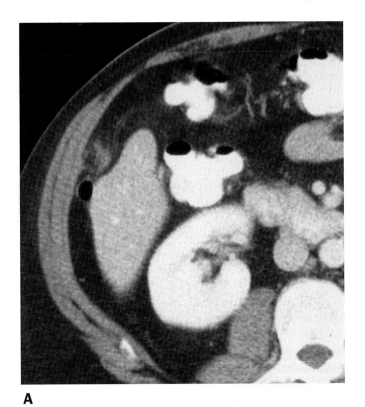

A

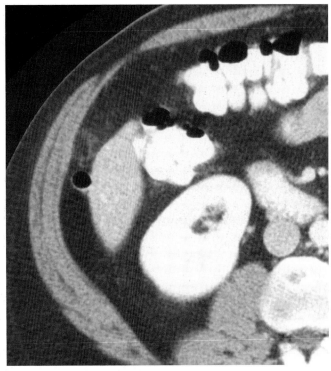

B

Findings

Contrast-enhanced CT. **A** and **B.** Focal inflammatory "stranding" is present in the fat of the right lateral abdominal cavity.

Differential Diagnosis

1. Diverticulitis
2. Omental torsion and infarction
3. Epiploic appendagitis

Diagnosis

Omental torsion and infarction

Discussion

Omental torsion with infarction is a rare acute abdominal condition, which is often clinically misdiagnosed as acute appendicitis. Middle-aged patients most commonly are affected, and they usually present with severe right lower quadrant pain and low-grade fever. Most omental infarcts are located on the right because the right side of the omentum is longer, heavier, and more mobile, and thus more likely to torque. Omental infarction is the final result of torsion that occurs from twisting of the omentum and its vascular pedicle along its long axis.

CT findings of omental infarction include a fatty mass with inflammatory stranding along the right inferior edge of the omentum. The adjacent colon should be normal. Omental torsion with infarction is considered a benign condition and has spontaneous resolution and disappearance of the CT abnormality over 1 to 2 months. This condition can be treated conservatively with analgesics once more common causes of acute right lower quadrant pain, including appendicitis, right-sided diverticulitis, and cholecystitis, are excluded. Epiploic appendagitis (case 5.56) usually presents as a smaller fatty mass with a hyperattenuating peripheral rim. Epiploic appendagitis is most common adjacent to the sigmoid colon, whereas omental torsion is usually in the right abdomen.

Miscellaneous Conditions of the Peritoneum and Mesentery

		Case
Pneumoperitoneum	Upright, air beneath diaphragm. Rigler sign (air on both sides of bowel wall), football sign (air outlining entire peritoneal cavity)	10.43
Misty mesentery	Diffuse or focal soft tissue stranding. Nonspecific findings: lymphoma, portal hypertension, hypoalbuminemia, inflammatory diseases, mesenteric panniculitis	10.44
Omental torsion with infarction	Inflammatory mass containing fat. Usually in right upper quadrant. Symptoms can resemble those of appendicitis. Conservative treatment	10.45

DIFFERENTIAL DIAGNOSES

Hernias

External

Groin, pelvic wall
Indirect inguinal
Direct inguinal
Femoral
Obturator
Sciatic
Perineal
Abdominal wall
Ventral or incisional
Spigelian
Umbilical

Internal

Paraduodenal
Foramen of Winslow
Pericecal
Intersigmoid
Transmesenteric
Paravesical

Diaphragmatic

Esophageal hiatus
Foramen of Bochdalek
Foramen of Morgagni
Traumatic

Peritoneal, Mesenteric Masses

Metastases
Malignant mesothelioma
Cystic peritoneal mesothelioma
Pseudomyxoma peritonei
Carcinoid
Retractile mesenteritis
Desmoid
Sarcoma
Lymphoma
Infectious lymphadenopathy
Abscess
Mesenteric cyst

Low-Attenuation Mesenteric Lymphadenopathy

Treated lymphoma
Necrotic metastases
Mycobacterial infection
(*Mycobacterium avium-intracellulare* or tuberculosis)
Whipple disease
Cavitary mesenteric lymph node syndrome

MESENTERIC AND PERITONEAL MASSES

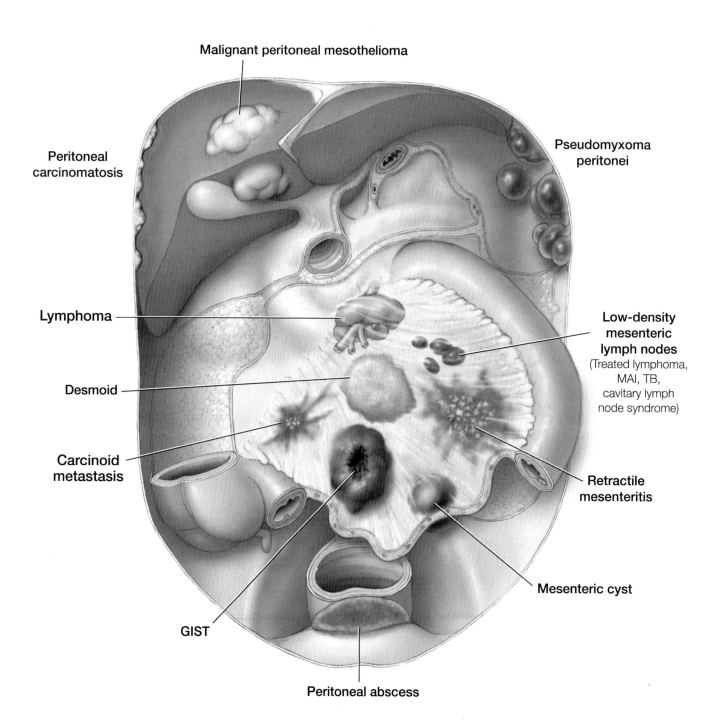

Malignant peritoneal mesothelioma

Pseudomyxoma peritonei

Peritoneal carcinomatosis

Lymphoma

Low-density mesenteric lymph nodes
(Treated lymphoma, MAI, TB, cavitary lymph node syndrome)

Desmoid

Carcinoid metastasis

Retractile mesenteritis

Mesenteric cyst

GIST

Peritoneal abscess

GIST, gastrointestinal stromal tumor; MAI, *Mycobacterium avium-intracellulare*; TB, tuberculosis

GROIN AND PELVIC HERNIAS

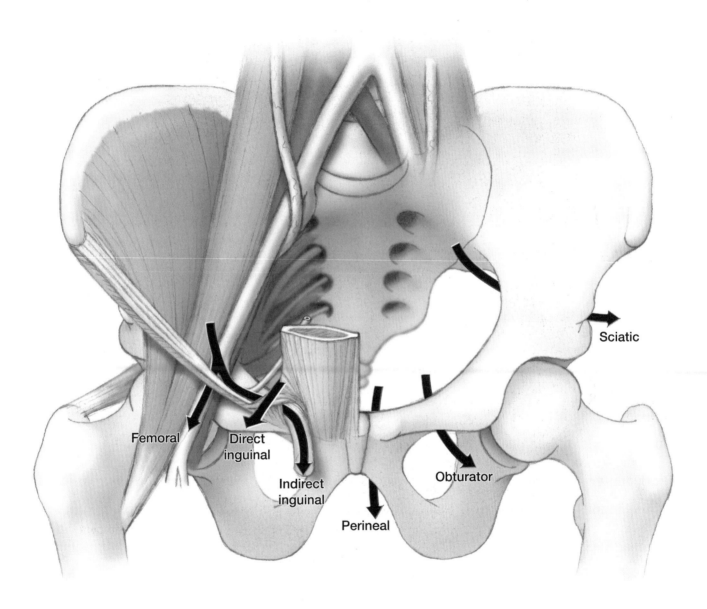

INTERNAL HERNIAS

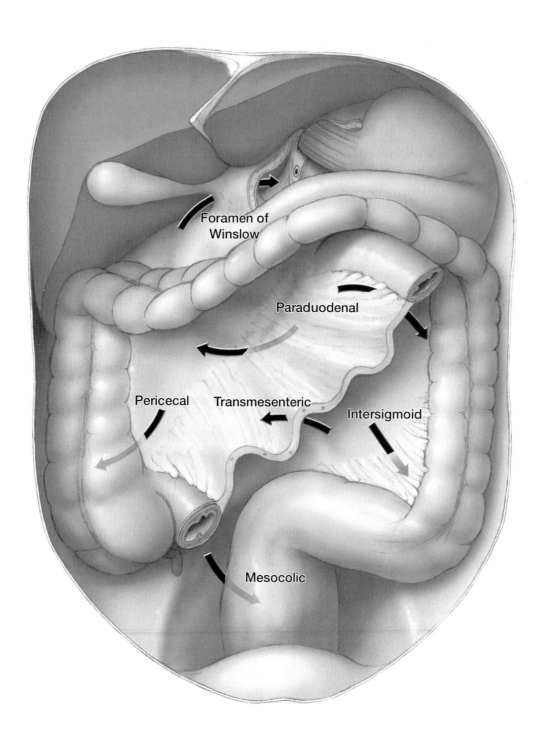

Abbreviations Used in This Book

CT, computed tomogram

ERCP, endoscopic retrograde cholangiopancreatogram

MRCP, magnetic resonance cholangiopancreatogram

MRI, magnetic resonance image

UGI, upper gastrointestinal series

SUBJECT INDEX

CASE INDEX

Esophagus

Esophagus (cont.)

Stomach

Duodenum

Peritoneum and mesentery